Oncology Nursing
SECRETS

Oncology Nursing
SECRETS

Third Edition

ROSE A. GATES, RN, PhD, ANP, AOCN®
Oncology Clinical Nurse Specialist/Nurse Practitioner
Rocky Mountain Cancer Centers
Colorado Springs, Colorado

REGINA M. FINK, RN, PhD, FAAN, AOCN®
Research Nurse Scientist
University of Colorado Hospital
Aurora, Colorado

SERIES EDITOR
LINDA J. SCHEETZ, EdD, RN, FAEN
Associate Dean for Student Affairs
Rutgers, The State University of New Jersey
College of Nursing
Newark, New Jersey

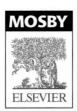

MOSBY

ELSEVIER

BP45

MOSBY
ELSEVIER

11830 Westline Industrial Drive
St. Louis, Missouri 63146

ONCOLOGY NURSING SECRETS, 3e   ISBN: 978-0-323-04457-8

Notice

Knowledge and best practice in this field are constantly changing. As new research and experience broaden our knowledge, changes in practice, treatment and drug therapy may become necessary or appropriate. Readers are advised to check the most current information provided (i) on procedures featured or (ii) by the manufacturer of each product to be administered, to verify the recommended dose or formula, the method and duration of administration, and contraindications. It is the responsibility of the practitioner, relying on their own experience and knowledge of the patient, to make diagnoses, to determine dosages and the best treatment for each individual patient, and to take all appropriate safety precautions. To the fullest extent of the law, neither the Publisher nor the Authors assumes any liability for any injury and/or damage to persons or property arising out or related to any use of the material contained in this book.

The Publisher

Library of Congress Control Number: 2007924813

ISBN: 978-0-323-04457-8

Senior Acquisitions Editor: Sandra Clark Brown
Senior Developmental Editor: Cindi Anderson
Book Production Manager: Gayle May
Project Manager: Tracey Schriefer
Senior Designer: Amy Buxton

Printed in the United States of America

Last digit is the print number: 9 8 7 6 5 4 3 2

2/17/10

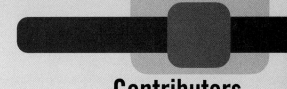

Contributors

NORMAN O. AARESTAD, MD, FACR
Radiation Oncologist
Rocky Mountain Cancer Centers
Denver, Colorado
  Chapter 5. Radiation Therapy

SUSAN ADNAN-KOCH, RN, MS, AOCN®
Clinical Case Manager
Department of Case Management—GynOncology
University of Colorado Hospital, Cancer Center
Aurora, Colorado
  Chapter 26. Gynecologic Cancers

TAUSEEF AHMED, MD
Professor of Medicine
Chief of Oncology and Hematology
New York Medical College
Chief of Oncology
Westchester County Medical Center
Valhalla, New York
  Chapter 19. Bladder Cancer

KATHERINE ALBERT, RN, MSN, AOCNP
Oncology Nurse Practitioner
Rocky Mountain Cancer Centers
Denver, Colorado
  Chapter 23. Colorectal Cancer (CRC)

MEGAN L. ANDERSEN, RN, MS
Advanced Practice Nurse
Rocky Mountain Blood and Marrow Transplant Program
Rocky Mountain Cancer Centers
Denver, Colorado
  Chapter 15. Leukemia and Myelodysplastic Syndrome (MDS)

MARGARET BARTON-BURKE, PhD, RN
Assistant Professor
School of Nursing
University of Massachusetts, Amherst
Amherst, Massachusetts
Associate Clinical Scientist
The Phyllis F. Cantor Center
Dana-Farber Cancer Institute
Boston, Massachusetts

Clinical Consultant
Department of Nursing
University of Massachusetts Memorial Medical Center
Worcester, Massachusetts
Adjunct Associate Professor
School of Nursing
University of Rhode Island
Kingston, Rhode Island
  Chapter 6. Principles of Chemotherapy

MICHELE BASCHE, MD
Rocky Mountain Cancer Centers
Denver, Colorado
  Chapter 25. Gastric, Pancreatic, Hepatocellular, and Gallbladder Cancers

CAROLYN BECKER, RN, MSN, APN, AOCN®
Advanced Practice Nurse
Rocky Mountain Blood and Marrow Transplant Program
Rocky Mountain Cancer Centers
Denver, Colorado
  Chapter 8. Blood and Marrow Stem Cell Transplant
  Chapter 52. Superior Vena Cava Syndrome

MAUDE BECKER, RN, MSN, OCN®
Oncology Clinical Nurse Specialist
Department of Cutaneous Oncology
University of Colorado Hospital
Aurora, Colorado
  Chapter 29. Malignant Melanoma

MONA BERNAICHE BEDELL, RN, MPH
Denver Health and Human Services
Department of Public Health
Denver, Colorado
  Chapter 2. Cancer Prevention and Detection

JEFFREY L. BERENBERG, MD
Clinical Professor of Medicine
John H. Burns School of Medicine
University of Hawaii
Chief, Hematology-Oncology Service
Department of Medicine
Tripler Army Medical Center
Honolulu, Hawaii
  Chapter 32. Testicular Cancer

ROCKY BILLUPS, RN, MS
Director of Oncology Program Development
Hospital Corporation of America
MidAmerica Division
Nashville, Tennessee
  Chapter 11. Blood Components

JANE SAUCEDO BRAATEN, RN, MS, CNS/ANP
Clinical Nursing Director
Department of Cardiovascular Services
Porter Adventist Hospital
Denver, Colorado
   Chapter 60. Advance Directives, End-of-Life Decisions, and Ethical Dilemmas

HARRI BRACKETT, RN, MS, OCN®, CRNI
Clinical Nurse Specialist, Palliative Care
University of Colorado Hospital
Aurora, Colorado
   Chapter 12. Vascular Access Devices (VAD)

CAROL BRUEGGEN, MS, AOCNS, APRN-BC
Assistant Professor of Nursing
Mayo Clinic College of Medicine
Oncology Clinical Nurse Specialist
Department of Nursing
St. Mary's Hospital
Rochester, Minnesota
   Chapter 4. Surgical Oncology

MARK W. BRUNVAND, MD
Rocky Mountain Blood and Marrow Transplant Program
Director, Unrelated Transplant Program
Rocky Mountain Cancer Centers
Denver, Colorado
   Chapter 8. Blood and Marrow Stem Cell Transplant

JOHN M. BURKE, MD
Rocky Mountain Cancer Centers
Colorado Springs, Colorado
   Chapter 14. Hodgkin Lymphoma

DAWN CAMP-SORRELL, MSN, FNP, AOCN®
Oncology Nurse Practitioner
Hematology Oncology Associates of Alabama
Sylacauga, Alabama
   Chapter 46. Cardiac Tamponade

MUHAMMAD CHOUDHURY, MD
Director of Urology
Department of Urology
Westchester Medical Center
Chief, Section of Urologic Oncology
Department of Urology
New York Medical College
Valhalla, New York
   Chapter 19. Bladder Cancer

ALLEN COHN, MD
Rocky Mountain Cancer Centers
Denver, Colorado
Chapter 23. Colorectal Cancer (CRC)

SUSANNE K. COOK, RN, BSN, OCN®
Oncology Nurse
University of Colorado Hospital, Cancer Center
Aurora, Colorado
Chapter 21. Brain Tumors

FRANCES CRIGHTON, RN, PhD
Coordinator, Tony Grampsas Urology Oncologic Clinic
University of Colorado Hospital, Cancer Center
Aurora, Colorado
Chapter 30. Prostate Cancer

DENISE M. DAMEK, MD
Associate Professor
Department of Neurology and Neurosurgery
University of Colorado at Denver and Health Sciences Center
Aurora, Colorado
Chapter 21. Brain Tumors

BARBARA I. DAMRON, PhD, RN
Director of Community Development & Advocacy
Cancer Therapy and Research Center
University of New Mexico
Albuquerque, New Mexico
President
Damron Oncology Consulting
Santa Fe, New Mexico
Chapter 34. Depression, Distress, and Anxiety

SUSAN A. DAVIDSON, MD
Chief, Gynecologic Oncology
Department of Obstetrics and Gynecology
University of Colorado Hospital, Cancer Center
Aurora, Colorado
Chapter 26. Gynecologic Cancers

GEORGIA M. DECKER, RN, MS, CS-ANP, CN, AOCN®
Founder and Advanced Practice Nurse
Integrative Care
Albany, New York
Chapter 13. Complementary and Alternative Medicine (CAM) Therapies

JANE M. DeSMITH, RN, BSN, OCN®
Rocky Mountain Cancer Centers
Colorado Springs, Colorado
Chapter 14. Hodgkin Lymphoma

DEBORAH A. DEVINE, RN, MS, AOCN®, CRNI
Director, Patient Services
Departments of Oncology and Bone Marrow Transplant
University of Colorado Hospital
Aurora, Colorado
  Chapter 12. Vascular Access Devices (VAD)

ANN MARIE DOSE, PHD(C), RN
Research Specialist
Department of Nursing
Division of Nursing Research
Mayo Clinic
Rochester, Minnesota
  Chapter 4. Surgical Oncology

CONSTANCE ENGELKING, RN, MS, OCN®
Oncology Nurse Consultant
The CHE Consulting Group, Inc.
Mount Kisko, New York
  Chapter 35. Diarrhea and Constipation

DAVID FARAGHER, MD
Medical Oncologist
Rocky Mountain Cancer Centers
Aurora, Colorado
  Chapter 18. AIDS-Related Malignancies

KYLE M. FINK, MD
Medical Oncologist, Retired
Rocky Mountain Cancer Centers
Denver, Colorado
  Chapter 20. Bone and Soft Tissue Sarcomas

REGINA M. FINK, RN, PHD, FAAN, AOCN®
Research Nurse Scientist
University of Colorado Hospital
Aurora, Colorado
  Chapter 42. Pain Management

THOMAS W. FLAIG, MD
Assistant Professor
Department of Medicine
Division of Medical Oncology
University of Colorado at Denver and Health Sciences Center
Aurora, Colorado
  Chapter 30. Prostate Cancer

MARY T. GARCIA, RN, BSN, MPH
Clinical Research Associate—Retired
University of Colorado Hospital, Cancer Center
Aurora, Colorado
  Chapter 10. Clinical Trials

ROBERT H. GATES, MD, FACP
Infectious Diseases Specialist
Colorado Springs, Colorado
  Chapter 49. Infections in Cancer Patients

ROSE A. GATES, RN, PhD, ANP, AOCN®
Oncology Clinical Nurse Specialist/Nurse Practitioner
Rocky Mountain Cancer Centers
Colorado Springs, Colorado
  Chapter 34. Depression, Distress, and Anxiety
  Chapter 42. Pain Management

CHRISTINE G. GATLIN, RN, OCN®, MHA
Director, Medicine and Oncology
Baton Rouge General
Baton Rouge, Louisiana
  Chapter 51. Spinal Cord Compression

COLLEEN GILL, MS, RD
Lecturer, School of Medicine
University of Colorado
Clinical Dietitian, Private Practice
Nutrition Foundation, LLC
Denver, Colorado
Clinical Dietitian, Outpatient Oncology Services
Department of Food and Nutrition Services
University of Colorado Hospital, Cancer Center
Aurora, Colorado
  Chapter 40. Nutritional Support

RENE GONZALEZ, MD
Associate Professor of Medicine
Director, University of Colorado Melanoma Research Clinic
Department of Medicine/Medical Oncology
University of Colorado at Denver and Health Sciences Center
Aurora, Colorado
  Chapter 29. Malignant Melanoma

BARBARA GRANT, MS, RD
Oncology Clinical Dietitian
Saint Alphonsus Cancer Care Center
Boise, Idaho
  Chapter 40. Nutritional Support

JULIE GRIFFIE, BSN, MSN, BC-APRN, CS, AOCN®
Adjunct Clinical Instructor
Health Maintenance Program
University of Wisconsin
Clinical Nurse Specialist
Froedtert Hospital
Milwaukee, Wisconsin
  Chapter 43. Palliative Care

GEORGIA A. HANSEN, RN, OCN®
Rocky Mountain Cancer Centers
Colorado Springs, Colorado
  Chapter 7. Tips for Administering Chemotherapy

LENORE L. HARRIS, MSN, RN, CNS
Educational Consultant
Oak Park, Illinois
  Chapter 27. Head and Neck Cancers

PAMELA J. HAYLOCK, RN, MA
Doctoral Student
University of Texas Medical Branch
Galveston, Texas
  Chapter 61. Caring for the Caregiver

IOANA HINSHAW, MD
Rocky Mountain Cancer Centers
Denver, Colorado
  Chapter 20. Bone and Soft Tissue Sarcomas

JOANNE ITANO, RN, PhD, OCN®
Director, Academic Planning and Policy
Associate Professor of Nursing
University of Hawaii
Honolulu, Hawaii
  Chapter 55. Culture and Ethnicity

R. LEE JENNINGS, MD
Clinical Assistant Professor
Department of Surgery
University of Colorado at Denver and Health Sciences Center
Aurora, Colorado
  Chapter 27. Head and Neck Cancers

GARI JENSEN, RN, BSN, OCN®
Oncology Nurse, Cancer Clinic
University of Colorado Hospital, Cancer Center
Aurora, Colorado
  Chapter 48. Hypercalcemia of Malignancy (HCM)

JAINE JEWELL, RN, OCN®
Assistant Nurse Manager
Department of Stem Cell Transplantation and Cellular Therapy
The University of Texas MD Anderson Cancer Center
Houston, Texas
  Chapter 50. Syndrome of Inappropriate Antidiuretic Hormone (SIADH)

PATRICK H. JUDSON, MD
Cancer Institute of New Mexico
Santa Fe, New Mexico
   Chapter 31. Renal Cell Carcinoma

LEIGH K. KASZYK, RN, MS
Nurse Consultant
Centennial, Colorado
   Chapter 50. Syndrome of Inappropriate Antidiuretic Hormone (SIADH)

KAREN KELLY, MD
Deputy Director
University of Kansas Cancer Center
Kansas City, Kansas
   Chapter 28. Lung Cancer

LINDA U. KREBS, RN, PHD, AOCN®, FAAN
Associate Professor
School of Nursing
University of Colorado at Denver and Health Sciences Center
Aurora, Colorado
   Chapter 54. Cancer and Pregnancy

SCOTT KRUGER, MD
Assistant Professor
Eastern Virginia Medical School
Sentara Williamsburg Hospital
Sentara Careplex Hospital
Riverside Regional Medical Center
Mary Immaculate Hospital
Norfolk, Virginia
   Chapter 17. Non-Hodgkin Lymphomas

SUSAN A. LEIGH, BSN, RN
Cancer Survivorship Consultant
Founding Member, National Coalition for Cancer Survivorship
Tucson, Arizona
   Chapter 58. Survivorship

KELLY C. MACK, RN, MSN, AOCNP, NP-C
Oncology Nurse Practitioner
Rocky Mountain Cancer Centers
Denver, Colorado
   Chapter 9. Biologic and Targeted Therapy
   Chapter 22. Breast Cancer
   Chapter 52. Superior Vena Cava Syndrome

BRENDA RONK MARTIN, MS, CRNP, OCN®
Nurse Practitioner
Cancer Center
Peninsula Regional Medical Center
Salisbury, Maryland
   Chapter 41. Organ Toxicities and Late Effects

DENNIS MARTIN, RN, BSN
Director of Oncology and Bone Marrow Transplant
Oklahoma University Medical Center
Oklahoma City, Oklahoma
   Chapter 11. Blood Components

JEFFREY V. MATOUS, MD
Associate Clinical Professor
Department of Medicine
Division of Oncology
University of Colorado Health Sciences Center
Department of Hematology and Bone Marrow Transplant
Presbyterian St. Lukes Medical Center
Physician, Medical Director
Rocky Mountain Blood and Marrow Transplant Program
Rocky Mountain Cancer Centers
Denver, Colorado
   Chapter 15. Leukemia and Myelodysplastic Syndrome (MDS)

ELLYN MATTHEWS, PhD, RN, AOCN®, CRNI
Assistant Professor
School of Nursing
University of Colorado at Denver and Health Sciences Center
Aurora, Colorado
   Chapter 45. Sleep-Wake Disturbances

MICHAEL T. McDERMOTT, MD
Professor of Medicine
Director of Endocrinology and Diabetes Practice
University of Colorado Hospital at Denver and Health Sciences Center
Aurora, Colorado
   Chapter 24. Endocrine Cancers

SANDRA L. MUCHKA, RN, MSN
Clinical Nurse Specialist
Department of Palliative Care
Medical College of Wisconsin
Milwaukee, Wisconsin
   Chapter 43. Palliative Care

TIMOTHY MURPHY, MD, FACP
Rocky Mountain Cancer Centers at the Pavilion
Colorado Springs, Colorado
   Chapter 3. Diagnosis and Staging

JAMIE S. MYERS, RN, MN, AOCN®
Medical Science Liaison
Oncology Scientific Operations
Novartis
East Hanover, New Jersey
   Chapter 33. Cancer of Unknown Primary Sites (CUPs)

LILLIAN M. NAIL, PhD, CNS, FAAN
Rawlinson Distinguished Professor and Senior Scientist
School of Nursing
Oregon Health and Science University Cancer Institute
Portland, Oregon
   Chapter 36. Fatigue

PAULA NELSON-MARTEN, RN, PhD
Associate Professor
School of Nursing
University of Colorado at Denver and Health Sciences Center
Aurora, Colorado
   Chapter 60. Advance Directives, End-of-Life Decisions, and Ethical Dilemmas

PATRICIA W. NISHIMOTO, BSN, MPH, DNS, FAAN
Adult Oncology Clinical Nurse
Department of Medicine
Tripler Army Medical Center
Honolulu, Hawaii
   Chapter 44. Sexuality
   Chapter 55. Culture and Ethnicity

JANELLE MCCALLUM OROZCO, RN, BSN, MSM, CHPN
Vice President, Clinical Operations
The Denver Hospice
Denver, Colorado
   Chapter 59. Hospice Care

DEV PAUL, DO, PhD
Department of Breast Oncology
Rocky Mountain Cancer Centers
Denver, Colorado
   Chapter 22. Breast Cancer

KELLY PENDERGRASS, MD
Clinical Professor of Medicine
University of Missouri—Kansas City
Oncologist
Kansas City Cancer Centers
Kansas City, Missouri
   Chapter 33. Cancer of Unknown Primary Sites (CUPs)

CAROLYN PHILLIPS, RN, BSN, OCN®
Oncology Nurse
New Mexico Cancer Care Associates
Santa Fe, New Mexico
   Chapter 31. Renal Cell Carcinoma

BRENDA MAUREEN RAJNIAK, AA, BSN, OCN®
Nursing Supervisor
Virgina Oncology Associates
Hampton, Virginia
Chapter 17. Non-Hodgkin Lymphomas

PAMELA A. ROSSÉ, MS, RN, CNS
Project Manager
Clinical Investigations Core, Cancer Center
University of Colorado at Denver and Health Sciences Center
Aurora, Colorado
Chapter 10. Clinical Trials

TINA RUSSELL, RN, OCN®
Clinical Nurse III
University of Colorado Hospital, Cancer Center
Aurora, Colorado
Chapter 28. Lung Cancer

DIANA L. RUZICKA, COL, AN, RN, MSN, CNS
Deputy Commander for Health Services and Nursing
Evans Army Community Hospital
Fort Carson, Colorado
Chapter 42. Pain Management

CARMEL SAUERLAND, RN, MSN, AOCNS
Oncology Clinical Nurse Specialist
Department of Nursing
Westchester Medical Center
Valhalla, New York
Chapter 19. Bladder Cancer

LISA SCHULMEISTER, RN, MN, CS, OCN®, FAAN
Oncology Nursing Consultant
New Orleans, Louisiana
Chapter 51. Spinal Cord Compression

MARY KAY SCHULTZ, MSN, NP
Instructor—Nurse Practitioner
Department Medical Oncology
University of Colorado Hospital, Cancer Center
Aurora, Colorado
Chapter 25. Gastric, Pancreatic, Hepatocellular, and Gallbladder Cancers

PAUL A. SELIGMAN, MD
Professor of Medicine
Department of Medicine/Hematology
University of Colorado at Denver and Health Sciences Center
Aurora, Colorado
Chapter 16. Multiple Myeloma

JEFFREY G. SHAW, MS
Oncology Genetic Counselor
Hereditary Cancer Service
Penrose Cancer Center
Colorado Springs, Colorado
Rev. Roger Dorcy Cancer Center
Pueblo, Colorado
Chapter 1. Carcinogenesis and Genetics

JEAN K. SMITH, RN, MS, OCN®
Clinical Nurse Specialist
Lymphedema & Cancer Complications
Penrose Cancer Center
Penrose St. Francis Health Services of Centura Health
Colorado Springs, Colorado
Chapter 37. Lymphedema

KAREN KAY SOUSA, RN, OCN®
Radiation Oncology Registered Nurse III
Department of Radiation Oncology
Rocky Mountain Cancer Centers
Colorado Springs, Colorado
Chapter 5. Radiation Therapy

KAREN J. STANLEY, RN, MSN, AOCN®, FAAN
Director of Institutional Advancement
The Connecticut Hospice
Branford, Connecticut
Chapter 57. Family and Caregiver Coping

JULIE R. SWANEY, MDIV
Assistant Clinical Professor
Department of Medicine
Clinical Faculty
Department of Psychiatry
University of Colorado at Denver and Health Sciences Center
Aurora, Colorado
Chapter 56. Religion and Spirituality

DANIEL T. TELL, DO, FACP
Rocky Mountain Cancer Centers at the Pavilion
Colorado Springs, Colorado
Chapter 3. Diagnosis and Staging

DEBRA THALER-DEMERS, RN, OCN®
Staff Nurse IV
Stanford University Hospitals and Clinics
Stanford, California
Chapter 58. Survivorship

SANDI VANNICE, MS, RN, AOCN®
Oncology Clinical Nurse Specialist
Division of Hematology/Oncology
Denver Health Medical Center
Denver, Colorado
    Chapter 38. Mucositis

CAROL S. VIELE, RN, MS, CNS
Clinical Nurse Specialist, Hematology-Oncology Bone Marrow Transplant
Department of Nursing
University of California San Francisco
San Francisco, California
    Chapter 47. Disseminated Intravascular Coagulation (DIC)

AMY WALL, RN, BSN, OCN®
Rocky Mountain Cancer Centers
Colorado Springs, Colorado
    Chapter 7. Tips for Administering Chemotherapy

RITA S. WICKHAM, PhD, RN, AOCN®, CHPN
Associate Professor
College of Nursing
Rush University College of Nursing
Chicago, Illinois
    Chapter 39. Nausea and Vomiting

GAIL M. WILKES, MS, RNC, AOCN®
Clinical Instructor
Oncology Nursing
Boston Medical Center
Boston, Massachusetts
    Chapter 6. Principles of Chemotherapy

PEG WISNER, RN, MN, AOCN®
Clinical Nurse Specialist
Menorah Medical Center
Overland Park, Kansas
Baptist-Lutheran Medical Center
Kansas City, Missouri
    Chapter 11. Blood Components

STACEY YOUNG-MCCAUGHAN, RN, PhD, AOCN®
Colonel, US Army Nurse Corps
Chief, Department of Clinical Investigation
Brooke Army Medical Center
Fort Sam Houston, Texas
    Chapter 36. Fatigue

ANNE ZOBEC, MS, RN, NP, AOCN®, AOCNP
Oncology Nurse Practitioner
Rocky Mountain Cancer Centers at the Pavilion
Colorado Springs, Colorado
  Chapter 53. Tumor Lysis Syndrome (TLS)

Preface

With over 50 years of combined oncology nursing experience, we were motivated to create this book to share knowledge that we wished had been at our fingertips when we began our careers. We have often heard new oncology staff nurses say: "I don't know enough to even ask a question"; "I don't know where to begin looking for the answers"; "I don't have time to look it up in something that weighs 50 pounds"; or "I'm embarrassed to ask a question." The Secrets Series® is an ideal format for presenting questions and answers, "tricks of the trade," and "oncology pearls" in a convenient, readable, and concise manner. This new third edition of *Oncology Nursing Secrets* includes questions and answers appropriate for novices as well as advanced practitioners. It also includes quick facts for cancer types, internet reference sites, and the most up-to-date evidence-based information.

Because oncology nursing derives "secrets" from many disciplines, we made full use of our collaborative ties with physicians and other care providers. The authors range from staff nurses to advanced practice nurses and nurse academicians to oncologists and other care providers, all of whom are actively contributing to the care of oncology patients. This book is not meant to be a complete reference or comprehensive textbook. Rather it is intended to focus on commonly asked questions and to stimulate further discussion and research. The reader is encouraged to make full use of the excellent textbooks, articles, and internet sites cited throughout the book. With so many facts to present, it is impossible to express the complex human dimensions and love that permeate every aspect of oncology nursing care. We hope that you will discover those secrets for yourself. We invite you to share your secrets and to always ask questions. May you find wisdom and compassion in the answers.

We are grateful to our patients and their families, who have been our best teachers. They have taught us to make the most of each day and to live even while we are dying. We would like to express our appreciation to all the contributors for taking time to write their chapters in the midst of busy professional and personal lives. We would also like to acknowledge the authors from previous editions who provided original and crucial contributions that were the foundation for this edition. We thank the oncologists, nurses, pharmacists, dieticians, social workers, and other health care providers who have been our partners, as well as our teachers. Finally thanks to the editorial staff, in particular Linda Scheetz, EdD, RN, CS, CEN for her thoughtful critique and the publishers at Elsevier for their assistance and support.

We offer this book to all those busy, committed oncology nurses who never have time to do everything that they want to do for their patients. We hope that this book will continue to provide quick answers to your questions and enhance nursing care and symptom management for patients with cancer.

ROSE A. GATES, RN, PHD, ANP, AOCN®
REGINA M. FINK, RN, PHD, FAAN, AOCN®

To my husband, Rob and my children, Melissa and Brandon, for their support and unselfishness, for enabling me to spend time away from them to work on this project. To the nurses, oncologists, and staff at the Rocky Mountain Cancer Center in Colorado Springs for their support and excellent care of cancer patients.
R.A.G.

To my husband, Kyle, for his love and understanding that sees me through each day. To my son, Brian, for his caring. To my dad who showed me how to live life to its fullest.
R.M.F.

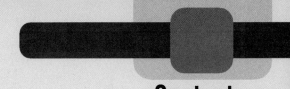

Contents

TOP SECRETS

- All cancer is genetic because cancer is caused by damage to genes that control cell division or cell growth.
- Most cancer is NOT due to an inherited cancer predisposition. Therefore, most people who get a specific type of cancer will not have a family history of it.
- Tumor markers are generally used to evaluate response to therapy and to monitor recurrence.
- Lower cancer rates have been associated with higher intake of fruits and vegetables.
- Excessive fat intake and obesity increase the risk of developing cancers of the breast, colon, and prostate.
- Heavy drinkers are at increased risk for cancers of the oral cavity, larynx, esophagus, breast, and liver.
- Altered hemostasis (hypercoagulability and thrombosis) can place the cancer patient at higher risk for postoperative complications.
- Certain types of chemotherapy can enhance tumor cell kill when given before or concurrently with radiation therapy.
- The sequence in which certain chemotherapy drugs are given may enhance efficacy and/or minimize toxicity.
- Cetuximab (Erbitux) and paclitaxel (Taxol) must be filtered during administration.
- Antioxidant use may compromise the effectiveness of cytotoxic agents.
- Drug resistance is one of the major barriers to cure.
- Performance status is one of most important factors that affect response to chemotherapy.
- Advances in cancer treatment are being made by using chemotherapy in combination with targeted therapy and using nanotechnology to target tumor flaws.
- Biologic and targeted therapy agents utilize and manipulate normal molecular pathways to treat cancer.
- Generally, tyrosine kinase inhibitors are oral agents and monoclonal antibodies are administered intravenously.
- Colony stimulating factors allow higher doses of chemotherapy to be given safely and facilitate administration of planned doses of chemotherapy on time.
- The severity of dermatologic reactions associated with the EGFR inhibitors appears to be dose related and may be an indicator of therapeutic efficacy.
- Graft-versus-leukemia effect refers to the potentially beneficial immunologic effect of mild GVHD (graft versus host disease) in eliminating residual leukemia in the host.
- The success of a clinical trial depends on the eligibility of participants and the evaluability of collected data.
- The most common transfusion reaction in the oncology patient is nonhemolytic febrile transfusion reaction.
- Recent research does not support the use of antithrombotic prophylaxis in most patients with central vein catheters.
- Tunnel infections usually and port infections always require catheter removal.
- Infection with fever is one of the most common presenting symptoms of acute leukemia.

- Although higher grade lymphomas are considered unfavorable, they are potentially curable.
- Reed-Sternberg cells are diagnostic of Hodgkin lymphoma.
- The most common malignancies in patients with HIV are Kaposi's sarcoma and non-Hodgkin lymphomas.
- Cigarette smoking is the greatest risk factor for bladder cancer.
- The common oncologic emergencies in patients with multiple myeloma are hypercalcemia, spinal cord compression, and hyperviscosity.
- Limb salvage surgery is now possible in close to 90% of osteosarcoma cases.
- Brain tumor size does not correlate with prognosis.
- Brain tumor recurrence is generally within 2 cm of the original tumor.
- Key breast cancer prognostic indicators include: lymph node involvement, estrogen (ER) and progesterone receptor (PR) status, HER-2/*neu*, and S-phase status.
- Papillary and follicular thyroid carcinomas have very low mortality rates, medullar carcinoma has an intermediate mortality rate, and anaplastic carcinoma has a very high mortality rate.
- Surgical resection is the primary treatment of choice for colorectal cancer.
- Upper GI cancers, such as pancreatic, gastric and gallbladder cancers, often have progressed to advanced stages at the time of diagnosis.
- Cervical cancer is preventable with early detection and quadrivalent human papillomavirus [HPV] recombinant vaccine administration in females 9-26 years, cervical adenocarcinoma in situ, cervical intraepithelial neoplasia, and genital warts caused by HPV types 6, 11, 16, 18.
- Intraperitoneal chemotherapy improves survival in women with optimally debulked stage III ovarian cancer versus intravenous chemotherapy.
- Ninety percent of patients with primary tumors of the oral cavity, pharynx, or larynx have a smoking history.
- For both SCLC and NSCLC, the single most common prognostic indicator for overall survival and response to treatment is weight loss.
- Lung cancer is the leading cause of death among men and women.
- There is no such thing as a "safe" tan.
- Sentinel node biopsy is the best predictor of survival for malignant melanomas.
- The Gleason score is based on the pathologic evaluation of the tumor's histology and correlates very well with the clinical behavior of prostate cancer.
- Approximately 50% of renal cell carcinomas are found serendipitously on imaging studies obtained for unrelated reasons.
- Even in advanced stages of testicular cancer, chemotherapy is often curative.
- Treatment decisions for cancers of unknown primary (CUPs) are based on the most likely primary site as indicated by cell type, geography of presentation, risk factors, and tumor markers.
- The biologic correlates, typically used for diagnosing depression in physically healthy adults, are frequently unreliable in patients with cancer.
- Diarrhea and constipation are relatively high incidence problems in cancer patients; both are underreported and often mismanaged.
- Exercise is effective in reducing cancer treatment-related fatigue.
- Consistent use of external compression products is crucial to optimal outcomes for patients with lymphedema of the extremities.
- Chlorhexidine is not recommended for the prevention of mucositis; the optimal rinsing agent for treating mucositis has yet to be identified.
- Serotonin subtype 3 ($5HT_3$) antagonists play less of a role in delayed than in acute chemotherapy-induced nausea and vomiting (CINV); patients are unlikely to achieve complete control of delayed CINV with a $5HT_3$ antagonist only.

- Since weight loss can adversely affect nutritional reserves, weight maintenance during cancer treatment, regardless of the extent of overweight, is recommended.
- "Chemo brain" or "chemo-fog" is a recognized condition and should be evaluated.
- Palliative care and "aggressive" disease management are not mutually exclusive paths.
- Pulmonary secretions may be minimized by the use of intravenous (IV) atropine or atropine 1% eye drops given sublingually.
- Approximately 10% of patients will experience pain that is resistant to traditional analgesic therapies.
- Opioid rotation is used when there is inadequate analgesia, unacceptable toxicity (e.g., myoclonus, agitation, hallucinations, pruritis, nausea/vomiting), the need for an alternative route of administration, to ensure patient adherence to the regimen, to decrease analgesic cost, or to comply with formulary requirements.
- Because of its unique pharmacodynamic properties, methadone is effective against neuropathic pain and hyperalgesia.
- The nurse's failure or hesitation to include sexuality counseling may add to the patient's anxieties and fears about future sexual activity.
- Sleep-wake disturbances, alone or as part of symptom clusters, occur twice as frequently in persons with cancer compared with the general population.
- Echocardiogram is the definitive diagnostic test for confirmation of cardiac tamponade.
- DIC is always a symptom of underlying disease.
- Osteonecrosis of the jaw has recently been associated with bisphosphonate therapy.
- Fever in a neutropenic patient is a medical emergency.
- The most important neutropenic precaution is strict handwashing.
- Diuretics, morphine, and antidepressant use may contribute to SIADH.
- Back pain in any patient with cancer should prompt a rapid evaluation for spinal cord compression.
- The most common **early** symptoms of superior vena cava syndrome (SVCS) include dyspnea, orthopnea (ability to breathe easily only in the upright position), and facial edema.
- There is no evidence that termination of pregnancy will stop/retard cancer growth and that hormonal/immunologic changes of pregnancy enhance cancer growth.
- Research has shown that metabolism of drugs is genetically determined (genetic polymorphism); thus, ethnicity or a person's race may affect responses to drugs.
- Patient/family-centered care supports open and honest communication.
- There is a correlation between spirituality and health.
- Decreased insurability and employment discrimination continue to impede full recovery from cancer for many survivors.
- Be truthful when patients ask if they are dying.
- A written advance directive, without a discussion of end-of-life wishes, will not ensure that a patient's wishes are followed.
- The impact of nurses' stress and burnout in oncology care settings affects patient satisfaction, patient outcomes, organizational outcomes, and nurses' health.
- To help grieving people – let them tell their story… every detail matters to them.

Unit I

Cancer Overview

Chapter 1

Carcinogenesis and Genetics

Jeffrey G. Shaw

CARCINOGENESIS

1. What are the chances of getting cancer?

In the United States, approximately one in three women and one in two men will develop a malignancy at some time in their lives. Cancer is second only to heart disease as the most common cause of death. In 2007 there will be an estimated 1,444,920 new cases of invasive cancer and 559,650 deaths due to cancer (1533 people per day).

2. Explain carcinogenesis. In other words, how do cancers get started?

Cancer is caused by mutations in a variety of genes responsible for controlling the growth of cells either directly (gatekeeper genes) or indirectly (caretaker genes).

3. Is all cancer genetic?

Yes, all cancer, the uncontrolled division of a cell, is genetic because cancer is caused by damage to genes that control cell division or cell growth. This damage is usually due to outside influences, or "carcinogens," damaging our genes over the course of a lifetime.

4. What is the difference between genetic and inherited?

People with a strong family history of cancer often say that cancer is "genetic" in their family, when probably they mean that the family has an inherited predisposition for cancer. The word *genetic* is not synonymous with *inherited*. Only a small percentage of cancers are inherited, which occurs when a damaged gene that confers a high susceptibility to cancer is passed down over many generations. We hear almost routinely now about genes that have been identified as being involved in some medical condition or trait. Hardly a day passes without the announcement of another gene being identified in those 3.2 billion letters of genetic code.

5. What is a carcinogen?

A carcinogen is any substance, situation, or exposure that can damage genetic material (DNA). The hundreds of known carcinogens include internal factors created in the body by metabolic processes (e.g., free radicals, hormones), viruses (e.g., hepatitis B, human papillomavirus), chemicals (e.g., tobacco, alcohol, industrial asbestos), and radiation (e.g., diagnostic radiation, ultraviolet light).

6. List the four stages of cancer cell growth.

The four stages are initiation, promotion, progression, and metastasis.

7. Describe the stages of cancer cell growth.

The **initiation stage** is the irreversible mutation of a gene that leads to malignant transformation. Although the cell appears somewhat abnormal, it is still able to carry out its original functions. The mutation must not impair the cell's ability to replicate, or the cell will die. To become malignant, the cell must enter the **promotion stage**. Usually there is a latency period between initiation and promotion, the length of which depends on many factors. The promoting agent does not act on the DNA but instead stimulates the growth and division of a cell. Promoting elements have a threshold, a minimal dose that is required before they stimulate the growth of the cancer cell. Promoting agents may be chemical carcinogens, endogenous hormones, ultraviolet light, or other factors. **Progression** refers to a series of changes that lead to the characteristics of an undifferentiated cell. The normal cell is transformed into a cell with malignant potential. Continued mutations in the cell lead to altered appearance, function, and growth rate. **Metastasis** is explained in Question 15.

8. How are cancer cells different from normal cells?

Unlike normal cells, the first rule for cancer cells is that they follow no rules; invasive cancer is complete anarchy. **Normal cells** reproduce in an organized, controlled, and orderly manner; do not divide when space or nutrients are inadequate; do not spread into parts of the body where they do not belong; become fully differentiated to perform a specific task; and have limited potential and lose their ability to replicate, eventually dying.

Cancer cells exhibit **dysplasia** (disorganized growth), **hyperplasia** (increased cellularity), **metaplasia** (abnormal appearance but not yet identified as malignant), and **pleomorphism** (variations in size and shape not seen in normal cell lines).

9. Summarize the basic features of malignant cancer cells.

- **Ability to grow uncontrollably**. Cancer cells grow and multiply uncontrollably, even when space and nutrients are lacking.
- **Ability to invade other tissues**. Cancer cells lack contact inhibition; they are not inhibited in either growth or movement by contact with other cells. Many metastatic cancer cells have altered surface enzymes and can secrete enzymes that dissolve their way through other cells.
- **Ability to remain in an undifferentiated state**. Well-differentiated cancer cells are more like the normal cells of the tissues in which they originate. Many cancer cells resemble normal, undifferentiated cells, retaining the ability to divide. Undifferentiated (anaplastic) cancer cells are disorganized and exhibit few features of the normal tissue, sometimes to the point that their site of origin cannot be determined. They also may express antigens (e.g., alpha-fetoprotein, CA-125) not normally expressed by the parent cell.
- **Ability to initiate new growth at distant sites**. Lack of contact inhibition and lack of adhesiveness allow cancer cells to grow and spread without the restraint exhibited by normal cells.
- **Ability to escape detection and destruction by the immune system**. Carcinogenesis and the metastatic potential of tumor cells may be a balance between the effectiveness of an individual's immunosurveillance and the ability of the tumor cells to evade destruction.

10. What is apoptosis?

Apoptosis is cellular suicide. It is a complex and extremely orderly process of cells killing themselves. It is so orderly that it is also referred to as "programmed cell death." Apoptosis is part of our normal development when the webbing between our fingers is removed during fetal stages. In the case of cancer, when a cell builds up enough DNA damage it has the ability to lose control and become cancer. This threat to the organism triggers cellular suicide to kill the cell before cancer can occur. The *P53* gene is a very important inducer of apoptosis. If this gene is damaged in a cell and cannot do its job, the cell is at risk for becoming cancer.

11. How can the concepts that underlie cancer cells be explained to patients?

Patients can be told that cancer cells have lost the ability to control their own growth and behavior. They do not recognize the "personal space" of neighboring cells in their tissue of origin and see no problem in spreading to other tissues of the body. They are selfish and continue to divide and multiply, even when there is a lack of adequate food or space to support them.

12. Why is it so difficult to detect cancer?

Once the cancer goes through about 30 doublings, it has reached roughly the size of a marble (about 1 cm in diameter). A tumor of this size contains approximately 1 billion cancer cells. This is about the earliest point at which screening x-ray studies can detect developing cancers. At this stage the cancer needs to go through only about 10 more doublings to reach 1 trillion cells, which is usually the number that leads to death. Thus much of the lifespan of the cancer is "silent" and takes place before the cancer is large enough to be detected.

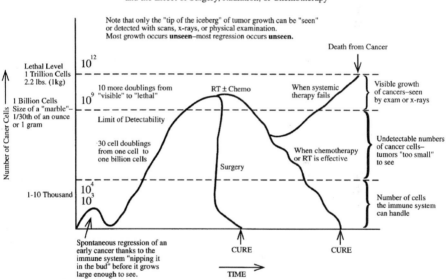

Growth curve for cancers. Adapted from DeVita VT, et al: Principles of chemotherapy. *(From DeVita VT et al, editors:* Cancer: principles and practice of oncology, *Philadelphia, 1982, Lippincott Williams & Wilkins).*

13. Explain the concept of tumor doubling time.

Tumor doubling time is the time required for the tumor to double in size. It varies from hours to months according to the type of cancer (primary or metastatic). It may take years for a tumor to double 20 times.

14. Explain tumor heterogeneity. Why is it important?

Tumor heterogeneity refers to the subpopulations of biologically diverse cancer cells in tumors. A key point is that not all of the cells that make up a malignant tumor are the same. A tumor mass may contain multiple clones with different chromosomal numbers and different characteristics. In addition, the genetic makeup of these cells can be quite different. Therefore, some cells within a malignant tumor may be sensitive to one chemotherapy drug, whereas other cells are resistant (hence the rationale for combination chemotherapy). Some cells are growing, whereas others are dormant and emerge years later. This lack of uniformity makes it difficult to eradicate every cell when treating cancers.

15. How does metastasis occur?

Usually a subpopulation of cells within the heterogeneous tumor has the properties needed to spread to other organs in the body. Certain cells in the tumor undergo genetic changes that allow them to "stick" in distant organs and establish a blood supply.

16. What steps are involved in cancer cells metastasizing to different sites?

The most unique characteristic of malignant cells that results in morbidity and mortality is their capability to invade tissues and to metastasize to other sites. The ability to metastasize requires multiple steps: (1) invasion of adjacent tissues through basement membranes, (2) entrance into nearby vessels (lymph or blood), (3) invasion of the immune system, (4) reentrance into distant tissues, and (5) implantation of malignant cell in new tissue.

Invasive tumor cells secrete enzymes that degrade basement membranes, which normally bar access to adjacent tissues. After access to adjacent tissue, malignant cells erode vessel walls and circulate as individual cells or small clumps of tumor cells (tumor embolus). These tumor cells may be coated by fibrin or circulate in clumps of platelets, thereby escaping the immune cells in the blood. This process is relatively inefficient, because only about 0.1% of tumor cells that enter the blood system survive more than 24 hours.

17. Define angiogenesis.

For tumor cells ultimately to develop into an organ metastasis, they must develop their own blood supply through a process called angiogenesis. The tumor cells and neighboring normal cells synthesize and secrete angiogenic molecules that produce capillary networks for tumors at least 1 to 2 mm in diameter.

18. What is homing?

It is not known why tumor cells of different malignancies prefer to metastasize to specific organs in a process called *homing*. In some cases, this process is simply a result of anatomic blood circulation—as in the spread of colon cancer to the liver via the portal venous circulation. In other cases, tumor cells home to specific target organs because of specific chemical signals released by certain cells. Specific receptors have been identified on the surface of certain circulating tumor cells that recognize sites on endothelial cells of specific organs.

19. How do you explain to a patient that cancer has spread to another site?

Patients and families frequently misunderstand the concept of cancer spreading to another site. For example, if breast cancer spreads to the bone, the patient may believe that she has a new bone cancer. It is important to explain to the patient that the bone cancer is still breast cancer that has spread to the bone (metastasized). Bone metastases from breast cancer are breast cancer cells that have spread through the body to another site. This process can occur long before the original tumor mass in the breast is large enough to be palpated on physical examination or detected on screening mammograms.

GENETICS

20. What is DNA?

DNA (deoxyribonucleic acid) is the molecule of life. All the information necessary to create a human is encoded in it. The human blueprint encoded in our DNA makes tens of thousands of different proteins which comprise all the tissue and molecules of the body. The achievement of the Human Genome Project (HGP) rests upon the work of two men, James Watson and Francis Crick, who in 1953 discovered the "double helix" structure of DNA. This double helix looks something like a twisted ladder. The long sides of the ladder are a repeating sugar-phosphate–sugar-phosphate polymer. The rungs of the ladder are formed by "base" pairs. The four bases are adenine (A), guanine (G), cytosine (C), and thymine (T). Each side of the helix is complementary to the other—that is, A will always match up to T, and C will always match up to G. The structure of DNA allows for: storage of vast amounts of information, an easy method of replication (each side of the double helix will separate, unwind, and copy itself), and protection against information loss from damage to the DNA.

21. What are some interesting facts about DNA?

- Less than 2% of the 3.2 billion letters of code make proteins.
- You could fit 5 million strands of DNA through the eye of a needle.
- If you were to pull all the chromosomes into long strands of DNA, there would be 6 to 7 feet of DNA in each cell.
- If all of the DNA in an average-sized adult were placed end to end, it would circle the globe about 114 million times.
- 99.9% of the letters of code are exactly the same in all human beings.

22. What is a gene?

A gene is a specific length of DNA that usually makes a protein product. The purpose of genes is to provide the blueprint to make all the proteins that constitute our bodies.

It is important to note that every human being has the same 20,000 to 25,000 genes (unless he or she has an inherited condition or a problem with chromosomes). It is the variations in these genes that give each of us our individual physical appearance and predispose us to certain diseases. For example, a patient may say, "My sister has *the gene* for breast cancer, and I want to be tested to see if I have it." By putting it this way, the patient makes it sound as if her sister has a unique gene causing breast cancer. In fact, the sister has the same genes as everyone else. We all have the same genes that control the growth of our breast tissue. What the patient is trying to say is that her sister has a mutation in one of these genes, that this mutation damages the gene, causing it to not make the protein correctly, and thus she has an increased risk for breast cancer.

23. What are chromosomes?

Chromosomes are the structures that "hold" our genes. The estimated 20,000 to 30,000 genes that make a human being are located on 46 chromosomes. Each chromosome is simply a long, tightly coiled strand of DNA. These 46 chromosomes occur as 23 pairs. We get 1 of each pair from our mother (in the egg) and 1 from our father (in the sperm). The first 22 pairs of chromosomes are labeled from 1 to 22, from the longest to the shortest. When it was first viewed under a microscope, the 21st chromosome looked longer than the 22nd. Improved technology revealed that the 21st chromosome was actually shorter than the 22nd. The 21st chromosome has 46 million letters of code, whereas the 22nd has 49 million letters. The longest chromosome, the 1st, has about 246 million letters of code. The last pair are the sex chromosomes, labeled X and Y. Females have two X chromosomes (XX), whereas males have an X and a Y chromosome (XY).

24. What is the difference between genotype and phenotype?

An individual's genotype is all of his or her genetic material, or every gene. If a person has a mutation in one gene, causing an increased risk for cancer, the mutation is part of that person's genotype. A genotype is passed down from generation to generation. It is always changing because half our genes are obtained from each parent. The phenotype is the outward appearance, or what is observed. It is what an organism looks like as a consequence of the interaction between the individual's genotype and the environment. A phenotype could refer to the entire physical appearance of an individual, or one specific trait, such as brown eye color.

25. Didn't the Human Genome Project find all of our genes?

The goal of the Human Genome Project, formally begun in 1990 and completed in 2003, was to map all 3.2 billion letters that make up our DNA. It opened the floodgates for other researchers to map out where the 20,000 to 25,000 genes were located in that 3.2 billion letters of code. Therefore, there are many genes yet to be discovered.

26. What genes are involved in cancer?

Hundreds of identified genes either directly or indirectly participate in a cell's ability to control growth. The list of genes involved in the control of a cell's growth is increasing daily. Currently the genes that control the growth of cells are divided into the following four major categories: oncogenes, tumor suppressor genes, mismatch repair genes, and "housekeeping" genes. All of these genes are undergoing substantial reclassification as we learn more about their exact functions.

27. Define oncogene.

Oncogenes originate from a mutation in normal genes called **proto-oncogenes**. Proto-oncogenes fall into four main classes with different functions, but all of them are involved with signaling the cell that it is time to divide. This process of normal cell replication is used to replace damaged or dying cells. **Activation** is the term used to describe a mutation in a proto-oncogene that transforms it into an oncogene. These mutations cause a gain of function, pushing the cell to divide uncontrollably. Therefore the mutation of one proto-oncogene of a particular pair (most genes occur in identical pairs, one from the mother and one from the father) can lead to the initiation of cancer. Examples of oncogenes include *abl, myc, ras,* and *ret.*

28. What are tumor suppressor genes?

Currently tumor suppressor genes are lumped into one category. They probably have a significant number of different functions and can be considered the opposite of oncogenes. Tumor suppressor genes are growth-suppressing and play an important role in the regulation of cell growth, either directly or indirectly. One functional copy of a particular tumor suppressor gene (either paternal or maternal) appears to be sufficient to control cell growth. Loss of function of both genes can lead to unregulated cell growth. Examples of tumor suppressor genes include *BRCA1, BRCA2, APC,* and *WT1.*

29. Explain the function of mismatch repair genes.

Every time a cell replicates itself into two daughter cells, all 3.2 billion letters of genetic code need to be duplicated exactly—a daunting task. Needless to say, errors are made. Mismatch repair genes function as "spell-checkers" after DNA replication is complete. If both pairs of a mismatch repair gene have mutated, resulting in loss of function, the cell can build up mutations, eventually affecting proto-oncogenes, tumor suppressor genes, and others involved with cell growth regulation. Examples of mismatch repair genes include *MLH1* and *MSH2*, which are mostly involved in controlling growth in colon, uterine, ovarian, and stomach tissues.

30. What are housekeeping genes?

This category is difficult to define because there are probably hundreds of different housekeeping genes, and researchers are just beginning to identify their existence and function. In general, housekeeping genes work to keep the cell clean and functional. For example, housekeeping genes: (1) break down the carcinogens in tobacco products, (2) regulate estrogen in the cell, and (3) protect against viral activation of cancer in the cervix. They include genes that code for metabolic activation enzymes, detoxification enzymes, and DNA repair enzymes.

31. What terms are used to describe the three patterns of cancer occurrence?

- **Sporadic** cancers are mostly caused by nonhereditary factors increasing risks to the general population.
- **Familial** or "multifactorial" cancer predispositions have moderate increases in risk.
- **Inherited** predispositions have a high degree of penetrance.

The following figure illustrates the different contributions between inherited susceptibility and mostly environmental risk. An example of a condition that has a very high genetic susceptibility (high penetrance) with a very low environmental component is familial adenomatous polyposis (FAP). This inherited predisposition, which is due to mutation in the *APC* tumor suppressor gene, causes a greater than 95% risk for colon cancer. In the middle of the diagram is hereditary breast ovarian cancer (HBOC). About 90% of individuals with this condition will have detectable mutations in either the *BRCA1* or *BRCA2* tumor suppressor genes. Those with HBOC have a wide variability in penetrance to breast cancer, anywhere from 44% to 87%. The risk for ovarian cancer can be well under 27% or as high as 44%. On the right side of the diagram is an example of what would be considered a sporadic occurrence of cancer due to being exposed to our make believe substance X. Substance X could be ultraviolet light, carcinogens from smoking, asbestos, or other potential carcinogens. In reality, we all have differing levels of susceptibility to different cancers based on our individual genetic variability. Therefore even sporadic cancer has some "inherited" aspect (albeit with very low penetrance).

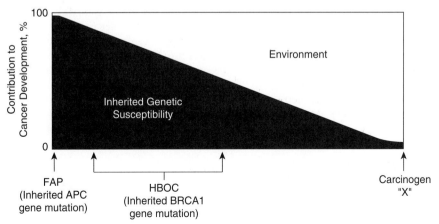

Inherited susceptibility vs. environmental contribution to cancer development. *(Courtesy of Penrose-St. Francis Health Services Cytogenetics Lab.)*

32. Describe the sporadic pattern of occurrence.

Most cancer occurs in a sporadic pattern. The patient has no unusual family history of cancer and the cancer appears to come from nowhere. The tumor suppressor, mismatch repair, and other important genes inherited from the parents are fully functional. Cancer is caused primarily from exposure to carcinogens. Sporadic cancers tend to occur later in life (after the age of 50 years), when many mutations are likely to have accumulated, and the immune system is not as proficient in protecting against cancer cells. However, many sporadic cancers occur in childhood or at a much younger age (e.g., testicular cancer). Realistically, we all have some increased risk for some types of cancer. Approximately 1 in 10 smokers will develop lung cancer. Not everyone exposed to asbestos will develop mesothelioma (a specific type of lung cancer).

33. What is meant by familial or "multifactorial" predisposition?

The patient has inherited several housekeeping genes that are functional but not doing a good job of protecting the patient from carcinogens. Affected families usually have an excess of cancer cases, but not necessarily at a young age. The cancer in the family does not have to be genetically related (e.g., the tumor suppressor genes that control the growth of cervical cells are different from those that control breast cells). Familial predispositions can be due to multifactorial inheritance. In other words, the patient must inherit several suboptimal housekeeping genes *and* be exposed to specific carcinogens. As a result, familial predispositions tend to dilute over each generation, because it is difficult to pass down several specific genes, and families do not tend to share the same environmental exposures from generation to generation. Therefore, familial predispositions tend to confer a small-to-moderate increase in the risk for cancer.

34. Define an inherited cancer predisposition.

The patient has inherited a faulty tumor suppressor, oncogene, or mismatch repair gene from one parent. Because the mutated (nonfunctional) gene was present in the egg or sperm, it is present in every cell of the body. An environmental insult is still necessary to mutate the other gene of the pair and possibly initiate cancer. Because of the inherited mutation, there is a significant increase in risk for malignancy, usually in specific organs. The cancer often has an early onset, and the risk for second primary tumors is increased significantly. Inherited cancer predispositions do not dilute. Either a child inherits the gene from a parent and has a significantly increased risk for cancer, or the child does not inherit the gene and is not at increased risk (based on the family history of cancer).

Inherited conditions tend to have a high penetrance of cancer risk. In other words, those that inherit a damaged gene have very high risks for a specific cancer. For example, those individuals with an inherited colon cancer predisposition called HNPCC (hereditary nonpolyposis colorectal cancer) have up to an 80% lifetime risk for developing colon cancer, and women with HNPCC have up to a 60% risk for developing uterine cancer. Therefore, the penetrance for cancer of these organs is high. However, they can also have a low increased risk for other types of cancer. For example, their risk for cancer of the kidney and ureter is 4%. Although this is 4 times higher than the average person, it is still a low penetrance level.

35. How common are inherited cancer predispositions?

There are hundreds of known inherited cancer syndromes, but luckily most are quite rare. For example, approximately 5% to 10% of all breast cancers are due to an inherited predisposition, 10% to 15% are due to familial predisposition, and the remaining 75% to 80% are sporadic. If a patient, family, or medical provider is concerned about a particular family history of cancer, a referral should be made to a health care professional specifically trained to evaluate family histories of cancer (e.g., genetic counselors).

36. What are common features seen in families with hereditary cancer?

- Cancer at earlier ages than normally seen in certain cancers
- Bilateral or rare cancers (e.g., male breast cancer)
- Second primary tumors in same individual
- Evidence of autosomal dominant inheritance
- Tumors in families consistent with specific cancer syndromes (e.g., breast and ovary in BRCA; colon, uterine in HNPCC)
- Specific ethnic background (e.g., Ashkenazi Jewish ancestry and family history of breast and/or ovarian cancer)

37. What are psychologic concerns about DNA testing?

Presymptomatic genetic testing can give individuals a significant psychological burden of knowing they have a high risk for a specific disease in the future. Genetic testing in this situation, without proper support, education, and pretest and posttest counseling, could potentially cause significant psychologic distress or anxiety and may also affect health care practices. Furthermore, genetic testing or DNA testing creates many unique medical concerns and rarely affects only the individual. For example, some genetic tests can reveal nonpaternity. As genetic testing usually deals with inherited disease, most test results affect an individual's children, siblings, parents, and even more distant family members.

38. What are the social concerns about DNA testing?

The biggest social concern regarding medical DNA testing has always been that presymptomatic genetic testing could be used by medical insurance companies to deny insurance coverage or to inflate the cost for those with an increased risk for disease. With over 12 years of this type of testing and hundreds of thousands of tests, we are still not aware of any cases of this type of discrimination in the United States. There is certainly a great deal of urban myth with no facts to back it up. Most states now have legislation protecting against this type of discrimination, and there is also federal law. However to date, none of these laws have been tested in court.

39. How is individual privacy protected?

Genetic records are protected the same as any other medical record. Some states have enacted laws that go further to protect the privacy of genetic testing information. The biggest problem with privacy issues is that if someone is found to have an increased risk for disease, this will affect medical management. Usually this medical management would need to be paid for by insurance, so you are in a catch-22 if you want to keep your records private, but also want to act on the information.

40. What is pharmacogenetics or pharmacogenomics?

The terms pharmacogenomics and pharmacogenetics tend to be used interchangeably, and precise definitions are still evolving. **Pharmacogenomics** refers more to the entire human genome with the possibility of developing new drugs based on an individual's genetic blueprint. **Pharmacogenetics** usually refers to one or two genes of interest that cause differing reactions to specific drugs. An example is the variation in genes that make enzymes to break down drugs into their active forms. Some individuals could have changes that cause them to metabolize a drug quickly, and others might not metabolize the drug at all, thus gaining no benefit from the drug.

41. What does the future hold in terms of understanding the biology and genetics of cancer?

Over the next decade the explosion of information about the basic processes of cancer derived from genetic research will continue to increase and holds great promise for cancer detection, tumor classification, and treatment.

An exciting new international study is the HapMap Project. The project's goal is to identify and catalog genetic similarities and differences in human beings. This information will help to identify genes that affect health, disease, and individual responses to medications and environmental factors, and should have a very significant impact on cancer prevention and treatment.

Key Points

- All cancer is genetic, because cancer is caused by damage to genes that control cell division or cell growth.
- Most cancer is NOT due to an inherited cancer predisposition. Therefore, most people who get a specific type of cancer will not have a family history of it.
- The most unique characteristic of malignant cells that results in morbidity and mortality is their capability to invade tissues and to metastasize to other sites.
- Currently the genes that control the growth of cells are oncogenes, tumor suppressor genes, mismatch repair genes, and "housekeeping" genes.

Internet Resources

International HapMap Project:
  http://www.hapmap.org
The Human Genome Project:
  http://www.ornl.gov/sci/techresources/Human_Genome/home.shtml
Gene Tests:
  http://www.genetests.org
National Society of Genetic Counselors:
  http://www.nsgc.org
The National Cancer Institute:
  http://www.cancer.gov
The American Cancer Society:
  http://www.cancer.org

Acknowledgments

The author wishes to acknowledge Richard Callahan, MD, and David Faragher, MD, for their contributions to the Biology of Cancer chapter published in the first edition of *Oncology Nursing Secrets* and Constance Engelking, RN, MS, OCN, and Rita Wickham, RN, PhD, AOCN, for their contributions to the Genetic Advances chapter published in the second edition of *Oncology Nursing Secrets.*

Bibliography

Aarnio M, Sankila R, Pukkala E, et al: Cancer risk in mutation carriers of DNA-mismatch-repair genes. *Int J Cancer* 81:214-218, 1999.

Bucholtz JD: Genetics. In Shelton BK, Ziegfeld CR, Olsen MM, editors: *Manual of cancer nursing,* Philadelphia, 2004, Lippincott Williams & Wilkins.

Bulow S: Familial polyposis coli. *Dan Med Bull* 34:1-15, 1987.

DeVita VT, et al: Principles of chemotherapy. In DeVita VT, et al, editors: *Cancer: Principles and practice of oncology,* Philadelphia, 1982, Lippincott Williams & Williams.

DeVita VT, Hellman S, Rosenberg SA, editors: *Cancer: Principles and practice of oncology,* ed 7, Philadelphia, 2004, JB Lippincott.

Ford D, Easton DF, Bishop DT, et al: Risks of cancer in BRCA1-mutation carriers. *Lancet* 343:692-695, 1994.

Human Genome Project Sequence Analysis. Available at: http://www.ornl.gov/sci/techresources/ HumanGenome/project/journals/insights.html. Accessed on 12/29/06.

Jemal A, Siegel R, Ward E, et al: Cancer statistics, 2007. *CA Cancer J Clin* 57:43-66, 2007.

Schneider KA: *Counseling about cancer: Strategies for genetic counselors,* New York, 2002, Wiley-Liss.

Chapter 2

Cancer Prevention and Detection

Mona Bernaiche Bedell

1. Which risk factors for cancer can be modified?

Over 70% of all cancers are associated with lifestyle choices. Adopting a healthy lifestyle and changing risky personal habits and behaviors can reduce the risk for cancer. Examples include eliminating both smoking and chewing tobacco, reducing alcohol intake, limiting exposure to ultraviolet light, adopting sexual practices that limit exposure to sexually transmitted viruses (e.g., abstinence, limited number of sexual partners, condom use), reducing stress, eating foods that are high in fiber and low in fat, and exercising regularly.

2. Elimination of which lifestyle factor would have the greatest impact on reducing the incidence of cancer?

Cigarette smoking is the most preventable cause of cancer-related death in the United States. Smoking not only contributes to 90% of lung cancer in men and 79% in women, but is also the leading cause of head and neck cancers. It is also associated with cancers of the stomach, bladder, kidney, pancreas, liver, and cervix. Smoking also contributes to deaths from cardiovascular disease, pneumonia, stroke, emphysema, and bronchitis.

3. Are vaccines available to prevent cancer?

Vaccine research looks promising. In 2006, the FDA approved a quadrivalent human papillomavirus (HPV) recombinant vaccine to protect females against cervical cancer, cervical adenocarcinoma in situ, cervical intraepithelial neoplasia, and genital warts caused by HPV types 6, 11, 16 and 18 (refer to Chapter 26). A highly effective vaccine is also available to prevent hepatitis B virus (HBV) infection, which increases risk for hepatocellular carcinoma. Approximately 30% to 90% of young children and 2% to 10% of adults who are infected with HBV develop chronic infection. At present there are over 1 million chronic carriers of HBV in the United States, or about 1 in every 250 Americans.

4. Describe primary and secondary levels of cancer prevention.

- **Primary prevention** refers to simple measures taken early to avoid the development of cancer. Primary cancer prevention can be achieved by making lifestyle changes that eliminate risky behavior before cancers occur. Examples of primary prevention activities include smoking cessation, dietary changes to reduce fat and increase fiber, and limiting exposure to ultraviolet light and sexually transmitted viruses.
- **Secondary prevention** targets specific populations and refers to activities, such as testing or screening, to identify high-risk groups with cancer or precursors to cancer. Mammography, Papanicolaou testing, sigmoidoscopy, and prostate-specific antigen (PSA) testing are examples of secondary prevention activities.

5. When is cancer screening most beneficial?

Screening produces the greatest benefit when a certain cancer is highly prevalent in the population, and early diagnosis and treatment would reduce the mortality rate. Screening tests must be simple, inexpensive, safe, and clinically acceptable to the patient.

Tests must be sensitive (able to identify cancer when it is present) and specific (able to determine when cancer is not present).

6. What is the most common cancer?

Skin cancer accounts for one third of newly diagnosed cancers in the United States, making it the most common cancer. Most patients develop nonmelanoma skin cancers, basal cell carcinoma, or squamous cell carcinoma. Basal cell carcinoma is the most common skin neoplasm worldwide, followed by squamous cell carcinomas. Malignant melanoma accounts for < 10% of skin cancers but is associated with higher mortality rates. Three quarters of all deaths associated with skin cancer are caused by malignant melanoma. An estimated 59, 940 new cases of invasive malignant melanoma will be diagnosed in 2007. Skin cancers are highly curable when diagnosed early and surgically excised.

7. Are tanning booths a safe way to obtain a tan?

Avoid tanning booths and salons! There is no such thing as a safe tan. Damage from sunlight or artificial sources of sunlight is cumulative over a lifetime and increases the risk for developing skin cancer. Tanning is the skin's response to injury. Excessive exposure to sunlight also contributes to skin changes that cause wrinkles, premature aging, and rough, leathery skin.

8. Are sunscreens effective in protecting against skin cancer?

Skin cancer is mostly preventable when sun protection measures are used consistently. The lifetime incidence of basal cell carcinoma and squamous cell carcinoma can be reduced by as much as 78% with regular use of sunscreen with a sun protection factor (SPF) of at least 15 during the first 18 years of life. Sunscreen use should begin in infancy, but it is never too late to start. Sunscreen preparations of at least SPF 15 should be applied liberally and frequently. Another simple precaution to protect against ultraviolet light damage is wearing protective clothing (e.g., closely woven long-sleeve shirts, pants, brimmed hats, sunglasses). Avoid or minimize outdoor activities between 10 AM and 4 PM, when ultraviolet light is most intense. Sun effects are also more intense at higher altitudes and when sunlight is reflected off snow, sand, or water.

9. How successful is screening for lung cancer in high-risk populations?

Extensive clinical trials have failed to show a significant decrease in lung cancer mortality, even when patients at high risk for lung cancer were screened with chest radiography and sputum cytology. However, a large collaborative study completed by the International Early Lung Cancer Action Program Investigators demonstrated that annual spiral CT screening can detect curable Stage I lung cancer. Routine screening in high risk patients to detect early lung cancer may now be indicated because of this data. Primary prevention through smoking cessation rather than smoking reduction still offers the best hope for reducing the incidence of lung cancer.

10. Does exposure to environmental tobacco smoke increase a nonsmoker's risk for lung cancer?

Passive cigarette smoke, involuntary smoke, and sidestream smoke are environmental exposures to tobacco smoke, which is responsible for about 30% of lung cancers. Risk of lung cancer is higher for nonsmokers who have lived or worked for years among heavy smokers. Secondhand smoke has significantly higher concentrations of carcinogenic compounds than mainstream smoke. A burning cigarette gives off at least 43 known carcinogens.

11. How useful is the Papanicolaou test?

The Papanicolaou (Pap) test is highly effective in detecting precancerous cells of the cervix. This simple, painless, and inexpensive test has reduced deaths from cervical cancer by

90% in the past 40 years, primarily through preventing invasive cancer. Screening efforts must be made to reach high-risk women in lower socioeconomic groups and older women who have not been previously screened. In both groups the incidence of advanced disease at diagnosis remains high. Over one half of all American women with newly diagnosed cervical cancer have never had a Pap test.

12. Explain the sharp increase in prostate cancer incidence, followed by a decline, in recent years.

Incidence of prostate cancer doubled shortly after prostate specific antigen (PSA) testing became available in 1986 and peaked dramatically in 1992. The rising incidence reflected extensive use of PSA screening in previously unscreened men and an increase in men diagnosed at an earlier age. PSA testing was originally developed as a tumor marker to measure treatment response, but in the 1990's it was widely adopted as a cancer screening test. The increase in incidence also reflected the start of mass screening programs, improved detection techniques, and increased public awareness. Incidence rates have generally declined since that peak in 1992.

13. What is the significance of PSA screening for early detection of prostate cancer?

Widespread PSA testing in asymptomatic men has led to the identification of earlier-stage prostate cancer (smaller and more localized lesions). Unfortunately, PSA testing cannot distinguish latent from aggressive prostate cancers that require treatment. In addition, it is not a specific test for cancer of the prostate; elevated levels are also found in men with benign hypertrophy, prostatitis, and prostatic trauma. Scientific evidence is insufficient to establish that PSA testing, alone or in combination with either digital rectal examination (DRE) or transrectal ultrasonography, has had any impact on reducing the mortality rates of prostate cancer. However, because appropriate use of PSA testing alone provides approximately 90% specificity for prostate cancer and offers a 5- to 10-year lead time in diagnosis, the American Cancer Society recommends that men 50 years and older, with a life expectancy > 10 years, should be screened annually with a PSA test and DRE.

14. Which tests are recommended to screen for colorectal cancer in asymptomatic people?

Screening tests include fecal occult blood testing (FOBT), DRE, sigmoidoscopy, colonoscopy, and double-contrast barium enemas (see Chapter 23 for American Cancer Society guidelines on screening for average-risk individuals). Screening for colorectal cancer clearly reduces mortality, and recommendations are that all men and women aged 50 years or older undergo screening. Fecal occult blood testing reduces colorectal cancer incidence and mortality, based on a review of randomized controlled trials, and sigmoidoscopy is associated with a reduction in mortality in a review of case-control studies. Despite the widespread endorsement of screening by medical organizations and the availability of effective screening tools, less than one third of eligible persons actually undergo screening. More effort is needed to raise awareness and promote colorectal screening at regular intervals.

15. Is virtual colonoscopy an option for colorectal cancer screening?

Also known as computed tomographic colonography, virtual colonoscopy is a noninvasive procedure that takes X-rays of the colon and rectum and views them multidimensionally by computer. Although the preparation for the procedure is similar to that of a colonoscopy, no scope is used, sedation is not necessary, and it is relatively safe. Air is pumped into the colon to distend it and the patient must ingest an oral contrast solution. If polyps are present, a colonoscopy must be performed to remove them. The use of virtual colonoscopy is controversial because small cancerous polyps may potentially be missed. Therefore, it should not be a substitute for routine optical colonoscopy screening. Further studies are needed.

16. **List foods and drugs that may give false-positive reactions to guaiac-based tests for fecal occult blood.**

Rare red meat, broccoli, turnips, cauliflower, parsnips, cabbage, horseradish, potatoes, and melons should be avoided for 3 days before and during testing. Aspirin, vitamin C, iron tablets, nonsteroidal antiinflammatory drugs, and cimetidine also should be avoided.

17. **What chemoprevention strategies are being studied that may decrease the risk of developing colorectal cancer?**

Chemoprevention is the use of natural or synthetic substances to reduce the risk of developing cancer or recurrence. The most widely studied agents in the prevention of colorectal cancer are aspirin and nonsteroidal antiinflammatory drugs (NSAIDs). Cyclooxygenase-1 (COX-1) and cyclooxygenase-2 (COX-2) (enzymes necessary for the synthesis of prostaglandins) are found in many tissues, and levels have been elevated in persons with colon cancer and adenomas. NSAIDs that have inhibitory effects on COX-1 and COX-2 also have been shown to decrease the number of intestinal adenomas and colon tumors. The mechanism by which this process occurs is not well understood but may involve an increase in apoptosis, regulation of angiogenesis, or both. In addition, calcium and folate supplementation in both men and women and hormone-replacement therapy (estrogen) in women have shown a chemopreventive benefit.

18. **What factors help to identify families at increased risk for hereditary forms of cancer?**

Hereditary cancer accounts for 5% to 10% of all cancers diagnosed. Families at high risk have some of the following features in their history and should be referred for genetic or cancer-risk counseling:
- Two or more generations diagnosed with the same or related forms of cancer
- Early age of onset
- Occurrence of rare tumors
- Bilateral, multifocal, or multiple primary tumors in one or more family members

19. **At what age should screening for breast cancer be started?**

Screening mammography is recommended by all major medical organizations in the United States for women 40 years of age and older, although recommended screening intervals may vary from 1- to 3-year intervals. Screening mammograms reduce breast cancer mortality for women ages 50 to 69 years by 20% to 35 %, and less so in women who are 40 to 49 years of age.

20. **What are the components of breast self-exam?**

The three essential components of breast self-exam (BSE) are: (1) visual examination using a mirror, (2) palpation in the shower, and (3) palpation in the supine position on the bed. Changes in breast appearance (including shape, size, or symmetry); skin discoloration or dimpling; sores or skin scaling in and around the areola; and nipple retraction, discharge, or puckering should be assessed.

21. **Should women be instructed to perform BSE?**

Clinical breast exams may detect some cancers missed by mammography; however, studies of BSE failed to show a reduction in breast cancer mortality. Women should be told about the benefits and limitations associated with BSE. Women who choose to perform BSE should be instructed on the proper technique. All women should be encouraged to promptly report breast symptoms, such as bleeding, discharge, pain, or if they notice a lump.

22. Are serum tumor markers useful for cancer screening?

Currently tumor markers are not sufficiently sensitive or specific enough to be used as screening tools in the general population, but they are helpful in monitoring response to therapy.

23. List the general dietary recommendations of the American Cancer Society to reduce cancer risk.

- Avoid overeating and maintain an ideal body weight.
- Reduce total fat intake to < 30% of caloric intake. Excessive fat intake and obesity increase the risk of developing cancers of the breast, colon, and prostate.
- Include a variety of fruits and vegetables that provide fiber, vitamins, minerals, and other chemicals known to have a protective effect. Lower cancer rates have been associated with higher intake of fruits and vegetables.
- Increase fiber intake by eating whole grain cereals, legumes, fresh fruits, and vegetables. Fiber decreases transit time of fecal material through the bowel and reduces contact between carcinogens and intestinal mucosa.
- Minimize the intake of foods that are salt-cured, smoked, or nitrite-cured, such as luncheon meats, bacon, and hot dogs. Stomach and esophageal cancers are associated with consumption of smoked and pickled foods. Nitrates and nitrites, used as food preservatives, are believed to enhance carcinogenic nitrosamine formation.
- Limit consumption of alcoholic beverages. Heavy drinkers are at increased risk for cancers of the oral cavity, larynx, esophagus, breast, and liver.

 Key Points

- Cigarette smoking is the most preventable cause of cancer-related death in the United States.
- There is no such thing as a safe tan.
- Mammography is the main screening tool for breast cancer.
- Screening for colorectal cancer clearly reduces mortality; however, less than one third of eligible persons undergo screening.
- Lower cancer rates have been associated with higher intake of fruits and vegetables.

 Internet Resources

Agency for Healthcare Research and Quality (AHRQ) Guide to Clinical Preventive Services 2006:
  http://www.ahrq.gov/clinic/uspstf/ uspstopics.htm
American Cancer Society Statistics for 2006:
  http://cancer.org/docroot/STT/stt_0.asp
American Cancer Society Guidelines for the Early Detection of Cancer, 2006:
  http://caonline.amcancersoc.org/cgi/content/full/56/1/11
Centers for Disease Control and Prevention: Cancer Prevention and Control:
  http://www.cdc.gov/cancer/index.htm#top
National Cancer Institute: The Cancer Trends Progress Report: 2005 Update:
  http://progressreport.cancer.gov/
National Guideline Clearinghouse:
  http://www.guidelines.gov
CA: A Cancer Journal for Clinicians:
  http://caonline.amcancersoc.org

Bibliography

Carter HB: Prostate cancers in men with low PSA levels—must we find them? *N Engl J Med* 350:2292-2294, 2004.

Clever H: Colon Cancer: Understanding how NSAIDs work. *N Engl J Med* 354:761-763, 2006.

Elmore JG, Armstron K, Lehman CD, et al: Screening for breast cancer. *JAMA* 10:1245-1256, 2005.

Frank-Stromberg M, Cohen RF: Assessment and interventions for cancer detection. In Yarbro CH, Frogge MH, Goodman M, editors: *Cancer nursing: Principles and practice,* ed 6, Boston, 2005, Jones and Bartlett.

Gangloff J: Screening for colorectal cancer. *Cure* 3:12-15, 2004.

Henschke CI, Yankelevitz DF, Libby DM, et al: Survivial of patients with stage I lung cancer detected on CT screening. *N Engl J Med* 355:1763-1771, 2006.

Janne PA, Mayer RJ: Chemoprevention of colorectal cancer. *N Engl J Med* 342:1960-1968, 2000.

Jemal A, Siegel R, Ward E, et al: Cancer statistics, 2007. *CA Cancer J Clin* 57:43-66, 2007.

Jerant AF, Johnson JT, Sheridan CD, et al: Early detection and treatment of skin cancer, *Am Fam Physician* 62:357-358, 2000.

Mahon SM: Principles of cancer prevention and early detection. *Clin J Oncol Nurs* 4:169-176, 2000.

Smith RA, Cokkinides V, Eyre H: American Cancer Society guidelines for the early detection of cancer. *CA Cancer J Clin* 56:11-25, 2006.

Walsh JME, Terdiman JP: Colorectal cancer screening: Scientific review. *JAMA* 289:1288-1296, 2003.

Diagnosis and Staging

Timothy Murphy and Daniel T. Tell

1. How is cancer diagnosed?

Cancer may be diagnosed clinically or by looking at a sample of tissue suspected of being cancerous under a microscope. A clinical diagnosis is the physician's best educated guess at the most likely diagnosis. A patient may be asymptomatic or present with a group of signs and symptoms that suggest a diagnosis of cancer. Most signs and symptoms, however, are nonspecific and can be seen in a wide variety of illnesses. A diagnosis of cancer requires a diagnostic test—and that test is the biopsy. A biopsy is a surgical procedure in which all or part of the tissue suspected of being cancerous is removed.

2. In addition to a biopsy, what other sampling method may be used?

Cytology specimens. Malignant cells can be found in body fluids (e.g., ascites, spinal fluid, pleural effusions) or exfoliated from organs (e.g., cervical Papanicolaou test, sputum).

3. Why is it important to establish a pathologic tissue diagnosis?

Cytology or biopsy specimens establish with certainty the diagnosis of cancer. A tissue diagnosis (tissue procurement and identification) eliminates all of the other diseases in the differential diagnoses originally considered by the clinician when the patient's signs and symptoms were first evaluated. With a firm diagnosis, accurate and specific treatment can be administered, and the patient can be given a prognosis.

4. What information does the pathologist report after doing the biopsy?

Specimens are sent to the laboratory to identify the histopathology (tumor type, classification, and grade) of the malignancy. Examples of tumor types are carcinoma, sarcoma, germ cell tumor, lymphoma, and glioma. Classification is the subtype of the malignancy, such as squamous cell or adenocarcinoma. Grade refers to the degree to which a malignant tumor is similar to normal tissue. For example, poorly differentiated or high-grade tumors contain few features of normal tissue.

5. How is biopsy tissue processed?

A biopsy sample may be processed in many different ways, depending on the suspected diagnosis. Initially all tissue is fixed in a preservative solution and embedded in wax (tissue block). This method of processing the tissue allows thin slices to be cut from the block for staining and subsequent viewing under a microscope. Standard stains allow the pathologist to identify features specific to the organ that the sample was removed from as well as individual cells, nuclei, and nucleoli. Results from a biopsy should be available in 24 hours.

6. What does the pathologist do if standard stains do not help?

If the pathologist cannot make a diagnosis with standard tissue stains, several stains and techniques are available to define the cancer further. In general, a pathologist is able to diagnose cancer from the standard fixation and tissue stains. It is not unusual for the pathologist to have some difficulty in giving a final diagnosis without further testing.

Additional testing often includes special stains and specialized studies (e.g., flow cytometry, monoclonal antibody testing, cytogenetics, and electron microscopy).

7. What are special stains?

Like the clinician, the pathologist generates a differential diagnosis when looking at the biopsy. The pathologist may not be sure of what he or she is looking at but usually has a good idea. Probabilities are ranked, and various tests are ordered to rule in (or out) the most likely diagnosis. The tests that the pathologist orders in this situation are collectively known as "special stains." The test may be as simple as a stain for mucin to differentiate squamous cell carcinoma from adenocarcinoma. Alternatively, immunoperoxidase techniques may be used to identify prostate-specific antigen in an otherwise nonspecific adenocarcinoma. Special stains generally take another 24 to 48 hours to complete. Considering the differential diagnosis obtained by looking at the biopsy, a pathologist generally orders several special stains at once.

8. What is flow cytometry?

Flow cytometry allows analysis of individual cells based on specific characteristics or characteristics identified by specific stains. The cells are placed in suspension and analyzed as they flow through a port or laser source that separates the cells according to the selected characteristic.

9. How is flow cytometry used in diagnosis?

As a diagnostic technique, flow cytometry is generally used to characterize the various types of lymphoma and leukemia. Cells can be labeled with antibodies directed at various antigens specific for certain types of lymphoma. The cells then are sorted by this characteristic. An example is the selection and sorting of the CD5 antigen, which is present in most cases of chronic lymphocytic leukemia. A suspension of lymphoma cells is exposed to an antibody to the CD5 antigen. The antibody is labeled to allow detection as the cells pass through the port. The CD5 cells are detected and counted separately, as is the total number of cells. The results are generally reported as a percentage of the number of CD5-positive cells relative to the total number of cells counted. It is, therefore, most useful in refining rather than establishing a diagnosis. Occasionally, an otherwise undiagnosable lymphoma may exhibit a characteristic flow cytometric pattern, thereby yielding a specific diagnosis.

10. How is flow cytometry used for solid tumors?

Flow cytometry is used to determine the chromosomal content and growth fraction of various tumors, most commonly breast cancer. Although neither a diagnostic nor a staging procedure, this ancillary test often is used to assess prognosis and guide treatment. Flow cytometry provides the clinician with the percentage of tumor cells in "S" phase (dividing cells) and it is an indicator of the presence of tumor cells with abnormal DNA content. High percentages of cells in S phase and with abnormal DNA content are generally believed to confer a worse prognosis in breast cancer, and often more aggressive treatment is prescribed.

11. Define ploidy analysis and its significance.

DNA ploidy analysis assesses the DNA characteristics of cancer cells in G1 phase. Cells are classified according to the amount of DNA in their nuclei. For example, cancerous cells that are more similar to normal cells are known as diploid; the cell's nucleus contains the appropriate number of human chromosomes. Aneuploid contains either too many or too few; tetraploid means the nucleus of the cell contains four times as many chromosomes as a healthy cell. Patients with diploid tumors (DNA index < 1, or normal DNA content) tend to have a better prognosis than those with aneuploid tumors (DNA index > 1, or abnormal DNA content). The incidence of subclinical dissemination and tumor recurrence is greater in patients with an aneuploid tumor having a high S-phase fraction. DNA ploidy analysis may be useful in determining tumor grade and response.

12. How are monoclonal antibodies used for the detection of cancer?

All cells possess surface antigens that may be detected by antibodies directed against them. The antibodies are labeled to facilitate detection. The label may be radioactive or designed to fluoresce or change color so that it can be seen. Cancer cells often possess antigens unique to that particular type of cancer. The pathologist may request a wide variety of monoclonal antibody tests to evaluate a biopsy, depending on the suspected diagnosis. Examples of commonly used monoclonal antibodies are antileukocyte common antigen (anti-LCA) and anticytokeratin. Both tests are often used to evaluate a poorly differentiated malignancy.

During routine staining, a pathologist may be able to say that a tissue specimen is malignant but unable to determine whether the cancer is lymphoma or carcinoma. This distinction is important for both treatment and prognosis. Such a biopsy probably would be tested for both LCA and cytokeratin. An LCA-positive biopsy is consistent with lymphoma, whereas a cytokeratin-positive biopsy is consistent with carcinoma.

13. What is electron microscopy?

Just as light is used to view microscopic structures, electrons can be used to visualize the extremely small cell components. Because the wavelength of electrons is much shorter than visible light, resolution and magnification are much greater. Electron microscopy (EM) can be used to visualize cellular organelles, cellular inclusions, and intercellular bridges, which are often characteristic of various malignancies. The limit of magnification with light microscopy is about 1000×. EM can enlarge into the tens of thousands and even higher with specialized techniques.

14. What are cytogenetic studies?

Some tumors are associated with specific genetic abnormalities, which often can be detected by cytogenetic studies. The chromosomes from individual cells are cultured and isolated during cell division. They are fixed, stained, and magnified so that rearrangements (translocations) and deletions can be seen. Probably the best known translocation is the Philadelphia chromosome, which is associated with and usually is diagnostic of chronic myelogenous leukemia. Further refinements of cytogenetic techniques have allowed the identification of individual mutations.

15. What is a FISH test?

FISH (fluorescent in situ hybridization) is a special method used to visualize chromosomal changes resulting from genetic differences and to detect gene amplification and genetic changes in specific cancers. A special probe helps to "light up" (fluoresce) mutated gene segments in chromosomes. In breast cancer patients, FISH is useful in confirming HER-2/neu status.

16. What is IHC?

IHC (immunohistochemistry) is currently the preferred standard for evaluating HER-2/neu status. A positive IHC test (2+ and 3+) suggests that the patient is a good candidate for trastuzumab (Herceptin) therapy.

17. What happens after the pathologist decides that the diagnosis is cancer?

Usually the pathologist calls the patient's physician, who has to tell the patient. In most cases the patient has been advised that a malignant diagnosis is likely and is mentally prepared to deal with the news. Preparing a patient to receive the news and actually delivering the news are an art that requires compassion, awareness of the patient's personality, and, to a certain extent, experience. The physician most qualified to inform the patient is the primary care physician; it is most important that he or she be involved. However, many physicians are uncomfortable in this role—which is why God made oncologists. Effective collaboration and communication between physicians and nurses are essential in assisting the patient through this initial crisis.

18. Describe the role of the nurse when the patient is told about a diagnosis of cancer.

The nurse's role in this setting is critical; it is not only supportive but also informative. The nurse should be able to address issues that invariably arise after the patient has been told the diagnosis. Because most patients are anxious, they hear little of the physician's discussion after they hear the diagnosis or are confused about what they did hear. Patients may not be comfortable questioning the physician or may believe they are taking up too much of the physician's time. The nurse should be prepared to address the patient's questions and have general information about the disease process, prognosis, further testing, potential complications, and available treatments. If a specific question cannot be answered, the nurse should say so and obtain the answer, or refer the patient to an oncology advanced practice nurse or other appropriate provider. It is always better to admit that the answer is not known than to provide incorrect information. The patient may not be interested in specific answers at this point. Listening to, supporting, guiding, and reassuring the patient may be more important than statistics and technical information. If the patient demonstrates emotional difficulty facing the diagnosis, the nurse should consider referral to a social worker, psychologist, or chaplain.

19. After the diagnosis of cancer has been made, what is the next step?

Patients must undergo a staging process or a series of tests to determine the extent of the disease. Patients need to be told why the tests are done and instructed about preparation procedures and possible complications. Other instructions include description of physical sensations or discomfort that may be anticipated, when results are available, and identification of who will report the results. Patients should be assessed for contraindications or hypersensitivities to iodine or other radioactive agents.

20. Why is staging important?

- The extent to which a disease has spread is prognostic.
- Extent of disease often dictates treatment.
- Accurate staging allows collection of data that eventually provides information about treatment outcomes for each type of cancer and each stage of disease. Staging information is collected and maintained by a tumor registry, which enables hospitals to make comparisons about their patients' treatments to those in hospitals around the country.

21. What tests are used in the staging of cancer?

All staging begins with a history and physical examination. More specific questions and more thorough physical testing may be performed after diagnosis to assess signs or symptoms peculiar to the diagnosed cancer. This information may make a physician suspect the presence of disease at another site, and other tests may be ordered to confirm such suspicions.

The physician generally orders a complete blood count, chemistry tests of liver and kidney function, and urinalysis when a patient is first suspected of having cancer.

These tests help to detect the presence of metastatic disease and to assess organ function in preparation for treatment. Tests for tumor markers may be ordered to serve as a point of reference for subsequent treatment. In some diseases, elevated tumor markers may suggest the extent of disease and tumor burden and have prognostic implications.

Additionally, several tests are available to evaluate the extent of a particular disease. The most commonly used tests are radiographs (plain film, computed tomography [CT] scans, magnetic resonance imaging [MRI], and nuclear medicine scans). Biopsies are sometimes used to confirm a suspicious radiograph or scan abnormalities and to evaluate tissue that cannot be evaluated in any other way (e.g., bone marrow).

22. What is the preferred staging system for solid tumors?

The tumor-node-metastasis (TNM) system of the American Joint Committee on Cancer (AJCC) is preferred for most solid tumors (e.g., breast, lung, colon), which are classified by the following:

T = characteristics of a given tumor (size, depth of invasion, involvement of surrounding structures)

N = presence or absence of involved lymph nodes and size or number of involved nodes

M = presence or absence of metastases

A typical TNM classification for a 3-cm breast cancer with one involved lymph node and bone metastases would be as follows: T2N1M1 (bone).

23. How are TNM results grouped?

TNM results can be incorporated into larger groupings, called stages, in which various Ts, Ns, and Ms with similar prognoses are collected. Most tumors proceed from stage I through stage IV. Prognosis worsens with stage progression for any given disease. Stage IV disease is generally metastatic, whereas stage I disease is generally confined to the organ of origin. A T2N1M1 breast cancer is stage IV, whereas a T2N1M0 breast cancer is stage II. Such a system allows the clinician to assign a prognosis and usually guides treatment. It also allows health professionals to discuss individual clinical situations and to exchange information about prognosis and management. The detail provided by such a system allows retrospective (or prospective) investigations, which may reveal differences in prognosis for certain situations. These differences may justify moving a particular TNM combination to a different stage or provide new information about its management.

The system is specific for all of the different anatomic sites with respect to T and many Ns; as a result, it is complicated. Fortunately, the *Cancer Staging Handbook*, published by the AJCC, lists all of the anatomic sites and the accepted staging schema for each. If a staging manual is not available, most oncology texts explain TNM staging in the chapter for each tumor.

24. Is the TNM classification always used to stage cancer?

No. Some cancers are staged using different classification systems. For example, the hematologic malignancies are staged differently. For example, Hodgkin and non-Hodgkin lymphomas are staged using the Ann Arbor classification, multiple myeloma is staged by the Durie-Salmon clinical system, and most of the leukemias are staged using the French-American-British system. The gynecologic malignancies are staged using the International Federation of Gynaecology and Obstetrics (FIGO) staging system.

25. Define tumor markers and how they are used.

Tumor markers are substances secreted by tumors that can be found in blood, urine, or other parts of the body. They may refer to proteins, DNA, genetic markers, oncogene receptors, hormone receptors, and enzymes. Tumor markers may be used diagnostically to help identify cancer in an individual, prognostically to estimate the risk of death or recurrence after surgical removal of the cancer without adjuvant therapy, and predictively to assess how patients may respond to a particular therapy. However, they are generally used to evaluate response to therapy and to monitor recurrence. Tumor marker tests are somewhat organ-specific, although overlap with other diseases is common. Many tumor markers also can be elevated in benign conditions.

26. What are the most commonly used serum tumor markers?

Many tumor markers are available to monitor various tumors; the most commonly used are listed in the table below. Tumor markers are more likely to be elevated in patients with metastatic disease and tend to rise progressively with worsening disease. No test is perfect, however, and some patients with metastatic disease may have normal tumor markers.

Common serum tumor markers

Tumor marker	Malignancies associated with elevated level of marker
Alpha-fetoprotein (AFP)	Hepatocellular carcinoma Choriocarcinoma, teratoma Embryonal cell tumors of ovary or testis
Carcinoembryonic antigen (CEA)	Colon, rectum, pancreas, gastric, lung, breast, ovary
CA-125	Epithelial ovarian neoplasms, breast, colorectal, gastric
CA-15-3	Breast
CA-19-9	Pancreas, colorectal, gastric, liver, biliary tract
CA-27-29	Breast
Human chorionic gonadotropin (HCG)	Choriocarcinoma, germ cell, testicular teratoma, hydatidiform mole
Prostate-specific antigen (PSA)	Prostate

27. Discuss the role of carcinoembryonic antigen testing.

Carcinoembryonic antigen (CEA) was the first tumor marker to be described and remains a useful test. CEA is a protein normally found in small quantities in the blood of healthy people. CEA is elevated in many tumors of epithelial origin but is used most commonly to evaluate colon malignancies. It is elevated in over 50% of patients who have cancer of the colon, pancreas, stomach, lung, or breast, but may be abnormal in patients who have noncancerous conditions, such as bronchitis, hepatitis, lung infections, and ulcerative colitis. It is mildly elevated in patients who smoke cigarettes. Thus CEA testing is not specific enough to be useful for screening or diagnosis. CEA testing is most useful for monitoring response to therapy and detecting disease recurrence.

28. What are CT scans?

CT (computed tomography) is a radiographic procedure in which a patient is exposed to x-rays, and an image is generated based on the differential absorption of x-rays by different tissues in the body. In this respect the technique is similar to plain radiographs. In CT scanning, however, the images are manipulated by a computer to provide cross-sectional images (or images in any plane, for that matter). The result is multiple cross-sectional images, usually several centimeters apart, depicted from head to toe.

29. How are CT scans used in patients with cancer?

CT usually is ordered for a general anatomic area, such as head, chest, abdomen, or pelvis. It allows visualization of most internal organs in great detail and may spare the patient a surgical procedure. It is useful in the staging of a wide variety of cancers. In patients with lung cancer, CT visualizes the mediastinum, which may show enlarged lymph nodes not apparent on plain chest radiograph. Such patients do not undergo surgical treatment; instead, they are treated with radiation and chemotherapy. In patients with pancreatic cancer, a CT scan of the abdomen may show liver metastases. Again, surgery is not an option; the patient receives chemotherapy. In either case, a biopsy probably would be performed to confirm the presence of disease in the lymph nodes or liver; the presence of disease in either location radically affects treatment and prognosis.

30. What is an MRI scan?

In MRI (magnetic resonance imaging), the area of the patient to be visualized is exposed to a strong magnetic field, which aligns all of the atoms of the organ in question in one direction. When the magnet is deactivated, the atoms return to their normal alignment and in so doing release energy. Different tissues with varying water content release energy at different times. This energy is monitored and can be imaged. The result is a scan that at first glance appears similar to a CT scan but provides different information.

31. How are MRI scans used in patients with cancer?

MRIs may be used to image a suspicious area on a CT scan, such as an area of fibrosis or an enlarged lymph node. A tumor within a scar or an enlarged lymph node emits a different signal, allowing the radiologist to detect its presence. MRIs also may be used to detect lesions that are isodense. Such lesions have the same density as the tissue in which they grow and may not be seen on CT scanning. Brain and liver metastases are occasionally isodense; when an MRI scan is performed, the lesions become obvious as bright white masses. Because isodense lesions are relatively uncommon, MRI scanning is not a routine part of staging. Generally a negative CT scan is accepted as normal, unless the patient displays symptoms suggesting the presence of disease. In this situation an MRI may be ordered to exclude isodense metastases.

MRI also has proved useful in the diagnosis of carcinomatous meningitis. Before the availability of MRI, patients often required myelography, which is invasive, uncomfortable, and potentially dangerous.

32. What are nuclear medicine scans?

Nuclear medicine scans are radiographic studies in which a radioactive isotope is administered to the patient intravenously. The radioactive isotope concentrates within the target organ, where it is temporarily trapped. The label emits radiation that can be imaged. Before the advent of CT scanning, brain and liver scans were commonly used for staging. However, CT scans have far better resolution and have largely replaced nuclear medicine scanning of the brain and liver.

33. How are nuclear medicine scans used in patients with cancer?

A bone scan is often used to stage patients with various solid tumors (e.g., lung and breast cancer). A **multiple-gated acquisition (MUGA)**, or heart scan, is often ordered during staging to assess cardiac function in patients who may need cardiotoxic chemotherapy. This scan provides information about cardiac wall motion, contractility, and ejection fraction; it is used to determine whether the patient's heart is functioning well enough to tolerate specific drugs (e.g., doxorubicin). It is not used for staging per se.

34. What is positron emission tomography?

Positron emission tomography (PET) is a special kind of nuclear medicine imaging tomography made possible by the unique fate of positrons. In contrast to CT scans that image the body's anatomy, PET provides imaging of the body's biochemistry and physiology. PET cannot be performed with conventional gamma cameras; a specially designed PET scanner is required. Malignant cells have an enhanced rate of glycolysis. FDG (fluorine-18 fluorodeoxyglucose), a positron emitter that mimics the increased rate of glycolysis in tumor cells, is used in most PET studies to give a rating of glucose metabolism in the cells. Active tumors show up as "hot spots" on the PET scan.

35. What is a PET/CT scanner?

A PET/CT scanner combines PET and CT imaging using precise calibration. PET and CT scan images are obtained consecutively and aligned, creating a more complete picture of the tumor's location and growth. Although PET scans are very accurate, the PET/CT is more accurate than PET alone in the staging of cancer.

36. How is PET/CT used in patients with cancer?

PET/CT is an imaging technique that takes advantage of unique metabolic characteristics of cancer cells, which allows for more accurate clinical staging of certain malignancies (e.g., non-small cell lung cancer and lymphoma). PET/CT is also being used to assess tumor response to chemotherapy and to detect recurrent disease before the patient develops clinical symptoms.

37. What is a bone marrow biopsy?

Bone marrow biopsy is a commonly used minor surgical procedure that determines the presence or absence of marrow involvement by tumor. The posterior iliac crest is the site most commonly chosen; when viewed from the back, it may be seen in most patients as two dimples on either side of the lower lumbar spine at the belt line. In most patients, the iliac bone is close to the surface at this point and separated from the surface of the skin only by fat.

38. How is a bone marrow biopsy performed?

The patient may be sedated for the procedure. After local anesthetic infiltration, a small stab incision is made. A needle is inserted through the bone cortex into the marrow cavity, and a small amount of liquid marrow is aspirated into a syringe. A biopsy needle then is inserted into the bone to remove a core or cylinder of bone marrow, usually about 2 cm long and a few millimeters wide. In patients in whom sedation is not possible, the procedure is moderately uncomfortable. The dominant sensation is an intense pressure punctuated by brief periods of toothache-like pain. In the bone marrow involved by tumor, collections of tumor cells may be seen in scattered areas throughout the marrow cavity, or the tumor may completely fill the space.

39. What are the complications of bone marrow biopsy?

The only major complication of a correctly performed bone marrow biopsy is the remote possibility of infection in the bone. Postprocedural pain is generally mild and resolves within a few days. Occasionally a patient develops a subperiosteal hematoma, which may cause point tenderness for several weeks.

40. How is bone marrow biopsy used in staging?

A bone marrow biopsy is a diagnostic procedure for leukemia, whereas it is generally a part of staging lymphomas. It also is used in patients with small cell lung cancer when the likelihood of marrow involvement is substantial, and when marrow involvement changes treatment. In most other diseases, marrow biopsy is used selectively. In patients with solid tumors and lymphomas, marrow involvement often changes treatment and always changes prognosis. As a result, bone marrow biopsy may be used to stage a patient in whom bone marrow involvement is suspected. For example, the complete blood count (CBC) of a patient with breast cancer may show mild anemia and thrombocytopenia. The differential may show a small number of immature white cells and an occasional nucleated red blood cell. This constellation of CBC findings is highly suspicious for marrow involvement by tumor. In the absence of another good explanation, bone marrow biopsy is recommended. Treatment and prognosis are affected dramatically if the bone marrow is involved.

41. Are there times when the type of cancer cannot be determined?

In some patients who have metastatic cancer, a careful search reveals no obvious primary tumor. This situation, known as adenocarcinoma–unknown primary (ACUP) or simply unknown primary, accounts for about 5% to 10% of all patients with cancer. Most commonly, such tumors are poorly differentiated carcinomas or adenocarcinomas (see Chapter 33).

42. What is scintigraphy?

In scintigraphy, a radioactive isotope is injected around a primary tumor and then imaged after it has traveled to the lymph node group that serves as primary drainage for the tumor site. This technique is useful in evaluating tumors with ambiguous lymph node drainage, such as melanomas on the trunk. A melanoma on the back, for instance, may drain to either the axilla or groin, or even the cervical region. Demonstrating lymph node involvement in melanoma has become very important because effective adjuvant treatment has been discovered for patients who have metastatic tumors in their lymph nodes.

Scintigraphy or sentinel lymph node mapping has gained popularity in the evaluation of breast cancer. Rather than dissecting the axillary lymph nodes, a biopsy is performed on the first lymph node, or sentinel node, draining the breast cancer. The assumption is that if the results of the biopsy on the sentinel lymph node are normal, the axillary nodes would also be normal (see Chapter 22).

43. Are there any controversies in the diagnosis of cancer?

No. A tissue diagnosis must always be made. Physicians may argue about the best way to obtain a diagnosis, but none would argue against making the diagnosis. The implications of a diagnosis of cancer and the potential for harm during the treatment of cancer are too great to assume the diagnosis. A clinical diagnosis, if incorrect, exposes the patient to great emotional, physical, and financial stress. The cardinal rule of oncology is simple— no DX (diagnosis), no RX (treatment).

44. Are there any controversies in the staging of cancer?

Yes. For most diseases, staging procedures and tests are standard. Controversy arises when technologic advances and new or ancillary tests become available. Patient risk, inconvenience, and cost must be considered, and there is a period of uncertainty until the new technology is perceived or proved to be indispensable or ancillary. In the future, advancing technology will clash with increasing cost consciousness, and the ways cancer is diagnosed and staged will change—hopefully for the better.

Key Points

- Cytology or biopsy specimens establish with certainty the diagnosis of cancer.
- Effective collaboration and communication between physicians and nurses are essential in assisting the patient through the crisis of receiving a cancer diagnosis.
- After the cancer diagnosis is made, patients must undergo a staging process or a series of tests to determine the extent of the disease.
- The tumor-node-metastasis (TNM) staging system of the American Joint Committee on Cancer (AJCC) is preferred for most solid tumors (e.g., breast, lung, colon).
- Tumor markers are generally used to evaluate response to therapy and to monitor recurrence.

Internet Resources

American Cancer Society:
   http://www.cancer.org/docroot/ETO/content/ETO_1_2X_Staging.asp
Lab Tests Online:
   http://labtestsonline.org

Bibliography

Greene FL, Page DL, Fleming ID, et al, editors: *AJCC cancer staging manual,* ed 6, New York, 2002, Springer.
Omerod KF: Diagnostic evaluation, classification, and staging. In Yarbro CH, Frogge MH, Goodman M, et al, editors: *Cancer nursing: Principles and practice,* ed 6, Boston, 2005, Jones and Bartlett.
Yamamoto DS, Viale PH, Lin A: The clinical use of tumor markers in select cancers: Are you confident enough to discuss them with your patients? *Oncol Nurs Forum* 32(5):1013-1025, 2005.

Unit II

Treating Cancer

Surgical Oncology

Ann Marie Dose and Carol Brueggen

1. What are the goals of surgery in the treatment of cancer?

- **Prophylaxis:** If an organ with potential for development of cancer is not crucial for survival, surgery may be necessary or desirable to prevent malignancy. Examples include colon cancer (in cases of familial polyposis), breast cancer, testicular cancer, or cervical cancer.
- **Diagnosis:** Tissue biopsy is necessary to validate the diagnosis and to identify the histologic markers or specific type of cancer.
- **Staging:** The extent of disease can be determined by surgical staging, which identifies tumor type, extent of growth, size, nodal involvement, and regional and distant spread. Exploratory surgery may be required to stage Hodgkin lymphoma or ovarian cancer. Sentinel node biopsy can be done for breast cancer or malignant melanoma.
- **Definitive or curative treatment:** Definitive or curative surgery involves removing the entire tumor, associated lymph nodes, and a 2- to 5-cm margin of surrounding tissue. Early diagnosis is essential when the goal is cure. Surgery for early-stage cervical, breast, skin, renal cell, prostate, and colon cancer may be curative. Surgical placement of brachytherapy for cervical and prostate cancers has curative intent.
- **Palliation:** Surgical intervention for palliation is most commonly done to minimize symptoms of advanced disease and relieve distress. For example, palliative surgeries include cytoreductive surgery; ablative procedures; surgery to relieve gastrointestinal, respiratory, and urinary obstructions or fistulas; and neurosurgical procedures for pain control. Decompressive laminectomy may be done to relieve spinal cord compression secondary to malignancy.
- **Adjuvant or supportive therapy:** Surgical procedures performed in addition to other treatment modalities are called adjuvant or supportive. Examples include surgery to implant a vascular access device, feeding tube, or tracheostomy.
- **Reconstructive or rehabilitative therapy:** Advances in plastic and reconstructive surgery have made it possible to repair anatomic defects and to improve function and cosmetic appearance after radical surgery (e.g., breast, head, and neck cancers). The goal is to minimize deformity and improve quality of life.
- **Salvage treatment:** Further surgery is done to treat local disease recurrence after use of a less extensive primary treatment. Examples include salvage radical cystectomy after primary radiation therapy for bladder cancer, and salvage mastectomy after primary lumpectomy and radiation therapy for breast cancer.

2. What patient and tumor factors need to be assessed before surgery?

Patient factors include overall health status and comorbidities, such as diabetes and cardiac, pulmonary, or kidney disease. General health habits, nutritional status, rehabilitation potential, and previous oncologic treatments are other issues to explore. Age may be a factor, but it is relevant only in the face of overall general health status and quality of life.

   Tumor factors include growth rate, invasiveness, metastatic potential, and location. In general, tumors that are slow-growing and have cells with prolonged cell cycles lend themselves best to local control by surgery. Surgeons need to know the pattern of local invasion for a specific tumor to remove it as an entire mass with adequate normal surrounding tissue to minimize seeding or local recurrence. Some tumor invasions may necessitate more radical surgery; other tumors may not need total resection if additional chemotherapy and radiation therapy have been demonstrated to improve survival. Metastatic potential of a tumor determines the amount and appropriate combination of multimodal therapies. Location of the tumor and spread into adjacent tissue and vital organs or structures also need to be considered in weighing the risks and benefits of surgical intervention and effect on functional status and overall quality of life.

3. Why are biopsies important in cancer care?

A biopsy is performed to confirm or diagnose cancer correctly. A biopsy consists of removing a tissue sample from an organ or other part of the body for histologic examination by a pathologist. Examination of the biopsy specimen may be abnormal and indicate the presence of cancer, whereas normal results of a biopsy may indicate that no cancer is present or that the biopsy specimen was not adequate. When a biopsy specimen does not show evidence of cancer but cancer is still suspected, further investigation is required.

4. What types of biopsies and surgical procedures are performed?

The ideal biopsy method should be relatively inexpensive and noninvasive, convenient for patients, easy to perform, and able to deliver a preliminary cancer diagnosis. The type of surgical procedure is determined by preoperative evaluation of tumor involvement and individual health considerations and preferences. Numerous types of biopsies and surgical procedures are available, each with different uses, advantages, and disadvantages.

Surgical procedures in patients with cancer

Type	Use	Advantages	Disadvantages
Incisional biopsy	Obtain tissue for pathologic exam	Simple method to obtain diagnosis	Additional, more extensive surgical procedure generally done to remove tumor
Excisional biopsy	Establish tissue diagnosis and tumor removal	Quick, simple removal of tumor at biopsy; may not require hospitalization; decreased cost; minimal cosmetic effects	Tumor cells may be implanted along surgical path and incision, resulting in local recurrence
Needle biopsy: fine-needle aspiration, core biopsy, sentinel node biopsy	Obtain tissue for pathologic exam; determine stage	Simple to perform, reliable, and inexpensive; performed under local anesthesia on outpatient basis; result obtained very quickly	Risk of injury to adjacent structures; risk of tumor cell implantation along needle track and recurrence
Diagnostic laparotomy	Determine stage and extent of disease	Provides more accurate information for treatment planning	Major surgical procedure with risk for postoperative complications;

Surgical procedures in patients with cancer—cont'd

Type	Use	Advantages	Disadvantages
			requires hospital stay; costly; multiple lifestyle disruptions
Local excision	Primary treatment Cytoreductive surgery Removal of solitary metastasis Palliative treatment	Minimal tissue removal with little effect on functional status and appearance; may not require hospital stay or require only short hospital stay	Risk of microscopic residual disease in tissue, resulting in local recurrence
Wide excision	Primary treatment Cytoreductive surgery Palliative treatment	Eliminates visible and microscopic disease locally and in adjacent tissue at increased risk for disease spread	Longer, more involved rehabilitation required; may cause major changes in functional ability and appearance; may require reconstructive procedures
Laser surgery	Primary treatment Cytoreductive surgery Palliative treatment	Can be used in all body systems; decreased blood loss and need for blood products; decreased local recurrence rates; minimal side effects, including minimal pain during and after surgery; decreased wound drainage; earlier return of functional ability; reduced incidence of functional disabilities; minimal preparation time and easy delivery; decreased procedure time; decreased or no hospital stay; may be repeated on recurrent tumor; immediate grafting possible; may be done when traditional surgery is contraindicated (e.g., because of tumor location, poor health status of patient)	None noted

Continued

Surgical procedures in patients with cancer—cont'd

Type	Use	Advantages	Disadvantages
Photodynamic therapy	Primary treatment	More precise in locating cancer cells, particularly when all sites of disease are unknown; decreased risks and variety of side effects compared with traditional surgery	Photosensitivity for 4-6 weeks, causing possible lifestyle disruptions
Stereotaxis	Obtain biopsy Primary treatment Cytoreductive surgery Implantation of radioactive sources, hyperthermia, or chemotherapeutic agents Perform thalamotomy for intractable pain or tremor	Minimizes exposed and affected tissue; less trauma to brain tissue than traditional approaches with decreased neurologic deficits; shorter hospital stay and reduced hospitalization costs; lower mortality and morbidity	Use depends on size and location of tumor and current expertise and technology in imaging modalities and computer technology; neurologic side effects depend on size and location of tumor
Laparoscopic and endoscopic surgery	Establish tissue diagnosis Determine stage Primary treatment	Decreased postoperative pain and procedure-related complications; earlier recovery and return to activities of daily living; shorter hospital stay with decreased treatment costs	Use depends on size and location of primary tumor and existence of regional disease; anatomic defects may limit access and use; inconclusive data on long-term effect on prognosis
Radiofrequency ablation	Primary treatment Cytoreductive surgery Palliative treatment	Performed on outpatient basis; decreased pain and postoperative complications; earlier recovery; used in clients unable to tolerate more invasive or traditional procedures	Use dependent on size and location of tumor

From Szopa TJ: Nursing implications of surgical treatment. In Itano JK, Taoka KN, editors: *Core curriculum for oncology nursing*, ed 4, St Louis, 2005, Elsevier Saunders, pp 737-739, with permission.

5. Why is surgery sometimes performed when metastasis is present?

In certain situations, when the primary tumor has been resected or is in remission, resecting solitary metastatic tumors may be appropriate. In patients with evidence of multiple metastatic lesions or aggressive tumors, resection is not indicated. The following factors must be considered before surgical intervention is attempted:

- Tumor histology
- Disease-free interval
- Tumor doubling time
- Tumor size and location
- Rate of metastasis
- Patient's performance status

Studies have reported successful resection of solitary metastatic tumors of the lung, liver, brain, and bone.

6. How does surgical staging differ from clinical staging?

Clinical staging includes findings acquired before definitive treatment, such as physical examination, imaging, endoscopy, biopsy, and some surgical exploration. Surgical evaluative and pathologic staging is done after surgery, including lymph node studies.

7. What topics should nurses include in preoperative and postoperative patient education?

Preoperative teaching should include discussion of the extent of the planned surgery and any expected functional limitations. Issues of concern should be clarified, and sources of support should be identified and discussed. Instructions about the use of any equipment, pulmonary exercises, coughing techniques, and pain management options should be provided. Because of shortened postoperative hospital stays, it is also beneficial to do an initial discharge assessment preoperatively. Factors that may influence discharge planning include home environment, financial status, self-care abilities, available family and agency support, employment status, and type of work. It is common for patients and families to experience anxiety. Patient and family concerns related to the uncertainty of long-term survival and the possible need for further treatment should be assessed and addressed. Because anxiety reduces a patient's ability to understand and retain information, teaching should be reinforced as appropriate.

Postoperatively, patients and families need to know about prescribed medications, ongoing wound care, signs and symptoms of infection, appropriate nutrition, proper balance of rest and exercise, care of catheters or ostomies, and where and when to return for postoperative examinations. Communication with agencies providing care after hospitalization, such as home care agencies or nursing homes, is key to ensuring continuity of care. If additional chemotherapy or radiation therapy is scheduled, baseline teaching can be done if the patient and family are ready and receptive.

8. Discuss the important aspects of physical care in the postoperative period.

Physical care centers on general surgical nursing principles, with specific focus on pain management, wound care, nutrition, hemostasis, and prevention of complications. Good pain control can improve patient satisfaction, promote healing, reduce recovery time, and decrease postoperative complications. Postoperative pain can be managed in many ways, including administering opioids by patient-controlled analgesia (PCA), continuous epidural analgesia, or regional nerve block; combining injectable nonsteroidal antiinflammatory drugs (NSAIDs), such as ketorolac (Toradol), with traditional intravenous opioids; and adding various nondrug methods to decrease anxiety and pain (see Chapter 42).

Complications after surgery for cancer

Complication	Contributing factors
Acute respiratory distress syndrome	Hemorrhage Deposition of platelets Aspiration Trauma to lung parenchyma Prolonged atelectasis Cardiopulmonary bypass Infection Pulmonary emboli Pulmonary edema
Aspiration pneumonia	Difficulty in swallowing Excessive sedation Mechanical obstruction from cancer
Bleeding	Prolonged cardiopulmonary bypass Coagulopathy Medications
Cardiovascular dysfunction	Congestive heart failure Arrhythmias Myocardial infarction
Infection	Neutropenia Splenectomy Cell-mediated deficiencies Transfusion-transmitted infections Humoral-mediated deficiencies Disruptions of mechanical barriers
Mucositis	Antimetabolite chemotherapeutic agents Head and neck radiation Dehydration
Obstruction/ileus	Immobility Opioids
Poor wound healing	Malnutrition Steroid therapy Neutropenia Local tumor invasion Chemotherapy Immune dysfunction Previous radiation therapy Pressure ulcer formation

Adapted from Polomano R, Weintraub FN, Wurster A: Surgical critical care for cancer patients, *Semin Oncol Nurs* 10:165-176, 1994; and Burke C: Surgery. In Liebman MC, Camp-Sorrell D, editors: *Multimodal therapy in oncology nursing*, St Louis, 1996, Mosby, pp 34-43.

9. What factors should be considered in the assessment and care of surgical wounds?

Wound assessment should include length, width, depth, location, direction of the wound, descriptions of the base and edges, and presence of any exudate. Factors that can delay wound healing include age, obesity, prior chemotherapy or radiation therapy, malnutrition, and diabetes. If the surrounding tissue is compromised, or a deep pocket of infection exists, wounds may be left to heal on their own (from the inside out). Dressings may be used to protect the wound, to promote comfort, to immobilize wound edges, and to maintain a moist environment.

10. Does nutritional status affect surgical outcome?

Protein and calorie malnutrition, a common problem in patients with prior treatment and compromised immune status, may lead to wound dehiscence, ileus, sepsis, and a longer hospital stay. Perioperative and postoperative support in the form of high protein and high calorie oral diets, enteral tube feedings, and total parenteral nutrition (TPN) can significantly decrease morbidity and mortality.

11. Are patients with cancer at increased risk for hemostatic or bleeding problems?

Altered hemostasis in the form of hypercoagulability and thrombosis can put the patient with cancer at higher risk for postoperative complications, particularly patients with adenocarcinoma of the lung, pancreas, and colon. Early postoperative ambulation is imperative to prevent deep vein thrombosis.

12. What factors should be considered in postoperative rehabilitation?

Rehabilitation centers on meeting physical, psychosocial, sexual, spiritual, educational, vocational, and financial needs. It begins preoperatively and continues postoperatively. Common nursing diagnoses include body image disturbance related to disfigurement, impaired tissue integrity, and decreased self-esteem. For example, some patients may have no desire to address workplace issues and concerns in the first few days after surgery; others may have increased pain, lack of sleep, or both that are related to anxieties about how they will continue to provide for their families.

13. How soon after surgery can adjuvant chemotherapy and radiation therapy begin?

Certain antineoplastic agents and radiation doses interfere with wound healing; thus special consideration must be given to the timing of adjuvant therapy. Adjuvant therapy can be started as early as a few days after surgery, but in many instances a recovery time of 3-6 weeks is standard.

14. If a tumor is exposed to air during surgery, will the cancer spread?

The myth that surgery may cause cancer to spread by exposing cancerous cells to air is not true. Cancer does not spread because it has been exposed to the air. Since early removal of all cancer cells provides the best chance of cure, people should not allow this myth to prevent them from seeking surgery.

15. What is "seeding"?

Seeding means that the cancer has spread, with the occurrence of small nodules in the peritoneum or wound. Seeding may occur in an area where a biopsy has been performed previously.

16. What types of reconstructive surgeries are indicated to improve quality of life?

After radical surgery, many wounds do not close adequately, or enough skin, muscle, or subcutaneous tissue may not be available for satisfactory results. Reconstructive surgery may be indicated to promote self-esteem and body image, to enhance quality of life, and to improve certain physical functions. Examples include breast reconstruction, facial reconstruction for head and neck cancers, and skin grafting after melanoma removal.

17. Should a surgeon say, "I got it all"?

In general, when a surgeon says, "I got it all," he or she means that the tumor was removed in its entirety, the margins were clean or free of cancer cells, and there was no evidence of lymph node or metastatic spread. This statement should be made with caution because approximately 70% of patients have evidence of micrometastases at the time of diagnosis. It may be less misleading to the patient if the surgeon says, "Apparently there is no evidence of cancer left behind. In 1 to 2 days we'll have a pathology report that will give us more information. If the pathologic results suggest that the margins are clear, there is a good chance that it's all been removed. There is a chance, however, that microscopic disease has already spread. That is why it is important to see a medical oncologist to talk about chemotherapy."

18. What does it mean when a surgeon says, "We got adequate margins"?

The surgeon should remove not only the tumor but also enough surrounding tissue to prevent local spread of disease. The amount of surrounding tissue that needs to be removed varies with the type of cancer and site of involvement. Margins range from 2 to 5 cm of "normal" tissue in solid tumors to wide excision for primary melanomas in the skin. How to define "adequate margins" is still under question.

19. What is a second-look procedure?

Second-look surgery is performed to stage cancer more accurately after completion of initial treatment, to determine treatment response, and to plan possible further therapy. Its use may be less common with advances in diagnostic imaging. It may be used in ovarian cancer and other solid tumors in the face of rising tumor markers and negative clinical work-ups for metastasis.

20. Why are radiopaque clips placed during surgery?

Radiopaque clips may be placed at the time of biopsy, staging, or during palliative procedures. The clips mark the areas of known tumor and are a guide to the areas where radiation therapy may be delivered.

21. What is robotic surgery and when is it used?

Robotic surgery is a variation of laparoscopic surgery, enhanced with the use of a system of robotics to mimic and potentially improve upon human surgical skills. The surgeon is seated at a special console in the operating suite and directs movements of interactive robotic arms, using a high-performance vision system and special instruments. Powered by robotic technology, the surgeon's hand movements are scaled, filtered, and translated into precise movements of these instruments. This technique has been used most for prostatectomies, but has also been attempted in some pulmonary and gynecologic procedures. Costs remain high for this technology and learning curves are steep for surgeons to achieve surgical and technical expertise.

As with any laparoscopic surgery, the intended benefits center around less invasive surgery. Potential advantages with robotic-assisted surgery include less pain and trauma, less blood loss, shorter hospital stay, faster recovery, and less scarring, but tightly controlled studies comparing laparoscopic procedures with open surgeries have not been done. Additionally, further research is still needed to determine if robotic procedures provide additional benefits regarding control of the cancer, urinary control, and sexual function for those with prostate cancer.

 Key Points

- Surgery plays many roles in treating cancer, including prophylaxis, diagnosis, staging, definitive or curative treatment, salvage treatment in the case of recurrence, palliative therapy, reconstruction, and rehabilitation.
- The ideal biopsy method should be the most cost-effective and least invasive procedure, and it should provide enough information to deliver a preliminary cancer diagnosis.
- Factors that can delay wound healing include: age, obesity, prior chemotherapy or radiation therapy, malnutrition, and diabetes.
- Altered hemostasis (hypercoagulability and thrombosis) can place the cancer patient at higher risk for postoperative complications.

 Internet Resources

Oncology Nursing Society, Surgical Oncology Special Interest Group:
   http://onsopcontent.ons.org/Interactive/VirtualCommunity/SIGDetail.asp?SigCode=SUR
World Oncology Network:
   http://www.worldoncology.net/surgical_oncology.htm
Society of Surgical Oncology:
   http://www.surgonc.org/

Bibliography

Burke C: Surgery. In Liebman MC, Camp-Sorrell D, editors: *Multimodal therapy in oncology nursing,* St Louis, 1996, Mosby.

Coleman J: Surgical therapy. In Shelton BK, Ziegfield CR, Olsen MM, editors: *Manual of cancer nursing,* ed 2, Philadelphia, 2004, Lippincott Williams & Wilkins.

Gettman MT, Blute ML: Critical comparison of laparoscopic, robotic, and open radical prostatectomy: Techniques, outcomes, and cost. *Current Urology Reports,* 7:193-199, 2006.

Gillespie TW: Surgical therapy. In Yarbro CH, Frogge MH, Goodman M, editors: *Cancer nursing: Principles and practice,* ed 6, Boston, 2005, Jones and Bartlett.

Greene FL, Page DL, Fleming ID, et al, editors: *AJCC cancer staging handbook,* ed. 6, Philadelphia, 2002, Lippincott-Raven.

Intuitive Surgical (2006). Patient resources: Minimally invasive surgery. http://www.intuitivesurgical.com/patientresources/robotic-assistedsurgery/index.aspx. Accessed January 10, 2007.

McGuire M: Nutritional care of surgical oncology patients. *Semin Oncol Nurs* 16(2):128-134, 2000.

Polomano R, Weintraub FN, Wurster A: Surgical critical care for cancer patients. *Semin Oncol Nurs* 10:165-176, 1994.

Rosenberg SA: Principles of surgical oncology. In DeVita VT, Hellman S, Rosenberg SA, editors: *Cancer: Principles and practice of oncology,* ed 7, 243-266. Philadelphia, 2005, Lippincott Williams & Wilkins.

Starnes DN, Sims TW: Care of the patient undergoing robotic-assisted prostatectomy. *Urologic Nursing,* 26: 129-136, 2006.

Szopa TJ: Nursing implications of surgical treatment. In Itano JK, Taoka KN, editors: *Core curriculum for oncology nursing,* ed 4, St Louis, 2005, Elsevier Saunders.

Wilke LG, Guiliano A: Sentinel lymph node biopsy in patients with early-stage breast cancer: Status of the national clinical trials. *Surg Clin North Am* 83:901-910, 2003.

Radiation Therapy

Karen Kay Sousa and Norman O. Aarestad

1. What is radiation therapy?

Radiation therapy is the treatment of disease with ionizing radiation. Normal tissues and tumors are both affected by ionizing radiation.

2. How does radiation work?

Radiation therapy delivers a precisely measured dose of ionizing radiation to a specific tumor volume, with the intent to kill the cancer cells but spare the normal tissues. Radiation treatment causes cellular damage that leads to biological changes in the DNA. Each radiation treatment causes permanent damage in the DNA of a tumor cell, which is then unable to divide and eventually dies. Radiation also damages the DNA of normal cells, but most of them are able to repair it and remain functional.

3. What does the term *radiosensitivity* mean?

All normal and cancer cells are vulnerable to the effects of radiation and may be injured or destroyed. Every cell has a different response or sensitivity to radiation. Rapidly dividing cells tend to be more sensitive to the effects of radiation than slowly dividing cells.

Tumor sensitivity

Degree of radiosensitivity	Types of malignancy
High	Lymphoma
	Seminoma
	Leukemia
	Ovarian germ cell tumor
Medium	Squamous cell cancer of the head, neck, and anus
	Astrocytoma
	Non-small cell lung cancer
	Colon cancer
	Breast cancer
	Prostate cancer
Low	Sarcoma
	Pancreatic cancer

4. How can radioresistance be overcome?

Most radiation treatments are given in daily "fractions" on Monday through Friday. The radiation oncologist prescribes a total dose of radiation, which is divided into daily fractions over 2 to 8 weeks. Radioresistance may be overcome by using alternative fractionation schedules. Treating twice per day with 6 hours between each radiation treatment may allow a higher total dose, or it may decrease the opportunity for the tumor cells to regenerate.

Using radiosensitizers and radioprotectors administered before daily radiation therapy is another way to overcome radioresistance. **Radiosensitizers**, usually given as chemotherapy, enhance cell death when given with radiation. **Radioprotectors**, such as amifostine, help to protect healthy cells during radiation treatments.

5. What is the role of amifostine in patients receiving radiotherapy?

Amifostine (Ethyol), a free-radical scavenger, has been shown to reduce the incidence of xerostomia (dry mouth) and mucositis in patients receiving radiation therapy to the neck, such as the parotid glands. It has also been shown to protect against late radiation reactions in skin, mucous membranes, heart, lungs, bladder, intestines, and pelvic structures. Amifostine can be given 30 minutes intravenously or 1 hour subcutaneously before daily radiation treatments. Side effects include nausea, vomiting, dehydration, and hypotension. Patients should be well-hydrated and premedicated with a serotonin-receptor antagonist antiemetic.

6. Explain the three roles of radiation in cancer treatment.

- **Curative.** Several cancers (e.g., early-stage cancer of the larynx, Hodgkin lymphoma, prostate and skin cancers) are curable with radiation alone.
- **Adjuvant.** When used after definitive surgery (e.g., orchiectomy for seminoma, lumpectomy for breast cancer), radiation is considered an adjuvant treatment.
- **Palliative.** When cure is not possible, symptom control with radiation therapy can substantially improve quality of life for many patients. Bleeding, ulceration, neurological symptoms, and obstruction due to tumor mass can be effectively controlled, often with a short course of treatment. Relief of pain, especially from bone metastases, can be quite dramatic.

7. How is radiation dose expressed?

Before 1985 the unit of radiation dose was the rad (radiation absorbed dose), and this term may still be found in the literature. However, the currently accepted term for the unit of radiation dose is the gray, or Gy; 1 Gy equals 100 centigray (cGy), and 1 cGy equals 1 rad.

8. What machines are used to deliver radiation therapy?

Treatment machines vary by institution. The linear accelerator delivers high-energy radiation to the tumor. Older machines required the creation of lead alloy blocks that shield healthy tissues from the beam of radiation. Newer linear accelerators have devices called multileaf collimators, or MLCs. The collimators' leaves are like tiny fingers that divide the field into narrow strips. Each finger can sweep across the field at a continuum of speeds ranging from very slow to very fast, adjusting the treatment field to the desired shape.

9. How is radiation therapy administered?

Radiation treatment can be delivered externally or internally. The radiation oncologist determines the method of treatment based on tumor type, tumor volume, tumor location, dosage needed to kill the cancer, and the availability of treatment equipment. Some tumors require both internal and external radiation.

- **Teletherapy (external beam therapy)** is radiation treatment delivered from a machine or source outside of the body. The teletherapy field encompasses the tumor site and may extend to cover regional lymph nodes or local extension of disease.

- **Brachytherapy** involves the use of radioactive sources placed in contact with the treatment target via implanted needles, wires, seeds, or intracavitary applicators. Brachytherapy delivers a full dose directly to the tumor or tumor bed.

10. How is brachytherapy delivered?

Brachytherapy can be delivered using low-dose rate (LDR) or high-dose rate (HDR) sources, with either temporary or permanent implants. There are many radioactive sources that can be used to deliver brachytherapy. These include: iridium-192, cesium-137, iodine-131 (oral), iodine-125, gold-198, phosphorus-32 (intravenous), radium-226, strontium-90 (intravenous), and palladium-109. Temporary implants, usually in place for 1 to 3 days, include needles, seeds, and ribbons that are loaded interstitially.

11. What is the difference between LDR and HDR brachytherapy?

LDR treatment generally requires hospitalization for several days, during which the patient is isolated to protect others from exposure to radioactivity. The patient also may be confined to bed to prevent dislodgment of the applicator. Disadvantages include potential complications of prolonged bed rest, discomfort, hospitalization costs, and radiation exposure to staff delivering bedside care. LDR brachytherapy is used for the following: oral cancer, sarcoma, prostate cancer (seeds), and uterine cancer.

HDR treatment has the distinct advantages of outpatient delivery and completion in several treatments, each lasting only a few minutes. Hospitalization and bed rest with its concomitant risks can be avoided. The staff is not exposed to radiation, because treatments are given with the patient inside a shielded room, using a remote delivery system. HDR brachytherapy is used in the following: cancers of the vaginal apex, esophagus, lungs, breast, and prostate.

12. How do nurses caring for patients undergoing brachytherapy protect themselves from radiation exposure?

Federal and state regulatory agencies govern the use of radioactive sources and have established maximum permissible doses for radiation workers. Each institution using radioactive materials must be licensed to do so under the watch of a radiation safety officer, who is responsible for ensuring that federal and state regulations are followed.

Radiation safety principals are based on the **ALARA** concept: exposure should be **A**s **L**ow **A**s **R**easonably **A**chievable. All who are involved in the care of radioactive patients must receive continuing education and wear a film badge that records exposure. Badges are checked regularly to ensure that the worker is practicing within safe parameters.

13. What are the three components of radiation safety?

Key components of radiation safety include understanding and following institutional guidelines and the three cardinal principles of radiation safety:
Time: minimize time spent near the source.
Distance: maximize distance from the source.
Shielding: use protective barriers between source and worker whenever possible.

14. How safe is it for others to be around patients who are being treated with seeds for prostate cancer?

It is safe for individuals to be in contact with these patients as long as certain safety precautions are followed. Patients are instructed to: strain their urine at home for 1 week, wear a condom during sexual activity for 1 week, stay approximately 6 feet away from children younger than 18 months old or women who are either pregnant or trying to get pregnant, and not allow children to sit on a their laps for at least 2 weeks.

Seed implants are generally out-patient procedures. The radioactive seeds stay in place permanently and gradually decay over time. The seeds are considered nonradioactive approximately 4 months after the implant. Some centers provide patients with a small card to carry in their wallets that states the date of the seed implant and the phone number of the physician who did the procedure. These cards are helpful in reducing panic in other health care providers who may see metal seeds in patients requiring pelvic imaging.

15. What happens during simulation?

Simulation is a special treatment planning session that helps determine the exact area of the body to be treated. The simulator is a special x-ray unit or CT scanner that assists the radiation oncologist and simulation therapist in planning the radiation fields of treatment. Each radiation center may have a different type of simulator. The newer machines have a CT scan capability that further assists the physician in designing the treatment plan.

Reproducibility is very important with every radiation treatment given. During simulation, patients will be given very tiny, permanent tattoos that assist the radiation therapist in setting up the treatment fields each day. To further ensure reproducibility, styrofoam casts are made to fit the patient's shape so that the patient is placed in the same position for each treatment. All of the information obtained during simulation is transferred to the radiation treatment planning computer.

16. What is the nurse's role during simulation?

The nurse or radiation therapist needs to ensure patient comfort and safety. Simulation typically takes 30 to 60 minutes and requires the patient to lie very still on a flat x-ray table. It is very important that patients who are in pain or claustrophobic be premedicated before simulation. It can be very difficult for patients and especially children to lie on a hard flat surface for any length of time. There may be other devices used during simulation to help immobilize the patient.

17. What is a dosimetrist?

A dosimetrist is a specially trained radiation therapist who assists the physician in fine tuning the treatment plan. Special 3-D treatment planning computers enable the physician/dosimetrist to look at a tumor from different dimensions so that they can spare normal tissue while giving the optimum radiation dose to the tumor. The physics staff also evaluates the plan of treatment.

18. What are port films?

"Port films" are a set of X-rays taken before the first treatment to ensure that the field set up in simulation is transferred exactly to the treatment machine. After the physician approves the port films, the patient has his first treatment. Weekly port films may be necessary to ensure consistency and accuracy.

19. How do patients feel during treatment?

Patients usually do not feel any discomfort during treatments. Patients may need to be premedicated to decrease anxiety before daily treatments, just as they were before simulation. Occasionally, some brain tumor patients see a blue light during treatment, which may happen if there are any scattered X-rays or photons that hit the retina. They may also say that they smell a burning odor. After patients are set up in the correct position on the treatment table, the therapist will then leave the room to deliver the treatment. The patient can be seen and heard via cameras in the room. The beam of radiation is on only for a few minutes, and then the patient is helped off the table and ready to go home.

20. How can the nurse help to prepare patients for radiation treatment?

The most powerful tool that nurses can offer to patients and their families is information. Radiation is poorly understood and surrounded by myths or horror stories from the past. Ask the patient or their family what they have heard about radiation therapy and clarify any misconceptions.

21. What effect does radiation therapy have on skin?

Acute skin reactions generally begin around the second week of treatment. Initially, dryness and faint erythema are common, but may progress to bright red erythema, rash, and desquamation as the dose increases. Patients should be reassured that skin effects are temporary. Mild skin reactions tend to heal and return to normal in about 2 weeks. More severe reactions may take 2 to 3 weeks before the reaction subsides and completely heals. Patients should be reminded that skin reactions can become more intense for several days after completion of therapy.

22. What is desquamation?

Desquamation is the sloughing of the top layer of skin. It usually starts with **dry desquamation**, which is peeling of the top layer of skin. Desquamation becomes uncomfortable because the nerve endings are exposed to the air. Dry desquamation in breast cancer patients usually occurs where two layers of skin rub against each other, such as underneath the breast or in the axilla. **Moist desquamation** is peeling of the skin with the addition of serous fluid leakage and is very uncomfortable.

23. What factors influence skin reactions to radiation therapy?

- Patient factors that influence skin reactions are: poor nutritional status, skin folds in the treatment field, sun exposure, exposure to heat, and the use of irritants in the treatment fields.
- Radiation-related factors that influence skin reactions are: use of electron beams, extra material (e.g., gel dressing) on the skin surface, and large treatment fields.

24. What is the nurse's role in skin care related to radiation therapy?

The nurse must perform frequent skin assessments and provide patient education about skin care. The nurse needs to inspect skin in the treatment area for any preexisting cutaneous conditions, including dryness, thinning, and infection (particularly fungal). Infections should be treated with antifungal or antibiotic creams as indicated.

25. What patient education should be provided to minimize skin reactions?

The nurse should provide patients with verbal and written instructions that include the following information to minimize skin reactions:
- Gently clean skin with mild soap.
- Avoid very hot water when bathing.
- Avoid friction from belts, collars, shoulder straps, bras, and so on.
- Avoid exposing treated area to the sun and extremes of heat or cold.
- Use only skin care products on the treated area that are recommended by the treating facility; avoid the use of extra lotions, creams, or powders in the treatment area.
- Moisturize prophylactically to decrease dryness and pruritus.
- Do not apply skin care products to the treatment site for several hours before daily treatment. Apply skin care products very gently. Do not rub in, because friction contributes to loss of skin integrity.

26. How do you treat skin care reactions from radiation treatment, and what types of products should be used on irradiated skin?

The goals of skin care management are patient comfort and the prevention of secondary infections. Every radiation center will have a particular skin care protocol. Some centers may restrict patients from applying anything to the irradiated skin.

Treatment of skin reactions to radiation therapy

Skin reaction	Intervention
Skin irritation	Apply a thin layer of a skin care product to the treatment area, 1-2 times per day, such as: Biafine RE, TheraCare cream, RadiaCare gel, Eucerin Aquaphor cream, or other OTC creams.
Dry desquamation	Use lotions and creams containing aloe, lanolin, petrolatum, vitamins A and D, and other moisturizing components. A light dusting of cornstarch may soothe erythematous skin. Do not use both cornstarch and an ointment or cream, because the resulting paste will be irritating, especially in skin folds and creases. Avoid preparations containing alcohol, witch hazel, or menthol ingredients, which will also dry the skin.
Moist desquamation	Apply antibiotic creams, such as silver sulfadiazine. A solution of hydrogen peroxide and saline (1:2) may be used to cleanse an area of moist desquamation before applying an antibiotic cream. Moisture-vapor-permeable dressings and gel-type dressings aid in healing larger areas of moist desquamation. Protective dressings that allow air to move through them, such as Vigilon dressings or RadiaCare Gel sheets, are soothing, especially when placed in a refrigerator before applying to the skin. The gel sheets also help to gently debride the dead skin cells and may also help keep the top layer of exposed skin from becoming infected.
Rash and/or pruritus	Apply 1% hydrocortisone cream. For severe pruritus, take diphenhydramine orally at bedtime.
Painful skin	Use topical anesthetics, oral NSAIDs, and/or opioids appropriate for the intensity of pain. For women who experience sore and tender nipples, use 2% viscous lidocaine jelly.

27. What are the acute and late side effects of radiation therapy?

Because radiation is a local, not systemic treatment, acute side effects will occur **only** in the site receiving treatment. For example, treatment to the head and neck will cause sore throat and dysphagia. Patients receiving concurrent chemotherapy and radiation therapy may have multiple side effects and require daily assessments. The severity of acute side effects does not predict the development of late side effects. Similarly, late effects can develop in tissues that showed no acute response. An example of a late effect is the increased risk of pelvic fractures in older women who received pelvic irradiation.

Acute and late side effects of radiation therapy

	Acute effects	Late effects
Duration	Usually transient reactions that occur during treatment and subside within 1 to 2 weeks	Usually permanent reactions that develop several months to years after treatment is completed
Affected areas	Tissues with rapid renewal characteristics, (e.g., skin, mucous membranes, and bone marrow)	Late-reacting tissues: skin, spinal cord, bone, and such organs as lungs, liver, and gonads
Predictive factors	Predicted from the volume of normal tissue exposed to the beam, total dose delivered, and sensitivity of the normal tissue to radiation Severity affected by: age, nutritional status, and prior or concomitant chemotherapy	Severity predicted by daily dose fraction. As daily dose increases, the normal tissue cannot maintain adequate repair, and chronic damage tends to be worse.
Examples	Site-specific: scalp alopecia, nausea, diarrhea, mucositis, dysphagia, xerostomia, taste alterations, pharyngitis, esophagitis, gastritis, cystitis, edema, lymphedema, cerebral edema, and sexual dysfunction General: fatigue, anorexia, and possible bone marrow depression	Site-specific: cataracts, xerostomia, dental caries, taste changes, head and neck flap necrosis, esophageal stricture or fistula, hypothyroidism, pneumonitis, pulmonary fibrosis, pericarditis, bowel adhesions, proctitis, enteritis, cystitis, vaginal fibrosis, infertility, osteoradionecrosis, myelopathies, permanent depilation, skin pigmentation changes, and second malignancies

28. How is radiation-induced second cancer defined?

The second tumor must be different histologically from the primary tumor, must arise within the previously irradiated tissue, and must occur from 10 to 15 years after the original tumor was treated. Approximately 5% of all patients treated with radiation develop second malignancies, such as high-grade sarcomas, meningiomas, and thyroid cancer.

Genetic factors, immune status, young age, and treatment with other modalities affect the probability of developing second cancers.

29. Can radiation treatment help manage pain?

Yes, radiation therapy is effective in providing long-term or partial relief of pain by stopping further extension of the cancer and relieving pressure by shrinking the tumor. Treatment for pain related to bone metastases permits bone to regrow after the tumor is destroyed and helps to prevent fractures.

30. How long does it take for radiation therapy to reduce pain?

Pain relief may occur in a few days or may take up to two weeks or longer. Improvement may continue even after treatment is completed. Some patients may have a "flare" pain (sudden increase or worsening of bone pain) that occurs after 1 to 3 treatments. Flare pain is temporary and will usually subside on its own or after a short course of steroid treatment to decrease the inflammation. Patients should be encouraged to take pain medications during radiation treatment until the pain is relieved.

31. Why is radiation so tiring?

The cause is unknown; however, it seems reasonable to assume that more energy is required to repair the radiation effects. Fatigue gradually increases over the course of therapy and can persist for a month or more after therapy is completed.

Variables that influence the degree of fatigue include: degree of fatigue before starting therapy, concurrent therapies, and age and general health of an individual. Constant reassurance that the fatigue will lessen over time is important. Patients may mistakenly believe that on their last day of treatment, the fatigue should be instantly gone.

32. Why do some radiation patients have nausea and vomiting?

Treatment fields close to the stomach area can cause nausea, such as radiation for stomach, pancreatic, and liver cancers. Treatments delivered to the mid or low spine can also cause nausea, because the radiation exits through the stomach area. These patients will be pre-medicated with antinausea medication, 45 minutes to an hour before daily radiation therapy. Patients should also be taught that an empty stomach before treatment increases nausea. Eating smaller meals more frequently is important.

33. What are the dietary concerns when a patient is receiving treatment?

Patients are encouraged to eat a well balanced diet. In general there are no foods to avoid. Patients prone to poor nutrition are encouraged to eat foods that are high in protein and calories. Increased protein intake leads to better healing and an overall sense of well-being. For patients with poor appetites, nutritional supplements and protein shakes between meals may help to maintain energy and weight.

Patients who experience diarrhea should eliminate fresh fruits and vegetables and follow a low residue diet. Patients who experience dysphagia will need to change to a soft or liquid diet, or a combination of the two.

34. Are tube feedings ever needed?

Yes. Early enteral nutritional support with a nasogastric or percutaneous endoscopic gastrostomy (PEG) should be considered in patients receiving head and neck or esophageal irradiation, when extended mucositis, dysphagia, or odynophagia is anticipated. Patients who are malnourished at consultation or have a large, obstructing tumor will need immediate referral for a feeding tube **before** starting radiation therapy. Patients who do not eat well generally do not drink well either. A feeding tube is a great way to give a large bolus of fluids versus having to receive daily IV fluids to prevent dehydration.

35. What happens when a course of treatment is completed?

During the final week of treatment a patient will see the radiation oncologist, who will reassess how well the treatment was tolerated. A follow-up appointment will be scheduled for approximately 1 month after the final treatment. Side effects of radiation therapy generally take 7 to 10 days to resolve. Lingering fatigue is probably the most frustrating side effect for patients and may persist for months after completing therapy. Just before returning for their follow-up appointment, most patients will have a CT scan or MRI to assess treatment response.

36. What is new in radiation therapy?

- **Intensity-modulated radiation therapy (IMRT)** allows patients to receive higher, more precise doses of radiation therapy with fewer side effects, less damage to normal surrounding tissues, and improved outcomes. Instead of using a single beam of radiation to deliver treatments, IMRT is administered with a single beam that has been broken up into thousands of tiny, thin beams of radiation to focus a higher dose of radiation on the tumor and spare surrounding healthy tissues. It is not recommended for every type of cancer, and not every center has the technology.

- A new way of delivering radiation therapy treatments will be the use of **image-guided radiotherapy (IGRT).** IGRT uses real-time imaging techniques to help the radiation oncologist locate and target moving tumors just before and during a daily treatment. This technology will be beneficial for lung cancers or other tumors that move with respiration.
- **Radioimmunotherapy** involves attaching a radioactive isotope to a tumor-specific antibody, such as ibritumomab tiuxetan (Zevalin), which is then injected into the patient, delivering its lethal radiation dose directly to the malignant cells.
- **Stereotactic radiosurgery (SRS),** a 3-D nonsurgical technique done as an outpatient procedure, delivers the radiation dose in one fraction to a targeted area. It is used most often to treat malignant and nonmalignant brain tumors, but can also be used to treat extracranial sites ("body radiosurgery"). Patients are imaged with a "halo" or other fixation device for stabilization. A high dose of radiation is delivered by narrow beams that come together at an isocenter, which spares surrounding tissues. After imaging, it generally takes several hours of radiation planning before the patient is treated. After the treatment is given (approximately 30 minutes), the halo is removed and the patient is monitored before going home.
- **Stereotactic radiotherapy (SRT)** is similar to SRS, but a few treatments are given instead of a single treatment. This causes less damage to normal tissue.

Key Points

- Both normal and cancer cells are vulnerable to the effects of radiation.
- Radioresistant tumors can be made more sensitive by the use of radiosensitizers. Certain types of chemotherapy can enhance the tumor cell death when it is given before or concurrently with the radiation.
- Advances in technology have lead to complex treatment planning, which yields precise radiation treatments that spare normal tissues and have fewer side effects.

Internet Resources

American Society for Therapeutic Radiology and Oncology:
  http://www.astro.org
OncoLink, Abramson Cancer Center of the University of Pennsylvania:
  http://www.oncolink.org
  http://www.penncancer.org
Radiation Oncology Online Journal:
  http://www.ROOJ.com

Acknowledgments

The authors wish to acknowledge Joan Foley, RN, BSN, Merle Sprague, MD, and Laura Hilderly, RN, MS, for their contributions to the Radiation Oncology chapter in the first and second editions of *Oncology Nursing Secrets*.

Bibliography

Baxter N, Mabermann E, Tepper J, et al: Risk of pelvic fractures in older women following pelvic irradiation. *JAMA* 294:2587-2593, 2005.

Gazda MJ, Coia LR: Principles of radiation therapy. In Pazdur R, Coia L, Hoskins WJ, et al, editors: *Cancer management: A multidisciplinary approach*, ed 9, Lawrence, KS, 2005, CMP United Business Media.

Hassey-Dow K, Bucholtz J, Iwamoto R, et al: *Nursing care in radiation oncology*, ed 2, Philadelphia, 1997, WB Saunders.

Itano J, Taoka K: *Core curriculum for oncology nursing*, ed 4, Philadelphia, 2005, WB Saunders.

Nystedt KE, Hill JE, Mitchell AM, et al: The standardization of radiation skin care in British Columbia: A collaborative approach. *Oncol Nurs Forum* 32(6):1199-1205, 2005.

Principles of Chemotherapy

Gail M. Wilkes and Margaret Barton-Burke

1. How has the role of chemotherapy changed in the treatment of cancer?

There has been a shift toward giving chemotherapy in earlier stages of cancer to prevent recurrences and to reduce micrometastases after primary treatment (**adjuvant**), or to shrink the tumor before giving other therapies (**neoadjuvant**). Adjuvant treatment with chemotherapy following surgery has demonstrated increased disease-free and overall survival for patients with breast, colon, and lung cancers. When cure and control of disease cannot be achieved, chemotherapy can provide **palliation** (comfort and symptom improvement) to improve quality of life.

2. How does chemotherapy work?

Chemotherapy drugs interfere with steps of the cell cycle specifically involved in synthesis of DNA and replication of tumor cells. The cell cycle, the process whereby both normal and cancerous cells replicate, involves five basic phases:

G0   Resting stage in which cells are out of cycle temporarily
G1   RNA and protein synthesis; the gap between resting and DNA synthesis
S   DNA synthesis
G2   Second gap, during which the cell constructs the mitotic apparatus
M   Mitosis

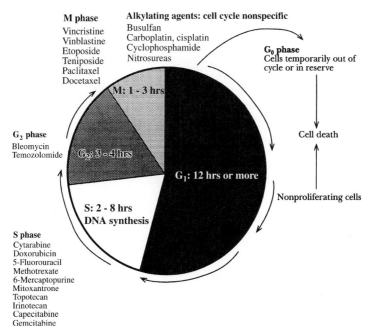

Cell cycle and cytotoxic targets of common antineoplastic agents. *(Adapted from Tannock IF: Biological properties of anti-cancer drugs. In Tannock IF, Hill RP, editors:* The basic science of oncology, *ed 2, New York, 1992, McGraw-Hill, pp 302-316.)*

3. How are chemotherapeutic agents classified, and by what mechanisms do they cause tumor cell death or prevent tumor growth?

Most antineoplastic agents are categorized according to their biochemical activity or origins. Many drugs are derived from natural products.

Classification of chemotherapy agents and mechanism of action

Category	Effect on cell cycle	Mechanism of action	Examples
Alkylating agents	Cell cycle nonspecific but are also effective against cells in the resting phase	Interacts with DNA bases, causing breakage of the DNA helix and prevention of DNA replication	Cyclophosphamide Ifosfamide Cisplatin Carboplatin Nitrogen mustard Nitrosoureas Busulfan
Antimetabolites	Cell cycle phase-specific, usually the S phase; most effective against highly proliferative cancers.	Inhibit enzyme production needed for DNA and RNA synthesis	Methotrexate 5-Fluorouracil Cytarabine Fludarabine Capecitabine Gemcitabine
Antitumor antibiotics (natural product)	Cell cycle phase-specific, S phase	Bind to DNA, causing partial unwinding of the DNA helix, and inhibiting DNA and RNA synthesis	Doxorubicin Idarubicin Mitomycin
Vinca alkaloids (natural product/microtubule agent)	Cell cycle phase-specific, primarily M phase	Bind to protein tubulin and disrupts mitotic spindle formation, so that cell dies as it attempts division	Vincristine Vinblastine Vinorelbine
Taxanes (natural product/microtubule agent)	M-phase–specific	Cause stabilization of the microtubule, which inhibits cell division	Paclitaxel Docetaxel
Podophyllotoxins (natural products)	M-phase–specific	Cause double-stranded breaks in DNA by inhibition of topoisomerase II	Etoposide Teniposide
Camptothecins (natural products)	S-phase–specific	Inhibit the formation of topoisomerase I, an enzyme responsible	Topotecan Irinotecan

Category	Effect on cell cycle	Mechanism of action	Examples
Classification of chemotherapy agents and mechanism of action—cont'd			
		for the prevention of DNA strand breakage during synthesis; DNA strands break and are not repaired	
Miscellaneous agents	Primarily phase-specific	Inhibit protein, RNA, or DNA synthesis	L-Asparaginase (enzyme) Hydroxyurea Procarbazine Dacarbazine

4. Discuss the role of chemotherapy in combination with a molecular or "targeted" agent.

Molecular or "targeted therapy" in combination with chemotherapy, has shown increases in response and survival (e.g., bevacizumab given with chemotherapy to patients with advanced colorectal cancers). Molecular "targeted" agents interfere with specific steps in the process of cancer development. Cancers can progress by becoming immune to the signals of apoptosis (programmed cell death that normally follows cellular damage). Chemotherapy kills cancer cells, often by damaging enough of the cell's DNA to cause apoptosis. Therefore it makes sense to combine a targeted agent which blocks molecular resistance to apoptosis with a chemotherapy drug that causes cell death through apoptosis. Other molecular agents stop cancer growth, development of new blood vessels, or invasion of other healthy tissues (see Chapter 9).

5. Describe the effect of tumor growth on responsiveness to chemotherapy.

The growth and size of a tumor is a product of the proportion of cells actively dividing (growth fraction), the length of the cell cycle (doubling time), and the rate of cell loss. The higher the growth fraction, the greater the cell kill will be. Chemotherapy is most effective on tumors with the highest proliferative rates. Tumors are most likely to be responsive to chemotherapy when they are small and vascular. Tumors are less responsive to chemotherapy later when cell proliferation slows because of crowding, poor vascularization with decreased blood flow to all the tumor cells, and limited nutrients.

6. Why are certain cancers resistant to chemotherapy?

Drug resistance, a major barrier to cure, may be intrinsic or acquired over time, because each cancer cell has the ability to mutate spontaneously. Many cancers (e.g., melanoma, renal cell cancer, pancreatic cancer) are intrinsically resistant to most, if not all, chemotherapeutic agents. Cancers that are intrinsically resistant to chemotherapy contain the multidrug-resistance (MDR) gene, known as the MDR pump, which contains P-glycoprotein. The MDR pump resides within the cellular membrane and actively pumps out certain drugs as they are given, thus preventing accumulation of the drug within the cell and resulting in little, if any drug effect. When the gene for P-glycoprotein is over expressed, chemotherapy drugs, such as doxorubicin, mitoxantrone, daunorubicin, vincristine, vinblastine, paclitaxel, etoposide, and dactinomycin, are readily extruded from the cell.

Cancer cells may be resistant to drugs by other mechanisms, such as decreased drug uptake, reduced drug activation, impaired drug transport into cells, increased catabolism of the drug, altered target enzymes that reduce drug binding, and increased DNA repair, all of which reduce therapeutic efficacy.

7. Describe the mechanism of increased DNA repair.

In the past decade, resistance to apoptosis and presence of telomerase have been described as significant properties that permit cancer cells not to die or age despite appropriate signals. When apoptosis cannot be induced in cancer cells, they survive despite damage from chemotherapy drugs or other mechanisms that normally initiate programmed cell death, thus contributing to malignant transformation and chemotherapy resistance. Normally, cell senescence (process of aging) results when telomeres shorten with each division and chromosomes are not able to replicate their DNA. Unlike normal somatic cells, most cancer cells possess telomerase, an enzyme that lengthens telomeres to sustain DNA replication. Telomerase permits cells to ignore the biologic clock, thereby promoting tumor cell growth and possible chemotherapy resistance.

8. How can drug resistance be overcome?

The use of combination chemotherapy given in a dose-intensive schedule is an important strategy to overcome resistance by killing the cancer cells before they have the chance to become drug resistant. Previous research on specific adjuvant agents (e.g., tamoxifen, cyclosporine, verapamil, and quinidine) that might reverse the MDR pump mechanism have not shown clinical benefit.

Certain molecular targeted agents can reverse some of the factors causing resistance, such as poor blood flow or the ability to avoid apoptosis. For example, when the molecular targeted drug cetuximab (Erbitux) is combined with chemotherapy in the second-line treatment of metastatic colorectal cancer, cancer cells that were resistant to irinotecan chemotherapy now become sensitive to it, and the tumors shrink. Cetuximab is a monoclonal antibody against the epidermal growth factor receptor (EGFR) and blocks its action, one of which is avoidance of apoptosis. The drug is believed to work by preventing the cancer cells from repairing the DNA damage from chemotherapy and radiotherapy, thereby making the cancer cells sensitive to the drug again.

9. What is dose dense chemotherapy?

Dose dense chemotherapy uses multiple cycles of chemotherapy with the shortest possible interval between cycles so that higher doses of drug are delivered. Because dose dense chemotherapy decreases blood counts more than standard therapy, patients need to take a growth factor to keep their white blood cell count up and to avoid infection.

10. What is metronomic chemotherapy?

Metronomic therapy is the prolonged, uninterrupted delivery of chemotherapy in small doses on a frequent schedule (daily, several times a week, or weekly). Whereas chronotherapy was first studied in the 1980s, metronomic therapy is being studied now to optimize the antiangiogenic properties of chemotherapy.

11. What tests are used to assess tumor response to chemotherapy?

- Flow cytometry is used to estimate the growth fraction, cell-cycle phase distribution, and kinetic properties of cell populations. Tumors that contain a higher percentage of proliferating cells (cells in S phase) are more sensitive to cycle-dependent chemotherapy, and patients with tumors of this type have a better prognosis than those who have tumors with a low S-phase fraction.

- Magnetic resonance imaging (MRI), positron emission tomography (PET), or computed tomography (CT) scan imaging are done following two to three cycles of chemotherapy and compared to a baseline image (before-treatment scan) to measure the change in the tumor size in response to the chemotherapy treatment.
- As nanotechnology emerges, we will see new tests that will reflect the changes in the DNA of tumor cells and provide a real-time estimation of the number of cancer cells killed by a specific treatment.

12. What factors affect response to chemotherapy?

- **Tumor burden** affects the probability that the cancer will spread. The larger the primary tumor, the greater the risk for metastatic disease.
- **Tumor growth rate** affects the proportion of cells that will be killed by chemotherapeutic agents. Rapidly growing tumors are usually the most responsive to chemotherapy.
- **Tumor cell heterogeneity** increases risk for primary and secondary resistance to chemotherapy. Unfortunately, malignant cells possess genetic mutations, and every time the cells divide, new mutations emerge. With successive mutations, the new cells become resistant to chemotherapy.

13. What other patient factors affect response to chemotherapy?

Performance status is one of the most important factors affecting response to chemotherapy. Patients with better performance—able to do all or most of their usual activities—may have less tumor burden, and thus are able to better tolerate and respond to chemotherapy. More tumor cells are actively dividing, so more cycling cells are responsive to chemotherapy. In a number of studies on patients with advanced cancer, performance status is also a predictor of survival. Two commonly used performance status scales are the Karnofsky performance scale (KPS) (0-100, with a higher score indicating better performance) and the Eastern Cooperative Oncology Group scale (ECOG) (0-4, with a higher score indicating poorer performance). Additional factors include stable weight, absence of significant concomitant illnesses, and optimal symptom management. A depressed immune system and weight loss decrease tolerance to the side effects of chemotherapy. In addition, dose reductions and treatment delays due to toxicity and patient adherence promote tumor resistance.

14. Can circadian rhythm affect the patient's response to chemotherapy?

Administering chemotherapy according to circadian rhythm may enhance response and minimize toxicity. For example, 5-fluorouracil (5-FU), which targets the gut and bone marrow, may be best tolerated if given in the evening, because the cells of the gut and the bone marrow divide most actively during the first half of the working day.

15. What are the advantages of combination chemotherapy?

- Maximizes tumor cell kill and results in higher response rates than when used alone (e.g., paclitaxel/trastuzumab and methotrexate/5-FU), because drug combinations are synergistic and act at different phases of the cell cycle
- Minimizes the proliferation of resistant tumor stem cells, thereby reducing the potential for drug resistance
- Produces differing toxicities while administering maximal doses of each drug

16. How does the combination of chemotherapy and radiotherapy increase responsiveness?

Certain drugs act as radiosensitizers (e.g., paclitaxel, 5-FU, capecitabine, carboplatin, oxaliplatin), allowing radiation therapy to be more effective. Unfortunately, they also increase the potential for toxicity. An advantage of combined chemotherapy and radiotherapy is that the patient can receive local (primary tumor) and systemic (micrometastatic disease) treatment simultaneously.

17. Does the sequence of administering certain drugs affect response to chemotherapy?

Yes, the sequence in which certain drugs are given may enhance efficacy, minimize toxicity, or do both (see Chapter 7).

18. What are the most common side effects of chemotherapy?

Generally, adverse effects from chemotherapy result from either damage to the rapidly dividing stem cells or drug toxicity to cells or tissues of specific organs unrelated to cell growth rate. The severity of effects varies according to dosage, timing, duration, route of administration, prior chemotherapy or radiation therapy, co-administration of other agents, condition of patient, and individual sensitivities. Acute, late, and chronic effects, ranging from mild to dose-limiting or fatal toxicities, may or may not be predictable. Additionally, interactions between chemotherapy agents and other drugs (refer to Chapter 7 for types of interactions). See the table on pages 59-69 for common side effects, toxicities, and drug interactions. Refer to Chapter 41 for specific organ toxicities and late effects.

19. What agents can be given to minimize the toxicity of chemotherapy?

Leucovorin, dexrazoxane, and mesna are examples of agents that protect normal cells. See the table on page 70.

20. What blood test is used to check for risk of increased toxicity in patients receiving irinotecan (Camptosar)?

The more that is learned about genetics, the more knowledge there is about how certain drugs are metabolized and whether the patient is at higher risk for toxicity. A genetic polymorphism occurs when there are different variations of one gene in different people. The active form of irinotecan is its metabolite SN-38, which is metabolized by the enzyme UGT1A1. Genes code for proteins, in this case an enzyme. If a person has a copy of the gene that makes a deficient enzyme, the metabolism of SN-38 is reduced. Thus, that person has increased serum drug levels and risk of toxicity, especially, grade 4 bone marrow suppression. This is the case in approximately 10% of people in the United States who have the UGT1A1*28 polymorphism. The "UGT1A1 Molecular Test" can detect whether the patient makes a normal UGT1A1 enzyme or the variant, UGT1A1*28 enzyme. If a patient has the gene for UGT1A1*28, then the dose of irinotecan should be reduced and the patient monitored very closely.

21. What are the two types of neurotoxicity associated with oxaliplatin?

Oxaliplatin, a heavy metal, may cause two types of sensory neuropathy:
- Acute oxaliplatin neurotoxicity is reversible, lasting less than 14 days, and characterized by cold-induced paresthesias and dysesthesias. This neuropathy appears to be caused by injury to the axonal ion channels, such as those for calcium and magnesium. Repletion of magnesium and calcium, given just before and after a dose of oxaliplatin, may prevent or lessen the signs and symptoms of peripheral neuropathy. Patients should be told to avoid cold drinks and exposure of hands and feet to cold during and for a few days following oxaliplatin administration.

Text continued on p. 71.

Cancer chemotherapy side effects and drug interactions

Drug	N/V	Mucositis	D/C	Alopecia	BMS	HSR	V/I	Organ and other toxicities	Drug interactions
L-Asparaginase (Elspar)	±	0	0	0	0	++	0	Hepatic, neurologic, hyperglycemia, pancreatitis	1) Prednisone: potential additive hyperglycemic effect 2) Drug may ↓ or ↑ effect of cyclophosphamide, vincristine, 6-MP 3) 6-MP enhanced hepatotoxicity 4) Methotrexate: antagonism if administered immediately before methotrexate 5) Cytosine arabinoside: synergy 6) Vincristine: additive neurotoxicity
Arsenic	++	0	D, C	0	++	Possible vasomotor symptoms	0	APL (acute promyelocytic leukemia), differentiation syndrome characterized by fever, dyspnea, weight gain, pulmonary infiltrates and pleural or pericardial effusions	Drugs that prolong QT interval or lead to electrolyte abnormalities ↑ risk of side effects and torsades de pointes

Continued

Cancer chemotherapy side effects and drug interactions—cont'd

Drug	N/V	Mucositis	D/C	Alopecia	BMS	HSR	V/I	Organ and other toxicities	Drug interactions
Azacitidine (Vidaza)	+	+	D, C	0	±	0	Injection site irritation	Rare coma and death in patients with extensive liver disease	Other myelosuppressive chemotherapy agents: ↑ myelosuppression
Bleomycin (Blenoxane)	±	+	0	±	0	+	–	Skin, fever, pulmonary, Raynaud's phenomenon	1) May ↓ digoxin effect 2) May ↓ phenytoin effect
Busulfan (Myleran)	±	0	D±	±	±	0	0	Skin, gonadal, hepatic, ocular, pulmonary	1) Phenytoin ↓ busulfan Area Under the Curve (AUC) by 15% 2) Other anticonvulsants may ↑ busulfan AUC 3) Itraconazole ↓ busulfan clearance by up to 25% 4) Acetaminophen before or with busulfan may ↓ busulfan clearance

							Toxicity	Drug Interactions
Carboplatin (Paraplatin)	±	0	0	0	+ delayed	—	Hepatic, neurologic, hypomagnesemia	1) Cisplatin: ↑ renal toxicity risk 2) Myelosuppressive drugs: ↑ bone marrow depression 3) Paclitaxel: give carboplatin after paclitaxel
Capecitabine (Xeloda)	+	D++	±	+	0	0	Hand and foot syndrome (may be severe), grade 3/4 hyperbilirubinemia	1) Warfarin: ↑ International Normalized Ratio (INR) 2) Phenytoin levels may be altered 3) Docetaxel: synergy 4) Leucovorin: synergy with potential ↑ toxicity
Carmustine (BCNU, BiCNU)	+	D±	0	++	0	—	Gonadal, hepatic, neurologic*, pulmonary*, renal	1) Cimetidine: may ↑ myelosuppression 2) Amphotericin B: may ↑ intracellular uptake of drug 3) Phenytoin: carmustine may ↓ effect of phenytoin
Chlorambucil (Leukeran)	±	0	0	±	0	0	Gonadal, pulmonary*	1) Barbiturates given at same time: possible ↑ chlorambucil toxicity
Cisplatin (CDDP, Platinol)	++	0	D±	±	+	—	Gonadal, neurologic, ototoxic, renal, hypo-magnesemia	1) Phenytoin: possible ↓ effect 2) Loop diuretics: possible ↑ ototoxicity 3) Aminoglycosides, amphotericin B: possible ↑ renal toxicity

*High doses.

Continued

Treating Cancer

Cancer chemotherapy side effects and drug interactions—cont'd

Drug	N/V	Mucositis	D/C	Alopecia	BMS	HSR	V/I	Organ and other toxicities	Drug interactions
									4) Etoposide: synergy 5) Paclitaxel: administer cisplatin after paclitaxel to prevent delayed paclitaxel excretion 6) Sodium thiosulfate, mesna: inactivates cisplatin
Cladribine (2-CdA, Leustatin)	±	0	0	0	+	0	0	Skin, neurologic, renal*	None known
Cyclophosphamide (Cytoxan, Neosar)	+	0	0	++	++	0	0	Cardiac*, gonadal, SIADH	1) Chloramphenicol: ↑ half life 2) Thiazide diuretics: ↑ duration of leucopenia 3) Anticoagulants: ↑ effect 4) Digoxin: ↓ digoxin level 5) Doxorubicin: potentiation of doxorubicin-induced cardiomyopathy 6) Succinylcholine: ↑ effect 7) Barbiturates: ↑ effect
Cytarabine (Ara-C, Cytosar-U)	+	++	D+	±	++	0	0	Skin, flu-like syndrome, neurologic,* ocular,* pulmonary	Digoxin: may ↓ bioavailability of digoxin when given together

Drug								Organ toxicity	Drug interactions
Dacarbazine (DTIC)	‡	0	0	±	0		I	Skin, hepatic, flu-like illness	1) Dilantin: ↑ drug metabolism with concurrent administration 2) Phenobarbital: potential ↑ toxicity with Imuran and 6-MP
Dactinomycin, actinomycin D (Cosmegen)	+	‡	D±	+	‡	0	V	Skin, fever, hepatic	Other myelosuppressive chemotherapy agents: ↑ myelosuppression
Daunorubicin, Daunamycin (Cerubidine)	+	+	0	‡	‡	+	V	Cardiac, red urine, skin	Heparin: forms a precipitate; do not use together
Docetaxel (Taxotere)	±	+	D±	+	‡	‡	I	Skin, neurologic, fluid retention syndrome, fatigue	Drugs that inhibit CYP3A4 may ↑ serum levels theoretically, and drugs that induce CYP3A4 may ↓ serum level
Doxorubicin (Adriamycin, Rubex)	+	+	0	+	‡	+	V	Cardiac, skin, red urine	Doxorubicin may potentiate toxicity of cyclophosphamide-induced hemorrhagic cystitis, hepatotoxicity of 6-MP
Epirubicin (epidoxorubicin)	+	+	D±	+	‡	+	V	Cardiac, red-orange urine	1) Calcium channel blockers: may ↑risk of congestive heart failure (CHF) 2) Cimetidine: ↑AUC by 50%
Estramustine (Emcyt)	+	0	D±	±	0	0	0	Cardiac, gynecomastia	None significant

*High doses.

Continued

Cancer chemotherapy side effects and drug interactions—cont'd

Drug	N/V	Mucositis	D/C	Alopecia	BMS	HSR	V/I	Organ and other toxicities	Drug interactions
Etoposide (VP-16, VePesid)	±	0	C±	+	+	+	–	Hypotension (rapid infusion), bronchospasm, neurologic	1) ↑ Warfarin action, ↑ INR 2) ↑ Toxicity of methotrexate
Floxuridine (FUDR)	±	+	D+	±	±	0	0	Skin, hepatic	None significant
Fludarabine (Fludara)	±	0	D±	±	±	0	0	Neurologic*, decreased T cell count	1) Pentostatin: ↑ risk of lung toxicity 2) Live vaccines: ↑ active viral disease
5-Fluorouracil (5-FU) (Adrucil)	±	++	D++	±	+	0	–	Cardiac, skin, neurologic, ocular	1) Cimetidine: ↑ 5-FU effect 2) Thiazide diuretics: ↑ risk myelosuppression 3) Leucovorin: ↑ 5-FU effect and toxicity 4) Warfarin: ↑ INR
Gemcitabine (Gemzar)	+	0	0	±	++	0	0	Skin, fever, flu-like syndrome, acute respiratory distress syndrome (ARDS); BMS may lead to cumulative thrombocytopenia	1) Cisplatin: administer cisplatin after gemcitabine 2) Paclitaxel: administer paclitaxel before gemcitabine
Hydroxyurea (Hydrea)	±	±	D±, C±	±	+	0	0	Skin, megaloblastosis	None significant

Drug								Toxicity	Interactions
Idarubicin HCl (Idamycin)	+	±	D±	+	+	0	V	Cardiac, skin	Heparin: incompatible, causes precipitate
Ifosfamide (Ifex)	+	±	D, C±	+	‡	0	I	Neurologic*, hemorrhagic cystitis, renal	1) Allopurinol, chloroquine, phenothiazides, potassium iodide, chloramphenicol, imipramine, vitamin A, corticosteroids, succinylcholine: ↑ toxicity 2) Mesna: inactivates ifosfamide metabolite
Irinotecan HCl (Camptosar)	‡	±	D+	+	+	0	I	Pulmonary	1) Carbamazepine, phenytoin, laxatives, phenobarbital, phenytoin, primidone, ketoconazole: ↑ drug toxicity 2) St. John's Wort: ↓ activity of irinotecan 3) Oxaliplatin, 5-FU/LV: synergy
Lomustine (CCNU, CeeNU)	+	±	D±	±	‡	0	0	Gonadal, hepatic, pulmonary, renal	Other myelosuppressive chemotherapy agents: ↑ myelosuppression
Mechlorethamine (HN2, Mustargen)	‡	0	0	+	‡	0	V	Skin, fever, gonadal	Other myelosuppressive chemotherapy agents: ↑ myelosuppression

*High doses.

Continued

Cancer chemotherapy side effects and drug interactions—cont'd

Drug	N/V	Mucositis	D/C	Alopecia	BMS	HSR	V/I	Organ and other toxicities	Drug interactions
Melphalen (L-PAM, Alkeran)	±	0	0	±	+	+(IV)	0	Skin, hepatic*, gonadal	1) Other myelosuppressive chemotherapy agents: ↑ myelosuppression 2) Cyclosporine: ↑ nephrotoxicity
Mercaptopurine (6-MP) (Purinethol)	±	+	D±	0	+	0	0	Hepatic, skin	1) Allopurinol: ↑ 6-MP levels 2) Hepatotoxic drugs: ↑ hepatotoxicity 3) Warfarin: ↑ or ↓ INR 4) Nonpolarizing muscle relaxants: ↓ neuromuscular blockage
Methotrexate (MTX, Folex, Rheumatrex)	±	++	D±	±	+	0	0	Skin, hepatic*, neurologic*, ocular, pulmonary*, renal*	1) Protein-bound drugs (aspirin, sulfonamides, sulfonylureas, phenytoin, tetracycline, chloramphenicol): ↑ toxicity 2) NSAIDs: ↑ and prolong MTX levels 3) Cotrimoxazole, pyrimethamine: ↑ MTX levels
Mitomycin C (Mutamycin)	+	+	0	+	++	0	V	Skin, hemolytic uremic syndrome, hepatic*, pulmonary	Other myelosuppressive chemotherapy agents: ↑ myelosuppression
Mitoxantrone HCl (Novantrone)	±	+	D±	+	++	0	I	Cardiac, blue-green discoloration (nails, sclera, urine)	Other myelosuppressive chemotherapy agents: ↑ myelosuppression

Drug								Unique toxicities	Drug interactions
Nelarabine (Arranon)	+	Rare	+	0	++	0	0	Rare severe neurologic events (e.g., confusion, seizures, peripheral neuropathy [PN])	↑ Risk of neurologic events if prior or concurrent intrathecal (IT) chemotherapy Other myelosuppressive chemotherapy agents: ↑ myelosuppression
Oxaliplatin (Eloxatin)	++	0	D	++	++	Delayed	–	Neuropathy: acute/cold-induced, lasting <14 days, and cumulative, persisting PN lasting >14 days	1) Incompatible with 5-FU, alkaline solutions, chloride, diazepam 2) Nephrotoxic drugs: ↓ renal excretion of oxaliplatin 3) High dose 5-FU: ↑ 5-FU plasma levels 20%
Paclitaxel (Taxol)	±	±	D±	+	+	++	–	Bradycardia, skin, neurologic	1) Cisplatin: administer after paclitaxel 2) Ketoconazole, other azole antifungals: may ↑ serum paclitaxel levels 3) Carboplatin: ↑ thrombocytopenia 4) Doxorubicin, liposomal doxorubicin: administer these drugs before paclitaxel 5) Doxorubicin: ↑ cardiotoxicity 6) Beta-blockers, calcium channel blockers, digoxin: additive bradycardia

*High doses.

Continued

Cancer chemotherapy side effects and drug interactions—cont'd

Drug	N/V	Mucositis	D/C	Alopecia	BMS	HSR	V/I	Organ and other toxicities	Drug interactions
Paclitaxel protein-bound particles; albumin-bound (Abraxane)	±	±	D±	++	++	0	0	Reversible PN	Same as paclitaxel
Pemetrexed (Alimta)	+	+	D+, C+	0	++	0	0		1) Nephrotoxic drugs: potentially delayed pemetrexed excretion 2) Probenecid: delayed pemetrexed excretion 3) Ibuprofen: 20% ↑ AUC pemetrexed in normal renal function 4) Long-acting NSAIDs: stop 5 days before drug
Procarbazine (Matulane)	+	±	D±	±	+	+	0	Gonadal*, neurologic, monoamine oxidase inhibitory effect	1) CNS depressants: synergy and ↑ CNS toxicity 2) Alcohol: disulfiram-like reaction 3) Tyramine-containing foods: hypertension (HTN), intracranial hemorrhage 4) Digoxin: ↑ bioavailability

Drug								Acute side effects	Drug interactions
Temozolomide (Temodar)	+	0	0	0	++	0	0	Headache, fatigue	Valproic acid: ↓ temozolamide clearance by 5%
Thioguanine (6-TG, 6-thioguanine) (Tabloid)	+ (Dose related)	+ (High dose)	0	0	+	0	0	IV use is investigational	Busulfan: ↑ hepatotoxicity
Thiotepa (Thioplex)	±	± (High dose)	0	0	+	0	0	Skin, gonadal, neurologic*	Other myelosuppressive chemotherapy agents: ↑ myelosuppression
Topotecan (Hycamtin)	+	+	D±	+	+	0	0	Skin, fever, flu-like illness, neurologic*	Other myelosuppressive chemotherapy agents: ↑ myelosuppression
Vinblastine (VLB) (Velban)	±	+	C+	±	+	0	V	Neurologic, jaw pain	Phenytoin: ↓ effects
Vincristine (VCR) (Oncovin)	±	±	C+	±	±	0	V	Neurologic, SIADH	1) Neurotoxic drugs: ↑ risk of neuropathy 2) Digoxin: ↓ digoxin bioavailability
Vinorelbine tartrate (Navelbine)	±	±	C+	±	+	0	V	Neurologic	1) ↑ neutropenia when given with cisplatin 2) Mitomycin C: ↑ possible pulmonary reactions

*High doses.

Disclaimer: This table illustrates principal or unique toxicities, but is not all-inclusive. It may not list rare, occasional, or late effects. Side-effect profiles change with dosage, route and duration of administration, prior chemotherapy or radiotherapy, coadministration of other therapies, and patient condition and sensitivities. N/V = nausea/vomiting, D/C = diarrhea/constipation, BMS = bone marrow suppression, HSR = hypersensitivity reaction, V/I = vesicant/irritant, SIADH = syndrome of inappropriate antidiuretic hormone, PR = peripheral neuropathy, 0 = none or rare, ± = mild, + = moderate to moderately high, ++ = severe.

Developed by Fink, R., Gates, R., Goodman, M., Petersen, J., 1997, 2001 revised by Wilkes, G.M. and Barton-Burke, M., 2006. May be reproduced for clinical use.

Cellular protectants: protecting normal cells from chemotherapy

Agent	Mechanism of action	Dosage	Key points
Leucovorin	Protects normal cells in the bone marrow and GI mucosa from effects of high dose methotrexate	Begin 24 hours after methotrexate dose; dose begins according to protocol and then is titrated according to serum methotrexate levels	Ensure that leucovorin is readily available before administration of high dose methotrexate
Dexrazoxane	Protects cardiac cells from effects of doxorubicin	Dosed at a 10:1 ratio (i.e., 1000 mg of dexrazoxane per 100 mg of doxorubicin), given IV push or IV bolus, 30 minutes before doxorubicin	Causes formation of free radicals, which may reduce chemotherapy effect
Mesna	Protects bladder epithelium from mechanical injury by ifosfamide and high dose cyclophosphamide metabolites (acrolein). Mesna binds directly to acrolein and blocks its ability to damage cells in the urinary tract, thus preventing hemorrhagic cystitis.	Oral mesna: dose is 40% of ifosfamide dose at 0, 4, and 8 hours after ifosfamide dose; IV push mesna: 20% of the ifosfamide dose given at 0, 4, and 8 hours after ifosfamide; Continuous infusion ifosfamide: give continuously together in the same bag, and continue mesna alone for 24 hours after the completion of the chemotherapy infusion	Ifosfamide should NEVER be given without mesna. Oral mesna tastes and smells of sulfur and may not be well tolerated by patients prone to nausea and vomiting. Taste may be masked in 7-Up or Coca-Cola. Advise patients to increase their fluid intake, empty their bladder frequently, and report symptoms of irritation, pain, or red urine. Patients unable to tolerate oral mesna may be taught to administer the drug intravenously at home, provided that they have a central line.

- Chronic, persistent, peripheral neuropathy lasts longer than 14 days and is related to increasing cumulative levels of oxaliplatin. The highest risk occurs when the cumulative dose is about 800 mg/m^2. It is primarily sensory (paresthesias, dysesthesias) and requires astute nursing assessment to identify when it interferes with patient's ability to function or perform activities of daily living. With functional interference, oxaliplatin may be dose reduced or stopped to prevent progression to worsening sensory or a motor disability. When oxaliplatin is used as adjuvant therapy, neuropathy was shown to be reversible. In studies underway that include patients with metastatic colorectal cancer, treatment with oxaliplatin/5-FU/leucovorin is alternated with 5-FU/leucovorin, so that patients enjoy the benefits of the drug with decreased neuropathy.

22. I know that nanotechnology is the new frontier, and albumin-bound paclitaxel (Abraxane) uses nanotechnology. How does nanotechnology make Abraxane an effective chemotherapy agent?

Paclitaxel is not soluble in water or blood, so it needs to be dissolved (e.g., in Cremophor EL) or bound to other carriers, such as albumin, that are soluble. Abraxane contains paclitaxel that is surrounded by an albumin sphere using nanotechnology. Nanotechnology capitalizes on molecular flaws or differences in cancer cells compared to normal cells, so that chemotherapy or other agents are delivered preferentially to tumor cells. A nanometer is a billionth of a meter, or 1/80,000 the width of a human hair. Malignant tumors use albumin for nourishment and have special mechanisms to transport albumin into the cell. Therefore, paclitaxel enters tumor cells with the albumin, like a Trojan horse. Higher intratumoral levels of paclitaxel accumulate and normal cells have lower drug levels, with theoretically less toxicity. Because of this, higher doses of albumin-bound paclitaxel can be given as compared to paclitaxel that is dissolved in Cremophor EL (Taxol). Abraxane is indicated for the treatment of patients with metastatic breast cancer after failure of combination chemotherapy (including an anthracycline) or relapse within 6 months of adjuvant chemotherapy.

23. What are the advantages of albumin-bound paclitaxel (Abraxane) over paclitaxel dissolved in cremophor EL (Taxol)?

- Because albumin-bound paclitaxel is given at higher doses, the incidence of sensory neuropathy is greater; however, the neuropathy is reversible in many patients (mean of 22 days). Whereas, the peripheral neuropathy experienced by patients receiving paclitaxel dissolved in cremaphor takes 2 to 3 times longer to reverse.
- Because albumin bound paclitaxel (a milky suspension) is not dissolved in Cremophor EL, there is no risk of hypersensitivity to the solvent. Patients do not require premedication with dexamethasone, diphenhydramine, or other drugs, as they do when receiving paclitaxel dissolved in Cremophor EL. Because of this, the drug can be given intravenously over 30 minutes, rather than the 1 to 3 hours required for paclitaxel dissolved in Cremophor EL.

24. What is meant by an off-label and expanded use of a chemotherapy drug?

Frequently, chemotherapy drugs are administered outside the original FDA-approved indication, usually when evidence, in the form of published clinical trials, supports their use for treatment of a particular disease. Because chemotherapy drugs are highly toxic, their use outside FDA-approved (off-label use) indications should be reserved for diseases in which there is strong supporting evidence of efficacy. Expanded FDA approval occurs when a drug that is already FDA-approved for one indication receives additional FDA approval for a different disease, based on supporting evidence.

25. What is the future of chemotherapy?

Clinical trials in the adjuvant setting are ongoing to determine if cure rates can be improved by using traditional chemotherapy agents with a molecular targeted agent, such as an angiogenesis inhibitor. Combining chemotherapy with various biologic agents that affect different aspects of tumor growth will allow more individualized, effective, and tolerable treatments. Improvements in cancer treatment will continue to focus on ways to reduce toxicities. Future chemotherapy may be developed to overcome cancer cell resistance to apoptosis and the presence of telomerase. The emerging field of nanotechnology promises development of minute nanodevices that can deliver a variety of therapies, including chemotherapy, to cancer cells, while sparing normal tissues.

 Key Points

- Advances are being made by using chemotherapy in combination with targeted therapy and using nanotechnology to target tumor flaws.
- The primary side effects of cancer chemotherapy result from damage to normal cells that divide frequently, principally bone marrow, gastrointestinal mucosa, gonads, and hair follicles. Each drug can also have specific organ toxicities.
- Drug resistance is one of the major barriers to cure.
- Performance status is one of most important factors that affect response to chemotherapy.

 Internet Resources

CancerSource:
> http://cancersource.com/

American Cancer Society Patient Drug Guide:
> http://search.cancer.org/search?client=amcancer&site=amcancer&output=xml_no_dtd&proxystylesheet=amcancer&restrict=cancer&q=drug+guide, or http://www.cancer.org

National Cancer Institute, Clinical Trials:
> http://www.cancer.gov/clinicaltrials, and http://www.clinicaltrials.gov

National Cancer Institute, Understanding Cancer Series: Nanodevices:
> http://www.cancer.gov/cancertopics/understandingcancer/nanodevices

National Comprehensive Cancer Network:
> http://www.nccn.org

National Cancer Institute, Chemotherapy and You: A Guide to Self-Help During Cancer Treatment:
> http://www.cancer.gov/cancertopics/chemotherapy-and-you

Center Watch Clinical Trials Listing Services:
> http://www.centerwatch.com/

Acknowledgments

The authors wish to acknowledge Matthew Kemper, PharmD, Irene Steward Haapoja, RN, MS, and Michelle Goodman, RN, MS, for their contributions to the Principles of Chemotherapy chapter published in the first and second editions of *Oncology Nursing Secrets*.

Bibliography

Abraxis Oncology. Abraxane (paclitaxel protein-bound particles for injectable suspension). [Package Insert]. Schaumburg, IL, 2005, Abraxis Oncology.

Antonadou D, Pepelassi M, Synodinou M, et al: Prophylactic use of amifostine to prevent radiochemotherapy-induced mucositis and xerostomia in head-and-neck cancer. *Int J Radiat Oncol Biol Phys* 52(3): 739-747, 2002.

Barton-Burke M, Wilkes GM: *Cancer therapies.* Sudbury, MA, 2006, Jones and Bartlett.

Chabner BA, Longo DL: *Cancer chemotherapy and biotherapy: Principles and practice,* ed 3, Philadelphia, 2001, Lippincott-Raven.

GlaxoSmithKline Oncology. Arranon package insert. Research Triangle Park, NC, 2005, GlaxoSmithKline.

Ellison NM, Chevlen EM: Palliative chemotherapy. In Berger A, Portenoy R, Weissman D, editors: *Principles and practice of palliative care and supportive oncology,* ed 2, Philadelphia, 2002, Lippincott Williams & Wilkins.

Hurwitz H, Fehrenbacher L, Novotny W, et al: Bevacizumab plus irinotecan, fluorouracil, and leucovorin for metastatic colorectal cancer. *N Engl J Med* 350:2335-2342, 2004.

Kerbel RS, Kamen BA: The anti-angiogenic basis of metronomic chemotherapy. *Nat Rev Cancer* 4(6): 423-436, 2004.

Moghimi SM, Hunter AC, Murray JC: Nanomedicine: Current status and future prospects. *FASEB J* 19:311-330, 2005.

Pharmion Corporation. Vidaza package insert. Boulder, CO, 2004, Pharmion Corporation.

Povlovich M, White JM, Kelleher LO: *Chemotherapy and biotherapy guidelines,* Pittsburgh, PA, 2005, Oncology Nursing Society.

Sengelov I, Kamby C, Geertsen P, et al: Predictive factors of response to cisplatin-based chemotherapy and the relation of response to survival with metastatic urothelial disease. *Cancer Chemother Pharmacol* 46(5):357-64, 2000.

Tortorice PV: Chemotherapy: Principles of therapy. In Yarbro C, Frogge M, Goodman M, editors: *Cancer nursing: Principles and practice,* ed 6, Boston, 2005, Jones and Bartlett, 2005.

Wilkes GM, Barton Burke M: *Oncology nursing drug handbook,* Sudbury, MA, 2006, Jones and Bartlett.

Winston T, Livingston R, Johnson D, et al: Vinorelbine plus cisplatin vs observation in resected non–small-cell lung cancer. *New Engl J Med* 352:2589-2597, 2005.

Tips for Administering Chemotherapy

Amy Wall and Georgia A. Hansen

1. What qualifications are needed to administer chemotherapy?

Only nurses and physicians with advanced educational preparation should administer chemotherapy. Preparation includes certification in chemotherapy administration, which consists of didactic instruction plus clinical application and skill supervision. The Oncology Nursing Society (ONS) has an exclusively didactic and official credentialing program. The practitioner should also be knowledgeable about the proper procedures for drug preparation, handling and alternate methods of drug delivery, including vascular access devices, ambulatory infusion pumps, and their associated complications.

2. What are the most important precautions for preventing errors in chemotherapy administration?

Nurses should take the following precautions to prevent errors in chemotherapy administration:

- Annually assess and document the competency of nurses who administer chemotherapy. Errors most likely occur when untrained personnel are asked to perform tasks beyond their expertise.
- Delay administration of chemotherapy until a properly trained practitioner is available. With rare exceptions (e.g., high-grade lymphoma), administration of chemotherapy is not an emergency procedure.
- Have two nurses double-check the preparation and administration of drugs.
- Have two nurses separately document the proper volume, dose, and programmed rate of all ambulatory pumps when patients receiving continuous infusion chemotherapy are discharged with the pump.
- Provide care to patients with the same one or two nurses who communicate and work together closely.
- Question any aspect of the order that is unclear, contrary to customary practice, or deviates from previous protocols for the patient, especially when unusually high doses or unusual schedules are used. If an unusual protocol is being used, a valid reference (e.g., recent journal article) should be available for review.
- Avoid distractions while checking an order or administering treatment.

3. Who should write chemotherapy orders? How should they be written?

Only the attending physician or oncology fellow (**order must be co-signed by the attending physician**) responsible for the patient's care and most familiar with the drug regimen and dosage should write the initial order for chemotherapy. Orders should be written according to the following guidelines:

- The order should be written clearly and without abbreviations or acronyms. Errors most often occur when the orders are written unclearly, allowing misinterpretation. Generic drug names should be used. Preprinted chemotherapy order sets or chemotherapy software ordering programs may be used to guide thorough and legible ordering. Although the treatment plan can be easily accessed and implemented by many members of the health care team, the original order remains the responsibility of the attending physician or oncology fellow.

- To clearly discern similar sounding chemotherapeutic agents, "tall man" (capital) lettering can be used to clearly distinguish the agents. Examples: CISplatin versus CARBOplatin, and VinBLASTine versus vinCRISTine.
- The dose should be written first as it is to be calculated (mg/m² or mg/kg), and the total dose should be indicated along with the administration route and length of time of the injection or infusion.
- Any dose modification requires a new written order. The original order should not be erased, crossed out, or tampered with in any manner.
- Multiday regimens should specify the dose per m² per day, dose per day, and number of days of therapy. This information should be followed by the diluent, route, and length of time of the injection or infusion.
- The distinction should be clearly indicated if one drug in a combination is to be given for 1 day only and the other(s) for more than 1 day.

4. Give an example of an appropriately written chemotherapy order.

Patient is 72 cm tall and weighs 150 lb; m² = 2.
Order: Cisplatin 75 mg/m² = 150 mg in 250 ml normal saline IV over 1 hour (day 1 only).
Etoposide 75 mg/m² = 150 mg in 250 ml normal saline IV over 1 hour on days 1, 2, 3.
Etoposide total dose = 450 mg over 3 days.

5. Why and how is dosing of carboplatin different from other chemotherapeutic agents?

Severe myelosuppression may result if the carboplatin dosage is not adjusted for patients with impaired renal function. The Calvert formula is used to adjust carboplatin dosage, based on glomerular filtration rate (GFR) and a desired serum concentration/area under the curve (AUC). The dose calculated using the Calvert formula is expressed as total milligrams, not milligrams per square meter (mg/m²). The target AUC depends on whether the patient has been previously treated.

AUC dosing for carboplatin is calculated with the Calvert formula:

$$\text{Total dose (mg)} = (\text{target AUC}) \times (\text{GFR} + 25)$$

Electronic carboplatin calculators are available online to ease the process of calculating a carboplatin dose. Calculation of a carboplatin dosage should be documented in the client's medical record.

Renal function can be estimated using several formulas. Refer to the following website to calculate carboplatin doses using these formulas for renal function: http://hcc1.musc.edu/hemonc/carboplatin_dose_calculator.htm

6. Should a nurse take a verbal order for chemotherapy?

No. Verbal orders for chemotherapy should not be given or taken. The risk of confusion about drug names and dosages is too great. Examples of look-alike and sound-alike drugs include: carboplatin and cisplatin, vincristine and vinblastine, taxol and Taxotere, doxorubicin and doxorubicin liposomal, leucovorin and Leukeran, and Myleran and Alkeran. Mitoxantrone may be easily mistaken for mitomycin, because both have a similar dosage range, are used for breast cancer, have an unusual color (mitomycin is light purple, mitoxantrone is dark blue), and can be given by the intravenous push method.

7. What is a chemotherapy acronym?

Chemotherapy regimens are often recognized by acronyms, which are abbreviations that represent particular agents to treat specific types of cancer. For example, patients with breast cancer may be treated with AC, which stands for Adriamycin and Cytoxan. The initial represents the first letter of the chemotherapy drug; however, the initials of some agents differ from the first letter in their generic name. For example, doxorubicin is usually represented with the letter *A* for Adriamycin, not the letter *D*. Vincristine is represented with the letter *O* for its brand name, Oncovin, in the acronym MOPP, or *V* in the acronym VAD. Several drugs are represented by the same letter. For example, the letter *D* represents dacarbazine and dexamethasone. *C* represents cyclophosphamide, cisplatin, and carboplatin.

8. What parameters should the nurse check before administering chemotherapy?

Parameters vary according to several factors, individual oncologists, clinical trials, drugs and regimens, and condition of the patient. Certain chemotherapy drugs require particular baseline and follow-up parameters. For example, a MUGA (MUltiple Gated Acquisition scan) or echocardiogram should be obtained before a client is given doxorubicin. A pulmonary function test should be performed before a client is given bleomycin. Liver function should be evaluated before a client is given 5-fluorouracil, particularly when it is used in conjunction with radiation therapy. Renal function should be evaluated before cisplatin is prescribed. Patients should have a complete blood count evaluated before each treatment, unless otherwise noted by the oncologist. The nurse should confirm that the patient's hemoglobin level, white blood cell count, absolute neutrophil/granulocyte count (ANC/AGC), and platelet count are within acceptable ranges.

9. Define ANC and how it is calculated.

The ANC is the absolute neutrophil count and is also known as the absolute granulocyte count (AGC). It is the number of mature white blood cells within the total white blood cell (WBC) count. Neutrophils are responsible for the phagocytosis and digestion of bacteria. The nadir of myelosuppression for most chemotherapy drugs is between 7 and 14 days after they are given. Neutropenia generally is defined as an ANC < 1000. The ANC is calculated by multiplying the percent of granulocytes (neutrophils + bands) by the total WBC:

Total WBC = 3.5 (3,500)
Neutrophils = 28%
Bands = 3%
28% (neutrophils) + 3% (bands) = 31% (0.31)
ANC = 3.5 × 0.31 = 1085

10. What special precautions should health care professionals take to minimize their exposure while mixing, administering, or handling chemotherapeutic agents?

All chemotherapeutic agents should be admixed in a biologic safety cabinet (BSC). While mixing chemotherapy agents, personnel should wear protective clothing, including surgical latex gloves and a disposable, lint-free, nonabsorbent gown. Careful handwashing is essential. Gloves should be replaced immediately if punctured. Spills should be cleaned up as soon as possible, and exposed garments should be replaced. If a BSC is not available, protective eye gear and a respirator mask should be worn in addition to the gloves and gown. An absorbent, disposable pad should be placed under the arm or body part where the chemotherapy drug is administered to catch any spills. For handling excreta, surgical latex gloves should be worn; a disposable gown should also be worn if splashing is possible. Staff who are sensitive to latex should follow alternative protocols outlined in their institution's policy and procedure manual.

11. What are the risks to health care professionals who mix, administer, or handle chemotherapeutic agents while pregnant, breastfeeding, or attempting to conceive?

The highest risk occurs when mixing drugs, the lowest risk when handling excreta. The Occupational Safety and Health Administration (OSHA) reports a lack of in-depth information available to quantify risks, which include possible spontaneous abortion and an increased incidence of ectopic pregnancy. Both women and men who are attempting pregnancy should minimize exposure to chemotherapeutic agents through the use of appropriate protective equipment, which should minimize, if not eliminate, potential risks.

12. When a patient receives multiple chemotherapy drugs, does the order in which they are given affect the patient's response?

Yes, in certain regimens, the order in which particular chemotherapy drugs are given may enhance efficacy, minimize toxicity, or do both. For example, paclitaxel is given first in combination with carboplatin or cisplatin because myleosuppression is increased if cisplatin is administered before paclitaxel. There is also possible increased cytotoxicity when carboplatin is given before taxol. When paclitaxel is combined with doxorubicin (or liposomal doxorubicin), it is administered *after* doxorubicin. If paclitaxel is given first, the clearance of doxorubicin may be reduced, resulting in dose-limiting neutropenia and mucositis.

13. Can small, frail veins that may have been adequate for methotrexate and 5-fluorouracil be used for doxorubicin, a known vesicant?

Small veins do not necessitate use of a vascular access device (VAD) to administer a vesicant. However, the vein must be properly selected and prepared before venipuncture is attempted. The nurse should avoid being rushed or distracted and remain focused on the patient.

14. Give guidelines for selecting the proper arm vein.

- Begin your exam at the dorsum of the hand and move upward.
- Avoid the antecubital fossa for vesicant administration.
- The distal forearm is the best site to avoid nerve and tendon damage.
- Avoid veins that have been accessed in the past 24 hours.
- Avoid veins with compromised circulation.
- Evaluate the need for a VAD if multiple cycles of chemotherapy are planned or if the above guidelines cannot be met.

15. What steps should the nurse follow before attempting venipuncture?

- Apply warm compresses to the potential venipuncture site.
- Have the patient squeeze a handball.
- Use gravity by lowering the patient's arm below the patient's heart.
- Offer the patient a hot drink.

16. Outline the safest way to administer a vesicant through a peripheral vein.

- Select the best vein, preferably one in the forearm, where soft tissue density is greater. However, a straight, supple, easily cannulated vein in the hand is preferable to a smaller, deeper vein in any other location that is more difficult to cannulate.
- Select a method of administration—either the direct push method or side-arm technique (infusion through the side-arm of a freely running IV line). The direct push method is used most often when fluids are not needed to hydrate the patient. A 23-gauge butterfly needle is large enough to permit both adequate dilution and minimal trauma to the vein. Both methods are equally safe.

- Flushing with a minimum of 3 to 5 ml of saline before and after vesicant administration is mandatory to ensure venous access and safe vesicant administration. When the direct push method is used, the nurse should aspirate immediately if extravasation is suspected.
- Injecting a vesicant through the side-arm of a freely running IV line when hydration is also needed or when the drug is known to cause vein irritation (e.g., nitrogen mustard).

17. What is the main problem with the side-arm technique?

The nurse has less control over fluid flow if extravasation occurs. Gravity propels the vesicant into the patient as the nurse clamps off the IV line and then attempts to aspirate the vesicant. The potential result is that a greater amount of drug infiltration would occur than if the direct push method was used.

18. How can you distinguish among extravasation, irritation, and flare reaction?

- **Extravasation**, although rare, is probably one of the most worrisome findings that a nurse encounters. It is characterized by swelling, erythema, pain at the IV site, and possible lack of blood return.
- Vein **irritation** manifests as complaints of achiness and tightness along the vein, and is accompanied by redness and darkness. Blood return is usually present.
- **Flare reaction is** almost always accompanied by blood return but not pain; it is associated with immediate appearance of blotches around the needle site and streaking or itching along the vein.

19. True or false: As long as you have blood return, you do not need to worry about extravasation.

False. Extravasations of vesicant agents may occur in the presence of perfect blood return. Evidence of good blood return is not the only measure of safe and trouble-free injection of a vesicant. If pain, swelling, or tension is evident in the surrounding tissue, the drug probably has infiltrated the tissue despite adequate blood return. Do not ignore the patient's complaint of pain—it may be the first sign of extravasation.

20. What should you do if you are giving a vesicant and lose blood return?

The main problem with small veins is that blood return may be intermittent during drug injection. The saying, "If in doubt, pull it out," is appropriate but sometimes not practical. Presumably the best vein already has been chosen, so removal of the needle without cause is not only unnecessary but also may diminish the chance of safe delivery of the drug. If either of the cardinal symptoms of extravasation (pain or swelling at the site) is present, the nurse should stop injecting the drug and attempt to aspirate. If it is not possible to aspirate blood or the drug, the needle is removed and the site is treated as an extravasation.

In cases involving flare at the site (redness or itching along the vein) and loss of blood return, the nurse should stop injecting the drug, switch to saline, and give 10 to 30 ml of saline through the line while observing for swelling and symptoms of discomfort. If the vein is determined to be patent, the vesicant is again connected and injected slowly. The blood return again may be evident as the drug is given. The nurse should not try to reposition the needle or press down on the cannula to obtain a blood return. This strategy may damage the vein and cause the drug to seep out of the vein (i.e., extravasation).

21. If extravasation is suspected, what should the nurse do?

1. Stop giving the drug.
2. Aspirate and leave the needle in place.
3. Call the physician.

4. Give an antidote (when appropriate) through the needle or by subcutaneous injection if the needle has already been removed.
5. Remove the needle and avoid undue pressure.
6. Apply cold or heat (depending on the extravasated drug) for 15 minutes, 4 times per day for 24 hours.
7. Arrange consultation with a plastic surgeon.
8. Photograph the IV site.
9. Document the incident, preferably on a preprinted form.

22. How often should a VAD be checked during continuous infusion of a chemotherapeutic agent or vesicant?

When VADs are used, extravasations are rare but may occur. Exit sites need to be inspected frequently for signs of edema, erythema, or fluid drainage. The site should be checked every 1 to 2 hours or more often, according to the patient's condition. Many nurses focus on checking blood return to ascertain catheter tip and needle placement; however, there is no consensus about how often this procedure should be done. It is probably reasonable to check blood return less frequently (every 4-8 hours) because of concerns about infection risk, catheter clotting, or needle dislodgements in implanted ports.

23. A patient with breast cancer needs only one more dose of doxorubicin. She has absolutely no usable veins in her good arm. Is it safe to use her other arm, even though she has had a node dissection?

If the patient has no evidence or history of swelling, if she is fully informed about the risks, and if an excellent vein is available, it is often safe to proceed, after you have consulted with a physician. More breast surgeons are now performing sentinel lymph node dissections (removal of only the first few nodes in the lymphatic chain), which significantly limit the incidence of lymphedema and other complications. Therefore the risk in accessing a vein in the arm on the side where the nodes have been dissected may be lessened. If the integrity of the vein appears questionable, a temporary central line may be considered.

24. What can be done to minimize the pain of needlesticks?

For many patients the pain of the needlestick (e.g., an implanted port, peripheral line, or Zoladex injection) is the most dreaded part of treatment. For some patients, ethyl chloride spray, ice cubes, or intradermal lidocaine is adequate to partially numb the site. The most effective solution is a topical anesthetic cream (e.g., Emla), which is placed over the port site 1 to 2 hours before the needle puncture. The topical anesthetic cream also may be used over peripheral veins. Patients often can identify their best veins by running the hand or forearm under warm water, observing for venous distention, and placing the topical anesthetic cream on the site before they come for treatment. An exception is the patient who will be receiving a vesicant or irritant agent; the topical anesthetic cream may numb the site sufficiently to mask the discomfort associated with extravasation or infiltration.

25. Define irritant.

An irritant is a chemotherapeutic agent that can cause a tissue reaction characterized by pain, venous irritation, and chemical phlebitis.

26. What special precautions should you take during administration of an irritant via a peripheral IV?

Slowing the drip rate, diluting the drug with extra fluids, or applying warm or cold compresses to the infusion site may relieve pain during the infusion. For administering an irritant peripherally, angiocaths are preferred over butterfly needles because they offer more stability and reduce the risk for infiltration. The patient should be instructed to report any pain, redness, or swelling around the IV site at any time. Only pressure-sensitive infusion pumps should be used, to avoid unnecessary delivery of the irritant in the case of an IV infiltration. Infiltration into surrounding tissue during an infusion may result in pain, inflammation, erythema, and possibly blistering, all of which resolve with time.

27. Why is the antecubital fossa avoided for chemotherapy administration?

The antecubital fossa is an extremely difficult site to heal if infiltration or extravasation occurs there. Infiltrations are also more difficult to detect in the antecubital fossa. Many nurses reserve this area for drawing blood or emergency use. Chemotherapy may cause venous thrombosis or fibrosis, making the antecubital fossa unusable for other purposes.

28. Define hypersensitivity reaction.

A hypersensitivity reaction (HSR) occurs when the immune system is over stimulated by a foreign substance (e.g., chemotherapy) or antigen, and forms antibodies that cause an immune response. Sensitization results, and subsequent exposures to the antigen cause a type I allergic reaction. HSRs may occur during the initial or subsequent administration of a chemotherapeutic agent.

29. Describe the symptoms of a hypersensitivity reaction.

Most HSRs occur within the first 15 minutes of infusion or injection, but they are not limited to this time frame. HSRs have been more commonly reported after several exposures. The patient may experience one or more of the following signs and symptoms: dizziness, flushing, nausea, generalized itching, hives, rash, rhinitis, abdominal cramping, chills, hypotension, dyspnea, bronchospasm, cyanosis, and feelings of agitation, uneasiness, or impending doom.

30. Which drugs are most often associated with HSRs?

Asparaginase, paclitaxel, and monoclonal antibodies, such as rituximab, are associated with a high risk of an immediate HSR. Drugs with a low to moderate risk of HSR include: anthracyclines, bleomycin, cisplatin, carboplatin, docetaxel, etoposide, melphalan, methotrexate, procarbazine, and teniposide. More HSRs may occur with the generic formulations than with brand-name drugs.

31. How can you minimize or prevent an HSR?

HSRs can be prevented or minimized by pretreatment with corticosteroids (dexamethasone), antihistamines (diphenhydramine), H_2-receptor antagonists (cimetidine, ranitidine), or a combination of these drugs. Although most HSRs occur with the first or second treatment, be aware that other agents, such as cisplatin and carboplatin, require repeated exposure (4 or 5 times). Pay attention to the duration of administration of the agent; for example, etoposide should be administered over a minimum of 45 to 60 minutes to prevent a hypotensive episode.

32. How should an HSR be managed?

First infusions of new chemotherapy regimens should be started slowly and increased gradually to the desired rate. In the event of an HSR, the first step is to call for help; then implement the following guidelines:
1. Stop the infusion immediately, stay with the patient, and notify the physician. Reassure the patient and family.
2. Maintain the IV line with normal saline.
3. Obtain all emergency drugs and oxygen therapy that may be needed to treat the patient.

4. Monitor vital signs, including blood oxygenation by pulse oximetry, and maximize rate of IV fluid infusion if the patient is hypotensive.
5. Administer emergency drugs according to policy and procedure or physician order.
6. Place the patient in supine position to promote adequate perfusion of vital organs.
7. Monitor vital signs every 2 minutes until the patient is stable, every 5 minutes for 30 minutes, and then every 15 minutes until a determination of the patient's condition is made.
8. Document the incident and patient reaction in the chart.
9. Pharmaceutical companies make note of incidents, such as an HSR; therefore it is important to provide information to the company about drug lot numbers, diluents, preservatives, and other factors that potentially caused the reaction. Adverse events and reactions to medications should be reported to MedWatch at: www.fda.gov/medwatch/

33. What emergency drugs may be used to treat HSRs?

- Epinephrine, 0.1-0.5 mg (1:10,000 solution) by IV push or subcutaneously every 10 minutes as needed
- Antihistamines: diphenhydramine HCl, 25-50 mg IV, and/or H_2-receptor antagonists: cimetidine 300 mg IV, ranitidine 50 mg IV, or famotidine 20 mg IV
- Aminophylline: 5 mg/kg (average dose: 300-500 mg) over 30 minutes, if the patient experiences bronchospasm or wheezing
- Steroids: methylprednisolone sodium succinate (Solu-Medrol) 30-50 mg IV, hydrocortisone sodium succinate (Solu-Cortef) 100-500 mg IV, or dexamethasone 10-20 mg IV, to ease bronchoconstriction and cardiac dysfunction
- Dopamine (Intropin): 2-20 µg/kg/min, to maintain blood pressure and organ perfusion

Note: All the above doses and drugs refer to adult, not pediatric, patients

34. Can patients who have had an HSR receive the causative drug again?

In most cases, patients should not receive the remainder of the drug on the day of the reaction or in the future, especially if the reaction was significant (bronchospasm, severe hypotension, or generalized urticaria). If the reaction is mild (e.g., a rash that resolves with diphenhydramine), the physician may choose to continue the drug once the patient's condition stabilizes. If the drug is absolutely necessary and no suitable substitute is available, rechallenge may be appropriate and safe. With subsequent doses, the patient may require preparation with antihistamines and corticosteroids; emergency drugs and personnel should be present during the rechallenge. The drug also may be further diluted to minimize an HSR.

35. What can be given to treat rigors during the administration of rituximab?

Rituximab is a monoclonal antibody that is given intravenously. It can cause rigors, which do not reflect an HSR. Rigors are often noted as the IV flow rate is escalated during infusion. Meperidine (Demerol) can be used effectively to treat rigors in patients receiving rituximab.

36. Does pain occur at tumor sites during infusions of anticancer agents?

Pain at the tumor site has been reported during infusions of vinorelbine tartrate (Navelbine), rituximab (Rituxan), and trastuzumab (Herceptin). The incidence is low; however, when it occurs it may be sudden, dramatic, and worrisome to patients. After ruling out more serious problems, patients need assurance that this reaction has been observed and is temporary. At this time the mechanism of tumor site pain is not understood.

37. What drug interactions may occur in the oncology setting?

A true drug interaction occurs when the effects of one drug are altered by concomitant administration of other medications. Drug interactions may be advantageous by producing synergy between drugs or detrimental by causing antagonism, enhanced toxicity, or inhibition of effects. Pharmacokinetic drug interactions are characterized by alteration in the absorption, distribution, metabolism, bioavailability, and elimination of a particular medication. Such interactions may occur directly at the cellular level; for example, co-administration of aspirin and methotrexate causes displacement of methotrexate from its protein-binding site, causing a higher blood level of methotrexate, decreased elimination of methotrexate, and increased toxicity (see Table of Chemotherapy Side Effects and Drug Interactions in Chapter 6, Principles of Chemotherapy).

Physical and chemical incompatibilities may occur when multiple drugs are mixed or administered together. A physical incompatibility occurs when the mixture of two or more agents changes the appearance of the solution (e.g., color, precipitation, or turbidity). Chemical incompatibility results in drug degradation, thereby diminishing their effectiveness. Interactions are not always visible in an IV bag or tubing; thus it is crucial to refer to compatibility data before administering IV chemotherapy.

38. What should be said to a patient who asks, "Can I drink alcohol while receiving chemotherapy?"

In most cases, patients are able to consume alcoholic beverages in moderation throughout their chemotherapy treatment. Patients should discuss alcohol consumption with their health care team before initiating treatment. The ingestion of alcohol may be contraindicated in certain patients while receiving chemotherapy. For example, patients who drink alcohol while taking procarbazine may experience an Antabuse-like reaction with facial flushing, headache, nausea, and hypotension. Similarly, the incidence of methotrexate-induced hepatotoxicity is increased in patients who consume alcohol.

39. Can a nurse administer chemotherapy through an Ommaya reservoir?

Yes—if she or he has demonstrated competency. An Ommaya reservoir is a small, plastic, dome-like device placed beneath the scalp. An attached catheter is threaded into the lateral ventricle for administration of chemotherapy intrathecally in patients with central nervous system leukemia, or into the spinal fluid in patients with metastatic disease. It is also used for obtaining samples of cerebrospinal fluid for examination. The following sterile procedure should be followed:

1. Wear a mask and sterile gloves.
2. Prepare the scalp area with Betadine or chlorhexidine scrub (parting the hair or shaving the area if necessary). Dry with sterile gauze.
3. Gently insert a small-gauge or butterfly needle attached to a syringe into the Ommaya reservoir. Local anesthetic is usually not needed before puncturing.
4. Withdraw the spinal fluid (the amount should equal the volume of the infusate).
5. Inject the preservative-free chemotherapeutic agent slowly into the reservoir.
6. Remove the needle, and gently pump the reservoir several times.
7. Place a bandage over the site, and ask the patient to lie supine for 15 minutes.

Patients should be instructed to notify the physician of signs and symptoms of infection, such as fever greater than 101°F; tenderness, erythema, or swelling at the site; neck stiffness; or headache.

40. What chemotherapy medications should be filtered during administration?

Cetuximab (Erbitux) and paclitaxel (Taxol) must be filtered during administration. Review the package insert before mixing to verify if an in-line filter is necessary.

41. What are some examples of oral chemotherapy agents and what should patients be taught about their administration?

- Patients should be educated about the treatment plan, proper administration schedule, storage, potential side effects, drug and food interactions, supportive medications to use, and when and how to contact their physician.
- To prevent altered serum drug levels, patients should restrict food and fluids that contain caffeine, avoid or limit alcohol consumption, and limit use of tobacco.
- Patients should keep a calendar of when they started and stopped their drugs. They also need to keep track of dates and reasons when drugs were missed.
- If a dose is forgotten, patients should not take a double dose; they should keep to their regular schedule and call their oncologist.
- Oral agents should not be crushed without a physician recommendation.
- Oral chemotherapeutics should be considered hazardous waste and should not be flushed down the toilet or disposed of with regular waste. Instruct patients to bring extra pills to their pharmacist.
- Oral agents should be stored in a cool, dry place.
- As with all medications, oral chemotherapy agents should be stored out of reach of children.

Oral chemotherapy agents: time of administration and food instructions

Agent (trade name)	Time of administration	With food?
Altretamine (Hexalen)	Take dose 2 hours after meals and at bedtime	No
Busulfan (Myleran)	Does not matter	Does not matter
Capecitabine (Xeloda)	Divide daily dose in half and take 12 hours apart	Yes, within 30 minutes after meals with plenty of water
Chlorambucil (Leukeran)	Does not matter	Does not matter
Cyclophosphamide (Cytoxan)	Take in morning or early afternoon	Yes
Etoposide (VP-16)	Single or divided doses	Does not matter
Hydroxyurea (Hydrea)	Take in the evening	Does not matter
Lomustine (CCNU)	Take in the evening	No, take on empty stomach (avoid consumption of alcohol for short time after administration)
Melphalan (Alkeran)	Does not matter	No, take on empty stomach
Procarbazine (Matulane)	Does not matter	Does not matter (avoid alcohol and foods with high tyramine level, such as beer, cheese, wine, brewers yeast, chicken livers, and bananas)
Temozolomide (Temodar)	About the same time each day	No, take on empty stomach with full glass of water
Thioguanine (6-TG)	Between meals	No, take on empty stomach

Key Points

- All staff administering chemotherapy should meet qualifications to ensure competency.
- Preprinted order sets or an electronic order entry system should be used to prevent errors.
- Sequencing plays an important role in the administration of certain chemotherapy regimens.
- All staff should have emergency drugs readily available and be familiar with institutional policies and procedures for extravasation and HSR.
- The use of central venous access devices should be considered for ongoing chemotherapy treatments in patients with frail veins.
- Patients should be educated on the proper use of oral chemotherapy agents in the home.

Internet Resources

Cancer Dictionary:
   http://dictionary.rare-cancer.org/
Carboplatin Dose Calculator:
   http://hcc1.musc.edu/hemonc/carboplatin_dose_calculator_htm
Clinical Pharmacology:
   http://www.clinicalpharmacology.com/
Drug Digest:
   http://www.drugdigest.org
Gold Standard:
   http://www.goldstandard.com/
Oncology Nursing Society
   http://www.ons.org
U.S. Food and Drug Administration, MedWatch:
   http://www.fda.gov/medwatch/

Acknowledgments

The authors wish to acknowledge Michelle Goodman, RN, MS, Jennifer Peterson, RN, MS, OCN, and Carol Blendowski, RN, BS, OCN, for their contributions to the Tips for Administering Chemotherapy chapter in the first and second editions of Oncology Nursing Secrets.

Bibliography

Hayden BK, Goodman M: Chemotherapy: Principles of administration. In Groenwald S, Frogge M, Goodman M, et al, editors: *Cancer nursing: Principles and practice,* ed 6, Boston, 2005, Jones and Bartlett.
Oncology Nursing Society: *Access device guidelines: Recommendations for nursing education and practice,* Pittsburgh, PA, 2004, Oncology Nursing Society.
Oncology Nursing Society: *Chemotherapy and biotherapy guidelines and recommendations for practice,* Pittsburgh, PA, 2005, Oncology Nursing Society.
Oncology Nursing Society: *Safe handling of cytotoxic drugs,* ed 2, Pittsburgh, PA, 2003, Oncology Nursing Society.
Oncology Nursing Society: *Cancer chemotherapy guidelines,* Pittsburgh, PA, 2001, Oncology Nursing Society.
Wilkes GM, Barton-Burke M: *Oncology nursing drug handbook,* Boston, 2006, Jones and Bartlett.

Blood and Marrow Stem Cell Transplant

Carolyn Becker and Mark W. Brunvand

1. **What is a hematopoietic stem cell transplant?**

   Hematopoietic stem cell transplant (HSCT) is the intravenous administration of hematopoietic stem cells to treat patients with malignancies, genetic diseases (sickle cell anemia), or autoimmune diseases. Hematopoietic stem cells are capable of long-term proliferation and differentiation into all of the blood cells (red and white blood cells and platelets). These cells can be driven to proliferate and circulate in the blood by administering hematopoietic growth factors (granulocyte colony-stimulating factors [G-CSF]), chemotherapy agents, and antiadhesion molecules. In adults and children the hematopoietic stem cells dwell primarily in the bone marrow, and in the fetus the hematopoietic stem cells reside in the spleen, liver, bone marrow, and umbilical cord. The hematopoietic stem cells are commonly stimulated to proliferate using chemotherapy when appropriate (autologous stem cell transplant for a malignant disease). The stem cells are "mobilized" to move into the blood by G-CSF or antiadhesion molecules, which increases the number of circulating stem cells by 100 to 1000 times to facilitate their collection from the peripheral blood where they can be concentrated by apheresis.

2. **What are the types of hematopoietic stem cell transplants?**

   The different types of transplants reflect the source of stem cells:
   - **Autologous transplant**. The stem cell donor is the patient. The patient's stem cells are harvested, processed, and frozen. The transplant consists of chemotherapy, radiation therapy, or both to eliminate malignant cells and then the frozen stem cells are infused to repopulate the marrow after the high-dose chemotherapy has been given. This process allows the administration of myeloablative chemotherapy to treat predominately malignant diseases.
   - **Allogeneic transplant**. Allogeneic stem cells come from a donor within the same species: related donor, unrelated volunteer donor, or placental blood (umbilical cord blood).
   - **Syngeneic transplant**. The stem cell donor is the patient's identical twin. This is essentially an autologous transplant with no chance of contamination of the stem cells by cancer cells.

3. **How common are bone marrow and hematopoietic stem cell transplants?**

   Statistics from the Center for International Blood and Marrow Transplant Research (CIBMTR) indicate continued annual growth in the number of transplants. It is estimated that more than 20,000 allogeneic stem cell transplants and 50,000 autologous (mostly peripheral blood stem cell) transplants are being performed annually worldwide.

4. **How is a hematopoietic stem cell donor selected?**
   - Family members are the most common source of stem cells for allogeneic transplantation. Based on genetics, each sibling has a 25% chance of being HLA-identical (human leukocyte antigen) with the patient. The donor for an allogeneic

transplant is chosen by determining the identity of the major histocompatibility genes sequences for both donor and host HLA genes. These genes are located on chromosome 6 and encode the HLA proteins, which are located on immune cell surfaces. These proteins present antigens to the immune system and ultimately define self versus nonself. Two classes of genes (class I and class II) have been identified within the major HLA locus on chromosome 6. The transplant-relevant class I molecules consist of HLA-A, HLA-B, and HLA-Cw, which are on many cell types in the body that present antigens to CD8-positive T cells. The transplant-relevant class II molecules, HLA-DR and HLA-DQ, are present on antigen presenting cells and present antigens to CD4-positive T cells. Suitable donors for most adult transplants usually must match at least 5 of the 6 loci.

- The pool of donors appropriate for allogeneic stem cell donation has been increased by using mismatched family members or volunteer unrelated donors through the National Marrow Donor Program (NMDP). Unrelated donors are HLA typed by DNA-based typing to choose the best genotypic match. Eighty percent of patients requiring transplant can identify donors for stem cell transplant if either unrelated volunteer donors or family members, including donors with mismatches at one or two antigens, are considered as donors. Unrelated donors do not share minor histocompatibility antigens with the recipient, causing higher rates of graft-versus-host disease (GVHD) and graft-versus-tumor diseases. Currently, HLA typing and recipient disease characteristics are used to identify a suitable donor.

- Recently, adult patients who require allogeneic stem cell transplant but lack a related or an unrelated donor have been successfully treated with cell transplantation from two umbilical cords. Each cord has 4 of 6 HLA antigens that match, and they are infused together after chemoradiotherapy conditioning. Recipients of these double cord transplants have experienced faster and more reliable engraftment and substantially improved survival. Transplants using two umbilical cords optimize the CD34+ cell count to improve engraftment in adults and provide another allogeneic stem cell option. The transplant-related mortality is about 20%, with one year disease-free survival of 71% for patients in remission at the time of transplant.

5. Is there an age limit for transplantation?

Using regimens that are more immunosuppressive and less cytoreductive have increased the age range of patients that can undergo transplantation up to 70 to 75 years in otherwise healthy patients. In patients with no co-morbid medical conditions, the transplant-related mortality is as low as 5%, regardless of whether stem cell donors are related, when immunosuppressive regimens (fludarabine/total body irradiation [TBI]) are followed.

6. How does a patient find a compatible unrelated donor?

If partially mismatched family members are included, 35% of patients have a suitable donor within their family. To address the paucity of family member donors, the NMDP maintains a registry of millions of volunteer marrow donors in the United States and coordinates searches for donors from registries around the world. The NMDP conducts donor drives, similar to blood drives, to attract more potential donors into the pool of volunteers. Blood is collected from the volunteer donors for molecular HLA typing. The results of the typing are entered into the NMDP computer registry that can be accessed by NMDP transplant teams during the search process. Special efforts are ongoing to recruit donors from racial minorities that are currently underrepresented in the U.S. registry.

If a patient does not have a suitable family member as a transplant donor, the physician may initiate a search for volunteer donors from the NMDP registry. It takes several months from the initial search request until the transplant can be scheduled. If a suitable unrelated donor is located, he or she is cleared medically for stem cell collection, undergoes an informed consent procedure, and has additional blood drawn for testing. All donor expenses are paid by the NMDP, and then billed to the patient, the transplant center, or both. NMDP donors are able to give either peripheral blood or bone marrow stem cells.

7. What are the functions of transplant conditioning regimens?

The pretransplant conditioning treatment performs two functions for the patient: (1) reduction in the number of malignant cells, and (2) immunosuppression of the host to prevent rejection of the donor graft. Patients who have a disease that is responsive to drug therapy but have a high risk of relapse may be treated with a conditioning regimen that is primarily immunosuppressive to facilitate engraftment of the allogeneic stem cells with minimal toxicity. Immunosuppressive regimens currently include fludarabine or another adenosine deaminase inhibitor, combined with either TBI or treatment with busulfan or melphalan. If graft rejection does occur, host hematopoiesis usually occurs with these regimens.

8. What is an umbilical cord blood transplant?

An umbilical cord blood transplant refers to the transplant of hematopoietic progenitor cells from umbilical cord blood. The fetal blood in the placenta is collected after delivery of the baby. The hematopoietic stem cells and naïve immune cells are present in this blood. The placental blood unit is then HLA typed and cryopreserved. Umbilical cord blood registries have been developed to facilitate transplantation using cord blood units. Most cord blood registries can be accessed via the NMDP.

9. What are the benefits and limitations of umbilical cord blood transplantation?

- Two advantages are associated with transplantation of umbilical cord progenitor cells: the units are typed and frozen so they are available for immediate use (within 1-2 weeks) and they are associated with lower likelihood of inducing graft-versus-host disease than transplants from adult unrelated donors with the same degree of HLA mismatch.
- A limitation of single cord blood transplantation is the limited number of CD34+ stem cells in the product. Recent data indicate that stem cell number is the most predictive factor for engraftment and survival. The threshold of 3.5×10^7 nucleated cells/kg patient body weight can be met in many more patients using two cords that are each matched at 4 of 6 HLA antigens. Many units were collected before CD34 determinations could be performed routinely, and therefore cell doses may be recorded as total nucleated cells rather than CD34+ cells. Both fully ablative and fludarabine-based primarily immunosuppressive conditioning can be used and yield high engraftment rates and low mortality in patients.

10. When are hematopoietic stem cell transplants indicated?

- Hematologic disorders and malignancies, including myelodysplasia/myelofibrosis, leukemias (acute and chronic), lymphomas, multiple myeloma, myelodysplasia, and severe aplastic anemia
- Certain genetic disorders, including sickle cell anemia, thalassemia, Hurler's syndrome; and autoimmune disorders, such as multiple sclerosis

11. What patient population undergoing hematopoietic stem cell transplantation has the best outcomes?

The best outcomes for most malignant diseases occur when the disease is responding to treatment or in remission. There are 30 years of data indicating that the use of allogeneic stem cells for transplants decreases the risk of relapse. This phenomenon is called graft-versus-leukemia or graft-versus-tumor effect. This lower relapse rate after allogeneic stem cell transplant is due to the immunological attack of the donor cells against the host malignant cells.

12. What criteria must be met for a disease to be treated by autologous bone marrow transplantation (BMT)?

In addition to consideration of the patient's age and general physical condition, the disease under treatment must meet four criteria for an effective transplant:
- The tumor must be responsive to chemotherapy.
- Myelosuppression must be the dose-limiting toxicity of effective chemotherapy.
- Stem cell transplantation can be performed when tumor burden is low and malignant cell drug resistance is minimal.
- Stem cells can be collected from the patient when the stem cells are healthy and relatively free of tumor cells.

13. Why are stem cell transplants performed for solid tumors?

Research has shown that many solid tumors cannot be eliminated by standard-dose chemotherapy. Stem cell transplants enable the use of potentially curative high-dose chemotherapy, radiation therapy, or both by reconstituting the hematopoietic and immunologic systems. Patients whose tumors respond to chemotherapy and who relapse (often in sites of initial bulk disease) after complete response are often considered for autologous stem cell transplantation. The stem cells are collected from the patient and stored before therapy and then returned to the patient after high-dose chemotherapy is delivered. At present patients with germ cell tumors and Ewing's sarcoma are the most likely among patients with a diagnosis of a solid tumor to receive a stem cell transplant.

14. Does autologous stem cell transplantation improve survival in women with breast cancer?

Data from prospective studies performed in the United States and Europe are too preliminary to determine whether autologous transplantation improves overall survival. A prospective, randomized study that was performed at multiple sites in the Netherlands included high-risk patients with primary breast carcinoma who also had malignancies in at least four lymph nodes. This study showed that autologous hematopoietic stem cell transplantation improved survival and disease-free survival compared with standard-dose therapy. So far, the first 285 patients in this study have been followed up for 7 years. U.S. studies have not shown a significantly improved survival in high-risk breast cancer patients treated with autologous transplant, but they have been plagued with methodological problems, such as high patient drop-out rates and high transplant mortality rates.

15. Describe the technique for harvesting marrow stem cells.

Marrow stem cells are collected by repeated bone marrow aspirations from the posterior iliac crest, the anterior iliac crests, or both, and occasionally the sternum of the donor. The procedure is performed in an operating room under general anesthesia. The amount of marrow collected is based on patient weight. During the 1 to 2 hour surgical procedure the marrow is removed, filtered to remove bone particles and large fat globules, and then transferred into transfusion bags for further processing and freezing (autologous marrow) or immediate infusion into the recipient (allogeneic marrow).

16. How are peripheral blood stem cells collected?

Peripheral blood stem cells (PBSCs) are collected from the patient/donor's peripheral blood through a technique called **apheresis**. The machine used in apheresis operates by density gradient centrifugation to select and separate stem cells based on the density of the cells. After the cells of desired density are removed, the remainder of the blood is infused back into the donor.

17. What is mobilization or priming and how does it occur?

- Before stem cells are collected, a procedure called mobilization is used to increase the number of primitive progenitor cells circulating in the peripheral bloodstream. Mobilization requires administering chemotherapy, colony-stimulating factors (CSFs), agents that block adhesion molecules, or a combination of these treatments, which synchronize the cells within the cell cycle and move the stem cells into the peripheral blood circulation.
- Allogeneic stem cell donors are not given chemotherapy to mobilize their stem cells.
- Protocols vary, but daily G-CSF is commonly given by subcutaneous injection. Stem cell collections begin on the fourth or fifth day of injections, when the CD34+ cell count in peripheral blood is at least 10 per µL of blood. Three to four collections, each lasting 2 to 4 hours and processing 3 to 5 blood volumes, are usually required to collect enough stem cells for transplantation. The stem cells are then processed and frozen for autologous transplantation. Often they are infused immediately into the patient in an allogeneic donation.

18. How do peripheral blood stem cells compare with bone marrow stem cells?

- Peripheral stem cell collection eliminates the need for a bone marrow harvest with the attendant risks of general anesthesia.
- A theoretical benefit of using PBSCs is less tumor contamination of peripherally-derived stem cells. Data from apheresis collection of autologous stem cells in patients with low-grade B-cell lymphoma have documented a 2 to 3 log decrease in tumor cell contamination with collection of PBSCs compared to marrow stem cells.
- The patient's hematopoietic function recovers more rapidly after transplant using G-CSF primed peripheral stem cells, probably because mobilization stimulates committed progenitor cells in addition to stem cells.
- PBSCs contain ten times more T cells that increase the risk of GVHD and decrease the risk of relapse in patients with a high relapse risk. Several studies have documented improved survival in patients with high-risk leukemia who receive transplanted PBSCs, because they have lower relapse rates.

19. What is "purging"?

The aim of purging is to remove contaminating malignant cells while leaving stem cells intact to reconstitute the hematopoietic system. Purging can be accomplished either in vivo or in vitro. Methods of eliminating malignant cells include the use of chemical agents and antibodies (monoclonal antibodies combined with complement, chemotherapy, or magnetic microspheres). Both antibody and chemical purging may damage stem cells and delay engraftment, resulting in prolonged neutropenia and delayed return of T- and B-cell function after transplantation. Research is ongoing to clarify the role and efficacy of purging in transplantation.

20. What is the role of colony-stimulating factors in transplant?

- Significantly decrease neutropenia sequelae
- Synchronize the hematopoietic stem cells to allow stem cell harvesting, which can be used for allogeneic or autologous stem cell transplantation
- Stimulate neutrophil recovery after the transplant, decrease the risk of bacteremia, and decrease the severity of mucositis

21. Is it safe to use growth factors in leukemia patients undergoing transplant?

Growth factor receptors are found on both normal progenitor cells and myeloid leukemia blast cells. Initially, clinicians were concerned that administration of growth factors might increase leukemia relapse rates by stimulating proliferation of residual leukemia cells. Studies using growth factors in patients with leukemia showed no increase in relapse; on the contrary, growth factors improved survival in select situations.

22. How are blood or marrow stem cells returned to the patient?

- Allogeneic marrow is harvested, filtered, and infused through a central line, much like a blood transfusion. The bone marrow product contains approximately 1×10^7 CD3+ T cells per kg and is associated with lower GVHD rates.
- Allogeneic peripheral blood progenitor cells are obtained with the red blood cells and plasma depleted. The cells may be directly infused through a central line. The peripheral blood infusions contain about 1×10^8 CD3+ T cells per product. Transplantation with PBSCs is associated with higher rates of chronic GVHD.
- With related, HLA-identical donors, the stem cells can be infused immediately. If the recipient is not at the same center as the donor, stem cells are transported by courier to the transplant center. Stem cells must be infused or frozen within 48 hours of collection.
- In autologous transplants, harvested bone marrow and blood stem cells are frozen in liquid nitrogen. Dimethyl sulfoxide (DMSO) is added before freezing to protect the cell membranes during freezing and thawing. At transplant, the frozen bags of blood or marrow stem cells are rapidly thawed in a 37°C water bath. They are infused directly by bag or syringe into a central venous catheter.

23. Discuss conditioning regimens.

Purine analogues or adenosine deaminase inhibitors (fludarabine or 2-CdA) and mycophenolate mofetil (MMF) have been integrated in the conditioning and GVHD prophylaxis regimens used for allogeneic transplantation. These drugs have increased the immunosuppression inherent in allogeneic transplantation regimens without the degree of damage to the patient's hematopoietic system seen with classical conditioning. MMF seems to enhance engraftment of allogeneic stem cells.

The integration of these drugs with nonmyeloablative doses of busulfan, melphalan, cyclophosphamide, or TBI (200-400 cGy) has allowed delivery of conditioning with 2% to 10% 100-day mortality rates and enough immunosuppression to allow engraftment of donor hematopoietic cells. Transplantation of allogeneic stem cells after one of these regimens is known as a nonmyeloablative or "mini" transplant. If engraftment fails after one of these regimens, the patient's autologous marrow function will return; hence, the designation of nonmyeloablative conditioning. Animal models of GVHD indicate that GVHD rates may be lower after a nonmyeloablative transplant. This finding, however, does not appear to be the case with humans who have a transplant 3 to 4 years after diagnosis.

24. What is the role of TBI in transplantation?

TBI is the exposure of the entire body to gamma radiation and is an important component of many BMT conditioning regimens. The LD_{50} (lethal dose) of a single dose of radiation is about 600 cGy; death often results from myeloablation. Radiation doses in fully ablative regimens are usually 2 to 3 times higher than the single-dose LD_{50}. Dose responses to malignancy occur up to 1575 cGy of fractionated total body irradiation. TBI doses in nonmyeloablative regimens typically are in the range of 200 to 400 cGy as one or two fractions. Coupled with fludarabine and posttransplant MMF, this dose of TBI is enough to allow engraftment of donor hematopoietic cells after transplant. Data from the treatment of relapsed severe aplastic anemia transplants have confirmed that TBI is profoundly immunosuppressive.

TBI has two additional advantages: it remains effective even in cancers that have become resistant to chemotherapy, and it treats sanctuary sites, such as the central nervous system and testes.

25. What are the side effects and complications of TBI?

Many normal tissues are affected by TBI. Potential acute side effects include nausea and vomiting, diarrhea, enlarged salivary glands, mucositis, and dry mouth. The most critical areas affected are the lungs (idiopathic interstitial pneumonia), gastrointestinal tract, reproductive system, central nervous system, and lens of the eye. As a result, some long-term side effects of TBI include sterility, cataracts, chronic pulmonary disease, leukoencephalopathy, endocrine dysfunction, sterility, and secondary malignancies. In addition to sterility, problems with sexuality, both physiologic (vaginal dryness and ejaculatory problems) and psychologic (body image and cancer survivor issues), may occur.

26. What are the major problems in the early posttransplant period?

The major effects of conditioning and marrow infusion for both autologous and allogeneic transplant are similar despite differences in preparative regimens and disease. GVHD and interstitial pneumonia are the major causes of death after allogeneic BMTs. Conditioning with chemotherapy, radiation, or both causes the following major side effects and complications in the immediate posttransplant period:

Hematologic effects include neutropenia, thrombocytopenia, anemia, and hemolytic uremic syndrome.

Infection due to neutropenia is the major cause of death during intensive chemotherapy. Bacterial and fungal infections and reactivation of viruses (e.g., herpes simplex and cytomegalovirus) are the most common problems immediately after BMT. Ninety percent of first fevers during the neutropenia that accompanies transplantation are caused by bacteria. Historically gram-negative bacteria accounted for the highest morbidity and mortality rates. However, since the widespread use of long-term, indwelling catheters, gram-positive organisms are the major pathogens responsible for most cases of bacteremias in the first 60 days after transplant.

Gastrointestinal effects include nausea, vomiting, mucositis, esophagitis, and severe diarrhea. Nausea and vomiting may result from the conditioning therapy as well as antibiotics. The combination of mucosal damage, nausea, and vomiting can make eating difficult or impossible, necessitating parenteral nutrition.

Pulmonary effects include noncardiogenic pulmonary edema, infection, and diffuse alveolar hemorrhage (serious).

Cardiac effects (less common) include cardiac arrhythmias, myocardial edema or fibrosis, and congestive heart failure.

Renal effects include hemorrhagic cystitis, renal insufficiency, and renal failure. Renal failure may result from chemotherapeutic agents administered with or without antibiotics, immunosuppression, and liver damage.

Neurotoxicity from drugs such as carmustine, thiotepa, and busulfan may cause seizures, dementia, confusion, and diplopia.

Dermatologic toxicity, which can be caused by many medications, may range from mild rashes to severe blisters and bullae.

Veno-occlusive disease (VOD) of the liver, an obstructive disease of the hepatic venules resulting in portal hypertension and liver failure, may occur in 10% to 60% of patients. Time of occurrence is usually between day 7 and day 28 after transplant.

VOD is a clinical syndrome consisting of hepatomegaly, discomfort in the right upper quadrant of the abdomen, fluid retention and weight gain, and elevated serum bilirubin level. Treatment is primarily supportive; 70% of patients recover spontaneously.

27. What causes GVHD?

GVHD, which is seen primarily in allogeneic transplants, results when the infused donor PBSCs recognize the recipient as foreign tissue. The donor's T lymphocytes mediate this response. The greater the degree of immunologic HLA disparity between donor and recipient, the more common and more severe the GVHD reaction. Donor-host sex mismatching, donor parity, and patient age also contribute to the incidence and severity of GVHD.

28. List the triad required for diagnosis of GVHD.

- The graft must contain immunologically competent cells.
- The host must possess important transplantation alloantigens that are lacking in the donor graft; therefore, the host appears foreign to the graft.
- The host must be incapable of mounting an effective immunological reaction against the graft.

29. What is the difference between acute and chronic GVHD?

Acute GVHD (aGVHD) occurs between engraftment and day 100 and is mediated by lymphokines. The organ systems targeted in aGVHD are the skin (dermatitis: ranging from minor rash to desquamation), gut (enteritis: severe diarrhea to painful ileus), and liver (hepatitis with elevated bilirubin and alkaline phosphatase levels).

   Chronic GVHD (cGVHD) occurs after day 100 and may be mediated by cellular immune cells, such as natural killer cells. Chronic GVHD affects the skin (syndrome similar to scleroderma), liver (elevated transaminases and bilirubin), oral mucosa (ulcerations, xerostomia, lichenoid changes), lungs (bronchiolitis obliterans), and gut (dysphagia, pain, and weight loss). Sicca syndrome (decreased eye lacrimation; vaginal vault ulceration, strictures, and atrophy) also may occur. Acute GVHD symptoms can also occur during the chronic GVHD phase.

30. What is the graft-versus-leukemia effect?

Graft-versus-leukemia effect refers to the potentially beneficial immunologic effect of mild GVHD in eliminating residual leukemia in the host. In allogeneic patients experiencing grade II acute GVHD with mild chronic GVHD, the relapse rate is one third the rate in patients without detectable GVHD. The lack of a GVHD reaction in autologous or syngeneic stem cell transplantation is thought to play a role in the higher relapse rate in autologous and syngeneic transplants. Thus some groups are attempting to induce GVHD in autologous marrow recipients.

31. How is GVHD prevented?

The most important way to prevent GVHD is to find an identically matched donor. Even in this case, however, prophylactic immunosuppressive drugs (e.g., cyclosporine, FK506, methotrexate, MMF, antithymocyte globulin, and steroids) are used singly or in combination to minimize the recipient's immunologic response to donor marrow. All of these drugs have side effects and toxicities.

   Another preventive method is T-cell depletion of the graft. Because T cells are believed to be responsible for the recognition and immunologic reaction in GVHD, reducing their number in the donor marrow may reduce the incidence and severity of the problem. However, because T cells also seem to play a role in engraftment of the marrow, reducing their number has potential risks. To date, T-cell depletion studies have reported lower GVHD rates but higher rejection and relapse rates, so that overall survival has not improved.

32. How is GVHD treated?

The severity of GVHD determines the treatment. Topical steroid creams, systemic steroids, and additional immunosuppressive medications may be administered to treat GVHD.

Intensive nursing interventions are needed to manage GVHD toxicities, such as skin (e.g., erythroderma, bullous formation, desquamation), gut (e.g., severe diarrhea, mucositis), and other organ toxicities. Patients with GVHD are even more susceptible to infections than during the period of neutropenia, because of the immunosuppressive effects of both GVHD and the drugs used to treat it.

33. What follow-up care is needed by patients who have had a BMT?

Important aspects of follow-up care in the early recovery period are the prevention and management of complications from the conditioning regimen and PBSC reinfusion. Blood counts may not have fully recovered, possibly causing fatigue, fever, infections, and bleeding. Close assessment and administration of antibiotics, blood products, and GVHD therapy also may be required. The gastrointestinal tract may not be fully recovered, necessitating antiemetics, antidiarrheals, fluids, electrolytes, and nutritional support. The intensity of needs depends largely on how early the patient is discharged after the conditioning therapy and bone marrow or stem cell reinfusion. Initially, the patient's condition may be assessed in the clinic 3 to 7 days per week.

As the acute toxicities of BMT resolve, outpatient follow-up is less frequent. Most transplant centers request follow-up visits annually to evaluate disease response, survival, disease-free survival, toxicities related to transplant, and quality of life.

34. How does chronic GVHD complicate follow-up?

Patients with cGVHD may require follow-up care at a transplant center for several years after BMT. Attention to immunosuppressive therapy, evaluation of response of GVHD, management of acute and chronic infections, and psychosocial and nutritional support require supervision from a multidisciplinary transplant team.

35. Describe the expected long-term physical effects of BMT.

Most physical effects occur within the first year and include toxicities or side effects from chemotherapy, radiation therapy, immunosuppressive drugs, or relapse of the original disease. Other potential delayed complications include immunodeficiency, autoimmune disorders, dental problems, and aseptic bone necrosis (steroid-induced). The rate of second malignancies appears to be 10% to 15% at 20 years after transplant.

36. Describe the long-term physical effects of chronic GVHD.

Effects from cGVHD may occur 5 years or more after transplant. Examples include skin changes, dry eyes and mouth, diarrhea, weight loss, anorexia, and pulmonary and liver involvement. Skin changes occur in 95% of patients who develop cGVHD. Symptoms consist of dryness, itching, and absence of sweating; skin tightness and contractures may develop later. The mouth and eyes are also frequently affected, with symptoms of dryness and pain. Extensive cGVHD can cause disability as a result of contractures, skin disfigurement, weight loss, and malaise. Patients with GVHD are also at risk for developing late infectious complications from encapsulated bacteria, varicella zoster virus, and *Pneumocystis carinii*.

37. How long does it take for patients to return to normal after BMT? How does BMT affect a person's quality of life?

The trauma of undergoing transplant usually affects all aspects of well-being and quality of life (physical, social, psychologic, and spiritual domains). The first year after transplant is often characterized by great emotional intensity and fear, as patients cope with continued treatment of transplant-related complications, including GVHD and infections. Many of the physical effects lessen over time, and most patients can resume a more normal life within 1 year after the procedure. A few patients (5%-15%) experience lasting physical effects that may not improve and require permanent adaptation or significant rehabilitation. Chronic GVHD, pulmonary problems, reproductive effects, and second malignancies are among the most devastating complications.

Many patients do not experience a linear recovery from the psychologic, social, and existential effects of transplant. Most BMT survivors report only mild to moderate psychological distress. Survivor guilt, changed relationships with family and friends, and changes in employability and insurability are unpredictable nonphysical effects. Because some patients encounter difficulties in returning to their previous work and level of functioning, vocational retraining may be an important element in full recovery. Long-term areas of concern include physical strength, sexual activity, fear of cancer recurrence, fear of secondary cancers, and uncertainty towards the future.

Informing patients of survivor groups and celebrations, networks, newsletters, and online computer resources is a first step to providing good follow-up care to the growing number of long-term survivors.

38. Is it difficult to get insurance coverage for BMT?

Because BMT is costly (approximately $75,000 to $250,000), obtaining insurance coverage is a complex and dynamic process. Of interest, studies at the University of Washington indicate that when the cost of transplantation is analyzed, the cost of transplant per year of life prolongation is the same as for treating moderate hypertension. Patients without insurance are not eligible for transplant unless they are able to pay for the procedure up front.

39. What are the likely directions for BMT in the future?

Hematopoietic stem cell transplantation is an ideal vehicle for gene therapy. Gene therapies are being developed to treat inborn errors of metabolism, such as sickle cell anemia. In vitro models are being developed to remove stem cells from animals with inborn errors of metabolism, replace the damaged gene, and transplant the stem cells. These strategies may allow autologous transplant with the patient's own stem cells, in which the damaged gene has been replaced. If the disease is manifested in hematologic cells or if small amounts of the gene product can correct the phenotype, autologous stem cells in which the defective gene is replaced may be used to correct the defect. With time, the modified autologous stem cells may take over a greater portion of hematopoiesis, correcting the gene defect for the remainder of the patient's life.

The use of nonmyeloablative transplants is an example of the power of immune-mediated antineoplastic treatment, or graft-versus-malignancy. Many centers are working to decrease the toxicity of conditioning by substituting immunosuppression for high doses of myeloablative chemoradiotherapy. These regimens decrease the toxicity of the transplantation conditioning, allowing the graft to eliminate the remaining malignant cells. We are finally entering a time when targeted chemotherapy (monoclonal antibody with conjugated chemo or radiotherapy) can be used to effectively treat patients while causing less damage to normal cells. Such new agents can be used to condition patients before transplant, allowing older patients to be treated with fewer toxic effects.

Key Points

- Autologous transplants, cells from self, are used to treat some solid tumors and hematological malignancies.
- Allogeneic transplant may be from a related donor, unrelated donor, or umbilical cord.
- Side effects of allogeneic transplant side include GVHD, infections, and the toxic effects of treatment.
- Graft-versus-host disease can occur soon after the transplant and continue for years, causing significant side effects.
- Quality of life after bone marrow transplant can be complicated by physical side effects, fear of recurring cancers, and role changes within the family and work environment.

Internet Resources

National Marrow Donor Program:
  http://www.marrow.org
National Institutes of Health:
  http://www.nih.gov
American Society for Blood and Marrow Transplantation:
  http://www.asbmt.org
National Bone Marrow Transplant Link:
  http://www.nbmtlink.org
Center for International Blood and Marrow Transplant Research:
  http://www.ibmtr.org

Acknowledgments

The authors wish to acknowledge Mary Roach, MS, RN, OCN, Marie Whedon, MS, RN, AOCN, FAAN, and Beth Mechling, RN, MSN, AOCN, APN for their contributions to the Blood and Marrow Stem Cell Transplant chapter in the first and second editions of *Oncology Nursing Secrets*. The authors thank Peggy Russell, Penny Odem, and Karrie Witkind for assistance with data gathering for this manuscript.

Bibliography

Barker JN, Weisdorf DJ, DeFor T, et al: Transplantation of 2 partially HLA-matched umbilical cord blood units to enhance engraftment in adults with hematologic malignancy. *Blood* 105:1343-1347, 2005.

Cornetta K, Laughlin M, Carter S, et al: Umbilical cord blood transplantation in adults: Results of the prospective Cord Blood Transplantation (COBLT). *Biol Blood Marrow Transplant* 11:149-160, 2005.

Crawley C, Szydlo R, Lalancette M, et al: Outcomes of reduced-intensity transplantation for chronic myeloid leukemia: An analysis of prognostic factors from the Chronic Leukemia Working Party of the EBMT. *Blood* 106:2969-2976, 2005.

Kim YJ, Kim DW, Lee S, et al: Comparison of 2 preparative regimens for stem cell transplantation from HLA-matched sibling donors in patients with advanced myelodysplastic syndrome. *Int J Hematol* 82: 66-71, 2005.

Kojima R, Kami M, Kanda Y, et al: Comparison between reduced intensity and conventional myeloablative allogeneic stem-cell transplantation in patients with hematologic malignancies aged between 50 and 59 years. *Bone Marrow Transplant* 36:667-674, 2005.

Kroger N, Zabelina T, Schieder H, et al: Pilot study of reduced-intensity conditioning followed by allogeneic stem cell transplantation from related and unrelated donors in patients with myelofibrosis. *Br J Haematol* 128:690-697, 2005.

Martino R, Caballero MD, Canals C, et al: Allogeneic peripheral blood stem cell transplantation with reduced-intensity conditioning: Results of a prospective multicentre study. *Br J Haematol* 115:653-659, 2001.

Ortega JJ, Diaz de Heredia C, Olive T, et al: Allogeneic and autologous bone marrow transplantation after consolidation therapy in high-risk acute myeloid leukemia in children: Towards a risk-oriented therapy. *Haematologica* 88:290-299, 2003.

Remberger M, Persson U, Hauzenberger D, et al: An association between human leucocyte antigen alleles and acute and chronic graft-versus-host disease after allogeneic haematopoietic stem cell transplantation. *Br J Haematol* 119:751-759, 2002.

Robin M, Guardiola P, Devergie A, et al: A 10-year median follow-up study after allogeneic stem cell transplantation for chronic myeloid leukemia in chronic phase from HLA-identical sibling donors. *Leukemia* 19:1613-1620, 2005.

Saleh US, Brockopp DY: Quality of life one year following bone marrow transplantation: Psychometric evaluation of the quality of life in bone marrow transplant survivors. *Oncol Nurs Forum* 28:1467-1464, 2001.

Shpall E, Adkins D, Appelbaum F, et al: Council on Education and Standards, Task Force on Guidelines for Clinical Centers and Training: American Society for Blood and Marrow Transplantation guidelines for training. *Biol Blood Marrow Transplant.* 7(10):577, 2001.

Sorror ML, Maris MB, Storb R, et al: Hematopoietic cell transplantation (HCT)-specific comorbidity index: A new tool for risk assessment before allogeneic HCT. *Blood* 106:2912-2919, 2005.

Biologic and Targeted Therapy

Kelly C. Mack

1. What are biologic response modifiers?

A biologic response modifier (BRM) is any substance capable of altering (modifying) the immune system with either a stimulatory or suppressive effect. These agents are usually made by human cells; however they are administered in a dose that is greater than physiologic levels. Biologic response modifiers can restore, augment, or modulate the host's immunologic mechanisms. They may also interfere with the ability of tumor cells to survive, metastasize, or differentiate. Biologic therapy involves the use of the following agents: colony-stimulating factors (includes hematopoietic growth factors), interleukins, interferons, and tumor necrosis factor. Recent additions to BRMs include gene therapy and immunomodulating agents (e.g., vaccines).

2. What is targeted therapy?

Molecular targeted therapy (MTT) uses agents that specifically target a known critical molecular pathway of tumor growth, rather than using a broad "shotgun" approach. MTTs prevent the usual signaling of growth, invasion, and metastasis signals used by malignant tumors. Four classes currently used are: (1) antibodies, (2) small molecule inhibitors (SMI) (e.g., tyrosine kinase inhibitors), (3) peptidomimetics or proteasome inhibitors, and (4) antisense therapies. Monoclonal antibodies are examples of targeted agents that used to be classed with the biologic modifiers.

3. What is the significance of cross talk in targeted therapy?

Cross talk occurs when a protein produced by one signal transduction pathway causes another unrelated reaction in another signaling pathway. For example, when the HER-2/neu pathway is stimulated, it sometimes causes down regulation of the estrogen receptor (the estrogen receptor "disappears" from the surface of the nucleus). The estrogen receptor is not normally associated with the HER-2 pathway, but one of the products of the HER-2 pathway interacts with the function of the estrogen receptor. This "side effect" is called cross talk.

4. Is there a difference between biologic response modifiers and targeted therapy?

It is largely a difference of semantics. Biologic response modifiers generally are broader in their spectrum of action (e.g., stimulate or suppress the immune system). The targeted agents work on a specific, small segment of the tumor growth pathway (e.g., inhibit a protein that signals the tumor to create its own blood supply).

TARGETED THERAPY

5. What are monoclonal antibodies?

Monoclonal antibodies (MOABs), often called "magic bullets," are antibodies generated against a specific antigen. Using hybridoma technology, developed in the mid 1970s, an antibody-secreting cell can be fused with a malignant cell, resulting in a single antibody that can recognize a single antigen. This technology allows the production of unlimited amounts of pure MOABs that are highly specific for a single antigen. MOABs tailored to recognize specific antigens on tumor cells can be used diagnostically to detect cancer cells or used therapeutically to enhance or cause the destruction of cancer cells. The MOABs are large molecule drugs given intravenously that work on the external domain of the receptor. They can be administered less often because they have a long half-life of many days. The most common side effects are hypersensitivity or allergic reactions.

6. How do monoclonal antibodies work?

Monoclonal antibodies target a specific protein on the surface of a tumor cell. The following are the four proposed mechanisms of action:
1. Direct tumor cell death via lysis or induction of apoptosis (programmed cell death)
2. Antibody dependent cytotoxicity (ADCC)
3. Complement dependent cytotoxicity
4. Neutralization of downstream signaling, possibly by blockage of receptor

7. What is meant by downstream signaling?

Downstream signaling and signal transduction describe the same process that begins outside the cell. A protein or ligand binds with a receptor on the cell membrane. The process of binding sends a signal through the receptor down a molecular pathway within the cell, ultimately delivering a message to the nucleus of the cell, telling it to divide, proliferate, invade, or metastasize. There are a variety of ligands, receptors, and signaling pathways; each has specific messages to deliver. The process can be interrupted at any of several points along the pathway. Interruption of this process will lead to stagnation of growth or cell death.

8. What are the different sources of MOABs, and why is it important to understand their origins?

Monoclonal antibodies are originally derived from mouse or human cells. Use of greater amounts of mouse antibody increases the likelihood of immunogenic reactions. Because monoclonal antibodies that contain mouse (murine) antibodies may be rejected by the human immune system as foreign, they may also be less effective. This reaction is known as "HAMA," for human antimouse antibodies. HAMA reactions are usually seen within

Monoclonal antibody nomenclature				
	Suffix -mab always stands for monoclonal antibody	**Clues to remember**	**Example**	**% Human**
Mouse/murine	-momab	Think mouse	Tositumomab (Bexxar)	0%
Chimeric	-ximab	Think cross ("X") species	Rituximab (Rituxan)	65%-70%
Humanized	-zumab	Remember Z in humanized and "zumab"	Trastuzumab (Herceptin)	95%-98%
Fully human	-umab		Panitumumab (Vectibix)	100%

the first 2 to 3 doses of therapy and can result in anaphylaxis. Conversely, allergic reactions are less likely with the presence of more human antibody. The suffix on the generic name of the antibody will indicate how much mouse and human antibodies are present (see table on opposite page). Other interesting facts about nomenclature of antibodies: presence of *tu* in the drug name means the target is on the **tu**mor (tras**tu**zumab targets the HER-2 protein on the tumor cell); presence of *ci* in the name means the target is in the **ci**rculation (beva**ci**zumab targets a serum ligand, not a cell surface antigen).

9. **What are the targets, indications, side effects, and precautions of treatment with MOABs?**

Monoclonal antibodies

Monoclonal antibody	Target	Indication	Side effects/precautions
Alemtuzumab (Campath)	CD52	Chronic B-cell lymphocytic leukemia Reduce the incidence of graft-versus-host disease in transplant patients	Infusion reactions (rigors, fever, nausea, vomiting, hypotension), most common the first week of therapy (Note: subcutaneous dosing is associated with fewer infusion-related reactions). Bone marrow suppression and increased incidence of opportunistic infections Consider prophylaxis against *Pneumocystis carinii* pneumonia (PCP) and herpes virus infections
Cetuximab (Erbitux)	EGFR (epidermal growth factor receptor) (external domain)	Metastatic colon-rectal cancer refractory to irinotecan Head and neck cancer	Infusion related reactions (airway obstruction, hypotension, urticaria) can be severe. (Note: monitor infusion reactions for longer than the standard one hour). Dermatologic reactions, diarrhea, constipation, nausea, malaise, headache, fever, and electrolyte depletion Rare: cardiopulmonary arrest or sudden death (2%) in head & neck cancer patients; interstitial lung disease (ILD) in less than 1% of patients Monitor for hypomagnesemia, hypocalcemia, and hypokalemia, during therapy and for up to 8 wk after completion of treatment.
Rituximab (Rituxan)	CD20	Refractory or relapsed, low-grade or follicular, CD20+, B-cell non-Hodgkin lymphoma. Diffuse large B-cell lymphoma (CD20+) Also used as maintenance therapy	Infusion-related fever, chills, and aches, usually with first infusion; myelosuppression; tumor lysis syndrome

Continued

Monoclonal antibodies—cont'd

Monoclonal antibody	Target	Indication	Side effects/precautions
Trastuzumab (Herceptin)	HER-2/neu	HER-2/neu-positive breast cancer in both adjuvant and metastatic setting	Infusion-related chills and fevers in 40% of patients with the first infusion, nausea, vomiting, pain at the tumor site, cardiomyopathy, congestive heart failure, anaphylaxis, dyspnea, cough, and pulmonary edema Caution: patients with history of cardiac dysfunction or prior anthracycline or cyclophosphamide exposure
Bevacizumab (Avastin)	VEGF (vascular endothelial growth factor) ligand	First line therapy for metastatic colo-rectal cancer in combination with 5-FU	Hypertension, proteinuria, asthenia, diarrhea, epistaxis, and leukopenia Rare: hemorrhage, wound healing complications, bowel perforation, and arterial or venous thromboembolic events Avoid starting for at least 28 days following major surgery.
Panitumumab (Vectibix)	Fully human antibody to EGFR (epidermal growth factor receptor) (external domain)	Second line therapy for metastatic colon cancer following progression on fluoropyrimidine, oxaliplatin, or irinotecan chemotherapy regimens	Infusion-related reactions (anaphylaxis, bronchospasm, hypotension, fever and chills) can be severe Dermatologic reactions may be severe and life threatening; ocular changes, diarrhea, fatigue, nausea, abdominal pain, and electrolyte depletion Rare: pulmonary fibrosis Monitor for hypomagnesemia and hypocalcemia during therapy and for up to 8 weeks after completion of treatment Advise patient to limit sun exposure (sunlight exacerbates skin reactions)

10. Are there any special dosing or administration considerations for MOABs?

Generally, infusion rates should be started low and gradually increased as tolerated by the patient (refer to local policies, Oncology Nursing Society guidelines, and other dosing references). Initial doses are generally infused over 90 minutes (trastuzumab) to 2 hours (alemtuzumab, cetuximab). Maintenance or subsequent doses may be administered over 30 minutes (trastuzumab) to 60 minutes (cetuximab). For initial or loading doses of rituximab, the rate of infusion is 50 mg/hr and is increased by 50 mg/hr every 30 minutes to a maximum of 400 mg/hr, provided the patient experiences no adverse effects; subsequent doses can be infused at 100 mg/hr to a maximum of 400 mg/hr. If therapy for alemtuzumab is interrupted for a period greater than 7 days, gradual escalation to the maintenance dose is required.

11. **Describe the rationale for antiangiogenesis agents.**

    Tumors are known to create their own blood supply. Antiangiogenesis agents target the process of blood vessel growth, which blocks the supply of oxygen and nutrients to a tumor. Paradoxically, because the vessels are less leaky, interstitial pressure is reduced, facilitating delivery of chemotherapy to the tumor. This causes cell death. These agents show clinical promise with minimal toxicity. In addition to bevacizumab (Avastin), other antiangiogenesis agents include thalidomide (Thalomid) for the treatment of multiple myeloma and lenalidomide (Revlimid) for the treatment of myelodysplasia.

12. **What are conjugated MOABs? List their indications and side effects.**

    Conjugated monoclonal antibodies are monoclonal antibodies that have been tagged to either a toxin or a radioactive molecule. They are able to increase cell kill by their monoclonal antibody action, as well as, the delivery of an associated toxin or radioactive molecule. Dosing of radioconjugates is calculated by a dosimetrist. The MOABs are administered in two steps over a course of 7 to 9 days (ibritumomab) or 7 to 14 days (tositumomab). The first dose is used to determine biodistribution, and the second dose is the therapeutic dose. Doses of gemtuzumab are separated by 14 days.

Conjugated MOABs

Monoclonal antibody	Target	Conjugated with	Indication	Side effects/ precautions
Tositumomab (Bexxar)	CD20, B lymphocyte antigen	Radioactive iodine-131	Relapsed or refractory CD20+ non-Hodgkin lymphoma	Infusion reactions, severe and prolonged hematologic toxicity (especially neutropenia and thrombocytopenia); nadir is 7-9 wk after administration. Long-term toxicity: hypothyroidism.
Ibritumomab tiuxetan (Zevalin)	CD20, B lympho-cyte antigen	Radioactive indium-111 or yttrium-90	Relapsed or refractory low-grade CD20+ non-Hodgkin lymphoma	Infusion reactions, severe and prolonged hematologic toxicity (especially neutropenia and thrombocytopenia); nadir is 4-7 wk after administration.
Gemtuzumab ozogamicin (Mylotarg)	CD33 antigen	Calicheamicin (a toxin that causes double-stranded DNA breaks)	Relapsed acute myeloid leukemia expressing the CD33 antigen	Infusion reactions, hypersensitivity, hepatotoxicity, and severe myelosuppression. Infuse over 2 hours; do *not* administer as an IV push or bolus.

13. **What are small molecule or tyrosine kinase inhibitors?**

    Small molecule inhibitors are low molecular weight targeted therapies. Tyrosine kinase inhibitors ([TKIs] also known as small molecule inhibitors) target on the internal domain of several receptors (e.g., epidermal growth factor receptor [EGFR]), by preventing a signal from being transmitted within a cell that would otherwise cause cell proliferation, growth, or metastasis. Their generic names end in the suffix *ib* (for **i**nternal **b**inding). Tyrosine kinase inhibitors are usually oral agents that are taken daily. TKIs have a shorter half-life than MOABs, which confers a reduced period of toxicity. A disadvantage of oral TKIs is their uncertain absorption, potential interference with the metabolism of other drugs, and interaction with targets other than those intended, such as the cytochrome P450 enzyme. Common side effects include an acne-like rash and diarrhea.

14. What are the targets, indications, and side effects of small molecule or tyrosine kinase inhibitors?

Small molecule inhibitors

Small molecule inhibitor	Target	Indication	Side effects/Precautions
Imatinib (Gleevec)	Bcr-abl (CML)	Chronic myelogenous leukemia (CML) in chronic phase: Philadelphia chromosome-positive	Fluid retention, nausea, vomiting, muscle cramps, fatigue, diarrhea, myelosuppression, transaminitis, and rash
	c-kit (GIST)	Gastrointestinal stromal tumors (GIST): c-kit/CD117-positive	Bullous dermatologic reaction, Stevens-Johnson syndrome, liver toxicity, anemia, thrombocytopenia, and leukopenia Drug/food interactions: take with a meal and a full glass of water
Erlotinib (Tarceva)	Epidermal growth factor receptor (EGFR)	Non-small cell lung cancer refractory to first-line chemotherapy Pancreatic cancer in combination with gemcitabine as first-line therapy	Skin rash, diarrhea, fatigue, transient elevation of liver enzymes Rare: interstitial lung disease, hemolytic anemia Contraindicated in squamous cell NSCLC because of fatal hemoptysis Drug/food interactions: take on an empty stomach
Gefitinib (Iressa)	Epidermal growth factor receptor (EGFR)	Restricted access for treatment of certain patients with non-small cell lung cancer who respond to Iressa therapy	Diarrhea, skin rash, transaminitis, mild nausea and vomiting Rare: interstitial lung disease and eye pain, corneal irritation/ulceration Drug/food interactions: may be taken with or without food

Small molecule inhibitors—cont'd

Small molecule inhibitor	Target	Indication	Side effects/Precautions
Sorafenib (Nexavar)	Raf kinase inhibitor	Advanced renal cell cancer	Hand-foot syndrome, rash, hypertension, diarrhea, fatigue, alopecia, nausea, vomiting, bleeding risk, and cardiac ischemia or infarction Drug/ food interactions: take on an empty stomach
Sunitinib malate (Sutent)	Multi-kinase inhibitor	Metastatic renal cell cancer; Gleevec-resistant GIST	Hypertension, CHF, left ventricular dysfunction, adrenal toxicity, and skin pigmentation Drug/ food interactions: may be taken with or without food
Dasatinib (Sprycel)	Multi-kinase inhibitor	Chronic myeloid leukemia in chronic, accelerated or blast phase after progression on previous therapy including imatinib	Fluid retention, bleeding secondary to thrombocytopenia and platelet dysfunction, nausea, vomiting, abdominal pain, fatigue, diarrhea, myelosuppression, and transaminitis Drug/drug interactions: metabolized by CYP3A4 pathway; H2 blockers and proton pump inhibitors interfere with drug absorption Drug/food interactions: may be taken with or without food. Do not crush or break tablets.

15. **Which oral targeted agents are associated with multiple drug/food interactions and why?**

Imantinib (Gleevec), erlotinib (Tarceva), gefitinib (Iressa), sunitinib malate (Sutent), bortezomib (Velcade) and thalidomide (Thalomid) are all metabolized through the cytochrome P-450 pathway (specifically by the CYP3A4 enzyme). Plasma concentrations of these agents may be increased by coadministration with CYP3A4 inhibitors (e.g., aprepitant, ketoconazole, clarithromycin, voriconazole, indinavir) or decreased by coadministration with CYP3A4 inducers (e.g. dexamethasone, phenytoin, carbamazepine, rifampin, phenobarbital, St. John's Wort). Therefore, decreased doses of these agents may be required when administered with CYP3A4 inhibitors, or increased doses when given with CYP3A4 inducers. Drugs (CYPP3A4 substrates) whose levels may have increased plasma concentrates when administered with oral targeted agents include cyclosporine, simvastatin, and warfarin. Patients should not consume grapefruit juice when taking these agents, because it is a potent inhibitor of the intestinal cytochrome P450 pathway for drug metabolism (specifically CYP3A4).

16. Describe the dermatologic reactions associated with the EGFR inhibitors (cetuximab, erlotinib).

Dermatologic reactions include rash, dryness, pruritus, inflammation around the nails (paronychial inflammation), and alopecia. The eyes may also be affected as evidenced by conjunctivitis, keratoconjunctivitis sicca (dry eye), trichomegaly (increased hair growth, particularly eyelashes and eyebrows), eye discomfort, and visual blurring. EGFR-associated rash, described as either a pustular, papular rash or follicular pustular eruptions, is usually confined to the face, scalp, upper torso, and arms. Although the rash looks like acne, it is not acne. The rash is not an allergic reaction and usually appears within the first 2 weeks of therapy, but can also occur later. The skin rash is generally mild and rarely (< 1%) requires an interruption in therapy. The severity of rash appears to be dose related and may be an indicator of therapeutic efficacy.

17. How is EGFR-associated rash treated?

EGFR-associated rash is possibly a new dermatologic entity. Precise classification is forthcoming and clinical trials are needed to determine the most effective treatments for this side effect. In most cases the rash resolves spontaneously without treatment. Retinoids and other acne medications are contraindicated, and the use of corticosteroids is controversial. The use of antibiotics is also controversial, because the underlying mechanism for the rash is not a bacterial infection. Moderate pustular rash may be treated with topical clindamycin gel or topical pimecrolimus. For more severe rash, oral antibiotics (erythromycin, tetracycline, minocycline, or doxycycline) may be used. Pruritic rash can be treated with topical or oral antihistamines and cool compresses. Ulcerative lesions may be treated with silver sulfadiazine ointment. Creams, such as Regenecare, which contains 2% lidocaine, help to relieve painful rashes and are also moisturizing. Self-care measures include:
- Washing with mild soap (e.g., Aveeno body wash, Neutrogena, Cetaphil, Dove)
- Moisturizing with water-based or bland emollients (e.g., Eucerin Aquaphor ointment, Udderly SMOOth Udder Cream, Sween cream)
- Avoiding sun exposure, heat, and humidity; using sunscreen
- For skin cracks and fissures, using liquid type bandage products

18. Give an example of a proteasome inhibitor.

Bortezomib (Velcade) targets the ubiquitin-proteasome pathway and is indicated for the treatment of multiple myeloma in patients who have received at least one prior therapy. Side effects include peripheral, sensory, or motor neuropathy; skin rash; asthenia; fever; hypotension; cardiac toxicity, including congestive heart failure (CHF) and decreased left ventricular ejection fraction (LVEF); nausea; vomiting; constipation; diarrhea; myelosuppression; and transient increase in liver enzymes. Serum levels of bortezomib may theoretically be affected by or may affect the serum levels of other drugs metabolized via the cytochrome P450 pathway.

19. What is antisense therapy?

Antisense therapy targets messenger RNA. A small segment of nonfunctioning RNA is designed to match up with the target mRNA. The nonfunctional segment of RNA blocks the translation of the RNA into protein. Unlike other agents that target the formed protein, antisense therapy prevents the protein from being formed in the first place. Oblimersen (Genasense) is an antisense agent being developed as an orphan drug.

It targets the bcl-2 protein that inhibits apoptosis (programmed cell death) and is under investigation for the treatment of a variety of malignancies.

BIOLOGIC RESPONSE MODIFIERS

20. What are colony-stimulating factors?

Colony-stimulating factors include hematopoietic growth factors (darbepoetin alfa, erythropoietin, and oprelvekin), granulocyte colony-stimulating factors (filgrastim, pegfilgrastim), and granulocyte macrophage colony-stimulating factor (sargramostim). These factors are hormone-like proteins endogenous to the human body. They are essential to the hematopoietic system for proliferation, differentiation, and maturation of blood cells. These factors bind to receptors on the hematopoietic cell membrane and regulate the growth and maturation of specific stem and precursor cells (white blood cells, red blood cells, and platelets). They all allow higher doses of chemotherapy to be given more safely. Palifermin (recombinant human keratinocyte growth factor) is a new agent that stimulates the growth and migration of epithelial cells and is approved for reducing mucositis in patients undergoing stem cell transplants.

21. What are the general indications for using granulocyte colony-stimulating factors to support chemotherapy?

Granulocyte colony-stimulating factors (G-CSFs) are used primarily to facilitate neutrophil recovery. Filgrastim and pegfilgrastim (granulocyte colony-stimulationg factors) are indicated to decrease the incidence of infections and febrile neutropenia in cancer patients undergoing myelosuppressive chemotherapy and bone marrow/ stem cell transplants, and to keep the chemotherapy treatments on schedule. They are also used in patients with HIV infection; myelodysplastic syndromes; aplastic anemia; and congenital, cyclic, and acquired neutropenia. Sargramostim (granulocyte macrophage colony-stimulating factor) is prescribed to enhance granulocyte and macrophage recovery and to decrease the incidence of severe or life-threatening infections after acute myelogenous leukemia (AML) induction therapy and stem cell transplants.

22. What are guidelines for the primary and secondary uses of G-CSFs?

NCCN (National Comprehensive Cancer Network) guidelines offer the most current evidence-based recommendations for the primary and secondary uses of myeloid growth factors:

- Primary prophylaxis: G-CSFs are prescribed after the first cycle of chemotherapy and before the occurrence of febrile neutropenia. They are recommended for patients receiving chemotherapy for the first time, in which the incidence of severe neutropenia is > 20% (e.g., adults with leukemia, patients undergoing bone marrow/stem cell transplant). CSFs are not recommended with the initial cycles of chemotherapy in regimens that do not cause severe neutropenia.
- Secondary prophylaxis: G-CSFs are prescribed in subsequent cycles of chemotherapy after a documented occurrence of febrile neutropenia in a prior cycle. Other indications for secondary administration include occurrence of pro-longed neutropenia that may delay chemotherapy or cause inappropriate dose reductions, a need for stimulation of hematopoietic progenitor cells, and recon-stitution of bone marrow elements after high-dose chemotherapy.

23. When should G-CSF and granulocyte macrophage colony-stimulating factor be initiated?

Granulocyte macrophage colony-stimulating factor (GM-CSF) and G-CSF should not be given within 24 hours before and no earlier than 24 hours after cytotoxic therapy, because they may enhance the myelotoxicity of chemotherapeutic agents by increasing cell turnover rate. Additionally, the therapeutic efficacy of the growth factors is improved with dosing on day 2 compared to dosing on the same day as chemotherapy. Beginning G-CSF or GM-CSF 24 to 72 hours after the completion of chemotherapy provides optimal neutrophil recovery.

24. Compare dosage and side effects of G-CSF and GM-CSF.

White blood cell colony stimulating factors

Growth factor	Dosage	Side effects
Filgrastim (Neupogen): G-CSF (granulocyte colony-stimulating factor)	5 mcg/kg/day, subcutaneously/IV, until ANC > 10,000 cells/mm^3 following expected chemotherapy nadir 10 mcg/kg/day for mobilization of progenitor cells and after bone marrow/stem cell transplant	Bone pain (20% incidence), flu-like symptoms Rare; leukocytoclastic vasculitis, manifested as a rash Minor elevations of lactate dehydrogenase (LDH) and alkaline phosphatase Hair thinning, splenomegaly, persistent bone pain, and, rarely, thrombocytopenia (long-term use > 1 year) (Note: store in refrigerator; do not freeze; do *not* dilute in any solution containing saline because of possibility of precipitate)
Pegfilgrastim (Neulasta): Peg G-CSF (granulocyte colony stimulating factor)	6 mg flat dose, subcutaneously/IV, once per chemotherapy cycle, 24 hours following chemotherapy but no sooner than 14 days before the next cycle	Same side effects as filgrastim (Note: store in refrigerator; do not freeze) Pegfilgrastim is contraindicated in patients with sensitivity to *E. coli-* derived proteins
Sargramostim (Leukine): GM-CSF (granulocyte-macrophage colony stimulating factor)	250 mcg/m^2, subcutaneously/IV, daily until ANC > 1500 cells/mm^3 is achieved for three days	Fever, bone pain Rare first-dose effect: flushing with hypotension, tachycardia, arterial oxygen desaturation, musculoskeletal pain, shortness of breath, and nausea; more common after intravenous than subcutaneous administration Dose-limiting side effects: fluid retention, pleural and pericardial inflammation and effusions, and venous thrombosis

25. Compare the hematopoietic growth factors, darbepoetin and erythropoietin.

Darbepoetin alfa (Aranesp) and epoetin alfa (Procrit, Epogen), a synthetic form of human erythropoietin, are erythropoietin (EPO) or red blood cell growth factors.

It usually takes 2 to 4 weeks to see an increase in hemoglobin and hematocrit values. Both factors are prescribed for patients with anemia associated with cancer chemotherapy and chronic renal failure. They have demonstrated effectiveness in decreasing blood transfusion requirements and have shown subjective improvements in fatigue, performance status, ability to work, and quality of life (QOL). Functional capacity and QOL were enhanced independently of tumor response. Darbepoetin is also used for chronic renal insufficiency (patients not on dialysis). Other indications for epoetin alfa include the treatment of other chronic anemias, anemia associated with neoplastic infiltration of the bone marrow, myelodysplastic syndromes, patients receiving zidovudine treatment, and the reduction of blood transfusions during elective, noncardiac or nonvascular surgery. Epoetin alfa is also being studied to determine if it improves cognitive function in cancer patients. Side effects of both include: flu-like symptoms, myalgias, pain at injection site, occasional headache, and hypertension. It in unclear whether the incidence of vascular access thromboses is increased with the use of erythropoietin.

26. What is an advantage of using darbepoetin?

The longer half-life of darbepoetin alfa (Aranesp) permits less frequent and more convenient dosing than epoetin alfa given weekly (QW) or three times a week. Darbepoetin may be administered every 2 weeks (Q2W), as well as QW. Recently, darbepoetin was approved by the FDA to be given at a higher dose (500 mcg) every 3 weeks.

27. What are NCCN guidelines for monitoring EPO growth factors?

The optimal hemoglobin level is 12 g/dl. If an adequate response (hemoglobin level > 1 g/dl from the patient's baseline value) does not occur after 4 weeks of therapy with epoetin, the dose can be increased from 10,000 units to 20,000 units three times per week, or increased from 40,000 units to 60,000 units QW. If there is no response to darbepoetin at 6 weeks, the dose can be increased from 2.25 mcg/kg QW to 4.5 mcg/kg QW, from 3 mcg/kg Q2W to 5 mcg/kg Q2W, or from 200 mcg Q2W to 300 mcg Q2W. If the hemoglobin level is > 13 g/dl or if the hematocrit rises above 40%, EPO should be held or discontinued. Additionally, the NCCN recently added a recommendation to continue erythropoietin therapy if the patient's hemoglobin level is stable (within 1-2 g/dl of baseline) while receiving chemotherapy.

- Iron is supplemented as indicated (ferritin level < 100 ng/ml, transferrin saturation < 20%) because stimulation of erythropoiesis by EPO causes a state of relative iron deficiency.

28. Describe a growth factor that stimulates production of platelets?

Interleukin-11 (IL-11), or oprelvekin (Neumega), which is derived from *Escherichia coli*, is the only platelet growth factor that has FDA approval. The recommended dose is 50 mcg/kg subcutaneously, daily, beginning 6 to 24 hours after completion of chemotherapy and continued until the postnadir platelet count is ≥ 50,000/mm^3 (dose is decreased to 25 mcg/kg for patients with renal impairment). Treatment should be discontinued at least 2 days before starting the next chemotherapy cycle. Dosing should not last beyond 3 weeks. Side effects include mild to moderate fluid retention, which may manifest as peripheral edema, dyspnea, or both. Caution should be used in patients with pre-existing pleural or pericardial effusions or ascites.

29. What is interleukin-2 and what are its indications?

Interleukin-2 (IL-2) is a glycoprotein produced by helper T cells after stimulation by antigens and IL-1. The primary function of interleukins (between leukocytes) is immunomodulation and immunoregulation of leukocytes. IL-2 promotes proliferation and differentiation of B cells, T cells, and monocytes, and also has many immunologic effects. The IL-2 receptor is present mainly on activated T cells. The effects of IL-2 include proliferation of various cytotoxic cells, including natural killer (NK) cells, lymphokine-activated killer (LAK) cells, and tumor-infiltrating lymphocytes (TIL), which aid in the destruction of tumor cells without damaging normal cells. FDA-approved aldesleukin (Proleukin), or IL-2, is produced by recombinant DNA technology (placement of human genes inside bacteria or yeast cells to produce large quantities of highly purified protein).

IL-2 causes tumor regression in patients with metastatic renal cell cancer and malignant melanoma that is resistant to conventional chemotherapy agents. Responses in patients with renal cell cancer have been ~ 20%. When used as a single agent in patients with malignant melanoma, IL-2 has shown response rates of ~ 15%.

30. How should IL-2 be administered?

IL-2 is administered most commonly by intravenous infusion; it also has been administered subcutaneously. The dosage of IL-2 should be adjusted carefully, according to patient tolerance, response, and route of administration. The potency of aldesleukin usually is expressed in international units (IU). Other units also have been reported, including Cetus units (CU) and Roche units (RU), but they are not equivalent (1 RU = 3 IU; 1 CU = 6 IU).

31. Discuss the toxicities associated with IL-2.

Most IL-2-induced toxicities appear to be dose-related and are reversible or manageable with appropriate supportive care. IL-2 may cause side effects in nearly every organ system. The most common dose-limiting toxicities of IL-2 are hypotension, fluid retention, and renal dysfunction. Patients receiving IL-2 may also experience thrombocytopenia, anemia, eosinophilia, and skin erythema with burning and pruritus (managed with a moisturizing cream such as Eucerin). Neurologic changes, hypothyroidism, and bacterial infections are also common.

A major side effect is a flu-like syndrome that occurs 4 to 6 hours after initiation of therapy. Another significant side effect is fatigue, which may be due to cytokine release. Other adverse effects include nausea, vomiting, and diarrhea, which can be managed with adequate antiemetic and antidiarrhea therapies.

A problematic side effect is **vascular leak syndrome** (VLS), for which the presenting symptoms are peripheral edema and weight gain (often > 10% of body weight). Ascites, with or without pleural effusions, and pulmonary edema may also occur. Patients with underlying cardiovascular or renal abnormalities may be more susceptible to these side effects. VLS is managed with vasopressors (e.g., dopamine), albumin, fluid support, diuretics, and oxygen.

32. What are the interferons?

The interferons (IFNs) are proteins belonging to the cytokine family. Three types have been described in humans: alpha (IFN-α), beta (IFN-β), and gamma (IFN-γ). Each type originates from a distinct cell and has different biologic and chemical properties. The IFNs have antiviral, immunomodulatory, and antiproliferative properties. Recombinant IFN-α-2a and IFN-α-2b are administered by intramuscular or subcutaneous injection.

33. What are the therapeutic uses of the interferons?

Labeled indications for recombinant IFN-α in the treatment of cancer include hairy cell leukemia, acquired immune deficiency syndrome (AIDS)-associated Kaposi's sarcoma, chronic myelogenous leukemia, follicular non-Hodgkin lymphoma, and malignant melanoma. Other uses of IFN-α include treatment of multiple myeloma and renal cell carcinoma. IFN-β is used to treat multiple sclerosis, and IFN-γ is used to treat chronic granulomatous disease.

34. Discuss the adverse effects associated with interferon use. How can they be managed?

Pharmacologic doses of IFNs have been associated with various side effects:

- Acute flu-like syndrome with fever, chills, malaise, myalgias, and headache that begins 2 to 8 hours after the first subcutaneous injection. Flu-like symptoms may be prevented or alleviated with administration of acetaminophen 650 mg before the IFN injection and every 4 hours thereafter, for 24 hours. Adequate hydration is important for decreasing many of the flu-like symptoms. Administration of IFN at bedtime enables the patient to sleep through the flu-like symptoms of initial therapy. Tolerance (tachyphylaxis) to the flu-like effects develops over several days to weeks.
- Fatigue and depression are the most common dose-limiting and dose-related side effects of IFN-α. Bedtime administration may help to minimize the fatigue, along with strategies to reduce activities and conserve energy. Severe fatigue, however, may require dosage decreases or discontinuation of therapy. Assessment of depression and use of selective serotonin reuptake inhibitors (SSRIs) often improve both fatigue and depression.
- Gastrointestinal symptoms, such as anorexia, nausea, vomiting, and diarrhea, are rare at low doses but increase in frequency and severity as the dose increases. Antiemetic and antidiarrhea medications help to control some of these symptoms. Hydration levels influence tolerance of therapy.
- Neurologic effects, such as vertigo, decreased mental status, confusion, depression, and paresthesias, occur at low doses but may increase in severity and incidence at increased doses.
- Hematologic effects include decreased leukocytes, granulocytes, and thrombocytes. Liver function tests and CBCs should be monitored at frequent intervals during interferon therapy.

35. What is tumor necrosis factor? What are its effects?

Tumor necrosis factor (TNF-α), also called cachexin, is a natural substance produced by activated macrophages, monocytes, and lymphocytes after exposure to endotoxin. As a type of cytokine, TNF-α causes tumor and healthy tissue necrosis by decreasing or stopping blood flow. It remains an investigational agent. To date, TNF-α has not shown significant palliative or curative results for any type of cancer. The clinical use of TNF-α has been limited by its severe systemic toxic effects (coagulopathy, cytopenia, and pulmonary failure).

 Key Points

- Biologic and targeted therapy agents manipulate normal molecular pathways to treat cancer.
- To be effective, the target has to be present on the cancer cell but not on normal cells. In most cases, the tumor will be tested for the presence of the particular target before treatment (e.g., HER-2/neu must be overexpressed on tumor cells of a breast cancer patient who is to receive trastuzumab).
- Tyrosine kinase inhibitors are given orally, and monoclonal antibodies are administered intravenously.
- Combining chemotherapy agents with colony-stimulating factors allows higher doses of chemotherapy to be given safely, and facilitates administration of planned doses of chemotherapy on time.
- NCCN guidelines offer the most current evidence-based recommendations for the primary and secondary uses of myeloid growth factors.

Internet Resources

Advances in Targeted Cancer Therapies:
   http://www.targetedtherapies.org
Amgen:
   http://www.amgen.com
Genentech BioOncology:
   http://www.biooncology.com
National Cancer Institute Fact Sheet, Targeted Cancer Therapies: Questions and Answers:
   http://www.cancer.gov/cancertopics/factsheet/Therapy/targeted
National Comprehensive Cancer Network:
   http://www.nccn.org

Bibliography

Camp-Sorrell D: Antiangiogenesis: The fifth cancer treatment modality? *Oncol Nurs Forum* 30(6): 934-944, 2003.

Iwata KK, Haley JD: *Molecular targeted therapy in oncology for the 21st century: Bench to bedside.* Tarrytown, NY, 2006, The Curry Rockefeller Group.

Lapka DM, Franson PJ: Antisense therapy. *Clin J Oncol Nurs* 7(4):441-443, 2003.

Lacouture ME, Basti S, Patel J, et al: The SERIES clinic: An interdisciplinary approach to the management of toxicities of EGFR inhibitors. *J Support Oncol* 4(5):236-238, 2006.

National Comprehensive Cancer Network: NCCN practice guidelines in oncology: Myeloid growth factors, vol 1,2006. Available at: http://www.nccn.org/professionals/physician_gls/PDF/myeloid_growth.pdf. Retrieved June 4, 2006.

Oncology Nursing Society: *Chemotherapy and biotherapy guidelines and recommendations for practice.* Pittsburgh, PA, 2005, Oncology Nursing Society.

Perez-Soler R, Delord JP, Halpern A, et al: HER1/EGFR inhibitor-associated rash: Future directions for management and investigation. Outcomes from the HER1/EGFR inhibitor rash management forum. *Oncologist* 10:345-356, 2005. Available at: http://www.TheOncologist.com/cgi/content/full/10/5/345

Schaal AD: Alemtuzumab (Campath 1-H). *Clin J Oncol Nurs* 9(5):630-632, 2005.

Viele CS: Keys to unlock cancer: Targeted therapy. *Oncol Nurs Forum* 32(5):935-940, 2005.

Vlahovic G, Crawford J: Activation of tyrosine kinases in cancer. *Oncologist* 8:531-538, 2003.

Wilkes GM, Barton Burke M: *Oncology nursing drug handbook,* Sudbury, MA, 2006, Jones and Bartlett.

Yamamoto DS, Viale PH, Zhao G: Severe acneiform rash. *Clin J Oncol Nurs* 8 (6): 654-656, 2004. Available at: http://www.ons.org/publications/journals/CJON/Volume8/Issue6/pdf/0806654.pdf

Clinical Trials

Pamela A. Rossé and Mary T. Garcia

1. Describe how a clinical trial differs from a protocol.

A **clinical trial** is a planned research investigation involving patients. It is designed according to accepted scientific methods and is intended to determine the most effective treatment for patients who develop a given medical condition in the future.

A **protocol** is the written plan for a clinical trial; it outlines the objectives of the study and summarizes research information that is relevant to the treatment under study. In addition, a protocol explicitly delineates criteria for inclusion and exclusion of participants. It also describes in detail the treatment that subjects will receive and specifies parameters for evaluating outcomes.

2. What types of clinical trials are the oncology nurse likely to encounter?

Studies may be designed as therapeutic or preventive, or they may address biologic or genetic questions by collecting and testing tissues or specimens. Therapeutic studies may include one or several modalities, such as chemotherapy, radiation therapy, surgery, hormonal therapy, immunotherapy, gene therapy, or alternative therapies for symptom management.

3. How are therapeutic studies characterized?

Every new chemotherapy drug is tested in three subsequent trials, called phase I, phase II, and phase III, before it is approved by the FDA for general use. Phase IV studies occur after initial approval. However, not all studies fall within the phase classification system (e.g., prevention, early detection, quality of life, and cost of treatment studies). Additional characteristics may be used to classify a trial, such as adjuvant or neoadjuvant.

4. Explain the purpose of phase I drug studies.

Phase I studies are dose-escalating clinical trials designed to determine the maximum tolerated dose (MTD) of a new drug, alone or in combination with another drug or modality. The phase I trial also helps to establish an optimal therapy schedule, determine pharmacokinetic properties, and identify toxicities associated with therapy. Frequently, a phase I study includes patients who have had extensive treatment, and who may have different types of cancer. Because the study is concluded once the MTD is reached, the number of patients included is often small (e.g., 20 patients) but may include 100 or more.

5. What are the goals of phase II studies?

Phase II studies evaluate antitumor activity in specific tumors and further define toxicities. The number of patients frequently ranges from 100 to 200, but several hundred may be involved.

6. Describe the primary goal of phase III studies.

Phase III studies compare a promising new treatment with established therapy in clinical practice to determine which one is superior for treating a specific disease. Large numbers of participants are required.

7. What is the purpose of phase IV studies?

After a treatment has been approved by the FDA and marketed, phase IV studies may be conducted to examine long-term effects, particularly risks versus benefits. Unlike the other phases, the general public has access to the treatment being studied without participating in a clinical trial.

8. What are adjuvant and neoadjuvant studies?

Adjuvant studies are designed to provide additional therapy to patients who have been deemed free of disease after treatment. The goal is to prevent recurrence.

Neoadjuvant studies are designed to treat patients before and after surgery, with the belief that no evaluable disease will remain after surgery. The goals are to optimize the success of surgery and to prevent recurrence.

9. In clinical trials with multiple treatment regimens, who decides which regimen a particular patient will receive?

In studies with multiple treatment regimens, each regimen is called an arm. Patients are often randomized to specific arms of a study or assigned to different treatments by a process similar to flipping a coin. Usually, the randomization schedule is generated by a computer. For some studies, assignment may be blind (the patient does not know which treatment he or she is receiving) or double-blind (neither the patient nor the health care team knows which treatment is administered). At times, patients who do not have a complete or partial response (CR or PR) to one treatment may cross over or switch to another arm of treatment.

10. Define equipoise and explain its significance in clinical trials.

Equipoise means "even balance." In clinical trials, it refers to a mind-set of approaching studies from an unbiased perspective. Because of the investigational nature of a study, it is important to impress on subjects that they may receive no direct benefit. It is also paramount in studies with more than one treatment option, or more than one arm, to present all treatments with equal enthusiasm. Sometimes this task is difficult for the health care team, because, based on professional experience, they may believe that one therapy is more promising than others.

Studies that compare therapy with no therapy or observation (which may be the standard of care in certain conditions) are particularly challenging. It is often difficult to do nothing novel or experimental when a patient is faced with the diagnosis of cancer. In such cases it is beneficial to remember that many investigational cancer therapies ultimately have been deemed ineffective and possibly significantly toxic to the study subjects.

11. Define eligibility and evaluability. Why are they important?

Eligibility refers to meeting the qualifications stipulated in the protocol for participation in the study. **Evaluability,** also known as treatment fidelity, refers to how well the protocol was followed once the patient was enrolled; it determines the usefulness of the patient's data. Both concepts are crucial to the integrity of the study. For example, regarding eligibility, if a patient does not have the same type, grade, or stage of cancer required in the protocol, the progress of disease may not be affected by the proposed therapy. Significant differences among patient characteristics make it difficult to include them in the same pool for analyses. Similarly, regarding evaluability, if patients are not treated for their disease in a standardized manner, it is difficult to generalize the results. Of equal importance, if a patient does not meet one of the eligibility criteria (e.g., adequate renal or cardiac function), he or she may experience serious toxic side effects.

12. In general, what information do investigators look for once a study has ended?

At the conclusion of a clinical trial the primary investigators concentrate on data that answer the following questions:

1. Were the original study questions (usually found in the objectives section of the protocol) answered? Most commonly these questions are endpoints, such as survival time, types of tumor responses, and time to recurrence.
2. What were the toxicities (in detail)? Do they outweigh the benefits?
3. Was each patient eligible and evaluable? If not, it may be difficult to generalize the data.

13. What are the implications if the treatment schedule stipulated in the protocol is not followed?

As a rule, the protocol schedule should not be violated because it is inconvenient or because the treating physician does not agree with the way the protocol is written. Such issues should be taken into consideration before the patient enters a clinical trial. Deviation from the stipulated protocol may be dangerous and may make the patient's data unevaluable. Compromise of treatment may jeopardize timely completion of select studies, may preclude some patients from participating in an innovative study, and may affect response to therapy.

14. What if a patient decides to discontinue treatment earlier than the protocol stipulates?

Every patient has the right to discontinue participation in a clinical trial at any time, and this right should be clearly stated in the consent form. In such cases, the patient, family, and health care team should thoroughly discuss appropriate alternatives, including no treatment. Even though the patient discontinues therapy, some of the early data may still be useful, for example, toxicities and early tumor response. In the final analysis, the principal investigators and biostatisticians decide whether the patient is evaluable.

Many clinical trials require follow-up of the patient's status until death to determine whether long-term survival was affected by the treatment. If the patient has chosen to discontinue participation, the type of long-term follow-up (i.e., the degree of intrusiveness) that may be continued must be clarified with and approved by the patient. In such cases, even if the patient has discontinued active participation in a clinical trial, the study remains open at an institution until all patients have died.

15. What role does pharmacokinetics play in clinical trials?

Often the drug tested in a clinical trial is reviewed for its pharmacokinetic properties. To measure absorption rates, duration of action, distribution within the body, and excretion, blood or other samples are collected at designated intervals before and after administration of therapy. Timing in obtaining samples is often critical to the reliability and validity of data. Patients and caregivers should adhere to established times for drawing blood or collecting other samples.

16. How does an institutional review board function?

An institutional review board (IRB) is entrusted with protecting the rights and welfare of human participants in research by asking the following questions:

1. Do the benefits outweigh the risks?
2. Is there adequate protection for the participants, including informed consent?
3. Is the selection of participants equitable?

All studies must be approved by an IRB before any subjects may be enrolled. The IRB also must be informed of changes and adverse events related to the studies. IRBs have the authority to suspend and close studies that previously have been approved, if regulations are not followed by the investigators and study personnel.

17. How are the members of an IRB selected?

Membership requirements for IRBs in the United States are established by the Office for Human Research Protections (OHRP), which is part of the U.S. Department of Health and Human Services. Other government agencies, such as the National Institutes of Health and the Food and Drug Administration (FDA), also regulate IRB activities. A minimum of five members of varied backgrounds, gender, racial, and cultural perspectives is required. A typical IRB may include physicians, pharmacists, nurses, scientists, lawyers, clergy, and community representatives. IRBs must include at least one member whose primary concerns are in scientific areas and at least one member whose primary concerns are in nonscientific areas. At least one nonmedical person and one person with no direct affiliation to the reviewing institution are mandated. Special expertise is required by regulation when studies involving vulnerable populations (e.g., children, prisoners, cognitively impaired people) are considered.

18. What is the purpose of a data and safety monitoring board?

In addition to the protection afforded by IRB review, some studies are monitored by an independent safety committee that periodically reviews the progress of a study. Data and safety monitoring boards (DSMBs) are composed of at least three highly qualified research professionals who have access to unblinded data and current study results. The committee makes recommendations regarding the continuation and conduct of a study to its sponsor, investigators and, ideally, to the IRB(s).

19. How does the federal privacy rule of April 2004 affect clinical research?

The HIPAA (Health Insurance Portability and Accountability Act) requires researchers to obtain written permission before a subject's protected health information can be collected and disclosed. This permission is different from the study consent, other study forms, and the typical HIPAA forms presented to patients by hospitals or other care providers. HIPAA regulations also define procedures for approaching, screening, and recruiting potential research participants. Many institutions require research and recruitment personnel to take educational courses on these regulations.

20. How can informed consent be ensured?

To inform potential participants adequately about the study, specific points must be covered:
  • Purpose of the study (and clear statement that it is research)
  • Expected duration of subject's participation
  • Specific procedures that will be followed, including those that are experimental
  • Alternative treatments that might be beneficial
  • Reasonably foreseeable risks, discomforts, and benefits of participation
  • A description of the extent to which confidentiality will be maintained
  • Clarification of compensation (or lack thereof) and any medical care available if injury should occur
  • An explanation that participation is voluntary and that the participant has the right to refuse participation or withdraw from the study at any time without penalty or loss of benefits
  • Information about who to contact if the patient has questions about the research and their rights as a research participant

Obtaining consent is a continuing process of discussing all of the preceding points with a potential subject. Information about the study may be provided by the physician, research nurse/data manager, pharmacist, or others knowledgeable about the clinical trial.

Researchers are strongly encouraged to provide consent forms written at a 6th-grade reading level using lay terminology. Frequently patients have just learned of their diagnoses; although seemingly aware of what they have heard and agreed to do, they have many questions later that require further clarification of the study process. Federal regulations require evidence that consent is provided in a manner that allows maximal comprehension and assessment of the subjects' understanding of the study. Participants must be given a copy of the written signed consent form.

21. Under what special circumstances may informed consent be waived?

According to federal regulations, the requirement for informed consent may only be waived if the study presents no more than minimum risk to participants. However, in cases where there is more than minimal risk and there is a prospect of direct benefit, for example, situations that involve emergency therapies, a number of conditions must be met for waiver of informed consent:

- The study could not practicably be carried out without the waiver.
- Consultation with community representatives must occur before starting the study.
- Public disclosure is made before and after the study.
- The researcher commits to try to locate a surrogate or legally authorized representative who can give consent within the defined therapeutic window before proceeding to waive consent.

22. Under what circumstance may eligibility criteria be waived?

On occasion, the IRB may approve participation in a study for a single patient on a compassionate basis, usually when no alternative treatment is available.

23. How is informed consent obtained from non-English speaking participants?

When non-English speaking subjects are enrolled in a study, an oral presentation may be given in the subject's native language, followed by a written "short form" stating that the elements of consent were presented orally in the subject's native language. A translator, fluent in the subject's native language as well as English, must translate the consent information to the patient or patient representative and obtain appropriate signatures on the short form.

24. Must subjects participate in all aspects of a study once they sign a consent form?

With the advent of multiple components requiring consent, IRBs are challenged with maximizing participation while preventing coercion. Some IRBs insist that, when feasible, the consent form be divided into sections, so that the subject has the opportunity to agree or refuse to participate in separate testing, additional follow-up, or secondary components to the main objectives of a study. Subjects always retain the right to withdraw from a study at any time without penalty or loss of benefits (for example, medical care).

25. What are the costs associated with participating in a clinical trial?

Studies may be sponsored by government sources, pharmaceutical companies, or individual institutions and investigators, and funding varies accordingly. Usually, patients participating in cancer treatment studies do not receive money, although study costs or drugs may be provided. In special circumstances reimbursement may be approved by the officiating IRB. It is specifically prohibited to charge subjects for research-specific costs. Typically, if the patient is insured, routine health care costs and standard of care costs are billed; remaining expenses are absorbed by the funding source. Similarly, Medicare covers routine patient care costs that are incurred in phase II and III government sponsored trials. However, some remaining costs may have to be paid by the patient. For-profit, nonprofit, and charitable organizations may contribute financially to defray patient's costs; nurses might suggest that patient seeks out these resources, as necessary.

With increasing frequency, payment incentives are offered to subjects who participate in prevention and early detection studies. These studies generally involve a healthier group of subjects than cancer treatment studies.

26. What information regarding study treatment should be shared with the patient whose condition precludes treatment at the full dose specified by the protocol?

A patient's condition may deteriorate once he or she has entered in a study. Rather than dropping the patient from the study, provisions may allow the patient to remain in the study at a reduced treatment dose. But in this case, is it is worthwhile for the patient to remain in the study? Because it is mandated that patients be adequately informed about participation in research studies, it seems logical to provide them with the facts necessary to make a truly informed decision. Therein lies the difficulty: the health care team does not typically know all of the facts. If they did, an investigational study would not be needed. One of the most honest approaches is to provide the facts that are known and to discuss issues for which the answers remain unknown.

27. How can the oncology nurse contribute to the validity of clinical trials?

- **Identification of potential study patients.** Oncology nurses know about cancer disease processes, understand the rationale for various treatments, and often have unique insights into whether a patient is likely to comply with a protocol.
- **Protecting the integrity of the study.** Most participants in an oncology clinical trial believe they are contributing to cancer research. Failure by the health care team to follow study rules undermines participants' efforts; adherence to the protocol is paramount. Because the nurse is frequently responsible for coordinating patient care, the nurse should be aware of protocol guidelines and remain in contact with trial coordinators. The treatment plan must be followed exactly, including drug administration, pretreatment and posttreatment hydration guidelines, antiemetic therapy, antibiotics treatment, and use of cell-stimulating factors. Various tests must be performed at specified times, and radiotherapy and/or surgery must be synchronized accordingly.
- **Documentation in the medical record.** In addition to their reliance on routine documentation, the reviewers of the study data greatly value additional notations, such as: (1) the patient's current performance status; (2) dose modifications or schedule changes and reasons for them; (3) specific symptoms of toxicity, including onset and duration, especially for serious adverse events; and (4) supportive care, particularly for symptom management.
- **Patient advocacy.** Often the oncology nurse can support patients' decisions to begin, continue, or discontinue treatment; nurses may be instrumental in helping patients feel comfortable with their decision or even to change their decision, if circumstances permit.
- **Patient education.** Patients may ask nurses about available study opportunities. Nurses should be aware of local, regional, and national resources, and how to access this information. For patients who are study participants but who are non-English speaking, low-level learners, or older adults, nurses can be especially helpful by reinforcing information that will promote study adherence, such as following appointment schedules and following treatment plans.

Key Points

- Mechanisms that safeguard patients while they participate in clinical research trials include informed consent, IRBs, DSMBs, and HIPAA.
- Clinical trials are identified by their phase (I, II, III) or purpose.
- Medicare and some insurance companies will reimburse specific patient care costs for particular types of clinical trials.
- The success of a clinical trial depends on the eligibility of participants, and the evaluability of data collected.
- Nurses are key to promoting patient participation and adherence in clinical trials.

 Internet Resources

General cancer trial information

http://www.cancernet.nci.nih.gov/pdqfull.html
http://www.cancer.gov/clinicaltrials
http://www.centerwatch.com
http://www.ctep.cancer.gov
http://www.cancer.org/docroot/ETO/ETO_6.asp

More specific cancer trial information

Many universities with medical schools provide websites that link to clinical trials. Type in the university's name followed by key words, such as "cancer trials," "cancer studies," or "cancer research." Also try substituting the word oncology for cancer.

Cooperative oncology groups have websites profiling their current trials (or use any search engine and type in the acronym of the group (e.g., SWOG, NSABP, ECOG, RTOG, CLAGB, etc.). Cooperative groups are also listed at the NCI website:
http://www.cancer.gov/clinicaltrials/finding/cooperative-group-web-sites/page2

Information about current regulatory updates

RGA Medical University of Ohio:
http://www.meduhio.edu/research/fed_regs.html
Office of Human Research Protections:
http://www.hhs.gov/ohrp/
Medicare and Medicaid Coverage:
http://www.cancer.gov/clinicaltrials/digestpage/medicare
http://www.cancer.gov/cancertopics/factsheet/support/medicare
http://www.cms.gov/medlearn/refctmed.asp

Bibliography

American Cancer Society: Clinical trials: What you need to know. American Cancer Society, 2004. Available at: www.cancer.org/docroot/ETO/content/ETO_6_3_Clinical_Trials_-_Patient_Participation.asp. Accessed January 3, 2006.

Ehrenberger H, Aikin JL: Making a mark in clinical trials nursing. *Clin J Oncol Nurs* 5(4):131-132, 2001.

HIPAA (Health Information Portability and Accounting Act) privacy rule and research. Society of Clinical Research Associates (SoCRA SOURCE) February:25-29, 2005.

Hochauser M: Informed consent reading, understanding plain English. Society of Clinical Research Associates (SoCRA SOURCE) November:24-26, 2004.

Jacobsen T: Adverse events and reporting ensuring safety during clinical research. Society of Clinical Research Associates (SoCRA SOURCE): February:30-32, 2005.

McCutchan JA: Data and safety monitoring. In Bankert EA, Amdur RJ, editors: *Institutional review board: Management and function,* ed 2, Boston, 2006, Jones and Bartlett.

Oncology Nursing Society: Cancer research and cancer clinical trials. ONS National Office, Pittsburgh, PA, 2004. Available at: www.ons.org/publications/positions/CancerResearch.shtml. Accessed January 3, 2006.

Schilsky RL: Conversations in care: Meeting the challenges of clinical trial enrollment. Available at www.conversationsincare.com/web_book/chapter07.html. Accessed January 3, 2006.

United States Code of Federal Regulations, Title 21 Food and Drugs, part 50, protections of human subjects; part 56, institutional review board. Rockville, M.D., 2002, U.S. Department of Health and Human Services.

University of California San Francisco: Human research protection program, consent guidelines. Available at: http://www.research.ucsf.edu/chr/Guide/chr10_ConsentGuides.asp#WaiverOne. Accessed May 9, 2006.

White-Hershey D, Nevidjon B: Fundamentals for oncology nurse/data managers: Preparing for a new role. *Oncol Nurs Forum* 17:371-377, 1990.

Blood Components

Rocky Billups, Dennis Martin, and Peg Wisner

1. **What are the four ABO blood types?**

   The four blood types are A, B, AB, and O. A and B are antigens present on the RBC membrane. A person may have both antigens and be AB, or neither antigen and be O. Individuals who lack these antigens on their RBC membranes may make antibody to the antigens when exposed to the A, B, or AB antigens. Individuals with a particular antigen on their RBC membrane will not make antibody to that antigen. Thus people with the blood type O are known as universal donors. Conversely, people with the blood type AB are universal recipients.

2. **What are the acceptable donor blood types for the eight ABO/Rh blood types?**

Acceptable donor blood type								
Blood type	A Positive	A Negative	B Positive	B Negative	AB Positive	AB Negative	0 Positive	0 Negative
A Positive	X	X					X*	X*
A Negative	X							X*
B Positive			X	X			X*	X*
B Negative				X				X*
AB Positive	X*	X*	X*	X*	X	X	X*	X*
AB Negative		X*		X*		X		X*
0 Positive							X*	X
0 Negative								X

   *If plasma is incompatible, reduce volume to 200 ml.

3. **What are the primary components of whole blood and their common indications for transfusion?**

   - **Whole blood:** not commonly used for transfusions because sound resource management requires that it be divided into its various components (e.g., RBCs, platelets, plasma) and used appropriately
   - **Packed red blood cells (PRBCs):** usually administered to oncology patients for intravascular volume expansion, support during hemorrhage, and treatment of symptomatic anemia
   - **Platelets:** transfused for significant thrombocytopenia or hemorrhage, with a platelet count threshold of < 10,000; or active bleeding with a threshold platelet count < 50,000; also may be transfused to boost a platelet count to > 50,000 immediately before or during a procedure
   - **Fresh frozen plasma (FFP):** contains clotting factors, albumin, globulins, and antibodies, and is administered to reverse the effects of warfarin; to correct coagulation abnormalities due to a deficiency of factors II, V, VII, IX, X, and XI or massive blood transfusions; and to treat thrombotic thrombocytopenic purpura

- **Cryoprecipitate:** portion of the plasma that is rich in certain clotting factors, including factors VIII and XII, von Willebrand's factor, and fibrinogen; most commonly used to prevent or control bleeding in patients with disseminated intravascular coagulation (DIC) or those with inherited coagulation abnormalities
- **Factor concentrates:** concentrates of individual plasma proteins that are used to replace specific factor deficiencies
- **White blood cells (WBCs):** granulocytes most commonly collected via apheresis and must be transfused within 24 hours; used in patients with prolonged neutropenia who have active infections, especially gram-negative bacterial or fungal infections, which are unresponsive to antibiotics or antifungal therapy; are generally irradiated and commonly cause febrile nonhemolytic reactions; may premedicate patients with acetaminophen and diphenhydramine; meperidine may be used to manage chilling; should be ABO compatible and infused via standard blood tubing without a leukocyte filter

4. What supplies and equipment are needed for a transfusion?

- Blood products can be administered through a peripheral or central catheter. Always check the patency of your access before obtaining the blood product from the blood bank. Catheters sized 18 or 19 gauge facilitate faster flow rates. A 22-gauge catheter can be safely used in an adult; however, the flow rate will be slow. Using small gauge catheters will not cause RBC hemolysis unless you try to increase the infusion rate by applying pressure to the product bag.
- Normal saline, 0.9%, is the only intravenous solution that is compatible with blood products. Agglutination or hemolysis may occur with use of other intravenous solutions. Only FDA-approved medications should be added to blood components.
- The appropriate tubing should be used for the specific blood product.
- The use of infusion pumps for blood product transfusions is a facility decision. If used, infusion pumps must be designated as compatible with the infusion of blood products. If information cannot be found about the pump's compatibility with blood products, the pump should not be used because of the risk of blood cell lysis.
- On rare occasion, a blood warmer may be needed to administer blood if a patient has a cold agglutinin disease.
- Equipment is needed to monitor the patient's vital signs for possible transfusion reaction. Emergency equipment and medications should be readily available.

5. Why are premedications administered before infusing PRBCs and platelets?

Pretransfusion medications are given to prevent nonhemolytic febrile and allergic transfusion reactions, especially if a patient had a previous reaction. Leukocyte-reduced blood products have decreased the number of these reactions. Prescribing practices may vary among physicians. Common premedications include acetaminophen (650-1000 mg), diphenhydramine (25-50 mg) and Solu-Cortef. The doses prescribed depend on the patient's clinical status.

6. What are the acceptable parameters for transfusion time of blood products?

- PRBCs are infused over 90 to 120 minutes, or 3 to 4 ml/kg/hr. The time of infusion depends on the age of the patient as well as clinical status. In the critical care unit, PRBCs may be infused in as little as 5 to 10 minutes to treat massive blood loss. To reduce the risk of bacterial contamination and sepsis, PRBCs must be transfused within 4 hours of leaving the blood bank.
- Platelets are infused over 20 to 60 minutes, or 10 ml/min. In emergent situations, such as exsanguination in a patient with thrombocytopenia, platelets can be infused

in less time. The longer platelets hang after being dispensed from the blood bank, the less effective they become. For patients who are refractory to platelet transfusion, some institutions give platelets by a continuous infusion, but for no longer than 4 hours per unit.

- FFP is usually infused over 15 to 30 minutes, or 10 ml/min.
- Cryoprecipitate is infused over 3 to 15 minutes, or 10 ml/min.
- Granulocyte transfusions begin slowly and increase to the rate ordered by the physician. The recommended length of infusion is 1 to 4 hours. Since granulocytes are suspended in plasma and will settle to the bottom of the bag, it is recommended that the bag be agitated every 10 to 15 minutes during infusion.
- Factor concentrates may be given as an intravenous bolus or as a continuous infusion.
  Note: It is important to evaluate the pulmonary status of each patient before rapid infusion of any blood product.

7. What parameters should be followed for monitoring vital signs during a patient's transfusion?

The frequency of vital sign monitoring depends on your facility's blood administration policy. According to common guidelines, complete vital signs should be monitored before beginning administration, at 15 minutes into the administration, and immediately after infusion is complete. The rationale for such standards is the increased risk of transfusion reactions associated with blood products. Remember that clinical symptoms, not changes in vital signs, are often the first indication of a transfusion reaction. Remain with the patient for the first 10 to 15 minutes, and monitor for fever or chills, hypotension, dyspnea, headache, or hives.

8. Is informed consent needed for a transfusion?

Many institutions and some states require that a patient give informed consent for blood product transfusions, except in emergencies. Patients should be informed of the benefits and possible immediate and delayed risks of a transfusion. They should also be informed of treatment alternatives and the possible consequences of not receiving a transfusion. All of the patient's questions regarding the transfusion should be answered to his/her satisfaction. Patient information is usually available from the community blood bank and from the American Association of Blood Banks (AABB) website. The patient has the right to refuse a transfusion. Some facilities require the patient to sign a form indicating their refusal is made with an understanding of the possible consequences.

9. Why should PRBCs and platelets be leukocyte reduced for patients who receive multiple transfusions?

The benefits of transfusing leukocyte-reduced products include reducing febrile nonhemolytic transfusion reactions and decreasing cytomegalovirus (CMV) risk. Using leukocyte-reduced blood products also decreases the risk for transfusion-associated graft-versus-host disease (TA-GVHD). Patients with hematologic malignancies and recipients of bone marrow transplants should receive leukocyte-reduced PRBCs and platelets.

10. What is the difference between random donor and single donor platelets?

Random-donor platelets are obtained from each unit of whole blood during processing. Platelets from several different donors are then pooled into a single pack for administration. Single-donor platelets are collected via apheresis from an individual donor and dispensed for administration. Use of single-donor platelets decreases sensitization (TA-GVHD) of the recipient and the risk of transfusion-transmitted diseases.

11. What techniques are used for leukocyte reduction?

The most common techniques available for leukocyte reduction are washing, centrifugation, freezing, and filtration. Currently, leukocyte filtration is the most common method of leukocyte reduction. Leukocyte reduction can occur at the blood center or at the bedside where leukofiltration is accomplished during transfusion with the addition of a commercially available filter that is attached to the blood product and intravenous tubing. Several commercially available filters consistently remove 95% to 99% of the leukocytes. Although bedside filtration is effective, the filtration becomes less effective as the blood warms during transfusion. The FDA permits blood products to be labeled "leukocyte-reduced" if they contain less than 5.0×10^6 WBCs.

12. Why are blood products irradiated?

Gamma irradiation of blood products is currently the most efficient and reliable method to decrease the incidence of developing TA-GVHD. Irradiation of blood products will interrupt lymphocytic mitosis and prevent TA-GVHD through inhibition of lymphocytic proliferation. Patients who have had a bone marrow transplant, Hodgkin or non-Hodgkin lymphoma, congenital immunodeficiency syndrome, neuroblastoma, glioblastoma, and patients receiving granulocyte transfusion or transfusions from relatives are at greatest risk for developing TA-GVHD.

13. Name the different types of transfusion reactions.

Transfusion reactions can be placed into two categories: acute reactions and delayed reactions. (See table on pp. 123-126.). Symptoms can range from mild to severe. Acute reactions can be seen within minutes to hours after the blood product is infused. Delayed reactions can occur days to years after the transfusion. Diagnosis may be complicated by the long period between the transfusion and the onset of reaction symptoms. See Question 15 for the common first actions to take for an acute reaction.

14. What is the most common transfusion reaction in the oncologic setting?

Nonhemolytic febrile transfusion reaction. The greater the number of antigens a person is exposed to through multiple transfusions, the higher the risk of reactions. As a result of antigen exposure, patients may develop allergic or febrile reactions to all erythrocyte and platelet transfusions. The symptoms of patients who develop hemolytic transfusion reactions are similar to those of nonhemolytic febrile transfusion reactions in the early stages. Hemolytic transfusion reactions account for 0.5% to 1% of all transfusion reactions and contribute to 70% of transfusion-related deaths.

15. What do you do if the patient develops symptoms of an acute transfusion reaction?

- Stop the blood component immediately.
- Keep the blood bag and IV tubing.
- Maintain your intravenous access with 0.9% normal saline solution.
- Monitor the patient and maintain his or her airway and blood pressure.
- Notify the physician and the blood bank.
- Follow your facility's policy for a transfusion reaction. You will usually need to send the blood and tubing to the blood bank in a transfusion reaction work-up.

16. Is it necessary to test blood products for cytomegalovirus?

Yes, the transmission of CMV via any blood product is of particular concern for patients with suppressed T-lymphocyte function. In patients with compromised immune systems, CMV infections may lead to life-threatening, multisystem disease. Clinical manifestations include hepatitis, pneumonitis (the most fatal complication),

Text continued on p. 127.

Acute and delayed transfusion reactions

Acute reaction	Cause and time of onset	Signs and symptoms	Treatment	Prevention
Allergic	Antigen–antibody reaction with release of histamine Results from sensitivity to plasma protein or donor antibody, which reacts with recipient antigen Onset: usually within 15 minutes into transfusion	**Mild reaction** • Urticaria, hives • Itching, rash • Swelling • Mild wheezing **Severe reaction** • Laryngeal edema • Bronchial asthma • Wheezing	**Mild cases** • Stop transfusion unless otherwise ordered • Antihistamines • Monitor for progressing reaction • If hives only, can sometimes continue transfusion **Severe cases** • Corticosteroids • Epinephrine	• No laboratory procedures available • Ask patient about past transfusion reactions • Premedication with an antihistamine may help prevent reaction
Anaphylaxis	Results from sensitivity to plasma protein or donor antibody, which reacts with recipient antigen and releases mediators of anaphylaxis Onset: usually within 15 minutes into transfusion	• Dyspnea • Pulmonary or laryngeal edema • Bronchospasm • Laryngeal spasm • Hypotension • Death	• Diphenhydramine • Corticosteroids • Epinephrine • Fluid therapy • Airway management	• Ask patient about past transfusion reactions
Febrile nonhemolytic	Action of antibodies against WBCs or action of cytokines in the blood product or produced by the recipient Onset: 30 min after initiation; up to 6 hours after completion of transfusion	• Rise in temp > 1°C or 2°F over baseline • Chills, rigors • Headache • Flushing • Anxiety	• Check temperature frequently • Antipyretics • Meperidine for rigors	• Premedicate with antipyretics • Use leukocyte-reduced blood products

Continued

Acute and delayed transfusion reactions—cont'd

Acute reaction	Cause and time of onset	Signs and symptoms	Treatment	Prevention
Febrile nonhemolytic —cont'd		• Muscle pain • Nausea • Shock		• Aseptic technique • Proper storage and handling • Complete infusions within established time frames
Bacterial sepsis/ septic shock	Endotoxin release due to contaminated blood product Can be Gram + or − Onset: anytime during or 2 hrs after transfusion	• Rapid onset of chills • Rise in temperature > 2°C or 3.5°F • Hypotension • Tachycardia • Abdominal pain • Vomiting • Diarrhea • Oliguria	• Obtain blood cultures • Treat septicemia as ordered: IV fluids, antibiotics, vasopressors	
Circulatory or volume overload	Pulmonary edema due to fluids administered at a rate or volume greater than what the cardiovascular system can tolerate Onset: anytime during or 1-2 hrs after transfusion	• Tachycardia • Hypertension • Increase in CVP & PAWP • JVD • SOB, cough • Crackles • Headache	• Slow or stop transfusion • Notify physician • Place patient in upright position with feet in dependent position • Diuretics, oxygen, and morphine as ordered	• Identify patients at risk • Minimize saline volume • Transfuse over maximum time frame; ask blood bank to divide units into smaller volumes if necessary • Monitor pulmonary status
Transfusion-related acute lung injury (TRALI)	Massive leakage of fluids and proteins into lungs Onset: within 6 hrs of transfusion	• Similar to ARDS • SOB • Hypoxemia • Tachycardia • Fever • Hypotension	• R/O heart failure, vol. overload, sepsis, MI • Treat symptoms to maintain VS and ventilation	• Ask patient about prior transfusion reactions • No known precautions

		Signs and symptoms	Treatment	Prevention
Acute hemolytic transfusion reaction (AHTR) NOTE: hemolytic reactions can be delayed	**Immunologic hemolysis** Transfusion of incompatible ABO blood products, causing intravascular destruction of the transfused RBC and release of Hgb and other substances into circulation **Nonimmunologic hemolysis** • Infusion of improper solutions or medications with the blood product • Improper processing or handling Onset: usually within 15 minutes into transfusion	• Fever • Chills • Tachycardia • Dyspnea • Chest or back pain • Pain at infusion site • Abnormal bleeding • Hypotension • Shock • DIC • Hemoglobinuria • Hemoglobinemia • Renal failure	• Treat symptoms to maintain VS and ventilation • Treat coagulopathy as needed • Promote and maintain urine output (may need dialysis)	• Follow proper steps in patient identification when drawing compatibility sample and when starting transfusion • Begin transfusion slowly and monitor patient closely for first 15 min
Delayed Reaction Delayed hemolytic reaction	**Cause and time of onset** Destruction of transfused RBCs by antibody not detectable during crossmatch, but formed rapidly after transfusion Onset: 2-14 days after transfusion	**Signs and symptoms** • Fever • Chills	**Treatment** • Generally no acute treatment needed • Recognition of reaction important as increased risk for acute hemolytic reaction with future transfusion	**Prevention** • Draw crossmatched blood sample within 3 days of transfusion
Hemosidererosis (iron overload)	Excess iron deposited in tissues after multiple RBC transfusions	• Diabetes • Impaired thyroid function • Arrhythmias • CHF • Other organ damage	• Monitor ferritin levels • Symptomatic treatment • Deferoxamine (Desferal) IV, IM or SC, to bind iron and promote iron excretion	• Use erythropoietin to reduce transfusion needs

Continued

Acute and delayed transfusion reactions—cont'd

Delayed reaction	Cause and time of onset	Signs and symptoms	Treatment	Prevention
Transfusion-associated graft-vs-host disease (TA-GVHD) Note: High mortality rate	Donor lymphocytes see transfusion recipient as foreign; immune response and attack on host tissues	• Erythematous skin rash • Abnormal liver function tests • Profuse, watery diarrhea • Fever	• Immunosuppression • Symptomatic treatment • Fluid and electrolyte replacement for diarrhea	• Transfuse with irradiated blood products to patients at risk
Hepatitis B and/or C, Epstein-Barr virus (EBV), cytomegalovirus (CMV), malaria, Chagas' disease, HIV/AIDS, human T-lymphotropic virus, types 1 & 2 (HTLV 1/2), Syphilis	Transmitted from donor to recipient via infected blood products	• Refer to signs and symptoms related to specific diseases	• Refer to treatment recommendations for specific disease processes	• Screen blood donors • Test blood donations
Posttransfusion purpura	Immunologic response that destroys natural and transfused platelets Onset: 7-10 days after transfusion	• Rapid drop in platelet count	• Monitor platelet count • Monitor for bleeding • High dose IGIV may help if patient is bleeding	

retinitis, central nervous system disease, gastrointestinal tract disease, and hematologic abnormalities. The risk of transfusion-associated CMV infection may be essentially eliminated by the use of leukocyte-reduced blood products or CMV-seronegative blood products. Either alternative is recommended for patients at risk for severe CMV disease.

17. What tests are performed on donated blood products to decrease the risk of a transfusion reaction or a transfusion-associated infectious disease?

Each unit of blood is tested for ABO group (blood type), Rh type, antibodies to human immunodeficiency virus (anti-HIV-I/II), hepatitis C virus (anti-HCV), human T-cell lymphotropic virus (anti-HTLV-I/II), hepatitis B core antigen (anti-HBc), and hepatitis B surface antigen (HBsAg). Additional analyses include a serologic test for syphilis, and nucleic acid tests (NAT) for HCV RNA, HIV-I RNA, and West Nile virus.

18. What are the estimated risks associated with transfusions?

VIRAL TRANSFUSIONS

HIV-I/II	1:1,900,000
HTLV-I/II	1:641,000
HAV	1:1,000,000
HBV	1:63,000
HCV	1:1,600,000

NONINFECTIOUS ACUTE RISKS

Fatal hemolytic reaction	1:1,300,000
Febrile nonhemolytic reaction	1:100
Minor allergic reaction	1:100
Anaphylaxis	1:20,000 to 1:47,000
Noncardiogenic pulmonary edema	1:5,000

19. Where can blood products be administered?

Blood products are generally administered in an outpatient or inpatient setting. Some home care agencies with infusion services provide home transfusions to patients who have had a prior transfusion without a reaction. Reimbursement of blood product administration in the home depends on the patient's insurance policy.

20. How much of an increase in hemoglobin should be expected in the patient who is not losing blood following a transfusion of one unit of PRBCs?

In the patient who is not losing blood by bleeding or destruction, an increase in the hemoglobin level of approximately 1 gm/dl and an increase of 3% to 4% in the hematocrit for each unit of PRBCs transfused can be expected.

21. What are "incompatible crossmatch" blood transfusions?

Patients who have been chronically transfused over a period of years have been exposed to many RBC antigens and may have developed numerous antibodies. There are circumstances under which compatible RBCs are not available, and the least incompatible units may be transfused with an order from the patient's attending physician. The units are ABO blood type compatible. Baseline plasma hemoglobin level is usually determined before administering these units, 15 minutes into the infusion, and after the infusion. An increase in the plasma hemoglobin level from baseline indicates a hemolytic reaction is occurring. Each institution should have a policy governing plasma hemoglobin results and the circumstances under which the unit must be discontinued.

22. What patient education about blood product transfusions should be provided? What educational resources regarding blood product transfusions are available?

Detailed education related to the process of blood administration and the warning signs of transfusion reactions should be provided to all patients. Discharge instructions must be given to the patient and family covering the signs and symptoms of adverse reactions, both immediate and delayed, and notification of physician. It is often very helpful to provide patients with educational materials to supplement the verbal information they have received.

 Key Points

- Always check the patency of your access before obtaining the blood product from the blood bank.
- Normal saline, 0.9%, is the only intravenous solution that is compatible with blood products.
- Pretransfusion medications are given to prevent nonhemolytic febrile and allergic transfusion reactions, especially if a patient has had a previous reaction.
- PRBCs are infused over 90 to 120 minutes, or 3 to 4 ml/kg/hr; platelets are infused over 20 to 60 minutes, or 10 ml/min; and FFP is usually infused over 15 to 30 minutes, or 10 ml/min.
- Complete vital signs should be monitored before beginning administration, 15 minutes into the administration, and immediately after the infusion is complete.
- Acute reactions may be seen within minutes to hours after the blood product is infused, and delayed reactions may occur days to years after the transfusion.
- The most common transfusion reaction in the oncology patient is nonhemolytic febrile transfusion reaction.

 Internet Resources

The American Association of Blood Banks:
  http://www.aabb.org
The Oncology Nursing Society:
  http://www.ons.org
The Association of Pediatric Hematology/Oncology Nurses:
  http://www.apon.org
Most local and regional blood centers have educational information available in their offices or on their websites.

Acknowledgments

The authors wish to acknowledge Lowell Anderson-Reitz, RN, MS, ANP, OCN, Beth Mechling, RN, MS, OCN, Tonya Cox, RN, BSN, and Marcia Maxwell, RN, BSN, for their contributions to the Blood Components chapter published in the first and second editions of *Oncology Nursing Secrets*.

Bibliography

American Association of Blood Banks: Circular of information for the use of human blood and blood components. Available at: http://www.aabb.org/Content/About_Blood/Circulars_of_Information/aabb_coi.htm. Accessed January 11, 2007.

American Association of Blood Banks: Facts about blood and blood banking. 2005. Available at http://www.aabb.org/Content/About_Blood/Facts_About_Blood_and_Blood_Banking/fablood Accessed January 11, 2007.

Brecher ME editor: *AABB Technical Manual,* American Association of Blood Banks, 15th edition, 2005.

Nettina SM, editor: The Lippincott manual of nursing practice, ed 7, Philadelphia, 2000, Lippincott Williams & Wilkins.

Puget Sound Blood Center: Blood components reference manual. Available at http://www.psbc.org/bcrm/index.htm Accessed January 11, 2007.

Suzama K, DeChristopher PJ, Dodd R, et al: Practice parameter for the recognition, management and prevention of adverse consequences of blood transfusion. *Arch Pathol Lab Med* 124:61-70, 2000.

Chapter 12

Vascular Access Devices (VAD)

Deborah A. DeVine and Harri Brackett

1. What is a central line?

A central line, commonly called a vascular access device (VAD) or central venous catheter (CVC), is a temporary or long-term intravenous catheter inserted into one of the major veins of the neck or chest (subclavian, superior vena cava, internal or external jugular) or peripherally through the basilic or cephalic vein. The distal tip of a central line terminates in or near the superior vena cava, just above the right atrium. The femoral venous system (leading to the proximal inferior vena cava) may be used if the superior vena cava cannot be catheterized.

2. How soon can a CVC be used after placement?

A central line may be used after the position of the radiopaque catheter tip in the superior vena cava is confirmed by fluoroscopy or radiography. Implanted ports may be used immediately after placement, perhaps even accessed during surgery. Some surgeons may request that the port not be accessed until postoperative swelling has decreased.

3. What are the advantages of a central line?

- The high blood flow of the vena cava promotes rapid dilution of intravenous (IV) fluids and concentrated solutions, thereby preventing an inflammatory response and the rapid thrombosis that occurs in smaller peripheral veins.
- It provides more stable access to the venous system, decreasing the risk of infiltration and tissue damage when irritating agents are administered.
- It allows infusion of incompatible solutions at the same time, through two or more lumens.
- Use of a central line may shorten hospital stays by providing access for therapy in an outpatient setting.
- Once the central line is placed, the negative physical or psychological factors associated with repeated venipuncture can be avoided.

4. Summarize the various uses of central lines.

- IV fluids, antibiotics, chemotherapy, blood products, total parenteral nutrition, analgesics
- Laboratory blood sampling, dialysis/pheresis
- Measurement of central venous or pulmonary capillary wedge pressure, determination of cardiac output, or rapid infusion of crystalloids
- Large-volume infusion (e.g., bleeding, trauma, surgery, sepsis) or hemodynamic monitoring

5. What materials are used to make central lines?

Central lines are made of several different materials, including polyvinyl chloride, silicone, and polyurethane. The stiffer nature of polyvinyl chloride catheters allows easier insertion but also may damage the tunica intima, leading to platelet aggregation and thrombus formation. Silicone is biocompatible, extremely soft and pliable, inexpensive, and hydrophobic (offering protection from bacterial growth). Polyurethane catheters are indicated for short-term use and placed percutaneously; they are stronger than silicone but become more pliable after insertion when warmed by blood.

Newer catheters, such as hydromer-coated polyurethane catheters, which are designed to prevent bacterial growth and adherence as well as platelet deposition and aggregation, have higher success rates for insertion. Recent meta-analyses demonstrated that bonded catheters, impregnated with antimicrobial substances, such as silver sulfadiazine and chlorhexidine, reduced the risk for catheter-related blood stream infection (CRBSI) when compared with standard uncoated catheters.

6. What are the major types of central lines?
- Nontunneled catheters
- Tunneled catheters
- Peripherally inserted central catheters (PICCs)
- Implanted ports

7. Which type of CVC is most commonly used? List its major advantages and disadvantages.
Nontunneled catheters are the most commonly used central lines. Available with 1 to 4 lumens, they are easily inserted into the subclavian, internal jugular vein, or external jugular vein. The right internal jugular vein is preferred, because it forms a straight line with the superior vena cava (SVC). Optional features include heparin, antibiotic, or antiseptic coatings along the catheter and addition of a Dacron cuff. Nontunneled catheters are associated with the highest incidence of catheter-related infections. Other disadvantages include the need for daily flushing, routine sterile dressing changes, and restrictions on physical activities, such as swimming, contact sports, and rough play for adolescents or children.

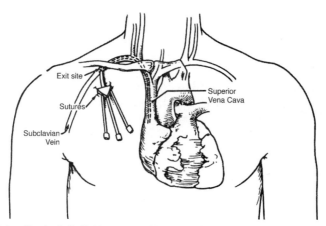

Nontunneled catheter. *(Drawing by Mel Drisko, courtesy of Educational Support Services, University of Colorado at Denver and the Health Services Center.)*

8. Discuss the advantages and disadvantages of tunneled catheters.
Tunneled catheters (Hickman, Broviac, Leonard, and Groshong) are indicated for long-term therapy (more than several months). Single-, double-, and triple-lumen catheters are available. Insertion costs are high if anesthesia is needed and the operating room is used; however, most tunneled catheters can be placed safely under fluoroscopy in the radiology department. After insertion in a central vein, the catheter is tunneled

several centimeters under the skin and brought out through the skin to a suitable exit site (anterior chest between the sternum and nipple, upper abdominal wall). Unlike most nontunneled catheters, the subcutaneous portion of the tunneled catheter includes a Dacron cuff that adheres to scar tissue, forming an internal anchor and barrier against the inward spread of microorganisms. A second antimicrobial cuff also may be present (e.g., VitaCuff, which releases silver ions as a deterrent to infection).

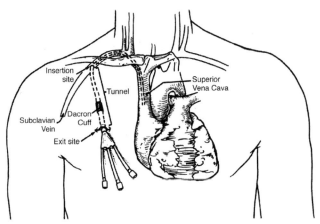

Tunneled catheter. *(Drawing by Mel Drisko, courtesy of Educational Support Services, University of Colorado at Denver and the Health Services Center.)*

The tunneling of the catheter offers the theoretical advantage of reducing the rate of infection. CVCs may be placed with minimal risk of catheter infections outside the operating room if maximal barrier precautions are used (e.g., sterile gloves, gown, drape, masks). Disadvantages include the need for site care with dressing changes for the first few weeks, activity restrictions, and regular flushing. Once the exit site of a tunneled catheter has healed (approximately 3-4 weeks), the sterile dressing change is modified to a clean technique, which decreases cost and time.

9. Discuss the advantages and disadvantages of PICCs.

PICCs are generally indicated for short-term use (> 5 days but usually < 1 year). Insertion costs are lowest of all CVCs. PICCs are easily placed by a trained nurse or physician into the cephalic or basilic veins of the antecubital space and are available with one or two lumens. The basilic vein provides the straightest, most direct route into the central venous system.

Advantages include reduced insertion risks (e.g., pneumothorax) and decreased rates of infection, in comparison to other nontunneled CVCs. Disadvantages include the need for daily flushing (weekly for the outpatient Groshong PICC), sterile dressing changes, and activity restrictions. Self-care may be difficult or impossible because the patient is required to change the dressing and flush the catheter with one hand.

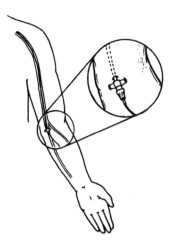

Peripherally inserted central catheter. *(Drawing by Mel Drisko, courtesy of Educational Support Services, University of Colorado at Denver and the Health Services Center).*

10. Describe the appropriate use of implanted ports. What are their advantages and disadvantages?

Implanted ports (e.g., mediport, portacath, infusaport, Cathlink 20) are made of stainless steel, titanium, or plastic and are indicated for long-term use. Port implantation is usually done under fluoroscopy in the interventional radiology suite or in the operating room at costs similar to those for tunneled catheters. Single- or double-lumen and low-profile (preferable in thin patients) ports are available. Ports are implanted entirely under the subcutaneous tissue and attached to a catheter that is threaded into the SVC. Smaller ports also may be implanted peripherally, like a PICC, in the forearm with the catheter threaded into the SVC. Advantages of the port include minimal site care with no dressing and infrequent flushing (once per month) when not accessed, which may decrease costs and infection rates. Implanted ports are associated with the lowest rate of infectious complications of all CVCs. Many patients prefer ports because they preserve bodily image and require no restrictions on activities, such as bathing or swimming. An advantage of the PowerPort™/PowerLoc system™, recently approved by the FDA, is the injection of contrast media. Identification of the PowerPort™ is aided by its unique shape (three sided port with three septum bumps).

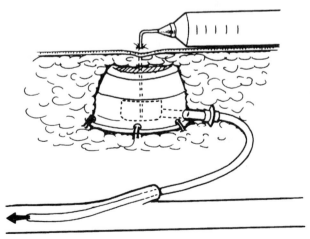

Implanted port. *(Drawing by Mel Drisko, courtesy of Educational Support Services, University of Colorado at Denver and the Health Services Center.)*

Disadvantages include discomfort related to accessing the port with a noncoring needle and the need for a surgical procedure for removal when the port is no longer needed or becomes infected. Ports are not recommended for patients undergoing treatment who will have prolonged nadirs, such as bone marrow transplant recipients or patients with leukemia.

11. Can a nurse assume that any line resembling a PICC is a central line?

No. If you do not have documentation of line placement, you should question the patient carefully. The line may be midline (with the tip resting in a vein below the shoulder) or mid-clavicular (with the tip resting in the subclavian vein). If the position of the line cannot be reliably obtained through history or documentation, a chest radiograph should be obtained.

12. How is a Groshong catheter different from other catheters?

A Groshong catheter is a silastic catheter with a two-way valve at the tip. Infusion of fluid opens the valve outward, and aspiration of blood opens the valve inward. When not in use, the pressure-sensitive two-way valve remains closed to prevent backward flow of blood or air into the catheter. The closed valve results in a potentially lower incidence of fibrin sheath formation and eliminates the need to clamp the catheter when injection caps are removed. Groshong valves are available for tunneled catheters, PICC lines, and implanted ports. Because blood clotting may be of less concern, normal saline is used instead of heparin for flushing; however, heparin is not incompatible with the material used to make Groshong catheters and can be infused, if needed, in patients with deep vein thrombosis.

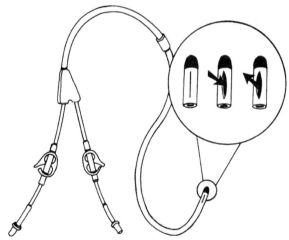

Groshong catheter and valves. *(Drawing by Mel Drisko, courtesy of Educational Support Services, University of Colorado at Denver and the Health Services Center.)*

13. What factors should be considered in choosing a central line?

- Costs
- Benefits and risks
- Length of therapy
- Patient preference (cosmetic appearance, activity/work limitations, anxiety associated with needle sticks)
- Treatment schedule (daily, continuous, intermittent)
- Type of drug or fluids to be infused (e.g., vesicant, pH < 5 or > 9, serum osmolality > 500 osm/L)

- Site care and flushing requirements
- Ability of patient or significant other to care for a central line at home
- Frequency of blood tests

14. What risks are involved with insertion of central lines?

- Bleeding and hematoma
- Air embolus
- Malpositioned tips and migration
- Nerve injury
- Pneumothorax
- Dysrhythmias
- Catheter embolism
- Introduction of bacteria
- Ulnar artery or nerve injury and puncture (rare complications of PICC placement)

15. The nurse observes bloody drainage at the insertion site of a newly placed central line. Is this a worrisome finding?

It is common for blood to saturate the dressing of a new exit site. Patients with a low platelet count should be monitored for increased bleeding, and bloody dressings should be changed as frequently as needed to prevent infection. Application of manual pressure or use of a sandbag helps to prevent development of a hematoma.

16. What are the signs and symptoms of malpositioned tips? What can be done to decrease this from happening?

Malpositioned tips are common and may be especially problematic with PICCs (4%-38% of patients). Catheters may be coiled in the superior vena cava, malpositioned in the jugular vein when the basilic vein is used, or malpositioned in the axillary vein when the cephalic vein is used. Should the PICC catheter migrate significantly, the catheter tip may move from the superior vena cava into a smaller vessel, such as the innominate or subclavian vein.

Catheter stabilization using aseptic technique should be instituted to prevent catheter migration and preserve the integrity of the VAD. Products used to stabilize a VAD may include manufactured catheter stabilization devices (e.g., StatLock®), sterile surgical strips, or sterile tape.

Symptoms associated with malpositioned CVCs

Site of malpositioned catheter	Symptoms
Internal jugular vein (ipsilateral or contralateral)	Sensation of ear gurgling, headache, swelling, or neck pain
Axillary vein	Hand and arm swelling, with arm and shoulder pain
Azygos vein	Vague back discomfort
Innominate vein or contralateral subclavian vein	Shoulder pain or swelling of contralateral arm
Internal thoracic vein	Anterior chest pain or tenderness
Right atrium or ventricle	Thrombosis, arrhythmia, or perforation of catheter, leading to pulmonary embolus

17. What causes catheter migration?

The cause of spontaneous migration is not completely clear; however, some reports describe forceful flushing, neck flexion, obesity, and extreme movements of the upper extremity; or changes associated with severe coughing, emesis, or constipation as possible causes of catheter migration. Untrimmed PICCs with excess catheter extending out from the site may cause the tip to migrate into the right atrium, which may lead to cardiac arrhythmias or thrombosis.

18. What should be done if catheter migration is suspected?

Suspected catheter migration should be reported to the physician, and radiographic studies to confirm PICC placement or flow should be performed. The catheter may then be pulled back or repositioned with a guide wire.

19. Should a PICC be removed for signs of phlebitis?

No. Immediate removal is not necessary. Sterile postinsertion phlebitis is the most common complication of PICCs (12.5%-23% of patients), occurring within 24 to 48 hours after insertion. It may be caused by trauma to the endothelial lining of the vein during insertion and consequent vasoconstriction. Powdered gloves also may irritate the vein and should not be used. A warm pack should be applied at the first sign of redness and swelling along the vein, palpable venous cord, skin temperature change, or tenderness. Rest, elevation of the affected arm, and administering nonsteroidal antiinflammatory drugs (NSAIDs) may benefit the patient. If symptoms do not improve within 24 hours or resolve in 72 hours, the catheter may need to be removed.

20. What is considered routine care and maintenance of a central line?

Routine care of a central line catheter includes cleansing the exit site, changing dressings and caps, and flushing the lumens to prevent clotting. Cleansing solutions, type of dressing, and frequency of dressing changes or flushing are controversial issues. Site-care protocols vary among hospitals. Refer to Oncology Nursing Society *Access Device Guidelines: Recommendations for Nursing Practice and Education* and the table on page 137 for common maintenance procedures.

21. What solutions or agents are recommended for cleaning the exit site?

- Isopropyl alcohol (70%) removes skin oils and squamous skin cells by denaturation of proteins and provides the most rapid and greatest reduction in microbial counts on the skin. However, it has no residual antimicrobial activity. Alcohol should be applied before iodine.
- Povidone-iodine (10%) or tincture of iodine (1%-2%) should be allowed to remain on the skin for at least 2 minutes, to enhance antimicrobial activity while it dries. It has minimal residual activity, and the duration of antiinfective effect is approximately 2 hours. To prevent skin irritation, it may need to be removed with alcohol after drying. It is effective for use before catheter insertion but has not been thoroughly evaluated for decreasing catheter colonization and infection.
- ChloraPrep (2% chlorhexidine gluconate in 70% isopropyl alcohol) results in a lower risk of catheter-related infection compared to povidone-iodine (Betadine), alcohol combinations or chlorhexidine gluconate (CHG).
- Chlorhexidine gluconate (CHG, also known as Hibiclens) kills microbes for a longer period than either alcohol alone or alcohol plus povidone-iodine (Betadine). It has excellent residual activity, with 4 to 6 hours of antiinfective effect after application.

University of Colorado Hospital central venous catheter maintenance procedures*

VAD	Flushing the catheter (each lumen)§	Changing the occlusive transparent dressing	Changing the positive pressure device
EXTERNALLY PLACED CVCs: Cook, Hohn, subclavian, internal jugular, femoral venous	Q day with 1 ml heparin (10 units/ml)	Inpatient: sterile dressing change Q week or PRN Outpatient: change Q week or PRN	Q week or with dressing change. Use sterile technique.
PICC LINE: Bard PerQCath or any open-ended PICC	Q day with 3 ml heparin (10 units/ml)	Inpatient: sterile dressing change Q week or PRN Outpatient: change Q week or PRN	Q week or with dressing change. Use sterile technique.
PICC LINE Groshong	Q week with 5 ml normal saline or more often if needed	Inpatient: sterile dressing change Q week or PRN Outpatient: change Q week or PRN	Q week or with dressing change. Use sterile technique.
TUNNELED: Hickman, Broviac	Q day with 3 ml heparin (10 units/ml)	Inpatient: sterile dressing change Q week or PRN Outpatient: clean technique daily	Q week or with dressing change. Use sterile technique.
IMPLANTED PORTS: Mediport, Pas-port	Q day with 3 ml heparin (100 units/ml) when in use Q month with 3 ml heparin (100 units/ml) when not in use	Inpatient: sterile dressing change Q week; change needle Q week (IV or catheter); no dressing change if needle/catheter is not in place	Q week or with dressing change. Use sterile technique.
TUNNELED: Groshong	Q week with 5 ml normal saline, or more often if needed	Inpatient: sterile dressing change Q week or PRN Outpatient: clean technique daily	Q week or with dressing change. Use sterile technique.

*Used with permission, University of Colorado Hospital Vascular Access Device committee, Denver, CO.
§After infusion of any medication, flush catheter with 10 ml normal saline (use 20 ml normal saline for groshong catheters).

22. Should antimicrobial ointments be used?

The Centers for Disease Control and Prevention (CDC) does not recommend routine use of topical ointments. Iodophor ointments have been proved ineffective; polymicrobial ointments have some benefit but may increase the frequency of candidal infection.

Some studies suggest that the Biopatch™ antimicrobial dressing absorbs exudate and reduces local infections by releasing chlorhexidene gluconate for up to seven days.

23. Are gauze dressings better than transparent dressings?

2002 CDC guidelines recommend use of either sterile gauze or sterile, transparent semipermeable membrane (TSM) dressing to cover the catheter site. There are advantages and disadvantages to both types of dressings; the decision is based on patient preferences, organizational policies and procedures, and other factors.

Advantages and disadvantages of dressing choice

	Advantages	Disadvantages
Transparent semipermeable membrane (TSM)	Easy visualization of exit site Occlusive Changed less frequently Allows for the ease of air exchange if highly permeable type used Provides protection against external moisture Assists in stabilizing the catheter	May trap, harbor bacteria, which may lead to infection in immunocompromised patients May not stay in place May irritate the skin
Sterile gauze + tape or TSM	Routine visualization if changed daily secondary to showering Allows for air exchange Not irritating to skin (preferred for diaphoretic or fragile skin)	Not occlusive when tape is used (but in tunneled catheters, this may not be needed, since the tunnel usually heals in 3-4 weeks) Does not provide a bacterial or water barrier (unless TSM is used) Limited visualization of the site

24. Are CVC dressings necessary?

Recent evidence in the literature has suggested that an occlusive dressing may not be necessary for tunneled central lines. Some investigators and clinicians still argue that a dressing is necessary for all patients in an inpatient environment to decrease the risk of nosocomial infection.

25. How often should dressings be changed?

According to the Infusion Nurses Society (INS) guidelines and the Centers for Disease Control (CDC), the following are recommended:

- Gauze and tape dressings that prevent visualization of the insertion site need to be changed routinely every 48 hours on central line catheter sites and immediately if the integrity of the dressing is compromised.
- Gauze used with TSM dressing should be considered a gauze dressing and changed every 48 hours.
- Frequency of changing transparent dressings continues to vary according to the patient population, neutropenic or transplant status, healthcare provider preferences and beliefs, and institution. The Infusion Nurses Society (INS)(2006) recommends that TSM dressings should be changed at least every 7 days.
- All types of dressings should be changed after showering or when damp, loose, or soiled.
- Tunneled catheters may not need a dressing after several weeks of healing. It may be preferable not to use a dressing for tunneled catheters because of a lower risk for infection.

26. What are the Infusion Nurses Society recommendations for flushing central lines?

- Use heparin (10 units/ml) for all CVCs except the Groshong, which requires flushing with saline.
- Use preservative-free saline before and after administering medications.
- Use a different syringe and needle for each lumen that is flushed.
- Use a flushing volume equal to two times the internal volume of the catheter and any add-on devices.
- Remove blood from the injection cap, if possible. New positive-pressure devices are designed to prevent backflow within the catheter and have replaced the use of the traditional cap.
- Avoid using syringes smaller than 5 ml, because smaller sized syringes generate pressure in excess of 25 to 40 PSI (pounds/square inch).

27. Is saline as effective as heparin for routine flushing?

Recent studies report that 0.9% saline solution is as effective as heparin in maintaining patency in peripheral lines; however, it is not yet routine practice to use only saline. Normal saline is more cost-effective than heparin and may cause less interference with laboratory tests. If only saline is used as a flush for central lines, the potential for occlusion, phlebitis, and formation of small clots or fibrin strands may be increased. Flushing the catheter with heparin not only prevents thrombosis but also may reduce infection because thrombi and fibrin deposits are potential sites of microbial growth.

28. Should I be concerned about the amount of heparin used for flushing?

Yes. Even low doses of heparin may cause thrombocytopenia and bleeding problems. Heparin-induced thrombocytopenia, which affects 1% to 2% of patients receiving heparin, is an allergic response in which the patient develops an antibody to platelets. The clumped platelets can cause clotting events, such as deep vein thrombosis or pulmonary embolism.

29. Should low-dose warfarin be used prophylactically to decrease the incidence of thrombosis in venous access devices?

No, research presented at the 2005 American Society of Clinical Oncology (ASCO) did not support the use of antithrombotic prophylaxis in patients with central vein catheters. In a multicenter prospective randomized controlled trial (WARP) of 1589 patients, there was no difference in the thrombosis-free interval between the group who took warfarin (1 mg) and the control group. In addition, there was a trend toward an increase in major bleeding events in the warfarin group. Further research is necessary to answer the question of whether patients with particular conditions warrant prophylaxis.

30. Can a registered nurse remove a central line?

In accordance with hospital policy and specific State Board of Nursing Practice Acts, nurses may discontinue a central venous catheter with a physician's order. The nurse should remember the following points when removing a catheter:

- To prevent pulmonary embolus, instruct the patient to perform a Valsalva maneuver while the catheter is withdrawn, or pull the line during the end of expiration if the patient is on mechanical ventilation, or during expiration for patients unable to bear down.
- To prevent air from entering the subcutaneous tract into the vein, apply digital pressure until hemostasis is achieved, then antiseptic ointment and a sterile occlusive dressing to the access site. The dressing should be changed and the access site assessed every 24 hours until the site is epithelialized.
- Contact the physician immediately if difficulty is encountered with removing the catheter or Dacron cuff. A cutdown procedure by the physician may be indicated to remove the cuff, particularly if a tunnel infection is suspected. A chest radiograph or venogram is recommended if there is any question about incomplete catheter removal.

31. What should be done if a PICC is resistant to removal?

Resistance to removal (5% rate of occurrence) may be caused by formation of a thrombus or fibrin sheath, or more commonly, venospasm. The following tips may facilitate removal of a resistant PICC:

1. Remove the catheter at a moderate rate, using gentle traction. Position the patient in an upright/sitting position with the arm held at 90° to the body. *Aggressive pulling is contraindicated.*
2. Do not apply pressure at or near the course of the vein.
3. Apply warm compresses to distend the vein.
4. Attempt removal again in 20 to 30 minutes after the spasm has abated.
5. If spasm is still present, wait an additional 12 to 24 hours.

If resistance is encountered when the catheter is being removed, it should not be forcibly removed, and the physician should be notified.

32. How are implanted ports accessed?

Sterile gloves, mask, and sterile technique should be used when accessing an implanted port. Locate the port by palpation. Clean the site with povidone-iodine or chlorhexidine 2%, starting over the port and moving outward in a circular motion. Using the fingers of one hand to stabilize the port, insert the needle through the skin, and push through the septum until the needle lightly touches the bottom of the port. Needle position is verified by blood return. If neither irrigation nor aspiration is possible, the needle may need to be pushed further into the septum or repositioned. In the absence of a positive blood return, infusion therapy should be withheld until the problem can be diagnosed and treated.

33. Are Huber needles necessary to access implanted ports?

Yes, except in emergencies. A Huber (noncoring) needle should be used to access an implanted port because it preserves the life of the septum. A port septum is good for 1,000 (using a 19-gauge needle) or 2,000 (using a 22-gauge needle) punctures. The gauge and length of the needle are determined by the viscosity of the infused solution, depth of port placement, and type of implanted port. Huber needles (90°) with extension tubing, wings, and foam pad attached are frequently used for continuous infusion. The Cathlink, however, is accessed with a straight angiocath. A straight Huber needle may be used for withdrawing blood samples or giving bolus injections. The smallest size, noncoring needle that can accommodate the prescribed therapy should be used. All needles and extensions should be primed with normal saline before use.

34. How often should Huber needles be changed?

To prevent skin breakdown, change the needle at least every 7 days. In the case of intermittent injections, some patients prefer that the port be accessed daily. Before needle removal at the end of the infusion, flush with normal saline followed by heparin.

35. How is discomfort decreased when ports are accessed?

Topical anesthetics, such as Emla cream (2.5% lidocaine and 2.5% prilocaine) covered with a transparent dressing, may be applied to the skin over the port at least 1 hour before needle placement. Application of ice over the site or ethyl chloride spray also may be helpful.

36. How much blood should be discarded before blood is sampled?

Approximately 5 ml of blood from adults and 3 ml from children are discarded before drawing the sample. There is no need to discard any blood when drawing blood cultures.

37. What is the procedure for drawing blood from a central line?

- Stop the infusion for at least one minute.
- Clamp all lumens not in use.
- Draw blood through the proximal lumen via the catheter hub or through the injection cap.
- Pull back slowly on the syringe to prevents catheter collapse.
- A Vacutainer may be used to decrease needlestick risk, except in the case of Groshong catheters and PICCs.
- Flush with 10 to 20 ml (20 ml for Groshong catheter) of preservative-free normal saline after blood withdrawal.

38. Can blood be drawn from a CVC for coagulation tests?

The literature does not support drawing blood for coagulation tests through a heparinized Hickman catheter if the results will be used to monitor anticoagulant therapy or evaluate coagulopathy. Heparin adheres to the catheter wall and can result in prolonged prothrombin time or partial prothrombin time. The literature does not support the use of Silastic catheters for sampling drug levels if the drug is being given via the same catheter. Consider drawing these tests from a peripheral vein.

39. What complications are associated with central lines?

- Infection
- Sepsis
- Occlusion
- Migration
- Pinch-off
- Extravasation

40. What are the signs of central line infection?

Erythema, pain, and purulence at the exit site or along the tunnel are the most consistent indicators of infection. Immunosuppression may diminish or completely mask these signs. A patient with an infection of a central lines may show symptoms of sepsis without another apparent source, or of thrombosis alone.

41. What are the four sources of catheter-associated infection?

1. Skin insertion site (most common)
2. Catheter hub
3. Secondary catheter infection from bloodstream seeding
4. Infusate contamination (rare)

42. How can I tell if a patient has an exit, tunnel, or pocket infection?

- Erythema, pain, swelling, and purulence at the exit site or along the tunnel are the most consistent indicators of infection. Keep in mind that immunosuppression may diminish or completely mask the following signs and symptoms:
- Exit-site infection: erythema that extends less than 2 cm from the exit site (up to the cuff) with warmth, tenderness, swelling, or purulence
- Tunnel infection: inflammation along the subcutaneous tract of the catheter, extending > 2 cm beyond the cuff from the exit site
- Port pocket infection: characterized by inflammation or necrosis of the skin over an implantable device or purulence in the pocket containing the device; closely resembles tunnel infections in treatment and response to therapy

43. How is infection in central lines treated?

Management depends on the causative organisms and extent of infection. Empiric treatment consists of an antimicrobial effective against gram-positive (e.g., methicillin-resistant *Staphylococcus aureus* [MRSA]) and gram-negative organisms. Specific antibiotic therapy is directed against organisms recovered from cultures. **Local site infections** may be treated by aggressive site care and oral antibiotics in the absence of neutropenia. Outpatient management may be successful for people with intact immune systems whose infection is localized to the exit site without fever or hypotension. **Tunnel infections usually and port infections always** require catheter removal. **Sepsis** requires treatment with parenteral antibiotics and removal of the catheter.

44. Which infections require catheter removal?

Because *S. aureus* infection is associated with serious complications, the catheter must always be removed. Catheters must also be removed if there is fungal or atypical mycobacterial infection (refer to Chapter 49, Infections in Immunocompromised Patients).

45. What can be done to prevent catheter infections?

Prevention strategies include hand washing, strict aseptic technique, and patient education. Special catheter designs include antimicrobial substances to prevent colonization, heparin coatings that may decrease formation of fibrin sleeves and thereby colonization of bacteria, or a collagen cuff impregnated with silver ions, which exerts an antimicrobial effect for 4 to 6 weeks and serves as a barrier to organisms that migrate down the catheter. The Centers for Disease Control supports the prophylactic use of antibiotics as a flush solution in combination with heparin only for patients requiring long-term access who repeatedly experience catheter-related bloodstream infections despite stringent catheter care.

46. What should be done if there is no blood return with aspiration?

If there is no blood return, the catheter may no longer be in the venous system. The site should be assessed for:

- Drainage due to catheter rupture, obstruction, or fibrin sheath
- Subcutaneous swelling due to catheter damage or infusate exiting backward out of the vein
- Stricture of sutures, kinking of the catheter
- Swelling of the neck, throat, or arm
- Loops of tunneled catheter under the skin

Ask the patient to change position (e.g.,Trendelenburg's position) to increase venous flow, and to cough or breathe deeply to help move the catheter away from the vein wall. Remove the injection cap and attempt to aspirate. Vigorously infuse 10 to 20 ml of normal saline while assessing for swelling. For implanted ports, try to reposition the needle. If catheter placement is still questionable, confirm position in the SVC by chest radiograph, dye study, or both. Do not infuse chemotherapy until tip placement is confirmed.

47. What causes central line occlusion?

Occlusion should be considered when the ability to infuse fluids is lost and blood return with aspiration is absent. Partial obstruction is indicated by resistance to flushing, absence of blood return with aspiration, or both. Causes include the following:

- **Intraluminal thrombus** may result from injury to the vein wall during insertion, contact with the catheter tip, or hardened blood in the catheter lumen.
- **Extraluminal fibrin sleeve** formed at the catheter entry site into the vein may impair ability to flush but not to withdraw, because it acts as a flap that blocks the tip during withdrawal but opens with injection.
- **Drug precipitate** may be caused by combination of incompatible solutions, inadequate flushing, or formation of calcium phosphorus complexes (as with total parenteral nutrition).
- **External occlusion** may occur when a catheter is clamped, twisted, or constricted by sutures or a nonpatent Huber needle.

48. How is an occluded line treated?

Alteplase (tissue-type plasminogen activator [t-PA]) is currently the agent of choice for clearing catheter-related thrombosis restoring function in 60–80% of thrombosed catheters. The standard concentration is 0.5 mg - 1 mg/ml. Using aseptic technique, instill an adequate volume that approximates the volume capacity of the catheter (usually 1 ml), and allow a dwell time of 30 to 120 minutes. Repeat if catheter function is not restored. Note: Because a Hickman's catheter capacity is usually 1.5 ml, follow alteplase instillation with 1.5 ml of preservative-free saline.

49. Helpful hints for administering alteplase

- Excessive pressure should be avoided when alteplase solution is injected into the catheter. Such force could cause rupture of the catheter or expulsion of the clot into the circulation.
- During attempts to determine catheter occlusion, vigorous suction should not be applied because of possible damage to the vascular wall or collapse of soft-wall catheters.
- Substances other than fibrin clots, such as drug precipitates, may occlude catheters. Alteplase solution is not effective in such cases and the substances may be forced into the vascular system.

- If alteplase is used for declotting the catheter and NOT only for restoring blood return, follow the alteplase dose with *preservative-free* normal saline if needed, until resistance is met. The volume of the catheter lumen should be filled with alteplase with or without added normal saline. If the volume of the catheter capacity is less than 1 ml, no additional saline is needed after the alteplase dose.

50. What serious complications can arise when declotting a catheter with alteplase?

- Bleeding can occur. If the patient's platelet count is less than 20,000/microliter, alteplase should only be administered once in 4 hours, unless otherwise ordered by a physician. Caution should be used with patients who have active internal bleeding or have had any of the following within the previous 48 hours: surgery, obstetrical delivery, or percutaneous biopsy of viscera or deep tissues,
- Side effects from alteplase include fever, bleeding, allergic reactions (dyspnea, flushing, rash), sepsis, venous thrombosis, and GI bleeding.
- Additional complications include potential release of an infected clot or septic emboli. Patients have demonstrated signs of hemodynamic instability (hypotension) and sepsis within a few minutes after flushing. This can also occur with routine catheter flushing.

51. Is extravasation a common complication of CVCs?

Although more common in peripheral IV access, extravasation is a potential complication of CVCs. Symptoms of extravasation may include pain, burning, stinging, and perhaps swelling or leaking. Blood return may or may not be present. If extravasation is suspected during infusion of a vesicant, the nurse should stop the infusion and aspirate the residual. If symptoms are present, a chest radiograph or dye study should be performed to confirm placement in the venous system.

52. What are the major causes of extravasation?

- The needle may be dislodged from the port.
- A fibrin sheath may form along the catheter tract, starting from the exit site and extending toward the catheter tip. When fluid infuses from the catheter tip, it backtracks along the catheter and leaks out of the exit site.
- Overly vigorous flushing may weaken or even perforate the catheter wall, resulting in catheter separation and embolism.
- The catheter tip may be dislodged or migrate from the venous system. Although the mechanism for spontaneous migration is unclear, coughing or sneezing may cause migration, especially when softer catheters are used.

53. What is "pinch-off syndrome"? How is it recognized?

Pinch-off syndrome results from compression and shearing of the catheter between the clavicle and first rib in about 1% of patients. It should be suspected when lack of blood return or inability to infuse occurs intermittently. It is worsened by sitting and relieved by raising the arms overhead. Pinch off is recognized on a chest radiograph by a narrowing of the catheter between the clavicle and first rib. It may cause embolization, and it is an indication for catheter removal and replacement. It may not be discovered until after the catheter fractures, when the catheter fragment must be retrieved from the central veins, pulmonary artery, or heart. Embolization of the catheter fragment into the pulmonary artery may produce patient complaints of chest pain, palpitations, and arrhythmias.

54. Can a central line be repaired?

A leaking catheter must be repaired or removed to prevent infection and formation of an air embolus. Catheter lumens are damaged by overly vigorous flushing, which weakens the catheter wall and eventually causes a hole. Instruct patients that if a catheter tears or breaks, they should fold the remaining end of the catheter in half, cover it with gauze, and secure it tightly with a rubber band. If a clamp is available, the patient should clamp the catheter above the leak and consult a doctor or nurse immediately. Some damaged central lines can be repaired, including tunneled catheters and PICCs. Using sterile technique, follow the manufacturer's instructions provided with the repair kit. Catheter guide wire exchange should be considered to replace a malfunctioning, nontunneled catheter if there is no evidence of infection.

Key Points

- The advantages of central venous catheters are that they allow for stable venous access, the simultaneous infusion of multiple solutions, and comfortable access for blood draws.
- A central line may be used only after the position of the radiopaque catheter tip in the superior vena cava is confirmed by fluoroscopy or radiography.
- Do not use a central line if it does not have a positive blood return, unless the position of the catheter tip has been confirmed.
- Sterile maintenance of central venous catheters includes routine flushing, dressing, and changing positive pressure caps.
- Drug precipitate may be formed by incompatible solutions and inadequate flushing.
- Signs of central line infection include: erythema, pain, and purulence at the exit site or along the tunnel. Immunosuppression may diminish or completely mask these signs.

Internet Resources

Association for Vascular Access:
    http://www.avainfo.org/website/article.asp?id=4
Center for Diagnostic Imaging:
    http://www.cdirad.com/Default.aspx?tabid=360
Centers for Disease Control and Prevention:
    http://www.cdc.gov/
Journal of Vascular Access:
    http://www.vascular-access.info/index.asp?a=current
Journal of Vascular and Interventional Radiology:
    http://www.jvir.org/
Infusion Nurses Society:
    http://www.ins1.org/
National Institute of Health:
    http://www.nih.gov/
Society of Interventional Radiology:
    http://www.sirweb.org/

Acknowledgment

The authors wish to acknowledge Charlene Trouillot, RN, MS, ANP, OCN, for her contributions to the Vascular Access Devices chapter published in the first and second editions of *Oncology Nursing Secrets.*

Bibliography

Alexander M, editor: Infusion nursing standards of practice. *J Infus Nurs* 29(1S):S1-S92, 2006.

Bagnall-Reeb H: Evidence for the use of the antibiotic lock technique. *J Infus Nurs* 27(2):18-122, 2004.

Camp-Sorrell D, editor: *Access device guidelines and recommendations for practice,* ed 2, Pittsburgh, PA, 2004, Oncology Nursing Society.

Frey A: Drawing blood samples from vascular access devices. *J Infus Nurs* 26(5):285-293, 2003.

Gorski L, Czaplewski L: Peripherally inserted central catheters and midline catheters for the homecare nurse. *J Infus Nurs* 27(6):399-409, 2004.

Hadaway LC: Skin flora and infection. *J Infus Nurs* 26(1):44-48, 2003.

Held-Warmkessel J: Catheter malfunction. *Clin J Oncol Nurs* 4(5):239-241, 2000.

Hibbard JS, Mulberry GK, Brady AR: A clinical study comparing the skin antisepsis and safety of chloraprep, 70% isopropryl alcohol, and 2% aqueous chlorhexidine. *J Infus Nurs* 25(4):244-249, 2002.

Infusion Nurses Society. *Policies and procedures for infusion nursing,* ed 3, Norwood, MA, 2006, Author.

Karamanoglu A, Yumuk P, Fulden MD, et al: Port needles: Do they need to be removed as frequently in infusional chemotherapy? *J Infus Nurs* 26(4):239-242, 2003.

Krzywada EA: Predisposing factors, prevention and management of central venous catheter occlusions. *J Intraven Nurs* 22(Suppl 6S):S11-S37, 1999.

LeBlanc A, Cobbett S: Traditional practice versus evidence-based practice for IV skin preparation. *Can J Infect Control* 15(1):9-14, 2000.

Levine MN, Lee AY, Kakkar AK: Thrombosis and cancer. In Perry MC, editor: *American Society of Clinical Oncology* educational book, Alexandria, VA, 2005, American Society of Clinical Oncology.

Mandell GL, Bennett JE, Dolin R, editors: *Principles and practice of infectious disease,* ed 6, New York, 2005, Churchill Livingstone.

National Association of Vascular Access Networks: The use of alteplase (t-PA) for the management of thrombotic catheter dysfunction: Guidelines from a consensus conference of the national association of vascular access networks. Clinician 18(2):1-14, 2000.

O'Grady NP, Alexander ME, Dellinger EP, et al: Guidelines for the prevention of intravascular catheter-related infections. Centers for Disease Control and Prevention. Available at: http://www.cdc.gov/ncidod/dhqp/gl_intravascular.html. Retrieved January 3, 2007

Ozer H: New developments in supportive care. Emerging trends in oncology: A post-ASCO update. Denver, CO, June 11, 2005, Physicians Education Resource Conference.

Power port, JUL 14: www.fda.gov/cdrh/pdf6/K060812.pdf, accessed December 29, 2006.

Timoney JP, Malkin MG, Leone DM, et al: Safe and cost effective use of alteplase for the clearance of occluded central venous access devices. *J Clin Oncol* 20(7):1918-1922, 2002.

Viale P: Complications associated with implantable vascular access devices in the patient with cancer. *J Infus Nurs* 26(2):97-102, 2003.

Chapter 13

Complementary and Alternative Medicine (CAM) Therapies

Georgia M. Decker

1. How are complementary and alternative therapies defined?

The interchangeable use of the terms *complementary* and *alternative* by clinicians has caused misunderstanding and miscommunication. Alternative medicine is an umbrella term that was used to describe therapies not taught in U.S. medical schools or provided in U.S. hospitals. Because many medical schools now include these therapies in their curricula and some are now provided in hospitals, the term is no longer appropriate or accurate. *Complementary* and *alternative* do not describe a particular therapy but rather the intent with which it is used. When a therapy is used as alternative it is used "instead of" when a therapy is complementary, it is used "with" a conventional therapy. The more contemporary terms, *integrative* and *integrated,* are more accurate when conventional and complementary and alternative medicine (CAM) therapies are used together.

2. What other words have been used to describe complementary or alternative therapy?

The following terms have been used inappropriately to describe complementary and alternative medicine (CAM) therapies:

Quackery: This term is used by some health care professionals and others to describe any therapy they disagree with. Proof of quackery requires scientific and legal documentation.

Unproven: The therapy has not been proven to be effective or ineffective.

3. How are CAM therapies characterized?

There are two main approaches to categorizing CAM therapies. The National Center for Complementary and Alternative Medicine (NCCAM), formerly known as the Office of Alternative Medicine (OAM), was established within the National Institutes of Health (NIH) to investigate the efficacy of alternative health care and to establish an information center on CAM therapies. NCCAM classifies CAM therapies into five domains: (1) alternative medical systems, (2) mind-body interventions, (3) biologically-based therapies, (4) manipulative and body-based methods, and (5) energy therapies. The National Cancer Institute (NCI) Office of Cancer Complementary and Alternative Medicine (OCCAM) expanded the NCCAM domains with additional categories for clarification: movement therapy, pharmacologic and biologic treatments, with a subcategory of complex natural products.

4. Describe CAM categories, examples, current clinical trials, and any controversies.

CAM categories, examples, current clinical trials, and controversies

Category/Description	Examples	Current clinical trials	Controversies/Comments
Alternative system of medical care: stresses prevention of disease and promotion of health, including emphasis on personal responsibility and self-healing	Traditional Chinese medicine Naturopathy Ayurvedic medicine	Acupuncture Acupressure Electroacupuncture Traumeel S	These systems are a way of being and a way of living. They are not meant to be parceled into individual or separate modalities.
Mind-body/behavioral medicine: unites bio-medical, behavioral, and psychological strategies for promotion of health	Meditation Guided imagery Visualization Relaxation Spirituality Art therapies Music therapy Biofeedback Yoga	Distance healing Exercise-based counseling Group therapy Healing touch Music therapy Spirituality Religiosity Standard counseling Stress management training	Controversies exist over whether mind-body interventions prolong survival or enhance quality of life and sense of being healed. There are concerns about the use of guided imagery in patients with a psychiatric history. Research has not proven that mental efforts after course of cancer and may induce feelings of guilt and inadequacy in patients whose disease progresses despite best efforts.
Bioelectromagnetic therapies: based on use of energy as healing modality	Acupuncture Magnet therapy Cymatics	Energy therapy	The contemporary use of magnets has stimulated research evaluating claims that magnets reduce pain. Acupuncture has proved helpful for various symptoms and is now accepted for pain relief.
Herbal medicine: based on Doctrine of Signatures, which states that a plant's appearance or characteristics provides a clue to medicinal implications	Herbs may be used as single agents or in combination Herbs used to treat cancer include Essiac tea and pau d'arco tea	Black cohosh Valerian officinalis Milk thistle Mistletoe St. John's wort	Patients believe that "natural means safe," and that "if a little is good, a lot is better." The concern for all patients is the risk for possible herb-drug or herb-herb interactions. Because herbs are not regulated or standardized, safety issues must be scrutinized.
Pharmacologic and biologic therapies: most often used as alternatives and have been described as having the "lure of cure"	Laetrile Shark cartilage Oxidative therapies Antineoplastons PC-SPES (combination of 14 herbs for prostate cancer)	Antineoplastons Pancreatic proteolytic enzymes	The concern has always been that patients will use these therapies instead of conventional therapies. Because many of the components of these therapies remain unknown, any risks associated with use are also unknown.

Manual healing methods: usually involve touch and often are viewed as complementary therapies	Reiki Chiropractic Reflexology Massage Therapeutic touch (a misnomer because touch is not involved) Energy healing Reiki Touch	The kind of touch has important cultural implications. Controversies have arisen, but therapeutic touch remains a popular complementary therapy.
Diet, nutrition, and lifestyle changes: use of food or other supplements to prevent and treat illness; appeals to patients because they can be initiated immediately and patients have control over them	Macrobiotics Kelley-Gonzalez High-dose vitamin therapies Antioxidants Creatine Curcumin Flax seed Folic acid Fruit and vegetable extracts Garlic Ginger Juven L-Carnitine Low-fat diet Lycopene Macrobiotic diet Noni fruit extract Pomegranate juice Selenium Soy protein isolate Vitamins C and E, Zinc sulfate, Chinese herbal extract Green tea extract (polyphenon E) Kanglaite injection Pycnogenol Shark cartilage Virulizin	Some controversies are related to risk of malnutrition with restrictive dietary programs, effects of antioxidants and/or vitamins during certain therapies, and effects of soy in certain cancers.

5. How often do patients with cancer seek CAM therapies?

Approximately 54% to 77% of cancer patients use CAM; breast cancer patients use more CAM than other cancer patients (Sparrebom, Cox, Acharya, and Figg, 2004).

6. Which CAM therapies have been helpful to patients?

Prayer and spiritual practices are the most commonly used CAM therapies. Mind-body therapies, including relaxation and imagery, and movement (physical therapies) are followed by vitamins, herbal medicine, diet, nutrition, and lifestyle. The following CAM therapies have been identified as helpful by cancer patients participating in clinical trials (Sparber et al., 2000):

Spiritual	94%
Imagery	86%
Massage	80%
Lifestyle/diet	60%
Relaxation	50%
Herbal/botanical	20%
High-dose vitamins	14%

7. What political and social factors affect the use of unproven CAM therapies?

Cancer patients often receive information about CAM therapies from well-meaning family members and friends, the media, internet, and health food stores. However, these sources can be fraught with misinformation. In addition, some practitioners promote themselves as having the cure for cancer. Such promotion is seductive and can be misleading to vulnerable patients. Increasing interest in CAM therapies led to the appointment of the White House Commission on Complementary and Alternative Medicine in March 2000 to address access to and delivery of CAM, priorities for research, and the need for consumer and health care provider (HCP) education.

8. Which mind-body technique can be used effectively in clinical practice?

Relaxation is a frequently used mind-body therapy that is simple to use and teach. Relaxation is an alert, hypometabolic state of decreased sympathetic nervous system arousal that can be achieved in various ways, from simple breathing exercises to hypnosis and biofeedback. The effects of relaxation exercises are gradual and cumulative.

9. Describe the steps of Benson's relaxation technique.

1. Select a focus word or phrase that is comforting to you.
2. Assume any comfortable position and close your eyes. (If preferred, eyes may be open.)
3. Relax your muscles.
4. Breathe slowly and naturally. As you exhale, silently repeat your focus word or phrase to yourself. (If you cannot think of a focus phrase, you can also count slowly from 1 to 10.)
5. If thoughts come to mind, let them go and return to the focus words. Continue for 10 to 20 minutes.
6. When you are finished, do not stand up immediately. Sit quietly for a minute or two, allowing the return of other thoughts. Then open your eyes and continue sitting for another minute before standing up.
7. Practice once or twice each day.

10. Are there any contraindications to massage therapy in patients with cancer?

Because massage stimulates lymphatic drainage and improves circulation, there was concern that it may support the spread of cancer. The general rule is to use gentle massage and to avoid sites of lymphatic drainage around the tumor. An exception is the use of a specific type of massage technique to treat lymphedema after mastectomy. No pressure massage should be used in patients with a low platelet count (e.g., patients with leukemia or severe marrow depression). Gentle, slow-stroke massage may enhance relaxation and increase feelings of well-being.

11. What is therapeutic touch?

Derived from ancient practices of laying on of hands, therapeutic touch is a systematic method for promoting healing or comfort through the use of hands. As described by Krieger, it involves the intentional use of the hands to direct energy to the patient. The three steps in the 15 to 20 minute therapeutic touch process are (1) centering oneself, letting go of busy thoughts and activities, and intending to be with the person; (2) scanning the person's body with the hands a few inches away from the body to assess personal energy and identify areas of heat or cold or other differences; and (3) moving the hands over the person ("unruffling") and then directing energy with the hands to places within the body that feel tense or distressed.

12. Is therapeutic touch effective?

Research has shown that therapeutic touch is effective in reducing pain, relieving anxiety, reducing behavioral distress in infants and toddlers, and decreasing headache pain. For patients with cancer, therapeutic touch may be used when massage is contraindicated for the general relief of anxiety and stress and for management of pain. Nurses throughout the United States can learn therapeutic touch in nursing schools, through continuing education classes, or from a video produced by the National League for Nursing.

13. What are the Gerson and Kelley-Gonzalez Programs?

These are restrictive dietary programs that claim to have therapeutic benefit for patients. Gerson suggests that cancer growth is supported by a potassium and sodium imbalance. Thus the Gerson program focuses on detoxification, cleansing, and juicing with specific supplements (low sodium and high potassium). The Kelley-Gonzalez program involves the use of restrictive diet, vitamin and mineral supplements, pancreatic enzymes, and coffee enemas. Both programs are under investigation in patients with various types of cancer.

14. What controversies surround the use of soy?

Some herbs (e.g., dong quai, ginseng) and soy contain phytoestrogens that may increase the risk of cancer and/or recurrence in women with estrogen-responsive tumors. Soy should not be consumed as a supplement but as a whole food. The American Dietetic Association recommends that soy intake should be limited to two servings a week in women who have an estrogen-responsive breast cancer treated with estrogen blocking pharmaceuticals. Further research is needed to determine the risks and benefits of phytoestrogen use.

15. Why should patients be cautious about using antioxidants while receiving chemotherapy or radiation therapy?

Some laboratory data show that antioxidant use may compromise the effectiveness of certain cytotoxic agents (e.g., taxanes and alkylating agents). Mechanistic considerations have illustrated that cancer cells take up more glucose and Vitamin C than normal cells, suggesting a protective effect, and the cancer cells may demonstrate resistance to the oxidative injury caused by chemotherapy and radiation therapy. Conversely, patients and some researchers believe that antioxidants may reduce toxicity associated with anti-cancer treatment. Other researchers suggest, based on in vitro and animal studies, that Vitamins A, C, and E, carotenoids, and other antioxidants can enhance the effects of chemotherapy and radiation therapy.

16. **What should nurses and other health care providers advise patients about taking antioxidants while receiving chemotherapy?**

Until more clinical trials are done in large patient populations, nurses and other health care providers should encourage their patients to avoid the use of antioxidant dietary supplements during chemotherapy and radiation therapy. However, if patients want to continue taking their antioxidants, they could be encouraged to avoid taking antioxidants 2 to 3 days before chemotherapy and for at least 3 to 7 days after the chemotherapy treatment or after the nadir of their chemotherapy drugs. Note: there is no research to substantiate the timing of antioxidants and chemotherapy.

17. **Why should oncology nurses be concerned about the use of herbs by their patients?**

- Herbal supplements do not have to undergo any federally regulated safety testing for purity or consistency. Furthermore, side effects are not required to be reported.
- The increased use of herbs has magnified the potential for herb-herb and herb-drug interactions and adverse events.
- Some herbs are unsafe, may affect platelet aggregation, and can promote or cause cancer.
- The leading cause of hepatotoxicity is related to the use of herbal medicines.
- Nurses, oncologists, and other health care providers lack knowledge and education about herbal medicine and other CAM.
- The majority of patients do not inform their health care providers that they are taking herbal supplements.

18. **What should the nurse do after learning that a patient is taking herbal supplements?**

- Assess or understand the patient's motive for taking the herb (e.g., advice from family members or friends, to boost the immune system, gain strength, and/or increase sense of control over treatments).
- Provide education about precautions, interactions, and possible side effects.
- Direct patients to reliable sources for information.
- Help patients sort through and understand information about herbs.

19. **List some precautions that patients should know about the use of herbs.**

Ten cardinal rules of herb use (Decker, 2006):

1. Do not take herbs at the same time as another drug. The actions of one or both agents may change. Patients should not take an herbal remedy and drug to treat the same condition.
2. "When in doubt, do without." Stop taking an herb immediately if you experience any unpleasant side effects.
3. Learn about herbs from qualified individuals who are knowledgeable about herbs and other medications.
4. Obtain an accurate diagnosis before starting *any* therapy.
5. Treat herbs as you would any other medicine.
6. Learn about contraindications related to the herbal medicine.
7. Take herbs in specific doses at specific times (e.g., pain-relief herbs should be taken between meals).
8. The effectiveness of herbs depends on a variety of factors, including proper dose, health status of the person, product, and purity.
9. When purchasing herbs, remember that the best values may be in herb shops or health food stores, but caution must be used about purity.
10. Fresh and dried herbs have near-equal advantages when purity is not questioned.

20. **Which commonly used herbs can affect platelet aggregation or increase the risk of bleeding?**

Patients undergoing surgery or cancer therapies, and/or taking anticoagulants should be aware that the following are examples of herbs that may increase the risk of bleeding or interfere with platelet development: alfalfa, angelica, anise, arnica, asafoetida, bogbean, boldo, capsicum, celery, chamomile, clove, danshen, feverfew, garlic, ginger, gingko, horse chestnut, horseradish, licorice, meadowsweet, onion, papain, passion flower, poplar, prickly ash, quassia, red clover, turmeric, wild carrot, wild lettuce, and willow.

21. **Which commonly used herbs are approved by the Food and Drug Administration?**

Aloe (laxative)
Capsicum (topical analgesic)
Cascara (laxative)
Psyllium (laxative)
Senna (laxative)
Witch hazel (astringent)

22. **What are some examples of commonly used herbs that are listed as unsafe by the FDA?**

American mistletoe, arnica, bittersweet nightshade, bloodroot, broom, chapparal, deadly nightshade, Dutch tonka bean, English tonka bean, ephedra, European mistletoe, heliotrope, horse chestnut, jimsonweed, lily of the valley, lobelia, Madagascar periwinkle, mandrake, mayapple, morning glory, periwinkle, snakeroot, spindle tree, St. John's wort, sweet flag, true alap, wahoo, wormwood, and yohimbine.

23. **What are examples of commonly used herbs that have sedative properties?**

Calamus, calendula, California poppy, catnip, capsicum, celery, couch grass, elecampane, Siberian ginseng, German chamomile, goldenseal, gotu kola, hops, Jamaican dogwood, kava, lemon balm, sage, St. John's wort, sassafras, skullcap, shepherd's purse, stinging nettle, valerian, wild carrot, wild lettuce, withania root, and yerba mansa.

24. **What are commonly used herbs/natural products that may affect cancer growth?**

The dose of the herb or natural product may affect whether it inhibits or promotes the growth of cancer. Note that there is overlap in certain categories in the following table because in vivo and in vitro evidence may be contradictory or literature is controversial (e.g., tannins have been described as both carcinogenic and having anticancer properties). Also keep in mind that this information may change as data is obtained from ongoing research.

Commonly used herbs and natural products that may affect cancer growth

Effect on cancer growth	Herbs/Natural products
May inhibit cancer growth in cancer patients	Astragalus, beta glucan, baikal skullcap, calcium-D-glucarate, cat's claw, cesium, chlorophyll, chrysin, *Cordyceps*, coriolus mushroom, diindolylmethane, European mistletoe, fish oils, gamma-linolenic acid, glossy privet, glutamine, gossypol, gotu kola, graviola, honey, IP-6, L-arginine, magnesium, marijuana melatonin, selenium, thymus extract, and tiratricol

Continued

Commonly used herbs and natural products that may affect cancer growth—cont'd

Effect on cancer growth	Herbs/Natural products
May protect against growth of cancer	Alpha-linolenic acid, American pawpaw, asparagus, barley, beta-sitosterol, bifidobacteria, black seed, blond psyllium, blueberry, cabbage, canthaxanthin, chaparral, choline, chrysanthemum, conjugated linoleic acid, cranberry, folic acid, forskolin, fructose-oligosaccharides, garlic, glucomannan, green tea, indole-3-carbinol, jiaogulan, lavender, lutein, lycopene, MGN-3, MSM, olive oil, peanut oil, propolis, quercetin, rice bran, shark cartilage, soy, spinach, tragacanth, turmeric, Vitamin A, Vitamin D, Vitamin K, wheat bran, whey protein, and yucca
May promote cancer growth in cancer patients	Alteris, alfalfa, androstenedione, anise, black tea, boron, chasteberry, coenzyme Q-10, cohosh, deer velvet, DHEA, dong quai, fennel, flaxseed, ginseng, glucosamine, hydrazine sulfate, kefir, star anise, *Lactobacillus*, licorice, milk thistle, pregnenolone, progesterone, raspberry leaf, red clover, resveratrol, scarlet pimpernel, soy, Vitamin C, and Vitamin E
May cause cancer	Alpha hydroxy acid, areca, *Aristolochia*, beer and alcoholic beverages, beta-carotene, bishop's weed, black and white pepper, calcium, marjoram, methionine, omega-6 fatty acids, pau d'arco, sassafras, shark liver oil, St. John's wort, and tannins (various types)

25. How do I know when a CAM therapy practitioner is properly credentialed?

Begin by contacting the state office responsible for professional licensing. The credentialing of each type of practitioner, as well as scope of practice, may vary from state to state. For example, some states license massage therapists and acupuncturists, whereas other states may license only acupuncturists who are physicians or nurses.

26. Can nurses provide CAM therapies as nursing interventions?

Scope of practice issues must be addressed through each state's Nurse Practice Act. In some states, certain interventions may be practiced only under the supervision of a medical doctor. Nurses are responsible for knowing the regulations in their state as well as the policies in their institutions. Before offering therapies to patients, you should know whether your institution has a policy about the provision of CAM therapies and practice accordingly to avoid liability.

Many nurses are trained in massage and therapeutic touch. Some nurses have private practices and often are listed in the directories of their professional organizations. To find nurses trained in massage therapy, contact the National Association of Nurse Massage Therapists (800-336-2668). Nurses experienced in therapeutic touch are often members of the Nurse Healers-Professional Associates (412-355-8476) or the American Holistic Nurses Association (919-787-5181).

27. What should patients with cancer expect from oncology nurses in relation to CAM therapies?

Patients must feel comfortable about confiding in nurses and other health care providers about the use of CAM therapies. A safe, nonjudgmental, caring atmosphere may facilitate this exchange of information. A primary wish of all patients with cancer is that doctors and nurses listen to their struggles with the diagnosis and treatment choices. Many patients look for guidance that makes them a full partner in designing their treatment. Patients may turn first to a nurse to explore his or her thoughts. The ethical dilemma facing nurses is to balance the patient's rights of free choice and personal control with the duty to protect the patient from harm. Nurses need to be knowledgeable about various CAM therapies or able to refer patients to appropriate, reliable references.

Key Points

- The interchangeable use of the terms "complementary" and "alternative" by clinicians has caused misunderstanding and miscommunication.
- A person with cancer often receives information about CAM therapies from well-meaning family members and friends.
- Antioxidant use may compromise the effectiveness of cytotoxic agents.
- Do not take herbs at the same time as another drug. The actions of one or both agents may change.
- Patients undergoing surgery or cancer therapies and/or taking anticoagulants should be aware that some herbs may increase the risk of bleeding or interfere with platelet development.

Internet Resources for Reliable Cancer CAM Information

Sponsored Websites

American Cancer Society:
  http://www.cancer.org
National Institutes of Health:
  http://www.nih.gov
Cancer Information Service:
  http://cis.nci.nih.gov
Office of Cancer Complementary and Alternative Medicine:
  http://www3.cancer.gov/occam
National Center for Complementary and Alternative Medicine:
  http://nccam.nih.gov
Office of Dietary Supplements:
  http://ods.od.nih.gov
Medline Plus:
  http://medlineplus.gov
Cancer Patient Education Network:
  http://cpen.nci.nih.gov
People Living with Cancer:
  http://www.plwc.org

Continued

Internet Resources for Reliable Cancer CAM Information—cont'd

Selected Peer-Reviewed Journals (Indexed in Medline)

Alternative & Complementary Therapies:
    http://www.liebertpub.com/publication.aspx?pub_id=3
Clinical Journal of Oncology Nursing:
    http://www.ons.org/publications/journals/CJON/index.shtml
Integrative Cancer Therapies:
    http://www.sagepub.com/journal.aspx?pid=286
Natural Pharmacy:
    http://www.liebertpub.com/publication.aspx?pub_id=47
Oncology Nursing Forum:
    http://www.ons.org/publications/journals/ONF/
Seminars in Oncology Nursing:
    http://www.elsevier.com/wps/find/journaldescription.cws_home/623110/
    description#description
The Journal of Alternative and Complementary Medicine:
    http://www.liebertpub.com/publication.aspx?pub_id=26

Selected Sponsored Databases

Alternative Medicine Foundation:
    http://amfoundation.org
American Massage Therapists Association:
    http://amtamassage.org
ClinicalTrials:
    http://clinicaltrials.gov/ct
Review of Natural Products Facts and Comparisons:
    http://www.factsandcomparisons.com/
Food & Drug Administration:
    http://www.fda.gov
HealthWorld Online:
    http://healthy.net
International Bibliographic Information on Dietary Supplements:
    http://dietary-supplements.info.nih.gov/databases/ibids.html
Natural Medicine's Comprehensive Database:
    http://www.naturaldatabase.com/
Natural Standard:
    http://www.naturalstandard.com/
PDQ:
    http://cancer.gov/cancerinfo/pdq/
The Cochrane Collaboration:
    http://www.cochrane.org/index0.htm

Bibliography

Cassileth B, Chapman C: Alternative and complementary cancer therapies. *Cancer* 77:1026-1034, 1996.
Cohen MH: Legal issues in complementary and integrative medicine: A guide for the clinician. *Med Clin North Am* 86:185-196, 2002.
D'Andrea GM: Use of antioxidants during chemotherapy and radiotherapy should be avoided. *CA Cancer J Clin* 55:319-321, 2005.

Decker GM: The ten cardinal rules of herb use. *Clin J Oncol Nurs* 10:279, 2006.

Decker G, editor: *An introduction to complementary and alternative therapies,* Pittsburgh, PA, 2007, Oncology Nursing Press.

Eisenberg DM, Kessler RC, Foster C, et al: Unconventional medicine in the United States. *N Engl J Med* 328:246-252, 1993.

Lee C: Herbs and cytotoxic drugs: Recognizing and communicating potentially relevant interactions. *Clin J Oncol Nurs* 9:481-490, 2005.

Montbriand M: Herbs or natural products that decrease cancer growth: Part one of a four-part series. *Oncol Nurs Forum* 31(4):E76-90, 2004.

Montbriand M: Herbs or natural products that increase cancer growth: Part two of a four-part series. *Oncol Nurs Forum* 31(5):E99-115, 2004.

Montbriand M: Herbs or natural products that protect against cancer growth: Part three of a four-part series. *Oncol Nurs Forum* 31(6):E128-146, 2004.

Montbriand M: Herbs or natural products that may cause cancer growth and harm: Part four of a four-part series. *Oncol Nurs Forum* 32(1):E21-29, 2005.

Oncology Nursing Society: Oncology Nursing Society position paper on complementary and alternative therapies, Pittsburgh, PA, 2006, Oncology Nursing Press.

Physicians' Desk Reference for herbal medicine, ed 2, Montvale, NJ, 2000, Medical Economics Company.

Smith A: Opening the dialogue: Herbal supplementation and chemotherapy. *Clin J Oncol Nurs* 9:447-450, 2005.

Sparber A, Bauer L, Curt G, et al: Use of complementary medicine by adult patients participating in cancer clinical trials. *Oncol Nurs Forum* 27:623-630, 2000.

Sparreboom A, Cox M, Acharya M, et al: Herbal remedies in the United States: Potential adverse interactions with anticancer agents. *J Clin Oncol* 22:2489-2503, 2004.

Unit III

Hematological Malignancies

Hodgkin Lymphoma

John M. Burke and Jane M. DeSmith

Quick Facts

Incidence	8190 newly diagnosed cases estimated in 2007 (4470 in men; 3720 in women)
Mortality	1070 deaths estimated in 2007
Risk factors	Human immunodeficiency virus (HIV) infection
	Epstein-Barr virus infection
	Environmental exposure to herbicides
	Occupational exposures (woodworking, livestock, meat processing)
	Small family size, having a high standard of living in childhood
Genetics	Monozygotic twin siblings of HL patients have a higher risk of developing HL than dizygotic twin siblings
Histopathology	Reed-Sternberg cells
	Pathological subtypes:
	• Classical HL: nodular sclerosis, mixed cellularity, lymphocyte-rich, lymphocyte-depleted
	• Nodular lymphocyte-predominant HL

Symptoms	Lymphadenopathy; B symptoms (fever, drenching sweats, weight loss), fatigue, pain in lymph nodes after drinking alcohol
Diagnosis and evaluation	Excisional biopsy of lymph node
	History and physical examination
	Lab workup: CBC, blood chemistry, ESR, LDH
	Imaging studies: CXR; CT of chest; abdomen and pelvis; PET scan
	Bone marrow biopsy
	Pretreatment tests: MUGA scan and pulmonary function tests (PFTs) if ABVD chemotherapy to be administered

Staging and Stage Grouping

Cotswold modifications of the Ann Arbor staging system for Hodgkin lymphoma

Stage	Description
I	Involvement of a single lymph node region (e.g. cervical, axillary, inguinal, or mediastinal) or lymphoid structure such as the spleen, thymus, or Waldeyer's ring (I) or localized involvement of a single extralymphatic organ or site (I_E)
II	Involvement of two or more lymph node regions or lymph node structures on the same side of the diaphragm (II) or localized involvement of a single associated extralymphatic organ or site and its regional lymph node(s), with or without involvement of other lymph node regions on the same side of the diaphragm (II_E)

Continued

Quick Facts—cont'd

Stage	Description
III	Involvement of lymph node regions on both sides of the diaphragm (III), which may also be accompanied by localized involvement of an associated extralymphatic organ or site (III$_E$), by involvement of the spleen (III$_S$), or by both (III$_{E+S}$)
IV	Diffuse or disseminated involvement of one or more extranodal organs or tissue beyond that designated E, with or without lymph node involvement

Designations applied to any disease stage

A	No systemic symptoms
B	Presence of fever > 38°C, drenching night sweats, or weight loss of at least 10% of body weight in the preceding 6 months
E	Refers to extranodal contiguous extension that can be encompassed within a radiation field appropriate for nodal disease of the same anatomic extent. More extensive extranodal disease is designated stage IV.
X	Refers to the presence of "bulky" disease. Bulky disease is defined as a mediastinal mass with a maximum width that is greater than or equal to one-third of the internal transverse diameter of the thorax at the T5-6 interspace, or a mediastinal mass that is greater than or equal to 10 cm in diameter.

1. What is Hodgkin lymphoma?

Hodgkin lymphoma (HL) is a malignancy thought to arise from B lymphocytes. HL is typically characterized by enlargement of lymph nodes and is defined by the presence of Reed-Sternberg cells or their variants on tissue biopsy. Alternative names for HL that have been used include lymphogranulomatosis and Hodgkin (or Hodgkin's) disease.

2. Who gets HL?

HL occurs with similar frequency in men and women, with a male to female ratio of 1.2:1. Compared with most other cancers, HL tends to occur in a younger patient population, with a median age of approximately 30 years. HL is more common in whites than in people of other races.

3. What are Reed-Sternberg cells?

When seen on tissue biopsy, Reed-Sternberg cells are diagnostic of HL. They are large, multinucleated cells that are usually scattered on a background of inflammatory cells and collagen fibers. The origin of the Reed-Sternberg cell is usually a B lymphocyte. In classical HL, the Reed-Sternberg cells express the proteins CD15 and CD30, but not CD20 or CD45.

4. What are the different pathological subtypes of HL?

The most commonly used system for classifying HL is the World Health Organization's (WHO) modification of the Revised European American Lymphoma (REAL) classification. In the WHO classification, HL is divided into 2 subcategories—**classical HL** and **nodular lymphocyte–predominant HL**—based on morphology (what the cells look like under the microscope) and immunophenotype (what proteins are expressed on the surface of the cells). Classical HL is further subdivided into 4 types: nodular sclerosis, mixed cellularity, lymphocyte depletion, and lymphocyte rich.

Immunophenotype of the two major subtypes of Hodgkin lymphoma		
Marker	Nodular lymphocyte predominant HL	Classical HL
CD15	–	+
CD20	+	–
CD30	–	+
CD45	+	–

5. Describe the four types of classical HL.

Classical HL accounts for 95% of HL cases. The most common sites of involvement are the cervical lymph nodes, followed by the mediastinal, axillary, and para-aortic lymph nodes. The spleen and bone marrow are involved in 20% and 5% of cases, respectively.

- **Nodular sclerosis:** Most common subtype, the lymph nodes contain cellular nodules surrounded by collagen bands.
- **Mixed cellularity:** Reed-Sternberg cells are scattered on a mixed inflammatory cell background without collagen bands or fibrosis.
- **Lymphocyte-rich:** Reed-Sternberg cells are scattered on a background of predominantly small lymphocytes, lacking neutrophils and eosinophils.
- **Lymphocyte depleted:** A very rare subtype, the Reed-Sternberg cells exist on a fibrillary matrix without lymphocytes.

6. Compare nodular lymphocyte–predominant lymphoma to classical HL.

Nodular lymphocyte–predominant HL (NLPHL) is less common than classical HL, accounting for only 5% of all HL cases. It occurs most commonly in men between the ages of 30 and 50 years. It usually involves cervical, axillary, or inguinal nodes; involvement of mediastinal nodes, spleen, and bone marrow is unusual. Morphologically, the lymph node is replaced by an infiltrate of small lymphocytes and histiocytes. Large cells with a large nucleus and scant cytoplasm—called "L&H cells" or "popcorn cells"—are scattered. In contrast to the Reed-Sternberg cells of classical HL, the L&H cells usually express CD20 and CD45 but do not express CD15 or CD30 proteins (see table in Question #4). Compared to patients with classical HL, those with nodular lymphocyte–predominant HL tend to experience symptoms at a younger age and survive longer after diagnosis.

7. What is the most common sign or symptom in patients with HL?

HL patients most commonly develop enlarged lymph nodes in the neck, mediastinum, or both. Patients may be asymptomatic but notice a "lump" in the neck or just above the clavicles. Mediastinal nodal enlargement may cause cough, chest pain, or shortness of breath. On examination, the lymph nodes are typically described as "rubbery." This is in contrast to lymph nodes involved with carcinomas, which often feel very hard. HL tends to spread in an orderly fashion to adjacent lymph node regions.

8. How often do "B symptoms" occur?

"B symptoms," defined as having a fever greater than 38° C, drenching night sweats, and weight loss of more than 10% of the body weight over the preceding 6 months occur in about 40% of patients with classical HL, and usually those with more advanced disease.

9. What other systemic symptoms can occur with HL diagnosis?

Other systemic symptoms include diffuse itching and pain in the lymph nodes after the ingestion of alcoholic beverages. Occasionally the disease will involve not only lymph nodes but also organs such as the lung, bone, bone marrow, skin, gastrointestinal tract, and central nervous system. The superior vena cava syndrome can occasionally occur in patients with bulky mediastinal disease.

10. How is HL staged?

The Ann Arbor staging system was developed at a conference in Ann Arbor, Michigan in 1974. In 1988 this staging system was modified at a conference in Cotswold, England. The staging description should contain a number and describe the presence or absence of B symptoms and "bulky" disease. For example, a patient with an enlarged left cervical node, no other evidence of disease, and no B symptoms has stage IA disease. A patient with a 10 cm mediastinal mass, para-aortic lymphadenopathy, and fever has stage IIIBX disease.

11. How is the diagnosis of HL made?

HL diagnosis is generally made by an excisional biopsy of the lymph node with appropriate immunohistochemical stains. Occasionally, core needle biopsy will be adequate to make the diagnosis, but fine needle aspiration is almost never sufficient. Pathological examination of the excised lymph node demonstrates the findings described in question 5.

12. Once the diagnosis of HL is made, how should patients be evaluated to determine the stage and extent of disease?

- Patients with HL should be asked about whether they have B symptoms, pain with drinking alcohol, itching, and fatigue.
- Level of functioning (i.e., performance status) should be determined.
- Physical exam should include careful examination of lymph nodes, liver, and spleen.
- Laboratory tests should include a complete blood count; electrolyte, blood urea nitrogen, creatinine, and liver enzymes levels; erythrocyte sedimentation rate (ESR); and lactate dehydrogenase (LDH) level.
- Imaging tests include a chest x-ray (CXR) and computed tomography (CT) scan of the chest, abdomen, and pelvis. Recently, positron emission tomography (PET) scanning has been found to be useful in determining the extent of disease and is now commonly performed.
- Bone marrow aspirate and biopsy should be done to determine HL marrow involvement.
- Historically, staging laparotomy with splenectomy, gallium scanning, and lymphangiograms were performed in the staging evaluation of HL patients, but these tests are rarely performed now.

13. What chemotherapy is used to treat HL?

HL is usually curable with chemotherapy and radiation therapy. The most commonly used chemotherapy regimen is ABVD (Adriamycin [doxorubicin], Bleomycin, Vinblastine, and Dacarbazine). One cycle is 28 days of therapy, with chemotherapy administered intravenously every 2 weeks, on days 1 and 15 (see Chapter 6 for common acute chemotherapy toxicities).

Other chemotherapy regimens that may be used in place of ABVD for various reasons include the Stanford V regimen (mechlorethamine, doxorubicin, etoposide, vincristine, vinblastine, bleomycin, and prednisone), BEACOPP (bleomycin, etoposide, doxorubicin, cyclophosphamide, vincristine, procarbazine, and prednisone), and MOPP (mechlorethamine, doxorubicin, procarbazine, and prednisone).

14. What potential long-term complications of chemotherapy can occur?

Potential long-term complications of therapy include cardiac toxicity or congestive heart failure from doxorubicin; pulmonary toxicity and Raynaud's phenomenon from bleomycin; peripheral neuropathy from vinblastine; infertility; and a risk of secondary malignancies, including myelodysplasia and acute myeloid leukemia. Avascular necrosis of the femoral heads may occur in patients treated with corticosteroids. Patients are also at risk for the development of herpes zoster.

15. What issues need to be addressed before therapy begins?

- Before beginning therapy with ABVD, patients generally undergo a test to measure cardiac function, such as an echocardiogram or a MUltiple Gated Acquisition (MUGA) scan (cardiac blood-pool imaging), and pulmonary function tests.
- Because of the potential for extravasation with ABVD chemotherapy, a central venous catheter may be inserted.
- If splenectomy or splenic radiotherapy is being considered, pneumococcal, *Haemophilus influenzae*, and meningococcal vaccines should be administered.

16. How is radiation therapy used to treat HL?

Radiation therapy can be used with or without chemotherapy to treat HL. The various fields to which radiation therapy can be targeted are described in the following table. If radiation therapy is used after a relatively short course of chemotherapy, the target of the radiation is usually the involved field. If radiation therapy is being used without chemotherapy to treat the disease, subtotal lymphoid irradiation is often used. Potential long-term toxicities of radiotherapy include pericarditis, pneumonitis, Lhermitte's sign (see question 17), hypothyroidism, infertility, coronary artery disease, and an increased risk of secondary malignancies, such as breast cancer, lung cancer, gastric cancer, skin cancer, sarcomas, and leukemias.

Radiation fields used in the treatment of Hodgkin lymphoma

	Field name	Description
Single fields	Mantle	Submandibular, cervical, supraclavicular, infraclavicular, axillary, mediastinal, and hilar nodes (i.e., all major lymph node areas above the diaphragm)
	Minimantle	Cervical, supraclavicular, and axillary nodes
	Para-aortic	Para-aortic nodes from the diaphragm extending down to the bifurcation of the aorta and including the spleen
	Pelvic	Iliac, inguinal, and femoral nodes
	Involved	Refers to radiation delivered after chemotherapy to initial sites of disease
	Subtotal lymphoid irradiation	Mantle plus para-aortic fields
Combination fields	Inverted-Y	Para-aortic plus pelvic fields
	Total lymphoid irradiation	Mantle plus para-aortic plus pelvic fields

17. What is Lhermitte's sign?

About 15% of patients treated with radiation to the neck develop an electric shock sensation radiating down the extremities when the neck is flexed. This symptom is called Lhermitte's sign. It usually occurs 6 weeks to 3 months after mantle-field radiotherapy. It resolves spontaneously after a few months and does not require specific therapy.

18. What fertility counseling issues should be included in this patient population?

Many patients with HL may want to have children after completing their treatment. Although therapy for HL may render patients infertile, many patients will still be fertile after receiving treatment. Men should consider semen cryopreservation (sperm banking) before the initiation of therapy. Women who may desire future pregnancy should consider ovulation induction, oocyte retrieval, and in vitro fertilization followed by cryopreservation of fertilized gametes, although this process may delay therapy by a few weeks. If pelvic radiotherapy is planned, oophoropexy (a surgical procedure to place the ovaries out of the radiation field) should be performed. Patients should be advised to use barrier contraception during their treatment, and are generally advised not to get pregnant for 1 year after the completion of therapy. Women of childbearing age should have a pregnancy test before the initiation of treatment.

19. How should early stage classical HL be treated?

Stages I and II HL are generally considered to be "early stage." Treatment of patients in these stages most commonly consists of 4 cycles of ABVD followed by involved-field radiotherapy. Patients with bulky disease or B symptoms may be considered for 6 cycles instead of 4 cycles of ABVD. Restaging usually takes place at the completion of chemotherapy. Assuming the patient has achieved complete remission, involved-field radiotherapy is then administered. Alternative treatment options include 6 cycles of ABVD alone, subtotal lymphoid irradiation alone, or an alternative chemotherapy regimen followed by involved-field radiotherapy.

20. How should advanced stage classical HL be treated?

Treatment of advanced (stage III or IV) HL usually consists of 6 to 8 cycles of ABVD alone. Patients with bulky disease may receive involved-field radiotherapy after chemotherapy completion. Restaging usually takes place after 4 to 6 cycles of chemotherapy. Assuming the patient has achieved complete remission, an additional 2 cycles of chemotherapy are then administered. Alternative options include other chemotherapy regimens, such as Stanford V or escalated doses of BEACOPP.

21. How is nodular lymphocyte–predominant HL treated?

Patients with early-stage NLPHL without B symptoms are usually treated with involved-field or regional radiotherapy alone. Patients with B symptoms or advanced-stage NLPHL are usually treated with chemotherapy with or without involved-field radiotherapy. The anti-CD20 antibody rituximab is an effective treatment for this subtype of HL, though its role in the management of the disease requires further study.

22. What is the prognosis of patients with HL?

Fortunately, 90% of patients with early stage disease will be cured with chemotherapy followed by involved-field radiotherapy. About 80% of patients with advanced stage disease are cured, either by their initial therapy or by their salvage therapy.

23. What are adverse prognostic indicators?

Factors with adverse prognostic implications include: age 45 years or older, male gender, white blood cell (WBC) count greater than or equal to 15,000/mcg; lymphocyte count less than 600/mcg, or less than 8% of total WBC count; hemoglobin level less than 10.5 g/dl; albumin concentration less than 4 g/dl; stage IV disease; bulky mediastinal disease; an elevated ESR; involvement of more than 3 sites; and the presence of B symptoms. The first seven of these factors have been incorporated into a prognostic index that has proven to be applicable to patients with advanced HL. Each factor decreases the survival rate by approximately 7% to 8%. However, even patients with five or more of these seven risk factors have a 5-year survival rate of about 50%.

24. How should patients with HL be followed after the completion of therapy?

Patients with HL are at risk for relapse and the development of secondary malignancies, coronary artery disease, and other medical problems. Patients undergo periodic physical examinations and laboratory work, including complete blood count, chemistry panel, ESR, and LDH level. In patients treated with radiation therapy to the neck, annual measurements of thyroid stimulating hormone (TSH) are recommended to detect hypothyroidism. Chest radiographs and sometimes CT and PET scans are often performed to monitor for recurrent disease. Women are advised to undergo annual mammography, beginning no later than 8 years after the completion of therapy or at age 40 years, whichever occurs earlier.

25. How are patients with relapsed HL treated?

Patients with suspected relapse should undergo repeat biopsy to confirm the diagnosis. The treatment of patients with relapsed HL depends on the prior therapy those patients have received. Patients initially treated with radiation therapy alone may be cured with conventional chemotherapy. Patients initially treated with combined modality therapy usually receive high-dose chemotherapy followed by autologous (or allogeneic) hematopoietic cell transplantation.

Key Points

- Reed-Sternberg cells are diagnostic of HL.
- The most common sign and symptom is lymph node enlargement in the neck, mediastinum, or both.
- 40% of patients with classical HL present with B symptoms (fever > 38°C, drenching night sweats, weight loss).
- HL is usually curable with chemotherapy and radiation therapy.
- Patients with HL are at risk for relapse and the development of secondary malignancies, coronary artery disease, and other medical problems.

Internet Resources

National Comprehensive Cancer Network, Clinical Practice Guidelines in Oncology, Hodgkin Disease/Lymphoma:

   http://www.nccn.org/professionals/physician_gls/PDF/hodgkins.pdf

National Cancer Institute, Hodgkin's Lymphoma:

   http://www.cancer.gov/cancertopics/types/hodgkinslymphoma/

Bibliography

Bonadonna G, Bonfante V, Viviani S, et al: ABVD plus subtotal nodal versus involved-field radiotherapy in early-stage Hodgkin's disease: Long-term results. *J Clin Oncol* 22(14):2835-2841, 2004.

Canellos GP, Niedzwiecki D: Long-term follow-up of Hodgkin's disease trial. *N Engl J Med* 346(18): 1417-1418, 2002.

Diehl V, Franklin J, Pfreundschuh M, et al: Standard and increased-dose BEACOPP chemotherapy compared with COPP-ABVD for advanced Hodgkin's disease. *N Engl J Med* 348(24):2386-2395, 2003.

Duggan DB, Petroni GR, Johnson JL, et al: Randomized comparison of ABVD and MOPP/ABV hybrid for the treatment of advanced Hodgkin's disease: Report of an intergroup trial. *J Clin Oncol* 21(4):607-614, 2003.

Ekstrand BC, Lucas JB, Horwitz SM, et al: Rituximab in lymphocyte-predominant Hodgkin disease: Results of a phase 2 trial. *Blood* 101(11):4285-4289, 2003.

Friedman DL, Constine LS: Late effects of treatment for Hodgkin lymphoma. *J Natl Compr Canc Netw* 4(3):249-257, 2006.

Greene FL, Page DL, Fleming ID, et al: *AJCC cancer staging manual,* ed 6, New York, 2002, Springer.

Hasenclever D and Diehl V: A prognostic score for advanced Hodgkin's disease. International Prognostic Factors Project on advanced Hodgkin's disease. *N Engl J Med* 339(21):1506-1514, 1998.

Hoppe RT, Advani RH, Bierman PJ, et al: Hodgkin disease/lymphoma: Clinical practice guidelines in oncology. *J Natl Compr Canc Netw* 4(3):210-230, 2006.

Jemal A, Siegel R, Ward E, et al: Cancer statistics, 2007. *CA Cancer J Clin* 57:43-66, 2007.

Lister TA, Crowther D, Sutcliffe SB, et al: Report of a committee convened to discuss the evaluation and staging of patients with Hodgkin's disease: Cotswolds meeting. *J Clin Oncol* 7(11):1630-1636, 1989.

Stein H: Hodgkin lymphomas: Introduction. In Jaffe ES, Harris NL, Stein H, et al (Eds.): *Pathology and genetics of tumours of haematopoietic and lymphoid tissues,* Lyon, 2001, IARC Press.

Stein H, Delsol G, Pileri S, et al: Classical Hodgkin lymphoma. In Jaffe ES, Harris NL, Stein H, et al (Eds.): *Pathology and genetics of tumours of haematopoietic and lymphoid tissues,* Lyon, 2001, IARC Press.

Stein H, Delsol G, Pileri S, et al: Nodular lymphocyte predominant Hodgkin lymphoma. In Jaffe ES, Harris NL, Stein H, et al (Eds.): *Pathology and genetics of tumours of haematopoietic and lymphoid tissues,* Lyon, 2001, IARC Press.

Straus DJ, Portlock CS, Qin J, et al: Results of a prospective randomized clinical trial of doxorubicin, bleomycin, vinblastine, and dacarbazine (ABVD) followed by radiation therapy (RT) versus ABVD alone for stages I, II, and IIIA nonbulky Hodgkin disease. *Blood* 104(12):3483-3489, 2004.

Leukemia and Myelodysplastic Syndrome (MDS)

Megan L. Andersen and Jeffrey V. Matous

LEUKEMIA

1. Define leukemia.

The leukemias are heterogenous groups of clonal disorders characterized by uncontrolled proliferation of white blood cells. Leukemias can be categorized as either acute or chronic. Acute leukemias primarily include acute myelogenous leukemia (AML) and acute lymphocytic leukemia (ALL). Chronic leukemias include chronic myelogenous leukemia (CML) and chronic lymphocytic leukemia (CLL).

2. How do acute leukemias differ from chronic leukemias?

Acute leukemias differ from chronic leukemias primarily on the degree of differentiation of the stem cell. In acute leukemia, there is a block in differentiation very early in the maturation process of the stem cell. This leads to an accumulation of "blasts," or immature forms of white blood cells in the blood, bone marrow, or other sites. The acute leukemias are aggressive, rapidly progressive diseases which, if untreated, are rapidly fatal. **Chronic leukemias** represent clonal disorders of differentiated and mature white blood cells. Cells accumulate in the bone marrow, spleen, blood and lymph nodes. Generally, chronic leukemias have a more gradual onset, but are usually progressive in nature.

3. How do lymphocytic leukemias differ from myeloid leukemias?

Lymphocytic leukemias are clonal diseases involving the lymphoid stem cell, while myelogenous leukemias develop from the myeloid stem cell.

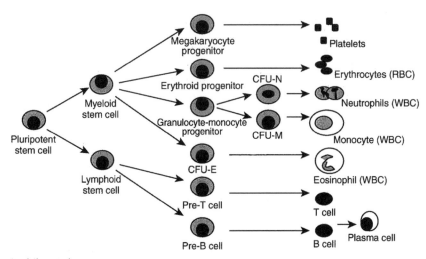

Hematopoietic cascade.

4. What causes leukemias?

The exact causes of leukemias are unknown.

- Several genetic disorders are associated with the development of AML. Chromosomal abnormalities associated with AML probably result from acquired genetic mutations over the person's lifetime. Environmental exposures have been implicated, including tobacco smoke, solvents, chemicals used in rubber and paint manufacturing, radiation, and alkylating chemotherapy agents. In older persons, myelodysplastic syndromes and myeloproliferative disorders often precede AML.
- There is no known causal factor for ALL.
- CML, one of the myeloproliferative diseases, is characterized by the presence of the Philadelphia chromosome, or t(9;22) translocation. There appears to be a link between incidences of CML with radiation exposure.
- CLL is more common in farmers and rubber and asbestos workers. In patients with CLL, there is a familial link in up to 8.8% of cases, indicating the possibility of genetic factors.

5. Discuss the incidence of leukemia.

- AML occurs more frequently in industrialized countries and has an overall incidence of 3.8 cases per 100,000 people. The incidence increases with age, and the median age at diagnosis is 68 years. AML is more common in men than in women. In 2007 it is estimated that 13,410 new cases of AML will be diagnosed in the United States.
- ALL is more common in boys, whites, and Hispanics than in girls and members of other races. It is the most common childhood malignancy. The overall incidence is 1.5 per 100,000 people, and the median age at diagnosis is 11 years. It is estimated that approximately 5200 new cases of ALL will be diagnosed in the United States in 2007, and approximately 64% of all cases are in persons younger than 20 years.
- CML is more common in men than women. The median age at diagnosis is approximately 60 years. The incidence is 1.6 in 100,000 people, with an estimated 4570 new cases diagnosed in the United States in 2007.
- CLL is the most common leukemia in North America, with an estimated 15,340 new cases in 2007. The incidence is higher in men and whites than in women and members of other races, and occurs most frequently with advancing age. The median age at diagnosis is 72 years.

6. Describe the signs and symptoms of acute leukemias.

Infection with fever is one of the most common signs because of the increased production of clonal white blood cells and decreased numbers of mature cells. Thrombocytopenia results from overcrowding of bone marrow space and causes increased bruising, petechiae, gingival bleeding, and epistaxis. Patients often experience significant malaise and fatigue from severe anemia. Less common signs and symptoms include swollen gums, bone pain, sweats, weight loss, and skin lesions. Adenopathy, hepatosplenomegaly, and involvement of the central nervous system (CNS) are more commonly seen in ALL.

7. Describe the signs and symptoms of chronic leukemias.

Nearly 30% to 40% of patients are diagnosed on routine hematologic evaluation before they experience any symptoms. The most common signs and symptoms are fever, sweats, bone pain, weight loss, early satiety, malaise, fatigue, bruising, and splenomegaly. Patients with CLL may experience diffuse lymphadenopathy.

8. **What diagnostic procedures are used during the evaluation and treatment of leukemia?**

Diagnostic tests include complete blood count (CBC) with examination of the peripheral blood smear, comprehensive metabolic panel, coagulation studies to look for disseminated intravascular coagulopathy (DIC), bone marrow biopsy and aspirate (for morphology), flow cytometry (to confirm the leukemic subtype), cytogenetic testing and fluorescence in situ hybridization (FISH) analysis (to evaluate chromosomal abnormalities), and often lumbar puncture.

9. **Describe the classification system for the leukemias.**

- AML has been historically classified according to the French-American-British (FAB) system, with subtypes based on cell origin and morphology, as well as flow cytometric and immunohistochemic differences. AML is also classified by molecular and cytogenetic differences rather than cell morphology alone.

FRENCH-AMERICAN-BRITISH CLASSIFICATION OF ACUTE MYELOGENOUS LEUKEMIA

M0	Acute myeloblastic leukemia, minimally differentiated
M1	Acute myeloblastic leukemia without maturation
M2	Acute myeloblastic leukemia with differentiation
M3	Acute promyelocytic leukemia
M4	Acute myelomonocytic leukemia
M5	Acute monocytic leukemia
M6	Erythroleukemia
M7	Acute megakaryoblastic leukemia

- For ALL, the FAB subtypes are L1, L2, and L3. They are based on cell size, nuclear shape, amount and appearance of cytoplasm, and number and prominence of nucleoli. Further differentiation of ALL subtypes is based on morphology, immunophenotyping of malignant cells, karyotype, and clinical features, such as age, tumor burden at diagnosis, presence or absence of splenomegaly, and presence or absence of CNS involvement.
- CML is characterized by a chromosomal rearrangement, the Philadelphia chromosome (t9;22 or BCR/ABL translocation), and has three phases. The chronic phase is normally associated with few symptoms. The accelerated and blast phases resemble acute leukemias and have a poor prognosis.
- Classification of CLL is based on clinical presentation. A modified version of the Rai system consists of three stages: low-risk, intermediate-risk, and high-risk. Prognosis is directly related to each stage. The low-risk group is associated with isolated lymphocytosis; the intermediate-risk group exhibits lymphocytosis with lymphadenopathy, splenomegaly, or both; and the high-risk group is identified by lymphocytosis with anemia, thrombocytopenia, or both. Because of the extremely variable course of CLL, survival can be measured from months to decades.

10. **How is the prognosis of acute leukemia determined?**

The most important prognostic factors for AML are patient age (> 60 years is associated with higher risk) and karyotype. Certain karyotypes confer a better survival in patients treated with chemotherapy: t(8;21), (inv16), and t(15;17). Others, such as deletion of chromosome 7 or presence of complex karyotypes, confer a very poor prognosis. A normal karyotype has an intermediate prognosis. In adults with ALL, advanced age, elevated white blood cell count, t(9;22) or t(4;11) translocations, and delayed attainment of complete remission (> 4 weeks) are poor prognostic factors.

11. How is the prognosis of chronic leukemia determined?

Prognosis for patients with CML correlates with the eradication of the Philadelphia chromosome. The development of specific tyrosine kinase inhibitors, such as imatinib, has revolutionized the care of CML patients. However, it is not known whether imatinib can cure CML. Allogeneic stem cell transplant is the only known curative treatment for CML, but its risks and requirement for a matched donor limit its application. Patients with a diagnosis of CLL in the low-risk stage with favorable cytogenetic analysis have a life expectancy measured in at least one to two decades. Higher risk patients may survive less than a decade. CLL can convert into more aggressive diseases, such as prolympho-cytic leukemia, diffuse large-cell lymphoma (Richter syndrome), acute leukemia, or multiple myeloma. Once this progression occurs, treatment is much more difficult, and mortality rates rise significantly.

12. Are the leukemias curable diseases?

Between 20% and 50% of adult patients with standard risk AML and ALL are cured with standard chemotherapy. Cure rates are generally higher in patients who undergo allogeneic stem cell transplant. Philadelphia chromosome positive ALL is only curable with allogeneic transplantation. CLL is currently considered incurable. CML is curable in 60% to 80% of patients who receive an allogeneic transplant while in the chronic phase.

13. What are the current treatment options for AML?

AML is treated most commonly with an intense chemotherapy induction and a tailored consolidation plan. Cytarabine and anthracycline-type agents (i.e., mitoxantrone, idaru-bicin, daunorubicin) are generally accepted treatments in the **induction** phase, which is often called the 7 and 3 treatment course. A repeat course of induction therapy is given if residual leukemia is seen on bone marrow biopsy performed one week after comple-tion of chemotherapy. Remission status is determined after recovery from induction chemotherapy. Patients in remission are then treated with **consolidation** treatment. This is tailored depending on the risk of relapse. Higher risk patients are normally referred for allogeneic transplantation, while lower risk patients are consolidated with chemotherapy. Sometimes high-dose chemotherapy and autologous stem cell transplan-tation are used as consolidation. **Maintenance** therapy is generally avoided. Allogeneic transplantation is the only curative option for patients with relapsed or refractory AML. It is extremely important when evaluating a patient with AML to determine if they have the promyelocytic subtype, also called M-3 AML. This subtype is associated with t(15;17) and PML/RARα rearrangement. PML-RARα, a fusion protein of promyelocytic leukemia (PML) and the retinoic acid receptor-α (RARα), causes acute promyelocytic leukemias (APL). AML has unique complications such as DIC with a risk of hemor-rhagic death. It requires distinct therapy, and has a better prognosis (cure rates > 80%) than other subtypes of AML.

14. What are the current treatment options for ALL?

The general treatment for ALL is divided into three phases: (1) **induction phase**, which is intended to result in first remission; (2) **intensification phase**, which has dramatically improved survival rates; and (3) **maintenance phase**, which begins once remission has been achieved and is continued for 2 to 3 years to preserve remission. A typical induction incorporates the drugs daunorubicin, L-asparaginase, prednisone, and vincristine. The L3 type of ALL is morphologically identical to Burkitt's lymphoma and requires a more aggressive therapy than "standard" ALL regimens. Diagnostic lumbar punctures are required. Even in the absence of CNS disease, prophylactic intrathecal (IT) chemotherapy with or without radiotherapy is required. Adult ALL patients with high-risk features should generally receive allogeneic transplants while in first complete remission (CR). Allogeneic transplant is the only curative strategy for relapsed or refractory ALL.

15. What are the current treatment options for CML?

Tyrosine kinase inhibitors; imatinib mesylate (Gleevec) and dasatinib (Sprycel) are the treatments of choice for CML. Imatinib works by inhibiting the enzyme, encoded by the Philadelphia chromosome, that is responsible for clonal proliferation leading to CML. Other treatment agents include hydroxyurea, (which alleviates symptoms but does not prolong survival) and alpha-interferon (which is associated with increased morbidity compared with hydroxyurea). Alpha-interferon does, however, provide some patients with both hematologic and cytogenetic responses. Allogeneic transplantation is the only known curative therapy for CML. However, because of a procedure-related mortality of 10% to 25% (depending on donor matching and patient age), and the excellent results from imatinib, transplantation is usually reserved for very young patients, for those who do not respond well to imatinib, or for patients who have become refractory to imatinib after a good initial response.

16. What are the current treatment options for CLL?

Treatment is based on stage and progression of disease. Because CLL is considered incurable, treatment is generally reserved for symptomatic patients. Patients in the low-risk stage who do not have progression are placed under close observation. Patients with intermediate- and high-risk stages are treated if symptoms are present. The nucleoside analogs, such as fludarabine, have excellent activity against CLL and are widely used to treat it, either alone or in combination with other chemotherapeutic agents or monoclonal antibodies. Patients generally respond to multiple rounds of various treatments. Allogeneic bone marrow transplantation is considered in some patients who are refractory to fludarabine and who have a good performance status.

17. What is the leading cause of death in persons with leukemia?

Infectious complications, which are common and serious in patients with leukemia, are the leading cause of death. Thrombocytopenia, DIC, and other clotting disorders can lead to hemorrhage and death. Most patients die from progressive leukemia.

MYELODYSPLASTIC SYNDROME (MDS)

18. Define MDS.

Myelodysplastic syndrome (MDS) is a heterogeneous stem cell disorder characterized by ineffective hematopoiesis, resulting in cytopenias.

19. Is there a relationship between MDS and leukemia?

MDS has a significant chance of evolving to AML, depending on a set of known risk factors. Patients in the **low** International Prognostic Scoring System (IPSS) risk group have a 19% lifetime risk of developing AML and a median survival of 5.7 years, whereas patients in the **high** IPSS risk group have a 45% lifetime risk and median survival of 0.4 years.

20. What causes MDS?

MDS can occur de novo (without any identifiable predisposing factors) or may develop after a patient has been treated with chemotherapy or radiation for another disease (therapy-related MDS). Acquired chromosomal abnormalities can be detected in

40% to 70% of cases of de novo MDS and 95% of therapy-related MDS. Deletions of the long arms of chromosome 5 or 7 are the most common chromosomal abnormalities.

21. Discuss the incidence of MDS.

MDS is a disease of older adults, with more than 80% of patients aged more than 60 years. Although it is difficult to determine the exact incidence (due to changing classification systems and frequent misdiagnosis), it is estimated that MDS affects between 12,000 and 20,000 people in the United States each year.

22. Describe the signs and symptoms of MDS.

The signs and symptoms of MDS are those related to cytopenias, although low-stage patients may be asymptomatic. Patients may develop fatigue, dyspnea, or pallor resulting from anemia. The anemia is frequently macrocytic. Frequent or difficult to treat infections may occur because of either neutropenia or dysfunctional neutrophils. Thrombocytopenia may manifest as easy bleeding or bruising, usually noted as gingival bleeding, epistaxis, petechiae, or ecchymoses.

23. What diagnostic tests and procedures are commonly used during the evaluation and treatment of MDS?

Diagnostic tests used for the evaluation and treatment of MDS, include complete blood count (CBC) and examination of the peripheral blood smear. A bone marrow biopsy and aspirate are necessary for diagnosis. Specialized tests on the bone marrow, which may be critical for diagnosis and prognosis, such as karyotype, fluorescence in situ hybridization (FISH) analysis, and flow cytometry, should be done. When considering the diagnosis of MDS, differential diagnostic considerations include vitamin B12 deficiency, aplastic anemia, drug toxicity, or severe infections.

24. Describe the classification system and list the types of MDS.

The classification system for MDS, up until 2001, relied on the French-American-British (FAB) system. In 2001, the World Health Organization (WHO) published new classification schemes for hematologic malignancies. See the following table for a comparison of the two systems.

FAB and WHO classification system for MDS

FAB		WHO
Disease	**Bone marrow findings**	**Disease**
RA (refractory anemia)	< 5% marrow blasts	RA (unilineage) 5q- syndrome RCMD (refractory cytopenia with multilineage dysplasia)
RARS (RA with ringed sideroblasts)	< 5% marrow blasts plus ≥ 15% ringed sideroblasts	RARS (unilineage) RCMD (with RS)
RAEB (RA with excess blasts)	5%-20% marrow blasts	RAEB-1 RAEB-2
RAEB-T (RAEB in transformation)	21%-30% marrow blasts	AML (acute myeloid leukemia)

FAB and WHO classification system for MDS—cont'd

	FAB	WHO
Disease	**Bone marrow findings**	**Disease**
CMML (chronic myelomonocytic leukemia)	≤ 20 marrow blasts plus monocytosis > 1000/mm^3	MDS (myelodysplastic syndrome)/ MPD (myeloproliferative disorder)
—	—	Unclassified

Modified from Vardimen JW, Harris NL, Brunning RD: The World Health Organization (WHO) classification of the myeloid neoplasms. *Blood* 100:7, 2002 and Greenberg PL, Young NS, Gatterman N: Myelodysplastic syndromes. *Hematology Online* 1:136-161, 2002. Available at: http://www.asheducationbook.org/cgi/reprint/2002/1/136. Retrieved on January 3, 2007

25. How is the prognosis of MDS determined?

The prognosis of MDS is best determined by the type of MDS the patient has, as well as the International Prognostic Scoring System (IPSS) score.

International Prognostic Scoring System (IPSS)

Prognostic variable (score)	0	0.5	1.0	1.5	2.0
Bone marrow blast (%)	< 5	5-10	–	11-20	21-30
Cytogenetics*	Good	Intermediate	Poor	–	–
Cytopenias	0-1	2-3	–	–	–

Prognosis

Score	IPSS subgroup	Median survival (yrs)	Lifetime AML evolution
0	Low	5.7	19%
0.5-1.0	Intermediate-1	3.5	30%
1.5-2.0	Intermediate-2	1.2	33%
> 2.5	High	0.4	45%

*Good = diploid, -y, del(5q), del(20q); Poor = chromosome 7 abnormalities or complex karyotypes; Intermediate = all others.

26. Is MDS a curable disease?

The only curative treatment for MDS is allogeneic stem cell transplant (SCT). The morbidity and mortality risk of allogeneic transplantation generally limits this treatment to higher risk and younger patients.

27. What are the treatment options for MDS?

Therapeutic options are tailored for patients based on disease risk, presence of cytopenias, and performance status.

- **Supportive care** options are appropriate for many patients and include red blood cell and platelet transfusion, as well as treating other complications, such as infections or secondary iron overload. Growth factors, such as erythropoietin, darbepoetin, or filgrastim may ameliorate cytopenias.

- **Chemotherapy or immune modulation** should be considered in higher stage patients who often have transfusion requirements and more aggressive disease. These agents include thalidomide, 5-azacytidine, arsenic trioxide, lenalidomide, decitabine, and antithymocyte globulin (ATG), possibly combined with cyclosporine.
- **Acute leukemia type inductions** are appropriate for better performance status patients with higher blast counts.
- Referral for **allogeneic stem cell transplantation** is indicated for selected higher risk patients.

28. What drugs have recently been approved by the FDA for the treatment of MDS?

Newer drugs, such as 5-azacytidine (Vidaza) and decitabine (Dacogen), have shown promise in treating MDS, which may be related to their epigenetic properties. Epigenetic modulation refers to potentially reversible changes to DNA and chromatin that regulate gene transcription not due to irreversible changes (mutations or deletions) and may be significant in the pathogenesis of MDS.

29. What are the leading causes of death in MDS patients?

The leading causes of death for MDS patients are transformation to AML and refractory cytopenias resulting in hemorrhage and infections.

30. How do MDS and aplastic anemia differ?

This is a very important distinction to make when faced with a patient with pancytopenia. Normally, the marrow is hypercellular in MDS and severely hypoplastic in aplastic anemia. The blast count is never elevated in aplastic anemia.

31. How do MDS and myeloproliferative diseases (MPD) differ?

Although both disorders share marrow hypercellularity (proliferation), in MDS the cells do not differentiate, or mature properly, whereas in MPD they do. Therefore, cytopenias are less common in patients with MPDs.

 Key Points

- The leukemias are characterized by uncontrolled proliferation of white blood cells and can be categorized as acute or chronic.
- Infection with fever is one of the most common symptoms of acute leukemia.
- Treatment options vary by leukemia type, but usually include chemotherapy. Allogeneic stem cell transplantation may also be necessary.
- Life-threatening complications of leukemia include infection, thrombocytopenia, disseminated intravascular coagulation (DIC), and other clotting disorders.
- Myelodysplastic syndrome can occur de novo or may develop secondary to chemotherapy or radiation therapy for another disease.
- The only curative treatment for MDS is allogeneic stem cell transplantation.

Internet Resources

National Cancer Institute Cancer Information Service:
  http://www.cancer.gov/cancertopics/factsheet/Information/CIS
Leukemia & Lymphoma Society:
  www.lls.org
The Myelodysplastic Syndromes Foundation:
  www.mds-foundation.org
Aplastic Anemia & MDS International Foundation, Inc.:
  www.aamds.org

Bibliography

Gore SD: Six (or more) drugs in search of a mechanism: DNA methyltransferase and histone deacetylase inhibitors in the treatment of myelodysplastic syndromes. *J Natl Compr Canc Netw* 4(1):83-90, 2006.

Greenberg P, Cox C, LeBeau MM, et al: International scoring system for evaluating prognosis in myelodysplastic syndromes. *Blood* 89:2079-2088, 1997.

Greenberg PL, Young NS, Gatterman N: Myelodysplastic syndromes. *Hematology Online* 1:136-161, 2002. Available at: http://www.asheducationbook.org/cgi/reprint/2002/1/136. Retrieved on January 3, 2007

Greer, JP, Foerster J, Lukens J, editors: *Wintrobe's clinical hematology,* ed 11. Philadelphia, 2004, Lippincott Williams & Wilkins.

Jemal A, Siegel R, Ward E, et al: Cancer statistics, 2007. *CA Cancer J Clin* 57:43-66, 2007.

Hoffman R, Benz EJ, Shattil SJ, et al, editors: *Hematology: Basic principles and practice,* ed 4, Philadelphia, 2004, Churchill Livingstone.

List AF, Vardiman J, Issa JJ, et al: Myelodysplastic syndromes. *Hematology Online* 1: 297-317, 2004 Available at: http://www.asheducationbook.org/cgi/reprint/2004/1/297. Retrieved on January 3, 2007.

Sawyers CL, Hochhaus A, Feldman E, et al: Imatinib induces hematologic and cytogenetic responses in patients with chronic myelogenous leukemia in myeloid blast crisis: Results of a phase II study. *Blood* 99:3530-3539, 2002.

Sekers MA: Myelodysplastic syndrome. Available at: http://www.clevelandclinicmeded.com/diseasemanagement/hematology/myelo/myelo.htm#table2. Retrieved December 21, 2005.

Vardimen JW, Harris NL, Brunning RD: The World Health Organization (WHO) classification of the myeloid neoplasms. *Blood* 100:7, 2002.

Wujcik D: Leukemia. In Yarbro CH, Frogge MH, Goodman M, et al, editors: *Cancer nursing: Principles and practice,* ed 6, Boston, 2005, Jones and Bartlett.

Chapter 16

Multiple Myeloma

Paul A. Seligman

Quick Facts

Incidence	19,900 newly diagnosed cases estimated in 2007 (10,960 in men; 8,940 in women); increasing age (median age: 50-70 yr)	**Diagnosis and evaluation**	History and physical examination
Mortality	10,790 deaths estimated in 2007		Complete blood count: test for anemia, neutropenia, and thrombocytopenia
Risk factors	Chronic exposure to low-level radiation		Chemistry screen: blood urea nitrogen (BUN), serum creatinine (Cr), albumin, lactic dehydrogenase (LDH) assess tumor burden
	Occupational exposure (agriculture, chemicals, rubber manufacturing, leather tanners)		Urinary and serum protein electrophoresis (UPEP/SPEP): test for presence of monoclonal proteins
	Chemical exposure (benzene, formaldehyde, hair dyes, paint sprays, Agent Orange)		Quantitative immunoglobulins (QIGs): evaluate amounts of different antibody types (IgG, IgA, IgM)
	Radiation exposure		Skeletal survey: evaluate degree of bone marrow involvement as indicated by percentage of plasma cells
Genetics	Abnormal genetic karyotypes are evident in 50% of patients		
Histopathology	IgG with kappa or lambda light chains, in 65% of patients		Bone marrow biopsy
	IgA with kappa or lambda light chains, in 20% of patients		$\beta2$ microglobulin: prognostic indicator reflecting tumor mass; increases with advancing disease
	Bence-Jones proteins, kappa or lambda light chains only, in 10% of patients		C-reactive protein: surrogate marker for IL-6, a growth factor for multiple myeloma
	IgM, IgD, IgE, rarely found		
Symptoms	The first symptoms are often complications of multiple myeloma, because the disease is a slow-growing neoplasm typified by a long prodromal or asymptomatic period		Cytogenetics and fluorescence in situ hybridization (FISH) tests: used to detect chromosomal abnormalities or deletions (worse prognosis)
	First symptoms, suggesting systemic involvement, include bone disease (back pain), renal disease, hypercalcemia, anemia, and infections		

Quick Facts—cont'd

	Staging* and Stage Grouping	
Stage	Durie-Salmon Staging System[†]	International Staging System (ISS)[‡]
I	< 0.6 myeloma cells × 10^{12}/m^2 (low burden) + all of the following:	β2 microglobulin < 3.5 mg/dl
	1. Hemoglobin value > 10 g/dl	Albumin ≥ 3.5 g/dl
	2. Serum calcium value normal (≤ 12 mg/dl)	
	3. On radiograph, normal bone structure (scale 0) or solitary bone plasmacytoma only	
	4. Low M-component production rates a. IgG < 5 g/dl b. IgA < 3 g/dl c. Urine light-chain M-component on electrophoresis (Bence Jones protein): < 4 g/24 hr	
II	0.6-1.2 myeloma cells × 10^{12}/m^2 (intermediate burden) fitting neither stage I nor stage III criteria	β2 microglobulin < 3.5 mg/dl, but serum albumin < 3.5 g/dl Or β2 microglobulin 3.5 to < 5.5 mg/dl irrespective of serum albumin levels
III	> 1.2 myeloma cells × 10^{12}/m^2 (high burden) plus one or more of the following:	β2 microglobulin ≥ 5.5 mg/dl
	1. Hemoglobin < 8.5 g/dl 2. Serum calcium value > 12 mg/dl 3. Advanced and multiple lytic bone lesions on radiograph (scale 3) 4. High M-component production rate a. IgG > 7 g/dl b. IgA > 5 g/dl c. Urine light-chain M-component on electrophoresis (Bence Jones protein): > 12 g/24 hr	
	Subclassification A = Normal renal function (serum creatinine < 2.0 mg/dl) B = Abnormal renal function (serum creatinine ≥ 2.0 mg/dl)	

*Criteria vary, and standard definitions are lacking. Some clinicians monitor serum levels of β2 microglobulin, which correlate with renal function and myeloma cell tumor burden. Although good indicators of prognosis and survival, current staging systems do not indicate treatment.

[†]Durie GB, Salmon SE: A clinical staging system for multiple myeloma. *Cancer* 36:852, 1975.

[‡]Greipp, PR, San Miguel J, Durie BGM et al: International staging system for multiple myeloma. *J Clin Oncol* 23:3412-3420, 2005.

1. What is multiple myeloma?

Multiple myeloma is a malignant proliferation of plasma cells that results in an overproduction of a specific immunoglobulin (e.g., IgG, IgA), generally detected in the blood or urine. Plasma cells are responsible for production of immunoglobulin (the basic unit of antibodies) and arise from stem cells in the bone marrow. Monoclonal "M" protein is produced excessively by the malignant plasma cell and interferes with effective antibody production. The presence of myeloma cells in the bone marrow and in the outer part of bones may cause multiple medical problems.

2. How is multiple myeloma diagnosed and classified?

Multiple myeloma is diagnosed in a few patients by chance, with the identification of abnormal protein in the blood or urine. In most patients, the first symptoms are one or more of the common complications of myeloma, and these patients are further evaluated using diagnostic studies (see Quick Facts).

Diagnostic criteria for various forms of monoclonal gammopathies

Old classification	New designation	Diagnostic criteria	Treatment plan
Monoclonal gammopathy of unknown significance (MGUS)	MGUS	1. Monoclonal gammopathy a. IgG < 3.5 gm/dl b. IgA < 2.0 gm/dl c. Urinary light chain < 1.0 gm/dl 2. Marrow plasmacytosis < 10% 3. No bone lesions 4. No symptoms	Observation and follow-up
Multiple myeloma*	Symptomatic myeloma	1. Plasmacytoma on tissue biopsy 2. > 30% marrow plasmacytosis 3. Monoclonal globulin spike (M protein) a. IgG > 3.5 g/dl b. IgA > 2.0 g/dl c. Urinary light chain > 1.0 g/24 hr 4. Additional features a. Lytic bone lesions b. Low residual immunoglobulins	Chemotherapy ± autologous or allogeneic stem cell transplant Biologic agents High dose and pulse steroids
Indolent myeloma	Asymptomatic myeloma	Same as for myeloma except: 1. 0-3 bone lesions, no fractures 2. Monoclonal spike < 7 g/dl IgG; < 5 g/dl IgA 3. No associated features: anemia, hypercalcemia, renal dysfunction, infection; good performance	Observation and follow-up Chemotherapy is withheld until disease progression or medical complication occurs

Diagnostic criteria for various forms of monoclonal gammopathies—cont'd

Old classification	New designation	Diagnostic criteria	Treatment plan
Smoldering myeloma	Asymptomatic myeloma	Same as for indolent myeloma except: 1. No bone lesions 2. Marrow plasmacytosis < 30%	Observation and follow-up Chemotherapy is withheld until disease progression or medical complication occurs

*Diagnosis requires 1, 2, or 3, plus either 4a or 4b if plasmacytosis and monoclonal spike are present but lower than above. Diagnosis can be made if 4a or 4b is present.
Modified from Gautier M, Cohen H: Multiple myelomas in the elderly. *J Am Geriatr Soc* 42:653-654, 1994; Jacobson J, Hussein M, Barlogie B, et al: A new staging system from multiple myeloma patients based on the Southwest Oncology Group (SWOG) experience. *Br J Haematol* 122:441-450, 2003; and the Multiple Myeloma Research Foundation website http://www.multiplemyeloma.org/about_myeloma/2.05.html. Accessed 01/03/07.

3. What is monoclonal gammopathy of unknown significance (MGUS)?

The diagnosis of MGUS is made when patients have no symptoms, no skeletal involvement, a marrow plasmacytosis that is less than 10%, and low M-protein production. Approximately 1% of the general population and 3% of persons over age 70 years have MGUS, which is relatively innocuous. However, patients with MGUS can slowly develop active myeloma at a rate of 1% per year. Because close to 20% of patients with MGUS eventually develop multiple myeloma, frequent evaluation is necessary.

4. What is a plasmacytoma?

A plasmacytoma is a single isolated collection of malignant plasma cells in the bone that can be treated with local therapy, such as surgery, radiation, or both. Because some of these patients eventually develop multiple myeloma, close monitoring is necessary.

5. What staging system is most often used for multiple myeloma?

The Durie-Salmon clinical staging system has been most commonly used since 1975 and is based on the measurement of four criteria: number of lytic bone lesions, and levels of hemoglobin, serum calcium, and M protein levels. Recently, however, a new International Staging System (ISS) sponsored by the International Myeloma Foundation (IMF) was developed by the International Myeloma Working Group (IMWG), composed of numerous physicians and researchers from around the world. The goal of the project was to develop an international staging system that can be used to more easily determine the extent and progression of disease in a simpler, more cost-effective way, using less testing. Using advanced statistical analyses on over 10,000 multiple myeloma cases, researchers were able to validate with significant accuracy two predictors of disease outcome: serum albumin and $\beta2$ microglobulin levels. Although the ISS may replace the more complex Durie-Salmon staging system, physicians are also relying more on the myeloma classification criteria to make treatment decisions. Research on DNA micro-array analyses and chromosomal abnormalities may be important predictors of response to treatment and survival.

6. What is the significance of Bence-Jones protein in the urine?

Some malignant plasma cells produce only the light-chain part of the immunoglobulin. These low-molecular-weight proteins are excreted in the urine; they allow the diagnosis of light-chain myeloma and may contribute to the development of renal failure (referred to as myeloma kidney).

7. Why are patients with multiple myeloma prone to the development of renal failure?

Renal failure in patients with multiple myeloma is multifactorial. The causes generally include an accumulation of Bence-Jones proteins, hypercalcemia, hyperuricemia, and dehydration. It is important that patients with multiple myeloma receive adequate hydration before receiving diagnostic dyes or contrast media. The degree of hydration depends on the patient's creatinine value and disease stage, but treatment generally involves the administration of at least 1 liter of normal saline and reevaluation of the patient's renal function and fluid status.

8. What are lytic lesions?

The first symptoms of many patients include skeletal involvement and bony destruction caused by the accumulation of plasma cells. Plasma cells also increase bone resorption, resulting in further bony destruction that may be seen as "punched-out" lesions on radiographs. A lytic lesion is a destructive loss of bone in an isolated area secondary to metastatic cancer infiltration. Diffuse osteoporosis also may result. Skeletal involvement may lead to pathologic fractures, increased serum calcium, and severe pain. The administration of intravenous bisphosphonates, such as pamidronate and zoledronic acid, which inhibit osteoclastic activity and decrease bone resorption, is currently recommended every 3 to 4 weeks to minimize bony destruction. Patients receiving bisphosphonates need to be informed about the associated risks of renal impairment and osteonecrosis of the jaw.

9. If patients with multiple myeloma have an increase in a specific immunoglobulin, why are they at increased risk for infection?

The elevated monoclonal protein is impaired and does not function normally to provide protection. Because it is produced in large quantities, it also results in a decrease in the levels of other normal and functional immunoglobulins. As the percentage of bone marrow infiltration by plasma cells increases, neutropenia further predisposes patients to infection.

10. What medical emergencies are patients with multiple myeloma prone to develop?

The common oncologic emergencies in patients with multiple myeloma are hypercalcemia, spinal cord compression, and hyperviscosity.

11. Define hyperviscosity. How is it exhibited?

The presence of high concentrations of M protein in the blood may lead to occlusion of blood vessels and circulatory problems. The patient may develop claudication, visual disturbances, and neurologic symptoms, such as headache, drowsiness, and confusion.

12. How is multiple myeloma treated?

Over the past 5 years there has been a marked change in the approach to the treatment of multiple myeloma. Once thought to be an incurable disease, treatment was usually reserved until the time that patients became symptomatic. Now, especially in younger patients, durable and long-term disease-free remissions of greater than five years can be achieved using one or more of the following approaches:

- High-dose chemotherapy combined with autologous peripheral stem cell transplantation (stem cell rescue)
- Disease-specific biologic agents including thalidomide which may be given in combination with high-dose dexamethasone and/or a proteasome inhibitor (bortezomib [Velcade])
- Traditional chemotherapy (e.g., vincristine, doxorubicin, and dexamethasone; melphalan and prednisone)

In general, patients older than age 70 years are treated symptomatically with traditional dose chemotherapy, often with some of the biologic agents listed previously. Even these patients can have prolonged survival and excellent quality of life for 3 years or more after diagnosis.

13. When is stem cell transplant indicated?

Up-front autologous stem cell transplantation is generally used in patients under the age of 60 years. However, depending on performance status, degree of medical complications at diagnosis (e.g., renal failure), patients older than age 60 may be considered. In some instances, patients with advanced disease can be pretreated to at least a partial remission with a combination of thalidomide and dexamethasone. Also, patients who receive thalidomide after transplantation as "maintenance therapy" have increased median survival when compared to those who do not receive thalidomide after transplantation. At the present time, when these therapeutic strategies are used, the median overall 5-year survival is greater than 50%; 25% to 30% of patients can achieve disease-free survival for longer than 5 years, suggesting they are cured.

14. What are the major complications of treatment?

In many instances, the problem with most treatments is drug resistance. However, even in these cases, especially if a patient is younger, a second stem cell transplantation may be efficacious. Side effects of treatment vary considerably and nurses should be aware of unusual side effects associated with some of the biologic agents, including severe weakness, neuropathy, and rash.

15. How has treatment improved prognosis in multiple myeloma?

A 5-year survival rate of greater than 50% is much higher than the 20% to 25% 5-year survival rates seen in the 1980s and 1990s.

16. What new approaches are used in the management of multiple myeloma?

Current studies are focusing on better support for patients receiving stem cell transplantation, because the mortality rate is still 2% to 3% in some studies. A newer biologic agent, that is a second generation thalidomide analogue, (lenalidomide [Revlimid]), appears to have similar if not better efficacy and fewer side effects than thalidomide. Recently approved by the FDA for use in patients with multiple myeloma who have received one prior therapy, lenalidomide can be administered orally in combination with dexamethasone.

17. When is radiation therapy used in the treatment of multiple myeloma?

Radiation therapy is used both for local control of solitary plasmacytomas of bone and for palliation of bone metastases (tumor infiltration of bone, pathologic fractures, spinal cord compression).

18. How can nurses promote safety and improve the quality of life in patients with multiple myeloma?

The nurse's role involves:

- Facilitating diagnosis and managing disease-related complications or treatment-induced side effects.
- Enabling patients with skeletal involvement to achieve optimal pain control while avoiding medication side effects. Education about positioning and ambulation also may help to prevent further pathologic fractures and continued bone destruction.
- Encouraging hydration to prevent hypercalcemia, and avoidance of drugs with renal toxicity to promote optimal renal function and prevent further damage.
- Preventing, recognizing, and treating infections, since infection is the leading cause of death in patients with multiple myeloma.

 Key Points

- Multiple myeloma, a common hematologic condition that occurs in older patients, is associated with bone involvement and increased immunoglobulins in serum, urine, or both.
- Complications of multiple myeloma include osteoporosis and bony fractures that can be extremely debilitating.
- Recent advances in the treatment of multiple myeloma not only improve quality of life but are also associated with improved survival and possible cure in some patients.
- Because of the bony complications, nursing care should be directed towards improvement in bone density and avoidance of pathologic fractures.

 Internet Resources

Multiple Myeloma Research Foundation:
    http://www.multiplemyeloma.org/about_myeloma
The Leukemia and Lymphoma Society:
    http://www.lls.org
American Cancer Society, Detailed Guide: Multiple Myeloma:
    http://www.cancer.org/docroot/CRI/content/CRI_2_4_1X_What_is_multiple_
    myeloma_30.asp
The International Myeloma Foundation:
    http://www.myeloma.org
National Comprehensive Cancer Network (NCCN), Clinical Practice Guidelines,
    Multiple Myeloma:
    http://www.nccn.org/professionals/physician_gls/PDF/myeloma.pdf
National Cancer Institute (NCI), Multiple Myeloma:
    http://www.cancer.gov/cancertopics/pdq/treatment/myeloma/HealthProfessional/page5

Acknowledgment

The author wishes to acknowledge Cathy Pickett, RN, OCN, for her contributions to the Multiple Myeloma chapter published in the first and second editions of *Oncology Nursing Secrets.*

Bibliography

Brinker BT, Waller EK, Leong T, et al: Maintenance therapy with thalidomide improves overall survival after autologous hematopoietic progenitor cell transplantation for multiple myeloma. *Cancer* 106:2171-2180, 2006.

Durie BGM, Salmon SE: A clinical staging system for multiple myeloma. *Cancer* 36:842-854, 1975.

Elice F, Raimondi R, Tosetto A, et al: Prolonged overall survival with second on-demand autologous transplant in multiple myeloma. *Am J Hematol* 81:426-431, 2006.

Greipp PR, San Miguel J, Durie BGM, et al: International staging system for multiple myeloma. *J Clin Oncol* 23:3412-3420, 2005.

Jacobson JL, Hussein MA, Barlogie B, et al: A new staging system from multiple myeloma patients based on the Southwest Oncology Group (SWOG) experience. *Br J Haematol* 122:441-450, 2003.

Jagannath S, Richardson P, Munshi NC: Multiple myeloma and other plasma dyscrasias. In Pazdur R, Coia L, Hoskins J, et al, editors: *Cancer management: A multidisciplinary approach,* ed 9, Lawrence, KS, 2005, CMP Healthcare Media.

Jemal A, Siegel R, Ward E, et al: Cancer statistics, 2007. *CA Cancer J Clin* 57:43-66, 2007.

Kyle RA, Vincent Rajkumar S: Treatment of multiple myeloma: An emphasis on new developments. *Ann Med* 38:111-115, 2006.

Shane KA, Shelton BK: Multiple myeloma. In Shelton BK, Ziegfield CR, Olsen MM, editors: *Manual of cancer nursing,* Philadelphia, 2004, Lippincott Williams & Wilkins.

Tariman JD, Estrella SM: The changing treatment paradigm in patients with newly diagnosed multiple myeloma: Implications for nursing. *Oncol Nurs Forum* 32:E127-E138, 2005.

Non-Hodgkin Lymphomas

Scott Kruger and Brenda Maureen Rajniak

Quick Facts

Incidence	63,190 newly diagnosed cases estimated in 2007 (34,200 in men; 28,990 in women); increased incidence associated with AIDS, immunosuppression and elderly; median age at diagnosis is over 50 years
Mortality	18,660 deaths estimated in 2007
Risk factors	**Infections:** human immunodeficiency virus (HIV), hepatitis C, Epstein-Barr virus (African Burkitt's and other lymphomas), human T-cell lymphoma virus (HTLV-1) (T-cell lymphoma), *Helicobacter pylori* associated with gastric lymphomas, mucosal-associated lymphoid tissue (MALT)

Environmental factors: pesticides, fertilizers, wood and cotton dust, early and prolonged use of some hair dyes, solvents, organic chemicals

Therapy-related factors: chemotherapy (alkylating agents), radiation therapy with latency period of about 5-6 years, immunosuppressants (azathioprine or cyclosporine), organ transplants

Congenital immune deficiencies: ataxia telangiectasia, Bloom's syndrome, Wiskott-Aldrich syndrome, severe combined immune deficiency, common variable hypogammaglobulinemia, acquired immunodeficiency states (e.g., HIV, organ transplantation)

Autoimmune disorders: Sjögren's syndrome, systemic lupus erythematosus, rheumatoid arthritis, celiac disease

Genetics	See Question 2
Histopathology	See Questions 2 and 4
Symptoms	Lymphadenopathy, B symptoms (fever, drenching sweats, weight loss), fatigue

Indolent lymphomas: painless, slowly progressive lymphadenopathy that may spontaneously regress in size and then grow later; extranodal involvement and B symptoms may be found in advanced disease

Aggressive lymphomas: sometimes first symptom is rapidly growing adenopathy; one third of patients develop extralymphatic disease in the GI tract, skin, sinuses, and central nervous system

Quick Facts—cont'd

(CNS); B symptoms are common; patients with lymphoblastic lymphoma may have a large mediastinal mass, superior vena cava syndrome, or cranial nerve involvement due to leptomeningeal disease; American Burkitt's lymphoma often starts with a large abdominal mass and obstructive symptoms, whereas African Burkitt's lymphoma often starts with a mass at the angle of the jaw or neck.

Diagnosis and evaluation
History and physical examination
Lymph node or tissue biopsy
Lab workup: CBC, blood chemistry, LDH
Imaging studies: CXR; CT of chest, abdomen, and pelvis; PET scan
Bone marrow biopsy

Staging and Stage Grouping

NHL is staged according to the Ann Arbor Staging System

Stage	Description
I	Involvement of a single lymph node region or lymphoid structure (spleen, thymus, or Waldeyer's ring)
II	Involvement of 2 or more lymph node regions on same side of diaphragm (the mediastinum is a single site, hilar nodes are lateralized); the number of anatomic sites should be indicated by a suffix (e.g., stage II$_3$)
III	Involvement of lymph node regions or structures on both sides of diaphragm
III$_1$	Splenic, celiac, or portal nodes
III$_2$	Para-aortic, iliac, or mesenteric nodes
IV	Multifocal involvement of extranodal sites, with or without associated lymph node involvement or isolated extralymphatic organ involvement with distant nodal involvement

Each stage is subdivided into **category A** (no symptoms) or **category B** (fever > 101.5°F, drenching sweats, loss of > 10% body weight within past 6 months)

X = bulky disease (> 1/3 widening of mediastinum and > 10 cm maximal dimension of nodal mass)

E = extranodal site, contiguous or proximal to known nodal sites. Sites are identified by the following notations: **P** = lung or pleura, **H** = liver, **M** = bone marrow, **S** = spleen, **O** = bone, **D** = skin.

Patients are also assigned: **Clinical stage (CS)**, based on node and bone marrow biopsy studies, physical exam, and radiologic evaluation; **Pathologic stage (PS)**, based on results of invasive procedures beyond initial biopsies

1. What are the non-Hodgkin lymphomas? How are they diagnosed?

The non-Hodgkin lymphomas (NHLs) are a diverse group of seemingly unrelated diseases arising from lymphoid tissues. NHL is caused by a malignant clonal expansion of one of the cell types in a lymph node. Because lymphatic tissue is present throughout the body, the disease may develop anywhere. It may begin in a lymph node, spleen, liver, or bone marrow as well as extralymphatic sites, such as skin, gastrointestinal tract, pharynx, and central nervous system. The diagnosis is established by biopsy of abnormal tissue and evaluation with histologic and immunophenotypic examination.

2. What are the most common cytogenetic abnormalities? How do they correlate with histology?

Chromosomal abnormalities are associated with oncogene expressions causing lymphoma.

World Health Organization classification of lymphoid malignancies

Cytogenetic abnormality	Oncogene expression	Histology
t(14;18)	bcl-2	Follicular and diffuse large cell
t(11;14)	bcl-1	Mantle zone
t(14;19)	bcl-3	B-cell chronic lymphocytic lymphoma (CLL)
t(8;14), t(2;8), t(8;22)	c-myc	Burkitt's and non-Burkitt's lymphoma
Trisomy 12		B-cell CLL and small lymphocytic lymphoma
14q11 abnormalities	tcl-1, tcl-2	T-cell acute lymphocytic lymphoma (ALL)
7q35 abnormalities	tcl-4	T-cell ALL and lymphoblastic lymphoma
t(2;5)	npm;alk	Anaplastic large cell

3. What characteristics of an enlarged node raise the suspicion of lymphoma?

A painless, enlarging lymph node that feels rubbery is suspicious for lymphoma. Infectious nodal enlargement is usually tender. Enlarged supraclavicular nodes are always suspicious for malignancy.

4. Why is the classification of NHLs so confusing?

The classification is confusing because the NHLs are a heterogeneous group of diseases that seem to have little relationship to each other. They are named according to growth pattern (follicular vs. diffuse) within the lymph node, cell size (large vs. small), and appearance (cleaved or noncleaved). Until the mid 1980s, the Rappaport classification was widely used in the United States, but it has been replaced by the Working Formulation, which attempts to simplify classification into risk categories of low, intermediate, and high grade. However, the Working Formulation does not include all lymphomas. The REAL (Revised European American Lymphoma) classification was proposed by the International Study Group in an effort to accommodate newly described lymphomas not included in the Working Formulation. Today the World Health Organization Classification of Lymphoid Malignancies is used, because it incorporates morphologic, genetic, and immunophenotypic characteristics for each lymphoma.

Working Formulation and WHO Classification of Lymphoid Malignancies

Working Formulation
Low grade

A Small lymphocytic (diffuse, well-differentiated lymphocytic)
B Follicular, small cleaved cell (nodular, poorly differentiated lymphocytic)
C Follicular, mixed, small cleaved cell, and large cell (nodular, mixed)

Intermediate grade

D Follicular, large cell (nodular, histiocytic)
E Diffuse, small cleaved cell (diffuse, poorly differentiated lymphocytic)

Working Formulation and WHO Classification of Lymphoid Malignancies—cont'd

F Diffuse, mixed, small cleaved and large cell (diffuse, mixed)
G Diffuse, large cell (diffuse, histiocytic)

High grade

H Immunoblastic (diffuse, histiocytic)
I Lymphoblastic (lymphoblastic)
J Diffuse, small noncleaved cell (Burkitt's and non-Burkitt's types)

WHO Classification
B-cell neoplasms

Precursor B-cell neoplasm
Precursor B-lymphoblastic leukemia and lymphoma
Mature (peripheral) B-cell neoplasms
B-cell chronic lymphocytic leukemia/small lymphocytic lymphoma
B-cell prolymphocytic leukemia
Lymphoplasmocytic lymphoma
Splenic marginal zone B-cell lymphoma (with or without villous lymphocytes)
Hairy cell leukemia
Plasma cell myeloma/plasmacytoma
Extranodal marginal zone B-cell lymphoma of MALT type
Nodal marginal zone B-cell lymphoma (with or without monocytoid B-cells)
Follicular lymphoma
Mantle cell lymphoma
Diffuse large B-cell lymphoma
Mediastinal large B-cell lymphoma
Primary effusion lymphoma
Burkitt's lymphoma/Burkitt's-like lymphoma

T-cell and NK-cell neoplasms

Precursor T-cell neoplasm
Precursor T-lymphoblastic lymphoma/leukemia (precursor T-cell acute lymphoblastic leukemia)
Mature (peripheral) T-cell neoplasms
T-cell prolymphocytic leukemia
T-cell granular lymphocytic leukemia
Aggressive NK-cell leukemia
Adult T-cell lymphoma/leukemia (HTLV-1+)
Extranodal NK/T-cell lymphoma, nasal type
Enteropathy-type T-cell lymphoma
Hepatosplenic $\gamma\delta$ T-cell lymphoma
   Subcutaneous panniculitis-like T-cell lymphoma
   Mycosis fungoides/Sézary syndrome
   Anaplastic large cell lymphoma, T-/null-cell, primary cutaneous type
   Peripheral T-cell lymphoma, not otherwise characterized
   Angioimmunoblastic T-cell lymphoma
   Anaplastic large cell lymphoma, T-/null-cell, primary systemic type

5. What are favorable and nonfavorable lymphomas? Are favorable lymphomas more curable?

- **Low-grade lymphomas** are considered "favorable," because of their relatively long natural history. Some patients can remain healthy for many years without treatment, whereas others require intermittent treatment with radiation or drugs to treat enlarged symptomatic adenopathy. Unfortunately, they are not considered curable. Most patients with low-grade lymphoma require treatment after a few years, but it is generally palliative rather than curative. The 5-year survival rate for patients with low-grade lymphomas ranges from 50 to 70%.
- **Unfavorable lymphomas (intermediate- and high-grade lymphomas)** are potentially curable with a combination of chemotherapy and immunotherapy. The high-grade lymphomas are considered "unfavorable" because without active treatment the natural history is poor. The 5-year survival rate for intermediate-grade lymphoma ranges from 33% to 45% of patients; for high-grade lymphomas, the rate is from 23% to 32%. Treatment may result in complete remission in 60% to 80% of patients with diffuse, aggressive NHL; however many patients relapse and will die of their disease.

6. What is the International Prognostic Index?

The International Prognostic Index consists of five adverse factors used by the major institutions and cooperative groups to predict overall survival in patients with unfavorable, aggressive lymphomas. As the number of risks increase, the 5-year survival rates decrease.

- Age (> 60 years)
- Elevated levels of serum lactate dehydrogenase (LDH)
- Performance status (levels ≥ 2)
- Stage III or IV disease
- Two or more sites of extranodal involvement

Degree of risk and survival rates—unfavorable, aggressive lymphomas

Degree of risk	Number of adverse risk factors	Five year survival rate
Low	0-1	73%
Low-intermediate	2	51%
Intermediate-high	3	43%
High	4-5	26%

7. Is there a prognostic model for low grade follicular lymphoma?

The Follicular Lymphoma International Prognostic Index (FLIPI) was developed to predict survival based on the following adverse factors:

- Age (> 60 years)
- Ann Arbor stage III or IV
- Hemoglobin level < 12 gm/dl
- Serum LDH level elevated
- Number of nodal sites involved > 4

Degree of risk and survival rates—low grade follicular lymphoma

Degree of risk	Number of adverse risk factors	Five year survival rate	Ten year survival rate
Low	0-1	91%	71%
Intermediate	2	78%	51%
High	3-5	53%	36%

8. What other prognostic factors are useful in unfavorable lymphomas?

- Tumor biology: Ki-67 (marker for cellular proliferation), abnormal cytogenetic findings, T-cell and null cell lymphoma
- Presence of B symptoms
- Tumor burden: bulky sites (diameter > 7 cm), elevated β2 microglobulin
- Drug resistance
- Persistent abnormal PET Scans
- Time to complete remission

9. How do Hodgkin lymphomas differ from non-Hodgkin lymphomas?

Pathologically, Reed-Sternberg cells, which are characteristic of Hodgkin lymphoma, are not found in NHLs. NHLs spread by skipping lymph node areas, whereas Hodgkin lymphomas are orderly and do not skip lymph node groups. NHLs are usually seen in older adults; Hodgkin lymphomas have a bimodal incidence with the first peak in young adults.

10. What is the treatment of favorable (low-grade) lymphomas?

Low-grade lymphomas are characterized by indolent behavior and median survival times of 6 to 12 years. Most patients are older adults and have advanced disease when their first symptoms appear. Only 10 to 20% have stage I or II disease.

Stage I or II. Involved field radiation therapy, which treats the entire involved lymph node group, can result in a 10-year disease free survival in 40% to 50% of patients. Since most relapses occur in nodes outside the radiation field, some physicians will also treat with a few cycles of chemotherapy. Better and more accurate staging techniques have allowed more accurate radiation therapy planning. Many patients who were thought to have early stage disease are found to have involvement of other nodal areas, their condition is assigned a higher stage, and chemotherapy is recommended.

Stage III and IV. Treatment options include watching and waiting. Various systemic chemotherapy regimens are begun when patients become symptomatic. Chemotherapy is usually started early in patients with unfavorable prognostic features, such as marrow involvement, bulky disease, high levels of serum LDH, many extralymphatic sites of disease, and decreased performance status. Treatment options include single agent alkylators, such as cyclophosphamide or chlorambucil; and combinations of drugs, such as cyclophosphamide, vincristine, prednisone, or fludarabine regimens. Rituximab used alone or with chemotherapy can result in long response rates.

11. Describe the treatment of unfavorable (intermediate-grade) lymphomas.

Intermediate-grade lymphoma is frequently diagnosed in early stages. High-grade immunoblastic lymphoma is treated like intermediate-grade diseases. Patients are usually treated with chemotherapy, using cyclophosphamide, hydroxydaunomycin (doxorubicin),

Oncovin (vincristine), and prednisone (CHOP). Patients are also treated with rituximab (R-CHOP), if cells are CD20-positive.

Stage I and II. A combination of chemotherapy with rituximab and radiation is the treatment of choice. The 5-year disease-free survival rate ranges from 78% to 95% for patients with stage I disease, and from 70% to 75% for patients with stage II disease. Patients usually receive 3 to 4 cycles of chemotherapy followed by involved-field radiation therapy. For patients who do not receive radiation, 6 to 8 cycles of chemotherapy are used.

Stage III and IV. Most patients are treated with 6 to 8 cycles of systemic chemotherapy. Radiation is sometimes added to sites of bulky disease to decrease the risk of local recurrence. Despite the availability of multiple chemotherapy regimens, the 5-year disease-free survival rate is approximately 40%.

12. What is rituximab (Rituxan) and how is it used?

This drug is a chimeric human-mouse monoclonal antibody that binds to the surface protein CD20, which is found on most B cells. This form of immunotherapy recruits the body's natural defenses to attack and kill the marked B cells (complement-mediated cellular toxicity, antibody-dependent cellular cytotoxicity, and direct apoptosis). Rituximab therapy is combined with chemotherapy to treat active disease and used alone as maintenance therapy. This drug has been bound with radioimmunotherapy agents (Zevalin and Bexxar) and used to treat relapsed and refractory disease by targeting the radiation to the lymph tissue.

13. What common oncologic emergency should be anticipated when lymphoma patients are treated with chemotherapy?

Tumor lysis syndrome should be anticipated. Typically this is seen in patients with acute leukemia and high grade lymphoma who are undergoing treatment. It occurs when the tumor cells are very sensitive to the chemotherapy and die rapidly. The best treatment is anticipation; appropriate measures should be taken to prevent this life-threatening complication (see Chapter 53 for more information on tumor lysis syndrome).

14. What is Richter's transformation?

Evolution of a low-grade lymphoma into a diffuse large cell lymphoma is called Richter's transformation. The term was first used in 1928 to describe a case of CLL (chronic lymphocytic leukemia) that developed into aggressive lymphoma.

15. Which lymphomas can be treated with antibiotics?

MALT (mucosa-associated lymphoid tissue) lymphoma in the stomach has been associated with infection by *Helicobacter pylori*. Treatment of this infection with antibiotics (Prevpac) can lead to complete remission of the lymphoma. Patients who do not respond to antibiotics can receive rituximab, chemotherapy, or both. Patients with systemic advanced disease require treatment with both chemotherapy and rituximab.

16. How is lymphoblastic lymphoma treated?

Lymphoblastic lymphoma is uncommon in adults, but in children it is the most common type of NHL. Treatment is the same as for acute lymphoblastic leukemia: high-dose chemotherapy, including treatment of the central nervous system (CNS) with intrathecal chemotherapy. Patients usually require several years of treatment. For patients with adverse prognostic features, autologous or allogeneic stem cell transplant can be considered after completion of induction therapy. Patients who relapse are offered salvage chemotherapy followed by stem cell transplant.

17. Which patients should receive CNS prophylaxis with radiation or intrathecal therapy?

All patients with Burkitt's, non-Burkitt's, and lymphoblastic lymphoma receive treatment for the CNS. Other patients with involvement of bone marrow, testes, nasopharynx, or sinuses should be evaluated for CNS disease. Epidural and brain disease is treated with intrathecal therapy, using methotrexate or cytarabine, or with radiation therapy.

18. How is mantle cell lymphoma different from the other lymphomas?

This lymphoma has an aggressive course with frequent relapses. At first diagnosis the disease is often widespread with bone marrow involvement and splenomegaly. Median survival is short at 3 years. The disease responds to standard chemotherapy, but relapses are common. Survival is not improved with standard chemotherapy. Because of its poor prognosis, patients are considered for stem cell transplant early in their treatment, or for very aggressive chemotherapy with such regimens as hyper-CVAD (cyclophosphamide, vincristine, Adriamycin, dexamethasone, methotrexate with leucovorin rescue, cytarabine, and rituximab). Bortezomib is also a useful chemotherapy agent for this disease. Patients with mantle cell lymphoma should be considered for inclusion in clinical trials.

19. What is the treatment of mycosis fungoides and other cutaneous T-cell lymphomas?

Topical chemotherapy with nitrogen mustard or carmustine (BCNU) and ultraviolet-A light activation of skin with psoralen (PUVA) are usually the initial therapies. Bexarotene, a retinoid that is available as a cream or a pill, has significant activity against the disease. Ontak, a monoclonal antibody, is a diphtheria toxin targeted to cells that express the IL2 receptor (CD25). Extracorporeal photopheresis and total skin electron beam therapy are used for more advanced disease. Systemic chemotherapy may be used to palliate symptoms.

20. What is the role of bone marrow transplant and stem cell transplant in NHLs?

- Stem cell and bone marrow transplants are considered in patients with aggressive lymphoma who have achieved first remission, have poor prognostic features, and have a high risk for relapse.
- In patients who have relapsed disease, high-dose therapy with autologous bone marrow or stem cell transplant can lead to remission, and in some cases even cure the disease. The stem cell or bone marrow support allows the patients to receive a more intense dose of chemotherapy.
- In patients who do not respond to high-dose therapy with stem cell transplant, an unrelated or related allogeneic transplant is sometimes considered, because of the added graft-versus-lymphoma effect on killing the cancer. This type of transplant has a higher risk of rejection, graft failure, and graft-versus-host disease than an autologous transplant.
- Reduced intensity transplants are being used (mini-allo transplant) to minimize the toxicity and still have the graft-versus-lymphoma effects. Patients who relapse within 1 year of diagnosis are less likely to benefit from transplant than patients who have a longer remission. Poor results have been obtained in patients with chemotherapy-refractory disease.
- In indolent disease, transplantation is usually reserved for younger patients who have relapsed or are in second or later remission. It is suggested that transplantation changes the natural history of the disease by providing more durable remissions and delaying relapses.

21. Describe the treatment for patients with CNS lymphoma.

Patients with CNS lymphoma have a poor prognosis. All tumors are high-grade; some are associated with HIV. The frequency of CNS lymphoma in HIV-infected patients is decreasing because of the effectiveness of antiviral therapy. Age and performance status are important prognostic factors. Treatment with combination chemotherapy seems to give the best long-term results. Chemotherapy includes drugs that cross the blood-brain barrier, such as high-dose cytarabine and methotrexate, with intrathecal treatments of the same drugs. High doses of steroids (e.g., dexamethasone) can be helpful in palliation of symptoms. It is important to make the diagnosis before initiating treatment with steroids, because the tumor can be highly sensitive to this treatment and may shrink before a diagnosis can be made. With treatment, the median survival time is 41 months. Radiation therapy is being used less often as the primary treatment for this disease because long-term neurotoxic effects includes dementia and leukoencephalopathy.

22. What precautions are needed in the follow up of long-term survivors?

In addition to monitoring for relapsed disease, it is important to evaluate patients for second malignancies. This includes all solid tumors, especially those in radiation fields; soft tissue sarcomas; skin cancers, including melanoma; acute leukemia; and myelodysplasia. Patients receiving brain radiation are at risk for dementia. Thyroid abnormalities are common in patients receiving head and neck radiation. Because their treatment includes cytotoxic agents, women should avoid pregnancy for at least 1 year after treatment; men should not father a child for at least 1 year after treatment.

 Key Points

- A painless, enlarging lymph node that feels rubbery is suspicious for lymphoma.
- The exact causes of NHLs are unknown.
- Non-Hodgkin lymphomas are named according to growth pattern (follicular vs. diffuse) within the lymph node, cell size (large vs. small), and appearance (cleaved or noncleaved).
- Favorable lymphomas are low-grade lymphomas; unfavorable lymphomas are intermediate- and high-grade lymphomas.
- Although higher grade lymphomas are considered unfavorable, they are potentially curable.
- In addition to monitoring for relapsed disease, it is important to evaluate patients for the development of second malignancies.

 Internet Resources

Leukemia & Lymphoma Society:
    http://www.leukemia-lymphoma.org
Lymphoma.com:
    http://www.lymphoma.com
Lymphoma Focus:
    http://www.lymphomafocus.org
National Cancer Institute:
    http://www.cancer.gov
American Cancer Society:
    http://www.cancer.org
Oncology Link, University of Pennsylvania:
    http://www.oncolink.com
National Comprehensive Cancer Network, Non-Hodgkin Lymphoma Practice Guidelines:
    http://www.nccn.org/professionals/physician_gls/PDF/nhl.pdf

Bibliography

Ansell SM, Armitage J: Non-Hodgkin's lymphoma: Diagnosis and treatment. *Mayo Clin Proc* 80(8):1087-1097, 2005.

Armitage J, Bierman P, Bociek R, et al: Lymphoma 2006: Classification and treatment. *Oncology* 20(3): 231-239, 2006.

Batchelor T, Loeffler JS: Primary CNS lymphoma. *J Clin Oncol* 24(8):1281-1288, 2006.

Celenetz AD, Buadi F, Ciligiuri MA, et al: Non-Hodgkin's lymphoma: Clinical practice guidelines in oncology. *J Natl Compr Canc Netw* 4(3):258-310, 2006.

Coiffier B: State-of- the art therapeutics: Diffuse large B-cell lymphoma. *J Clin Oncol* 23(26):6387-6393, 2005.

Fisher R, Mauch PM, Harris NL, et al: Non-Hodgkin's lymphoma. In DeVita V, Hellman S, Rosenberg S, editors: *Cancer: Principles and practice of oncology,* ed 7, Philadelphia, 2004, JB Lippincott.

Foon KA, Fisher R: Non-Hodgkin's lymphoma. In Beutler E, Lichtman M, Coller B, et al, editors: *Williams hematology,* ed 7, New York, 2005, McGraw-Hill.

Greene FL, Page DL, Fleming ID, et al: *AJCC cancer staging manual,* ed 6, New York, 2002, Springer.

Hiddemann W, Buske C, Dreyling M, et al: Treatment strategies in follicular lymphoma: Current status and future perspectives. *J Clin Oncol* 23(26):6394-6399, 2005.

Jemal A, Siegel R, Ward E, et al: Cancer statistics, 2007. *CA Cancer J Clin* 57:43-66, 2007.

Rosen ST, Winter JN, Gordon LI, et al: Non-Hodgkin's lymphoma. In Pazdur R., Cola LR, Hoskins WJ, et al, editors: *Cancer management–a multidisciplinary approach,* ed 9, Lawrence, KS, 2005, CMP Media.

Rizvi MA, Evens AM, Tallman MS, et al: T-cell Non-Hodgkin's lymphoma. *Blood* 107(4):1255-1264, 2006.

Witzig TE: Current treatment approaches for mantle-cell lymphoma. *J Clin Oncol* 23(26):6409-6414, 2005.

Zintzaras E, Voulgarekis M, Moutsopoulos HM: The risk of lymphoma development in autoimmune diseases: A meta-analysis. *Arch Intern Med* 165(20):2337-2344, 2005.

Unit IV

Solid Tumors

AIDS-Related Malignancies

David Faragher

1. What are the AIDS-defining malignancies?

The AIDS-defining malignancies are Kaposi's sarcoma (KS), non-Hodgkin lymphoma (NHL), and invasive cervical cancer. KS and NHL account for the majority of malignancies in patients with HIV. In one international series, these malignancies accounted for up to 90% of cancers in patients with HIV. In a second series, the total incidence of malignancies in patients with HIV was 4% per year.

2. Why are malignancies included in the Centers for Disease Control and Prevention list of AIDS-defining conditions?

Malignancies are a relatively common complication of a broad range of immunodeficiency states. There have been many reports of malignancies in patients with organ transplants as well as various congenital immunodeficiency conditions. Immunosuppression may predispose people to malignancies for several possible reasons: (1) absence of protective immune surveillance that usually eliminates abnormal clones, (2) deregulation of cell proliferation and differentiation, and (3) chronic antigenic bombardment of the immune system by various infections. KS was one of the first recognized conditions in AIDS. Epidemiologic studies subsequently showed that NHL and, most recently, invasive cervical cancer in women are much more common in patients with AIDS than in age-matched controls. The greater than expected frequency of these malignancies led to their inclusion as AIDS-defining conditions.

3. Have other malignancies been associated with AIDS?

Several malignancies that are not used to define AIDS have nevertheless been described in patients with AIDS, including Hodgkin lymphoma (HL) (relative risk = 18-fold increase), squamous cell carcinomas (SCC) of the head and neck, SCC of the anus (relative risk = 31.7-fold increase), germ cell cancer (relative risk = 2.9-fold increase), lung cancer (relative risk = 3.8-fold increase), melanoma, basal cell carcinomas of the skin, colon cancer, and plasmacytoma/multiple myeloma (relative risk = 12-fold increase). There are also several reports of myelodysplastic syndrome (preleukemia) and acute myeloid leukemia (relative risk = 3-fold increase) in patients with AIDS. Some of these malignancies, such as HL and germ cell cancers, are more common in 30- to 45-year-old people, which is the age group most often afflicted with AIDS. The results of epidemiologic studies to determine whether these cancers have a higher incidence in patients with AIDS than in age-matched controls are conflicting. There is also some controversy about different biologic behavior of malignancies in patients with AIDS compared with immunocompetent patients. Many malignancies are significantly more aggressive and more advanced in patients with AIDS.

4. Does KS occur with equal frequency in all groups of patients with AIDS?

KS is much more frequent in homosexual and bisexual men with human immunodeficiency virus (HIV) than in other risk groups. Studies from the early 1980s revealed that up to 50% of homosexual/bisexual men presented with KS as the initial manifestation of AIDS. In 1991 this percentage had decreased to 11%. Over 90% of all AIDS-related KS occurs in homosexual/bisexual men. KS also has been described in homosexual men who are not infected with HIV. It is uncommon in intravenous drug users, heterosexual men, and women. Compared with the general population, the risk for developing KS is increased approximately 100,000-fold for homosexual men with AIDS and approximately 13,000-fold for others with AIDS.

5. Does KS occur only in patients with AIDS?

No. KS initially was described by Moricz Kaposi in 1872 in older men of eastern European or Mediterranean descent. It was limited primarily to skin involvement of the legs and was rarely life threatening (classic type). Cases of lymph node involvement or visceral disease were rare. An endemic form also has been described in younger men and women of sub-Saharan Africa. The endemic form is more aggressive, with visceral and lymph node involvement as well as cutaneous disease. A third category of non–HIV-related KS occurs in patients who are immunocompromised from organ transplantation or autoimmune diseases.

6. What causes KS?

There have been multiple theories about the cause of KS in AIDS. Because KS was seen primarily in homosexual and bisexual men, it was hypothesized that KS was caused by an infectious agent such as cytomegalovirus (CMV), Epstein-Barr virus (EBV), or human papillomavirus (HPV). These viral DNA sequences were reported in some, but not all, samples of KS tumors. It is known that various soluble factors (cytokines) stimulate growth of KS in tissue culture systems as well as in the human body. These cytokines include interleukin-1 (IL-1), IL-6, tumor necrosis factor-beta (TNF-β), platelet-derived growth factor (PDGF), and oncostatin M. In addition to cytokines, KS production and growth are stimulated by a protein product of the HIV virus. The HIV-*tat* protein induces and stimulates KS in animal systems. In the search for a sexually transmissible KS agent, Chang, Moore, and colleagues discovered a previously unknown herpes virus—KS-associated herpes virus (KSHV), also known as human herpes virus-8 (HHV-8). HHV-8 has been isolated from almost 100% of AIDS-KS tumor cells by polymerase chain reaction, but it is not found in normal cells from the same patients. HHV-8 has numerous genes capable of deregulating mitosis, interrupting apoptosis (programmed cell death), increasing angiogenesis, and blocking presentation of antigens. It is thought that HHV-8 may be the agent that transforms normal mesenchymal cells into pre-KS cells. In patients with HIV who are positive for HHV-8, the incidence of KS is as high as 50% in 10 years. Further activation by cytokines (e.g., IL-1, HIV-*tat*, TNF-β) may trigger a true monoclonal malignant condition.

7. How is KS staged?

Most malignancies are staged by parameters developed and standardized by the American Joint Committee on Cancer (AJCC). This system uses the tumor-node-metastasis (TNM) classification. However, KS has a unique presentation, prognosis, and natural history. Many staging systems modeled after the TNM classification have been proposed, but none accurately predicts the prognosis of AIDS-associated KS. The Oncology Subcommittee of the NIH-sponsored AIDS Clinical Treatment Group (ACTG) proposed a new staging scheme based on factors that more accurately predict the natural history and prognosis of KS:

GOOD RISK (ALL OF THE FOLLOWING):
- Tumor confined to the skin and/or lymph nodes
- CD4 cell count > 200/mm^3

- No opportunistic infections, thrush, or "B" symptoms (fevers, night sweats, and weight loss)
- Karnofsky performance status greater than 70%

POOR RISK (ANY OF THE FOLLOWING):
- Extensive oral, GI, or other visceral disease
- Tumor associated with edema or ulceration
- History of opportunistic infection or B symptoms
- Karnofsky performance status less than 70%

8. What are the indications for treatment of AIDS-associated KS?

The primary indications for treatment include: (1) cosmetic control; (2) painful, bulky lesions; (3) oral lesions interfering with eating or swallowing; (4) lymphedema from lymph node or lymph vessel infiltration; (5) pulmonary involvement; (6) extensive GI involvement, causing obstruction; and (7) rapidly progressive disease.

9. Which treatment modalities are used for AIDS-associated KS?

The many options for treatment of KS include local and systemic therapies.
- Local treatments include radiation therapy, intralesional therapy, and cryotherapy with liquid nitrogen. Intralesional therapy is usually the direct injection of dilute solutions of vincristine, but other agents have been used.
- Systemic treatment includes single-agent chemotherapy, multiagent chemotherapy, and alpha-interferon (with or without concomitant antiretroviral therapy). Life-threatening disease, usually pulmonary disease, requires aggressive treatment with multiagent chemotherapy. Response rates have ranged from 70% to 100%. The response rate to alpha-interferon is up to 65% in a select subset of patients with good prognosis (CD4 cell count > 200/mm^3, no opportunistic infection, or B symptoms). Highly active antiretroviral therapy (HAART) has had a dramatic impact on KS, with regression of some lesions when HAART is used alone. All patients with AIDS and KS should be given a trial of HAART. Although many older chemotherapy agents have had response rates of 15% to 30% with KS, the current systemic chemotherapy treatments for KS generally include liposomal formulations of anthracyclines and paclitaxel. The liposomal coating allows long circulation time, higher intralesion drug levels, and high response rates (up to 70%) with lower toxicity. Paclitaxel, a microtubule toxin, has response rates up to 70%. Hematopoietic growth factors have helped to minimize cytopenia and infections while maximizing the chemotherapy dose that can be tolerated by the patient. All treatment for KS is palliative; therefore risks and benefits must be weighed before initiating therapy. Future research in the treatment of KS will target HHV-8 as the etiologic agent.

10. Which of the NHLs occur in patients with AIDS?

The predominant types of NHL in AIDS are high-grade B-cell NHLs, such as immunoblastic, Burkitt's lymphoma, non-Burkitt's small noncleaved lymphoma (70%), intermediate-grade large cell lymphomas (30%), and primary NHLs of the central nervous system (CNS). Epidemiologic studies have shown a sharp rise in the incidence of NHL since 1983, predominantly in men aged 20 to 54 years. In a study of 100,000 patients with AIDS from 1981 to 1989, 3% had NHL—a 150- to 250-fold increase in incidence compared with the general population. Herpes virus infections play a distinct role in NHL in patients with AIDS. HHV-8 was discovered in almost every case of the newly defined clinicopathologic condition currently termed *primary effusion lymphoma*. EBV can be detected in close to 100% of primary CNS lymphomas in patients with AIDS.

11. Does HIV-related NHL follow the same natural history as NHL in immunocompetent patients?

AIDS-associated NHL is significantly more aggressive than NHL in immunocompetent patients. Typically, it is more extensive and frequently involves extranodal sites (central nervous system, bone marrow, gastrointestinal tract). Patients also frequently have B symptoms (fevers, night sweats, and weight loss). Lymphomas of the central nervous system may occur as mass lesions or with leptomeningeal involvement only. The risk for developing NHL rises significantly as immunosuppression worsens. The incidence of NHL is much greater in patients with CD4 lymphocyte counts greater than $50/mm^3$. Opportunistic infections are likely in people with CD4 cell counts less than $200/mm^3$. Another unique finding in AIDS-associated NHL is the presence of polyclonal malignant cells. Monoclonality is generally considered a hallmark of malignancy. However, the patient with AIDS is exposed to repeated infections and subsequent polyclonal B-lymphocyte activation and transformation to a polyclonal malignancy.

12. Describe the treatment for HIV-associated NHL.

Because AIDS-associated NHL is an aggressive disease that usually involves multiple organs, chemotherapy is generally the standard of care. However, patients most likely to develop AIDS-associated NHL are severely immunocompromised and frequently have active opportunistic infections. A complete evaluation must be done to determine whether any treatment is appropriate. If treatment is chosen, multiagent chemotherapy is necessary. In immunocompetent patients, multiagent chemotherapy yields response rates as high as 80% and long-term survival rates of approximately 40%. However, in patients with AIDS-associated NHL, response rates are 50% and median survival is approximately 5 to 6 months. Survival is significantly better in subgroups of patients, including those with CD4 cell count greater than $100/mm^3$, Karnofsky performance status greater than 70%, no opportunistic infections, and no extranodal disease. Furthermore, randomized studies have confirmed the safety of concurrent use of HAART with combination chemotherapy in patients with NHL. The overall rates of response and survival may be favorably affected by the use of HAART along with chemotherapy.

The current standard treatment for aggressive lymphoma is CHOP (cytoxan, doxorubicin [Adriamycin], vincristine, and prednisone). Rituxan is a standard treatment of patients with lymphoma who do not have HIV, but has not been found to be beneficial in patients with both lymphoma and HIV. Because the risk of leptomeningeal involvement is extremely high, the use of meningeal prophylaxis is strongly encouraged. Overall survival is still very poor, with average survival of approximately 1 year. Treatment for HIV-CNS lymphoma is generally radiation therapy combined with steroids. Overall survival is only 2 to 3 months without therapy and 6 to 8 months with therapy.

13. Why is it more difficult to complete a full course of chemotherapy for AIDS-associated NHL?

Completing full courses of chemotherapy may be more difficult because of frequent dose reductions and delays due to prolonged bone marrow suppression and opportunistic infections. The likelihood of morbidity increases as the degree of immunosuppression increases. Current recommendations to reduce morbidity and mortality include use of attenuated doses and/or use of hematopoietic growth factors if CD4 cell count is less than $100/mm^3$ and standard chemotherapy doses (with or without G-CSF [granulocyte colony-stimulating factor] or GM-CSF [granulocyte-macrophage colony-stimulating factor]) if CD4 count is greater than $200/mm^3$. Such patients also should be treated with HAART and prophylaxis against PCP (*pneumocystis carinii* pneumonia).

14. Has the incidence of HIV infection increased in women?

Yes. The percentage of women infected with HIV has risen significantly. HIV infection in women now accounts for 40% of all infections worldwide and for up to 12% in the United States. In selected regions in the United States, such as New York City, up to 25% of patients with HIV are female. Most HIV infections in American women result from heterosexual transmission. It is also known that the incidence of cervical neoplasia is significantly higher in congenital immunodeficiencies, autoimmune diseases, and acquired immunodeficiency states (e.g., organ transplantation). Reported rates of cervical neoplasia in such patients reach as high as 40%; the risk of anogenital neoplasia is increased 9- to 14-fold compared with matched controls.

15. Why has invasive cervical squamous cell cancer been included as an AIDS-defining malignancy?

The association of HPV and cervical neoplasia is well known. The oncogenic HPVs have been identified in 80% to 90% of invasive cervical cancers as well as high-grade cervical intraepithelial neoplasia (CIN). Several studies have reported a high incidence of HIV in women under 50 years of age with invasive cervical cancer. Furthermore, cervical cancer in patients with HIV appears to be much more biologically aggressive, less responsive to conventional therapies, and associated with a poorer prognosis. Because of these findings, CDC revised the AIDS-defining criteria in 1993 to include invasive cervical cancer.

16. Is preinvasive neoplasia of the cervix included in the revised AIDS-defining CDC list?

The risk of abnormal cervical cytology is increased by as much as 10-fold in HIV-positive women; some studies report abnormal cervical cytology in 30% to 60% of women with HIV. However, a high degree of discordance between results of cytology and biopsy has been found in HIV-positive women with normal cytological findings and abnormal results of a cervical biopsy. Although preinvasive cervical neoplasia is not included in the AIDS definition, cervical dysplasia and CIS are considered AIDS-related conditions. The degree of cervical neoplasia is positively correlated with the degree of immune suppression. Women with CIN (cervical dysplasia, carcinoma in situ, preinvasive neoplasia) tend to have lower CD4 counts than HIV-positive women without CIN.

17. Describe the proper screening for cervical neoplasia in HIV-positive women.

Papanicolaou tests should be done every 6 months, in addition to baseline colposcopy or cervicography. There is also an extremely high association between HPV and anal neoplasia. All HIV-positive women with HPV or cervical dysplasia should have a thorough anal examination, including visual and digital exam, anal cytology smear, and anoscopy.

18. Describe the appropriate treatment for invasive malignancy of the cervix in women with AIDS.

Patients with AIDS-associated cervical cancer have a more advanced disease at diagnosis than age-matched controls. Incidence of high-grade tumors, lymph node involvement, and aggressive biologic behavior is more common in women with AIDS. In addition, risk of recurrence is higher and survival times are shorter for patients with AIDS. Therapy for invasive disease should be based on the patient's condition and stage of malignancy. Patients with relatively good immune function tolerate surgery quite well. Patients with advanced inoperable disease should be considered for chemotherapy or radiation therapy. Patients with poor immune function do not tolerate pelvic radiation treatment or chemotherapy because of depressed hematologic reserve.

19. Are any nursing considerations different in patients with AIDS-related malignancies and other patients with cancer?

Nursing care and symptom control are similar in patients with AIDS-related malignancies and other patients with cancer, except that even more vigilance may be required for early identification of life-threatening infectious complications and assessment of neurologic abnormalities. Patients need to be well educated about prevention of infection and signs and symptoms of opportunistic infections, particularly PCP. Symptoms of PCP include shortness of breath with or without exertion and a dry, nonproductive cough. In addition to other neutropenic precautions, HIV-infected patients should be instructed not to handle or eat raw meat, to avoid eating raw shellfish because of the risk of *Vibrio* infection, and to wear gloves when handling litter boxes because of the potential for contracting toxoplasmosis. Assessment of neurologic abnormalities can be complicated, because mental status changes may be associated with HIV-related dementia, CNS involvement, drug side effects, viral or opportunistic infections, or depression.

20. What problems are associated with medications for people with AIDS and cancer?

A particularly difficult nursing challenge in patients with AIDS-related malignancies is keeping track of various drug interactions and incompatibilities in patients who are on multiple drug regimens to treat malignancy, underlying HIV disease, and opportunistic infections. Patients need to be encouraged to inform health care providers if they are taking any other drugs, supplements, or homeopathic agents that may interact with prescribed therapies. The large potential for drug interactions may be synergistic or antagonistic and result in increased effect, decreased effect, or enhanced toxicity.

21. Are there additional psychosocial issues in patients with AIDS and cancer?

Yes. Even in communities that are accepting of people with AIDS, the patient with AIDS and cancer may experience more social isolation, particularly as the illness progresses.

Key Points

- HIV-infected individuals have an increased risk of developing malignancies that may be the AIDS-defining component of their immunodeficiency.
- The most common malignancies in HIV-infected patients are Kaposi's sarcoma and non-Hodgkin lymphomas.
- Lymphoma that occurs with HIV infection should be evaluated and treated in a unique way.
- Women with HIV infection need intensive screening for cervical neoplasia, with awareness of the high risk of preinvasive and invasive cervical cancer.

Internet Resources

HIV/AIDS Malignancies Link:
  http://www.malignancies.hiv-aids-poz.com
National Cancer Institute, PDQ Cancer Information Summaries, Adult Treatment:
  http://www.cancer.gov/cancertopics/pdq/adulttreatment

Bibliography

Burgi A, Brodine S, Wegner S, et al: Incidence and risk factors for the occurrence of non-AIDS-defining cancers among human immunodeficiency virus-infected individuals. *Cancer* 104:1505-1511, 2005.

Carbone A, Gloghini A: AIDS-related lymphomas: From pathogenesis to pathology. *Br J Haematol* 130:662-670, 2005.

Eltom MA, Jemal A, Mbulaiteye SM, et al: Trends in Kaposi's sarcoma and non-Hodgkin's lymphoma incidence in the United States from 1973 through 1998. *J Natl Cancer Inst* 94:1204, 2002.

Friedman-Kien AE, Laubenstein LJ, Rubinstein P, et al: Disseminated Kaposi's sarcoma in homosexual men. *Ann Intern Med* 96:693-700, 1982.

Goedert JJ: The epidemiology of acquired immunodeficiency syndrome malignancies. *Semin Oncol* 27:390-401, 2000.

Kirk O, Pederson C, Cozzi-Lepri A, et al: Non-Hodgkin's lymphoma in HIV-infected patients in the era of highly active antiretroviral therapy. *Blood* 98:3406-3412, 2001.

Robinson W: Invasive and preinvasive cervical neoplasia in human immunodeficiency virus-infected women. *Semin Oncol* 27:463-470, 2000.

Bladder Cancer

Carmel Sauerland, Tauseef Ahmed, and Muhammad Choudhury

Quick Facts

Incidence	67,160 newly diagnosed cases estimated in 2007 (50,040 in men; 17,120 in women); average age at diagnosis is 65 years
Mortality	13,750 deaths estimated in 2007
Risk factors	Cigarette smoking and tobacco use (aromatic amines contained in cigarettes)
	Exposure to aniline dyes (benzidine) used in a variety of industrial trades Occupations at risk: dry cleaners, printers, painters, hair dressers (hair dyes), janitors, and workers in leather, rubber, aluminum, and textile industries
	Chronic urinary tract inflammation
	Schistosoma hemotobium parasite
	Chronic phenacetin use
Genetics	Genetic basis for familial clustering of transitional cell (urothelial) cancers is undefined
Histopathology	Transitional cell (urothelial) carcinoma: most common (90%); 75% are noninvasive (superficial) at diagnosis
	Squamous cell carcinoma (8%)
	Adenocarcinoma (1%)

Symptoms	Painless hematuria (80%-90%) which can be persistent, microscopic, or gross at presentation
	Irritative symptoms (20%), such as urgency, frequency, and dysuria
	Late symptoms: lymphadenopathy, pain (flank, back, suprapubic)
Diagnosis and evaluation	History and physical examination
	Urine cytology
	Intravenous pyelography
	Cystoscopy
	Bimanual examination
	Transurethral resection of the bladder tumor (TURBT) (+ sampling of surrounding tissue if tumor is high grade)
	Computed tomography (CT)/MRI of abdomen and pelvis (if tumor is high grade or muscle invasion present)
	Chest x-ray (PA and lateral)

Quick Facts—cont'd

Staging and Stage Grouping

Stage	Description

Tumor, node, metastasis (TNM)*

Primary tumor (T)

TX	Primary tumor cannot be assessed
T0	No evidence of primary tumor
Ta	Noninvasive papillary tumor
Tis	Carcinoma in situ: "flat tumor"
T1	Tumor invades subepithelial connective tissue
T2	Tumor invades superficial muscle
T2a	Tumor invades muscle
T2b	Tumor invades deep muscle
T3	Tumor invades perivesical tissue
T3a	Tumor invades perivesical tissue microscopically
T3b	Tumor invades perivesical tissue macroscopically (extravesical mass)
T4	Tumor invades any of the following: prostate, uterus, vagina, pelvic wall, abdominal wall
T4a	Tumor invades prostate, uterus, vagina
T4b	Tumor invades pelvic wall, abdominal wall

Regional lymph nodes (N)

NX	Regional lymph nodes cannot be assessed
N0	No regional lymph node metastases
N1	Metastasis in a single lymph node, ≤ 2 cm in greatest dimension
N2	Metastases in a single lymph node, > 2 cm or ≤ 5 cm; or multiple lymph nodes, none > 5 cm in greatest dimension
N3	Metastasis in a lymph node, > 5 cm in greatest dimension

Distant metastasis (M)

MX	Distant metastasis cannot be assessed
M0	No distant metastases
Ml	Distant metastases

Stage	Primary Tumor	Regional Lymph Nodes	Distant Metastasis
0a	Ta	N0	M0
0is	Tis	N0	M0
I	T1	N0	M0
II	T2a	N0	M0
	T2b	N0	M0
III	T3a	N0	M0
	T3b	N0	M0
	T4a	N0	M0
IV	T4b	N0	M0
	Any T	N1-3	M0
	Any T	Any N	M1

*The TNM staging system is preferred over the Jewett-Strong staging system.
Used with permission of the American Joint Committee on Cancer (AJCC), Chicago, Illinois. The original source for this material is the AJCC Cancer Staging Handbook, Sixth Edition (2002) published by Springer New York, www.sprinfleronline.com.

1. What is the greatest risk factor for bladder cancer?

Cigarette smoking. Smokers are two times more likely to develop bladder cancer. In men, 50% of bladder cancers are attributed to smoking. Some early research has shown that the cessation of smoking following diagnosis can improve survival.

2. What type of bladder cancer is related to chronic irritation and infection?

Squamous cell carcinoma, the second most common type of bladder cancer, is usually seen in the bladder following chronic irritation secondary to infection, bladder stones, and chronic indwelling Foley catheters. An example is infection from *Schistosoma hemotobium* parasite, which causes chronic bladder irritation.

3. Are there any new diagnostic tests for bladder cancer?

In 2002 the U.S. Food and Drug Administration (FDA) approved a new urine assay called the NMP22 (nuclear matrix protein 22) BladderChek Test. This test appears to be more sensitive than cytology but still must be performed in combination with cystocopy. Other tests, such as fluoroscence in situ hybridization (FISH), used to identify chromosomal abnormalities in exfoliated cells in urine is under investigation.

4. What are important prognostic features?

Bladder cancer can be divided into two groups, noninvasive (stages Ta, Tis, and T1) and invasive (stages T2–T4).

- **Noninvasive** cancers tend to recur throughout the patient's life but remain superficial; they require continued monitoring and local treatment. The most important prognostic factor in superficial or noninvasive bladder cancers is the tumor grade (level of cell differentiation). Tumors are typically graded as low (G1), moderate (G2), and high (G3). The presence of multiple tumors, invasion of the stroma, and a history of recurrence within the first 3 months in addition to the grade indicate a high rate of recurrence with likely progression to muscle invasion. About 25% of superficial bladder tumors can eventually invade muscle tissue, requiring more aggressive therapy, such as cystectomy.
- In patients with **invasive** cancers (almost all are G3), the stage, not the grade, is the most important prognostic factor. These patients usually require radical surgery and have a higher probability of developing metastatic disease.

5. What new areas are being investigated for prognostic value?

The key to increasing survival is early identification of patients at high risk for progression of disease followed by choice of the appropriate initial therapy. Tumor behavior patterns show there are factors in addition to grade and stage that influence the response to treatment. The presence of changes in certain proteins may serve as an early indication of a more aggressive disease process. Proteins that may have predictive value are p53 (tumor suppressor gene), pRB (retinoblastoma gene-control cell proliferation), and p21 (inactivates the cell cycle). Understanding the relationship between the functions of these proteins and disease progression could lead to development of less invasive or toxic treatments. Additionally, nomograms (statistical models to predict patient outcome) are now being used by some clinicians.

6. What are the most common sites of metastases?

Invasive bladder cancer tends to directly invade the ureters and prostate (in men); ureters, uterus, and vagina (in women) locally. The most common distant metastatic sites are lymph nodes, bones, liver, and lungs.

7. How are superficial tumors treated after cystoscopy and transurethral resection of bladder tumor?

TaG1 or G2 following a transurethral resection of bladder tumor (TURBT) can be managed with surveillance (cystoscopic and cytologic evaluation every three months), with or without receiving a single dose of mitomycin C intravesically within the first 24 hours after surgery.

TaG3 and Tis or T1 with either G1, G2, or G3 should receive adjuvant treatment with intravesical agents, such as BCG (Bacillus Calmette-Guérin, an attenuated strain of *Mycobacterium bovis*), doxorubicin, mitomycin, thiotepa, or interferon alpha-2a.

The agent with the best response rate is BCG; however, intravesical chemotherapy using mitomycin, doxorubicin, or thiotepa may be a better choice for certain patients because these drugs have low side-effect profiles. Also, BCG should not be used to treat patients who are immunosuppressed, have active urinary tract infections, or have exhibited previous sensitivity to BCG.

The goal of intravesical treatment is to decrease both the risk of recurrence and the rate of progression. Patients who relapse after an initial response to BCG may respond to a combination of BCG and interferon alpha-2a.

8. How often is intravesical BCG administered?

The standard regimen is weekly intravesical BCG for 6 weeks with cystoscopic evaluation approximately 6 weeks after the last treatment. Evidence suggests that maintenance BCG treatment improves results.

9. What are the local effects of intravesical instillation of BCG?

Three to four hours following instillation, patients may experience dysuria, hematuria, urinary frequency, and urgency.

10. What systemic reactions may occur in some patients treated with BCG?

Approximately 3% of patients receiving BCG develop fever greater than 103° F. These patients require immediate attention and may need to be hospitalized and treated with cycloserine, isoniazid (INH), and rifampin, especially if the high fever occurs within the first 2 hours of BCG therapy. BCG therapy should not be reinstituted unless other causes for fever are identified. Some patients experience low-grade fevers between 4 to 8 hours after the BCG treatment. These usually resolve in response to antipyretics and do not recur past 24 hours. In this case INH or rifampin is not necessary, and BCG treatment may be continued with close monitoring. Patients with low-grade fevers lasting longer than 24 hours can be pretreated with INH. BCG sepsis rarely occurs.

11. What about intravesical chemotherapy?

It is usually given weekly for 6 to 8 weeks with a 2-hour holding time. Myelosuppression is a common side effect. Mitomycin C and doxorubicin should not be administered if there is possibility of bladder perforation. Both drugs may cause irritative bladder symptoms; mitomycin C may cause a skin rash.

12. How is muscle-invading transitional cell carcinoma treated?

Radical cystectomy is the treatment of choice for muscle invading transitional cell carcinoma (TCC) (T2 or greater, recurrent high grade T1 or Ta, or multiple recurrence of low grade Ta). This procedure involves removal of the local pelvic lymph nodes and performing a radical cystoprostatectomy in men and anterior exenteration in women.

Patients have urinary diversions (e.g., ileal-conduit with external bag, or continent urinary diversions that do not involve external drainage).

13. Bladder preservation—is it possible?

Yes. Bladder preservation may be possible in a select patient population. The decision is based on the location of the lesion, depth of invasion, size of tumor (T2 or T3a), absence of hydronephrosis, and status of the patient. The goals are to achieve a complete resection with clean, adequate margins and to maintain sufficient bladder capacity. Following transurethral resection of the bladder tumor (TURBT), the patient will receive neoadjuvant treatment with chemotherapy or chemotherapy plus radiation, then a second TURBT. The use of neoadjuvant treatment with combinations, such as M-VAC (methotrexate, vinblastine, doxorubicin, cisplatin), have increased survival for patients with tumors that have invaded muscle. If there is no evidence of disease, the patient will be closely monitored with follow-up cytology and cystoscopy. If strict surveillance is not possible, a radical cystectomy should be performed.

14. What factors determine who is eligible for a neobladder (continent urinary diversion) versus an ileal conduit?

The absence of impaired renal function, dilated ureters, and bowel disease; absence of disease at bladder neck and prostate; no contraindications to a prolonged surgery; and a patient's performance status are all factors that make a patient eligible for a neobladder.

15. What is an ileal conduit?

It is an incontinent diversion that requires an external drainage bag. The ureters are not brought to the skin directly after removal of the bladder because of the high rate of occurrence of stomal stenosis, which may lead to renal obstruction and failure. By placing a segment of ileum between the ureters and skin, this complication is virtually eliminated. The ileal conduit maintains its blood and nerve supply, peristalsis continues, and urine is eliminated. An ileal conduit may have less morbidity when compared with continent diversions.

16. Describe an Indiana pouch. How is it formed?

An Indiana pouch is a continent, catheterizable pouch. It is made from the terminal ileum and proximal colon. The colon portion is opened, then folded back on itself to decrease the pressure and increase the volume within the pouch. The terminal ileum is left attached to the colon and is brought to the skin. The ileal-cecal valve keeps the urine from leaking out of the colonic pouch and can be catheterized through the stoma to drain the pouch. A bag is not required over the stoma because it should not leak. The pouch should be catheterized every 4 to 6 hours, using clean technique. Only a 4 × 4 gauze pad is necessary to cover the stoma.

17. What is a Studer pouch? How is it formed?

A Studer pouch is a neobladder made entirely from ileum. It can be connected to the urethra in both men and women, so that they can void through the urethra and maintain continence.

18. What changes in urine and urine flow should nurses expect after cystectomy?

- Because the bowels normally make mucus, neobladders and ileal conduits will continue to make mucus. Mucus passes freely through ileal conduits, but continent neobladders may need to be irrigated to remove mucus.
- Urine cultures are always positive because of intestinal colonization by bacteria. True infections, manifested by fever and possible flank pain, are managed with antibiotics.

- Reflux of urine to the kidneys may contribute to development of pyelonephritis and late renal deterioration.
- Stones may develop in the kidney or pouch if urinary stasis is present.

19. What metabolic alterations may patients experience after surgery for bladder cancer?

Patients may develop metabolic disturbances depending on the type of urinary diversion and segment of intestine used. Since the intestine is responsible for absorption, urine that is in prolonged contact with the intestine may cause metabolic disturbances.

Ileal conduits probably have the least amount of metabolic abnormalities because of the short time of urine contact. Continent diversions using ileum and colon may cause hyperchloremic metabolic acidosis, which in turn may cause osteoporosis over the long term. Patients may have frequent loose bowel movements after an intestinal urinary diversion. This symptom may resolve in the following 3 months. A few patients have persistent change in bowel habits, especially if the ileal-cecal valve is removed. Patients with presurgical renal dysfunction (creatinine > 2.0 mg/dL) may have a problem compensating for any metabolic alteration; therefore they are probably candidates for ileal conduits only.

Patients with neobladders and patients with resection of large amounts of terminal ileum are at risk for vitamin B12 deficiency, possibly leading to megaloblastic anemia. Blood levels should be monitored.

20. Can adjuvant systemic chemotherapy significantly retard or eliminate disease progression?

Patients with extravesical tumor extension, evidence of vascular invasion in the resected specimen, and evidence of nodal involvement are often offered the option of adjuvant chemotherapy. Unfortunately, poor enrollment in clinical trials has inhibited finding the most effective regimen and identifying any real benefits. Chemotherapy combinations, such as gemcitabine and cisplatin, or methotrexate and cisplatin, have been shown to be beneficial with less toxicity than standard M-VAC. Current research is focusing on identifying effective and less toxic regimens.

21. Is there an effective treatment for metastatic transitional cell carcinoma?

Cisplatin-based chemotherapy is effective in patients with metastatic transitional cell carcinoma. M-VAC is still considered the standard; unfortunately its considerable toxicity has limited the number of patients who can tolerate it. MCV (methotrexate, cisplatin, and vinblastine) and gemcitabine plus cisplatin have been used as combination alternatives to M-VAC. Carboplatin has been substituted for cisplatin to reduce the toxicity of treatment. The use of taxane-based regimens is still under investigation. Use of other agents, such as ifosfamide and gemcitabine, have been explored in combination with regimens based on cisplatin or other chemotherapy agents. The goal of finding a balance between managing side effects and improving outcomes has yet to be achieved.

22. What role does radiation therapy play in the treatment of bladder cancer?

Radiation therapy can be used in combination with surgery and chemotherapy to achieve bladder preservation. If the patient is not a candidate for surgery or chemotherapy, radiation therapy can be used as the primary treatment. The use of multiple fields from high-energy linear accelerators is recommended. In the presence of bone metastatis, radiation may be used palliatively for pain relief.

Potential acute reactions to bladder irradiation include: cystitis, stress incontinence, diarrhea, local skin inflammation, and fatigue. Late reactions include decreased bladder capacity and chronic cystitis. Radiation therapy may also affect sexual function.

23. How can radiation therapy–induced cystitis symptoms be managed?

Symptoms of cystitis can be controlled by increasing fluid intake (2-3 liters/day), avoiding caffeine-containing beverages, and using analgesic agents, such as phenazopyridine hydrochloride. Urinary frequency and urgency can be controlled with parasympatholytic agents, such as oxybutynin chloride, tolterodine tartrate, and flavoxate hydrochloride.

24. What teaching points should be included in patient and family education about intravesical treatment?

The patient and family should understand that this treatment requires weekly visits to the clinic or physician's office for 6 to 8 weeks. At each visit, a bladder catheter will be placed, immunotherapy or chemotherapy will be instilled, and the catheter will be removed. The patient will be encouraged to retain the intravesical agent in the bladder for approximately 2 hours.

Patients should be instructed to avoid drinking an excessive amount of fluids and caffeine-containing beverages for 6 to 8 hours before and a few hours after treatment (approximately 12 hours total). Good hygiene (hand washing after voiding, cleansing of toilet with bleach) should be practiced at home to avoid exposing household members to BCG or chemotherapy agents. Men receiving BCG therapy should be instructed to use a condom and women should be instructed to avoid vaginal contact for 1 week after the treatment.

25. How is quality of life assessed in patients with bladder cancer?

Understanding a patient's perception of quality of life (QOL) can assist in making treatment decisions, particularly about the type of urinary diversion. A QOL instrument, specific to the patients with bladder cancer, is the Functional Assessment of Cancer Therapy for Bladder Cancer (FACT-Bl). Open discussion about the patient's perceptions, understanding of disease process, impact of treatment choices, and overall goals will allow the provider to achieve a better understanding of the patient's values.

26. How is sexuality affected by bladder cancer?

Body image changes associated with diagnosis and treatment may affect the patient's sexuality. For men undergoing a radical cystectomy, there is a possibility of impotence, even with the nerve-sparing technique. Most women experience discomfort during intercourse because of vaginal shrinkage. Intravesicular instillation therapy, chemotherapy, and radiation therapy may further alter the individual's sexual function. Education about these potential side effects and interventions available to assist the patient should take place throughout the care continuum. The nurse may have to directly question the patient about this issue and its impact on his or her sexuality.

27. What is on the horizon for bladder cancer?

- A change in the grading system will take place over the next 3 years—the WHO (World Health Organization) 1973 histological classification of urinary tract tumors will be replaced by the new WHO system.
- The term *urothelial* will be used instead of *transitional cell.*
- The use of fluorescent rather than white light with cystoscopy (standard in Europe) will be introduced. White light cystoscopy is not adequate to detect all urothelial neoplasia.
- Ongoing research should identify proteins that signify the initial onset of disease as well as reveal resistant disease, allowing for patient-specific treatment options.
- Early studies using intravesical gemcitabine as adjuvant treatment show promise.
- Areas of interest are dose dense chemotherapy and application of newer targeted agents in combination with chemotherapy.

Key Points

- Cigarette smoking is the greatest risk factor for bladder cancer.
- Radical cystectomy is still recommended, but bladder preservation can be considered when the disease and patient status permit.
- The search continues to find the most effective and least toxic chemotherapy regimen for the treatment of metastatic disease.
- Initial patient education regarding the disease process and treatment options is important in addressing quality of life.

Internet Resources

National Comprehensive Cancer Network, Clinical Practice Guidelines in Oncology, Bladder Cancer:
  http://www.nccn.org/professionals/physician_gls/PDF/bladder.pdf
National Comprehensive Cancer Network, Bladder Cancer Treatment Guidelines for Patients:
  http://www.nccn.org/patients/patient_gls/_english/_bladder/contents.asp
National Cancer Institute, Bladder Cancer:
  http://www.cancer.gov/cancertopics/types/bladder
American Urological Association Foundation:
  http://www.auafoundation.org/
United Ostomy Associations of America:
  http://www.uoaa.org/

Bibliography

Boyer M, Petrylak DP: Adjuvant chemotherapy for transitional cell carcinoma of the bladder: Paradigms for the design of clinical trials. *Curr Oncol Rep* 7(3):207-214, 2005.
Carrion R, Seigne MB: Surgical management of bladder carcinoma. *Cancer Control* 9(4):284-292, 2002.
Chen YC, Su HJ, Guo YL, et al: Interaction between environmental tobacco smoke and arsenic methylation ability on the risk of bladder cancer. *Cancer Causes Control* 16(2):75-81, 2005.
Del Muro XG, Munoz J, Condom E, et al: p21 and p53 as prognostic factors for bladder preservation and survival in patients with bladder cancer treated with neoadjuvant chemotherapy. Program and abstracts of the American Society of Clinical Oncology 38th Annual Meeting, May 18-21, 2002; Orlando, FL, Abs 712.
Engelking C, Sauerland C: Maintenance of normal elimination. In Watkins-Bruner D, Moore-Higgs G, Haas M, editors: *Outcomes in radiation therapy (multidisciplinary management)*, Sudbury, MA, 2001, Jones and Bartlett.
Galsky M: The role of taxanes in the management of bladder cancer. *Oncologist* 10:792-798, 2005.
Gray M, and Sims T: NMP-22 for bladder cancer screening and surveillance. *Urol Nurs* 24(3):171-172, 177-179, 186, 2004.
Greene FL, Page DL, Fleming ID, et al: *AJCC Cancer staging manual*, ed 6, New York, 2002, Springer.
Grossman HB, Natale RB, Tangen CM, et al: Neoadjuvant chemotherapy plus cystectomy compared with cystectomy alone for locally advanced bladder cancer. *N Engl J Med* 349:859-866, 2003.
Herr HW. Transurethral resection of muscle-invasive bladder cancer: 10-year outcome. *J Clin Oncol* 19:89-93, 2001.
Jemal A, Siegel R, Ward E, et al: Cancer statistics, 2007. *CA Cancer J Clin* 57:43-66, 2007.
Jichlinski P, Leisinger H: Fluorescence cystoscopy in the management of bladder cancer: A help for the urologist. *Urol Int* 74:97-101, 2005.
Karakiewicz PI, Shariat SF, Rogers CG, et al: A prognostic tool to identify patients at high risk of relapse at 2, 5, and 8 years after cystectomy for transitional cell carcinoma of the urinary bladder: Nomogram development and internal validation. Program and abstracts of the American Urological Association Annual Meeting; May 21-26, 2005. San Antonio, TX, Abs 1116.

King CR: Introduction: Improving oncology nursing through advances in quality-of-life issues. *Oncol Nurs Forum* 33(1supp):3-12, 2006.

Lamm D, McGee W, Hale K: Bladder cancer: Current optimal intravesical treatment. *Urol Nurs* 25(5): 323-332, 2005.

Lehmann J, Retz M, Wiemers C, et al: Adjuvant cisplatin plus methotrexate versus methotrexate, vinblastine, epirubicin, and cisplatin in locally advanced bladder cancer: Results of a randomized, multicenter, phase III trial (AUO-AB 05/95). *J Clin Oncol* 23(22):4963-4974, 2005.

Meliani E, Lapini A, Serni S, et al: Gemcitabine plus cisplatin in adjuvant regimen for bladder cancer: Toxicity evaluation. *Urol Int* 71(1):37-40, 2003.

National Comprehensive Cancer Network (NCCN). Clinical practice guidelines in oncology –v.1.2006 Bladder cancer. Available at: www.nccn.org/professionals/physician_gls/PDF/bladder.pdf. Retrieved November 9, 2005.

O'Donnell MA, Krohn J, DeWolf WC: Salvage intravesical therapy with interferon-alpha 2b plus low dose bacillus Calmette-Guerin is effective in patients with superficial bladder cancer in whom bacillus Calmette-Guerin alone previously failed. *Journal of Urology* 166(4):1300-1304, 2001.

Pashos CL, Botteman MF, Laskin BL, et al: Bladder cancer: Epidemiology, diagnosis, and management. *Cancer Pract* 10(2):311-322, 2002.

Pectasides D, Pectasides M, Nikolaou M: Adjuvant and neoadjuvnat chemotherapy in muscle invasive bladder cancer: Literature review. *Eur Urol* 48(1):60-7, 2005.

Porter MP, Wei JT, Penson DF: Quality of life issues in bladder cancer patients following cystectomy and urinary diversion. *Urol Clin North Am* 32(2):207-216, 2005.

Serretta V, Galuffo A, Pavone C, et al: Gemcitabine in intravesical treatment of Ta-T1 transitional cell carcinoma of bladder: Phase I-II study on marker lesions. *Urology* 65(1):65-69, 2005.

Shariat SF, Tokunaga H, Zhou J, et al: p53, p21, pRB, and p16 expression predict clinical outcome in cystectomy with bladder cancer. *J Clin Oncol* 22(6):1014-24, 2004.

Sternberg CN, Calabro F: Adjuvant chemotherapy for bladder cancer. *Expert Rev Anticancer Ther* 5(6):987-92, 2005.

Tolley DA, Parmar MK, Grigor KM, et al: The effect of intravesical mitomycin C on recurrence of newly diagnosed superficial bladder cancer: A further report with 7 years follow-up. *Journal of Urology,* 155:1233-38, 1996.

Torres-Rocca JF: Bladder preservation protocols in the treatment of muscle-invasive bladder cancer. *Cancer Control* 11(6):358-363, 2004.

Wu X: Urothelial tumor genesis: A tale of divergent pathways. *Nat Rev Cancer* 5(9):713-725, 2005.

Bone and Soft Tissue Sarcomas

Ioana Hinshaw and Kyle M. Fink

Quick Facts

Incidence	**Rare tumors**: < 1% of all cancers
	2370 newly diagnosed bone sarcoma (1330 in men; 1040 in women) and 9220 newly diagnosed soft tissue sarcoma (5050 in men; 4170 in women) cases estimated in 2007
Mortality	1330 bone sarcoma and 3560 soft tissue sarcoma deaths estimated in 2007
Risk factors	Prior radiation therapy, exposure to certain herbicides, prior treatment with alkylating agents, cumulative chemotherapy associated with secondary malignant neoplasms (osteosarcoma and soft tissue sarcomas); chronic lymphedema (angiosarcoma)
Genetics	Rarely, genetically inherited diseases such as von Recklinghausen's disease (increased risk [7%-10%] for neurofibrosarcomas), Paget's disease (increased risk for osteosarcoma), familial retinoblastoma (increased risk of osteosarcoma)
Histopathology	Bone sarcomas (tissue of origin)
	Osteosarcoma (bone)
	Ewing's sarcoma (bone marrow)
	Chondrosarcoma (cartilage)
	Malignant fibrous histiocytoma (MFH) of bone (spindle cell connective tissue)
	Soft tissue sarcomas (at least 70 histologic subtypes)
	Liposarcoma (fat)
	Rhabdomyosarcoma (striated, skeletal muscle)
	Leiomyosarcoma (smooth muscle)
	Malignant fibrous histiocytoma (fibrous, soft tissue)
	Angiosarcoma (blood vessels)
Symptoms	Local pain, soft tissue swelling, palpable mass
Diagnosis and evaluation	History and physical examination
	Alkaline phosphatase, LDH
	CT
	MRI
	Bone scan
	Chest x-ray
	Biopsy (open incisional)

Continued

Quick Facts—cont'd

Staging and Stage Grouping	
Stage	**Description**

Tumor, node, metastasis (TNM)

Primary tumor (T)

TX	Primary tumor cannot be assessed
T0	No evidence of primary tumor
T1	Tumor confined within the cortex, ≤ 8 cm (bone); ≤ 5 cm (soft tissue)
T2	Tumor invades beyond the cortex, > 8 cm (bone); > 5 cm (soft tissue)

Regional lymph nodes (N)

NX	Regional lymph nodes cannot be assessed
N0	No regional lymph node metastases
N1	Regional lymph node metastases

Distant metastasis (M)

MX	Presence of distant metastasis cannot be assessed
M0	No distant metastases
M1	Distant metastasis

Histopathologic grade

GX	Grade cannot be assessed
G1	Well differentiated
G2	Moderately differentiated
G3	Poorly differentiated
G4	Undifferentiated

NOTE: Ewing's sarcoma is classified as G4

Stage	Histopathologic Grade	Primary Tumor	Regional Lymph Nodes	Distant Metastasis
IA	G1, 2	T1	N0	M0
IB	G1, 2	T2	N0	M0
IIA	G3, 4	T1	N0	M0
IIB	G3, 4	T2	N0	M0
III	Any G	T3	N0	M0
IVA	Any G	Any T	N1	M1a (lung mets)
IVB	Any G	Any T	Any N	Any M

Used with permission of the American Joint Committee on Cancer (AJCC), Chicago, Illinois. The original source for this material is the AJCC Cancer Staging Handbook, Sixth Edition (2002) published by Springer New York, www.sprinfleronline.com.

1. What are sarcomas?

Sarcomas are a group of malignant tumors that originate from a common embryologic ancestry, the primitive mesoderm. During embryogenesis the mesoderm gives rise to soft tissues (e.g., muscles, tendons, fibrous tissue) as well as bone and cartilage. Sarcomas are tumors derived from any of these structures.

2. When do sarcomas related to previous radiation therapy occur?

Radiation therapy-related sarcomas, more common after high doses of radiation, tend to be high grade and occur more than 10 years after the exposure. Their distribution includes the sternum, sternoclavicular joint, cervical and thoracic spine, and soft tissue areas in the radiation fields used for treatment of lymphomas, seminomas, and Hodgkin lymphoma.

3. What are the most common sarcomas in adults and children?

In adults the most common sarcomas are malignant fibrous histiosarcoma, liposarcoma, leiomyosarcoma, and osteosarcoma. Children most often have rhabdomyosarcoma, osteosarcoma, or Ewing's sarcoma.

4. Describe the importance of histologic grade in sarcomas.

Histologic grade is of paramount importance in evaluating the aggressiveness of sarcomas and is included in the pathology report along with the histopathologic type. The grade may be low, intermediate, or high (most aggressive). High-grade tumors more often have distant metastasis and are associated with a lower survival rate. Low-grade tumors, in general, have a better prognosis. The histopathologic grade is based on the degree of differentiation, cellularity, number of mitoses, pleomorphism, and amount of necrosis.

5. Describe the clinical presentation of patients with sarcomas.

The early symptoms of sarcomas are nonspecific and include mild pain and mild soft tissue swelling; they are often attributed to local trauma, which leads to frequent delays in diagnosis. Eventually they grow to form palpable masses. Of interest, in osteosarcoma the pain precedes the soft tissue swelling and is caused by stretching of the periosteum by the tumor.

6. What steps are necessary in the diagnosis and staging of sarcomas?

- **CT and/or MRI of the affected area.** MRI is the most sensitive imaging modality because the images have very high resolution, which facilitates accurate distinctions between normal and abnormal tissues.
- **Open incisional biopsy.** Although fine-needle aspiration (FNA) and core biopsy can give a diagnosis of malignancy, they rarely provide the exact histopathologic type and grade of the tumor. The incision should be made (by the surgeon who will excise the tumor) in a direction that allows incorporation into the subsequent excision, which prevents local recurrence.
- **Complete staging to define the extent of disease.** CT of the chest and bone scan are most commonly done to exclude metastases in these two most frequent sites of distant spread.

7. How does staging differ between bone and soft tissue sarcomas?

Bone sarcomas are staged using the TNM system, with the additional factor of presence of discontinuous tumor in the primary bone site. The staging of soft tissue sarcoma depends on tumor size, pathologic grade, location (superficial vs. deep), presence or absence of lymph node involvement, and distant metastasis. The grade and size of the malignancy have greater bearing on treatment planning and prognosis than any other characteristic of the disease.

8. What are the most important prognostic factors in sarcomas?

The TNM stage has direct influence on 5-year relative survival:

Stage I	90%
Stage II	70%
Stage III	20-50%
Stage IV	< 20%

High-grade tumors that are greater than 5 cm in diameter have a more than 50% chance of recurrence, whereas tumors less than 2 cm in diameter have an excellent prognosis, with a cure rate of approximately 90%. It is important to emphasize the poor prognosis of local recurrence, which almost always correlates with the presence of systemic disease.

9. Describe the prognosis and management of pulmonary metastasis from sarcomas.

The lung represents the most common site of distant spread of sarcomas. It is important to recognize a subset of patients who benefit from surgical resection of pulmonary metastasis. This subset includes patients whose primary tumors have been controlled, who lack extrapulmonary disease, and who have adequate cardiac and pulmonary function. Important prognostic factors are number of pulmonary nodules (preferably < 5), disease-free interval (> 1 year), and completeness of resection. Resection of up to 5 nodules or aggressive repeated removal of metastases results in a long-term disease-free survival rate of 20% to 35%.

10. Which age group and gender are most often affected by osteosarcoma?

Osteosarcoma usually affects young patients, 10 to 20 years of age, with a peak incidence around the adolescent growth spurt. The second peak occurs during the sixth decade of life. Osteosarcoma affects men more than women (male to female ratio = 1.5:1).

11. Which sites does osteosarcoma most often involve?

The knee is most often affected, and the distal femur is the most frequent primary site. The proximal tibia is second in frequency, followed by the proximal humerus.

12. What is the recommended management of osteosarcomas?

In the past osteosarcomas were treated by amputation one joint above the location of the primary tumor. Despite this mutilating surgery, survival was poor (in the range of 20%), with patients succumbing to metastatic disease. The modern approach involves preoperative (neoadjuvant) chemotherapy, followed by limb-sparing surgery and more adjuvant chemotherapy. Preoperative chemotherapy decreases the size of the tumor and permits limb-sparing surgery; most importantly, however, response to chemotherapy is a significant prognostic factor and correlates with survival. Limb salvage surgery is now possible in close to 90% of cases. Some institutions use preoperative treatment with intraarterial cisplatin with great success.

13. What is considered a good histologic response to chemotherapy in osteosarcoma? What are the clinical implications?

The response to preoperative chemotherapy, as assessed by the pathologist through examination of the surgical specimen, is correlated with long-term survival. A good pathologic response is defined as necrosis of more than 90% of the specimen. In general, patients without metastasis who have a good response to chemotherapy have a 10-year survival rate approaching 90%; the rate is much lower in patients without such a response.

14. What are the most effective drugs for treatment of osteosarcoma?

The most active drugs are high-dose methotrexate with leucovorin rescue, cisplatin, doxorubicin, cyclophosphamide, and ifosfamide. The combination of docetaxel and gemcitabine appears promising as salvage therapy and is now being evaluated in clinical trials.

15. What is the long-term prognosis for osteosarcomas?

With modern therapy the long-term survival rate is approximately 60% to 80%. The local recurrence rate is approximately 5% to 10%.

16. What is Ewing's sarcoma? How does it differ from osteosarcoma?

Ewing's sarcoma is a rare tumor of the bone that affects mainly adolescents. It differs from osteosarcoma morphologically by the presence of small, round, blue cells, as opposed to the typical spindle cells of osteosarcomas. It also has a preference for the diaphysis (midshaft) of the bone rather than the metaphysis, and tends to involve the flat bones of the pelvis, scapula, and spine in addition to the femurs. Bone metastases are more common than in osteosarcoma.

17. Describe the usual plan of therapy and prognosis in Ewing's sarcoma.

Therapy should involve a multimodal approach; the initial step is preoperative chemotherapy followed by limb-sparing surgery and adjuvant chemotherapy. The usual treatment program involves extended periods (9-12 months) of chemotherapy (ifosfamide/etoposide) and VAC (vincristine, doxorubicin, cyclophosphamide). With this approach, the long-term disease-free survival rate is approximately 70%.

18. How do you choose between limb-sparing surgery and amputation in the surgical treatment of sarcomas?

In experienced hands, limb-sparing surgery is considered safe and routine for a large number of carefully selected patients. Use of neoadjuvant chemotherapy increases the number of patients who undergo this procedure. Because limb-sparing surgery offers local control rates similar to amputation and provides better quality of life, it is the procedure of choice. However, in large and poorly differentiated tumors, the risks and benefits must be carefully weighed by the surgeon, keeping in mind that local recurrence is almost always fatal.

19. What are contraindications for limb-salvage surgery?

- Bone tumors with major neurovascular involvement
- Pathologic fracture with hematoma at tumor site
- Infection
- Muscle involvement (extensive)
- Inappropriate biopsy site
- Immature skeletal age (< 10 years; rare)

20. Where and when do soft tissue sarcomas most commonly arise?

Soft tissue sarcomas most often arise in the extremities, with more frequent involvement of the lower (38%) than upper extremities (11%); rarely are they seen in other parts of the body, such as the retroperitoneal area (15%), trunk (13%), viscera (5%-10%), and head and neck region (5%). Soft tissue sarcomas commonly appear in adults; 20% are in adults younger than age 40 years; 28% in adults aged 40 to 60 years; and 52% in adults older than 60 years.

21. To what sites do soft tissue sarcomas metastasize?

The lungs are the most frequent site (33%), followed by bones (23%) and liver (15%).

22. Describe the current therapy for soft tissue sarcomas of the extremities.

For low-grade sarcomas, the treatment is complete surgical excision with negative margins, a prerequisite for local control and cure. Low-grade sarcomas are relatively resistant to chemotherapy and radiation; therefore, these two therapies play no role in their management. High-grade sarcomas show higher response rates to chemotherapy and radiation. For small high-grade tumors, the preferred modality is still surgery; however, for larger tumors (> 5 cm in diameter) a multimodality approach that involves surgery, adjuvant chemotherapy, and radiation therapy is preferred.

23. Which chemotherapy agents are most effective against soft tissue sarcomas?

The most effective drugs are doxorubicin and ifosfamide, which have response rates of 15% to 25% when used as single agents. The preferred approach is a regimen that includes both agents; response to this regimen is positive in 40% to 50% of patients. Taxol is an effective agent for angiosarcomas. A new chemotherapy combination with docetaxel and gemcitabine has shown a high response rate in the subset of leiomyosarcomas and is currently being studied for refractory sarcomas.

24. What is GIST? How is it treated?

GIST tumors are mesenchymal tumors of the GI tract, most often arising from the stomach. They have a common precursor with the interstitial cells of Cajal (the pacemaker cells of the gut), since they both express c-kit (CD117), a transmembrane tyrosine kinase receptor. These unusual sarcomas are refractory to systemic chemotherapy, and the prognosis of patients with metastatic disease was uniformly fatal. The new drug Gleevec (imatinib mesylate) has revolutionized the treatment of this disease. The drug is a tyrosine kinase inhibitor, which targets c-kit and induces a response in the majority of patients. The drug is given orally and is generally well tolerated by patients.

 Key Points

- Histologic grade is important in evaluating the aggressiveness of sarcomas.
- Early symptoms of sarcomas include mild pain and mild soft tissue swelling.
- The lung is the most common site of distant metastasis in sarcomas.
- Limb salvage surgery is now possible in close to 90% of patients with osteosarcoma.
- For large soft tissue sarcomas, a multimodal approach involving surgery, adjuvant chemotherapy, and radiation therapy is preferred.

 Internet Resources

Sarcoma Foundation of America:
  http://www.curesarcoma.org
Medline Plus, Soft Tissue Sarcoma:
  http://www.nlm.nih.gov/medlineplus/softtissuesarcoma.html

Bibliography

Brennan MF, Singer S, Maki RG, et al: Sarcomas of the soft tissues and bone. In De Vita VT, Hellman S, Rosenberg SA: *Cancer: Principles and practice of oncology,* ed 7, Philadelphia, 2005, Lippincott-Raven.

Frustaci S, Gherlinzone F, DePaoli A, et al: Adjuvant chemotherapy for adult soft tissue sarcomas of the extremities and girdles: Results of the Italian randomized cooperative trial. *J Clin Oncol* 19(5):1238-1247, 2001.

Greene FL, Page DL, Fleming ID, et al: *AJCC Cancer staging manual,* ed 6, New York, 2002, Springer.

Hensley ML, Maki R, Venkatraman E, et al: Gemcitabine and docetaxel in patients with unresectable leiomyosarcoma: Results of a phase II trial. *J Clin Oncol* 20(12):2824-2831, 2002.

Jemal A, Siegel R, Ward E, et al: Cancer statistics, 2007. *CA Cancer J Clin* 57:43-66, 2007.

Malawer MM, Helman LJ, O'Sullivan B: Sarcomas of bone. In De Vita VT Jr, Hellman S, Rosenberg SA: *Cancer: Principles and practice of oncology,* ed 7, Philadelphia, 2005, Lippincott-Raven.

Pisters PWT, Casper ES, Mann GN, et al: Soft-tissue sarcomas. In Padzur R, editor: *Medical oncology: A comprehensive review,* Huntington, NY, 2005.

Wilkins RM, Cullen JW, Camozzi AB, et al: Improved survival in primary nonmetastatic pediatric osteosarcoma of the extremity. *Clin Orthop* 438:128-136, 2005.

Yaski AW, Chow W: Bone sarcomas. In Padzur R, editor: *Medical oncology: A comprehensive review,* Huntington, NY, 2005.

Brain Tumors

Susanne K. Cook and Denise M. Damek

Quick Facts

Incidence	20,500 newly diagnosed cases estimated in 2007 (11,170 in men; 9330 in women)
Mortality	12,740 deaths estimated in 2007
Risk factors	High-dose radiation exposure
Genetics	Familial syndromes comprise 5%-10% of cases
Histopathology	Glial tumors
	Low grade
	Astrocytoma
	Oligodendroglioma
	Mixed neuronal glial (ganglioglioma)
	High grade (anaplastic, diffuse)
	Glioblastoma multiforme
	Gliosarcoma
	Anaplastic astrocytoma
	Anaplastic oligodendroglioma
	Ependymomas
	Medulloblastoma
	Primitive neuroectodermal tumors (PNETs)
	Pineoblastoma
	Neuroblastoma
	Extraaxial tumors
	Meningioma (benign or malignant, rare)
	Acoustic neuroma (vestibular schwannoma)
Symptoms	Headache, nausea, vomiting, lethargy, confusion, disorientation, seizures, papilledema, focal neurological deficit (weakness, language dysfunction, sensory loss, personality change, cognitive dysfunction, aberrant behavior), endocrine dysfunction
Diagnosis and evaluation	History and physical examination (including neurological examination)
	CT or MRI
	Biopsy and/or resection

Staging and Stage Grouping

TNM, classification is not applicable to primary brain tumors because they are locally invasive and do not spread to regional lymph nodes or distant organs.

WHO 2000 Classification (see Question 6).

1. What causes brain tumors?

The causes of most primary brain tumors are unknown. The only environmental factor clearly associated with brain tumor development is high-dose radiation exposure. The lay press frequently implicates electromagnetic fields, power lines, and cell phones in brain tumor development, but to date this remains unsubstantiated. These and other possible environmental factors, familial tendencies, and viral causes remain under investigation.

2. Who gets brain tumors?

Primary brain tumors occur in people of all ages, whereas metastatic brain tumors are more commonly diagnosed in adults.

3. Is the incidence of primary brain tumors increasing?

The incidence of primary brain tumors appears to be increasing. However, this trend may reflect improved diagnostic studies and an aging population, rather than a true increase in incidence.

4. What is the difference between benign and malignant brain tumors?

Most patients have a preconceived notion of the distinction between benign and malignant tumors that is generally correct. However, this is frequently not the case with primary brain tumors. From a clinical perspective, the location of the tumor within the brain is often a more important determinant of outcome than tumor grade alone, especially when symptom burden or clinical aggressiveness is considered. Because of their slow growth rate, histologically benign tumors may reach substantial size prior to detection. Frequently these tumors are located near critical brain structures or within eloquent brain areas, where injury causes disabling neurologic deficits. Location and size often limit surgical resection, and slow growth rate limits benefit from radiation and chemotherapy. As a result, these histologically benign tumors may cause more neurological deficits, more functional disabilities, and potentially a significantly shorter life expectancy than a malignant brain tumor.

5. How are brain tumors classified?

The World Health Organization (WHO) brain tumor classification system classifies brain tumors in groups according to their cell of origin. In most cases the tumor name reflects its cell of origin. For example, the most common group of primary brain tumors in adults, the gliomas, arise from glial cells, which include astrocytes, oligodendrocytes, and ependymal cells. Uncontrolled growth of these cells gives rise respectively to astrocytomas, oligodendrogliomas, and ependymomas. However, in some cases the tumor name is not based on the cell of origin, but on location of the tumor. Examples include such tumors as craniopharyngiomas and medulloblastomas.

6. What is the grading system for brain tumors?

Brain tumor size does not correlate with prognosis, and lymph node involvement and presence of metastases are exceedingly rare. The WHO 2000 classification system, the most commonly used grading system for primary brain tumors, provides an estimate of tumor malignancy using a scale from one to four, with four being the worst. This system reflects the degree to which a tumor's cells are different from normal cells, its growth rate, and its tendency to spread or invade surrounding tissues. Not surprisingly, the natural history of many primary brain tumors is amenable to only a benign or malignant behavior designation, not a four point scale. In these cases, the grading is generally based on the tumor subtype itself rather than a specific scale.

7. Are brain tumors hereditary or genetically linked?

Only 5% to 10% of brain tumors result from a genetic predisposition. The most common familial syndromes and the chromosomal abnormalities that may predispose a person to the development of a brain tumor are listed in the following table.

Possible predisposing factors to CNS tumor development

Familial syndrome	Chromosome/gene associated with syndrome	CNS tumor type
von Hippel-Lindau	3p 25-26/VHL	Hemangioblastomas
Neurofibromatosis 1	17q11/NF 1	Neurofibromas, optic gliomas
Neurofibromatosis 2	22q12/NF 2	Bilateral acoustic schwannomas, multiple meningiomas, ependymomas, astrocytomas
Li-Fraumeni	17p13/p53 suppressor gene	Malignant glioma, primitive neuroectodermal tumor (PNET)
Turcot's I/II	3p21, 7p22/5q21	Glioblastoma, medulloblastoma

8. What are the survival rates for the more common brain tumors?

CNS tumor survival rates

Tumor type	5-year survival (%)	10-year survival (%)
Anaplastic astrocytoma	29.4	22.2
Glioblastoma	3.3	2.3
Anaplastic oligodendroglioma	40.1	30.1
Diffuse astrocytoma	46.9	38.7
Oligodendroglioma	70.5	53.9
Medulloblastoma (PNET)	55.7	47.1
Lymphoma, CNS	16.9	11.4
Meningiomas, benign	70	Data unavailable
Meningiomas, malignant	55	Data unavailable

9. What are the prognostic factors associated with brain tumors?

The prognosis of brain tumors varies widely and depends on the tumor type, grade, and location; the patient's performance status and age; the extent of surgical resection; and whether cancer cells have spread to other parts of the central nervous system. In malignant gliomas, factors associated with a better prognosis include age younger than 50 years, good performance status, presence of an oligodendroglial cell component within the tumor, and surgical resection of at least 80% of the tumor. More recently, the genetic profile of tumors has been correlated with prognosis in some cases. The presence of p53 mutations in malignant astrocytomas may be associated with a better prognosis. In oligodendrogliomas, the combined allelic loss of chromosome 1p and 19q is associated with chemosensitivity, recurrence-free survival, and longer overall survival.

10. What are the most common symptoms of brain tumors?

Clinical presentation and associated symptoms are determined by a tumor's location and its growth rate. Signs and symptoms may be nonlocalizing or focal. **Nonlocalizing** signs and symptoms are most commonly seen with a rapidly-growing space-occupying lesion, causing either increased intracranial pressure or obstructive hydrocephalus. These include headache, nausea, vomiting, lethargy, confusion, disorientation, generalized seizures, and papilledema. **Focal** signs and symptoms are caused by tumor invasion or compression of normal brain tissue. These include seizures, focal neurological deficit (weakness, language dysfunction, sensory loss, etc.), and endocrine dysfunction.

11. Describe headaches that occur in patients with brain tumors.

Headache is initially present in approximately 20% of the patients and will occur at some time in the disease course in 70% of patients. Headaches worrisome for increased intracranial pressure are described as an intermittent pressure sensation at the top of the head or behind the eyes, which increases in severity over days to weeks. These headaches are more prominent in the early morning and with supine body positioning, and are often precipitated by maneuvers that can increase intracranial pressure, such as exertion, coughing, sneezing, or Valsalva maneuvers. They are frequently accompanied by nausea, vomiting, and lethargy.

12. What is the significance of seizures?

Seizures commonly herald the diagnosis of slow growing or superficially located tumors, such as oligodendrogliomas, brain metastases, and meningiomas. Seizures can also occur following a neurosurgical procedure. The first symptoms in 15% of all patients with brain tumors are seizures, and approximately 30% will eventually develop seizures. Focal seizures and complex partial seizures are most commonly reported; but primary and secondarily generalized seizures are also seen (see Question 32).

13. How is a brain tumor diagnosed?

Diagnosing a brain tumor involves a thorough neurological exam. A CT or MRI scan will be performed. MRI provides better definition between intracranial tumors and normal brain tissue, and can better depict edema or swelling surrounding the tumor. However, calcification in the brain and acute hemorrhage is better delineated by CT. Some patients may have contraindications to MRI, such as a cardiac pacemaker or metal fragments in the eye. Tissue procurement is necessary to make an accurate diagnosis and assessment of tumor grade. This can be achieved by brain biopsy or tumor resection.

14. What additional imaging modalities are used to visualize brain tumors?

- **Positron emission tomography (PET) scan** allows visualization of the metabolic rate of different areas of the brain. Areas of abnormal metabolism can be identified by comparing a PET scan to a CT or MRI. Low-grade gliomas are generally hypometabolic, showing very little uptake of the metabolic marker during a PET scan. A high-grade tumor that is present within a low-grade tumor can be visualized with a PET scan. Occasionally there is question as to whether enhancement seen on MRI or CT is recurrent tumor or radiation necrosis. Recurrent high-grade tumor is usually hypermetabolic, showing increased uptake of the marker, whereas radiation necrosis is hypometabolic. Spectroscopy and blood flow studies are also useful when there is a question of recurrent tumor versus necrosis. The drawback to this study is the false negative and positives.

- **Perfusion imaging studies** measure the rate of blood flow into the brain. Cerebral blood volume, or the volume of blood passing through a portion of the brain, is the most commonly used measure of perfusion. Magnetic resonance perfusion may localize higher grade components of a tumor to guide stereotactic biopsy, and may differentiate tumor recurrence from tumor necrosis.
- **Functional MRI** is a faster-paced MRI and shows the tumor's use of oxygen. It is most often used for brain mapping, which delineates the areas of the brain that control speech, movement, or memory, so that the neurosurgeon may perform a procedure that produces maximum results and minimal injury to functioning brain.
- **Angiography and MRI angiography (MRA)** are both done to map cerebral blood vessels. Angiography is more invasive than MRA because it consists of injecting dye into a deep artery, whereas MRA uses a rapid succession of MRI scans to trace the blood flow.
- **Magnetic resonance spectroscopy (MRS)** evaluates function rather than image and measures metabolites. MRS shows patterns of activity that can be used to diagnose specific tumors, distinguish between tumor recurrence and necrosis, and determine degree of tumor malignancy.
- **Single photon emission tomography (SPECT)** is similar to PET. A camera measures the rate of radioactive material as it is emitted through the brain. SPECT is also helpful in making distinctions between low-grade and high-grade tumors, or between recurrent tumor and necrosis.

15. What is the standard therapy for brain tumors?

Treatment varies according to the biologic behavior of the tumor. Generally, the higher the tumor grade, the more aggressively the tumor is treated. Therapy is also determined by tumor location and the symptoms the patient is experiencing because of tumor effects. For benign or slow-growing tumors, a watch and wait approach is appropriate when the patient is asymptomatic. However, if detrimental consequences are imminent because of the tumor's location, or the symptoms the patient is experiencing are unacceptable, combinations of surgery, radiation, and chemotherapy may be offered. Malignant brain tumors are treated at the time of tumor detection with combinations of surgery, radiation, and chemotherapy.

16. What is the role of surgery in the management of brain tumors?

The purpose of surgery is to establish a tumor diagnosis, provide a cure, minimize tumor bulk, and decrease an area that requires further treatment. Total or partial tumor resection can also relieve mass-related symptoms, which helps decrease the need for steroids. Surgery can also be used to provide other treatments, such as chemotherapy-impregnated wafers and vaccine therapy.

17. What neurosurgical procedures are performed for tumor diagnosis or treatment?

- **Open biopsy** removes a small piece of tissue during surgery to make a diagnosis.
- **Needle biopsy** involves making a skin incision, drilling a small hole through the skull, and inserting a hollow needle to draw up a sample of the tumor for pathologic analysis.
- **Stereotactic needle biopsy,** useful for deep or multiple tumors, is a needle biopsy achieved using a combination of computers and MRI/CT equipment to help the neurosurgeon accurately target the lesion.
- **Stereotactic surgery** (see Question 21)

- **Craniotomy** is done to surgically remove a tumor. The tumor is exposed by penetrating the scalp and bone with saws and drills. The dura is opened, the tumor removed, the bone is replaced, and the scalp is sutured.
- **Ventriculoperitoneal (VP) shunt** is placed to relieve increased intracranial pressure caused by a blockage of cerebrospinal fluid flow through the brain. Excess fluid is drained through a tube that is placed into a ventricle and then threaded into a body cavity, where the fluid drains and is absorbed.

18. What surgical tools do neurosurgeons use to perform these procedures?

Brain mapping tools provide additional benefit to presurgical scans. The computer-assisted techniques allow real-time intraoperative guidance by linking image data to the surgical area. This allows for a more aggressive surgery, sparing eloquent areas of the brain, and identifying the easiest access to the tumor.

- **Direct cortical stimulation** electrically stimulates a specific area of the brain and a body part may visibly move in response.
- **Somatosensory evoked potentials (SSEP)** measures the electrical response of a stimulated area. This can be used to map the eloquent areas of the brain, which can then be avoided during surgery, and allows for the most extensive surgery possible.
- **Functional MRI** (see question 14)
- **Intraoperative ultrasound imaging** uses sound waves to determine the depth and diameter of the tumor. In addition to images being displayed on a TV screen that the surgeon uses for assistance during the procedure, this ultrasound imaging also shows blood flow, and is helpful in distinguishing between tumor, necrosis, cysts, edema, and normal brain tissue.
- **Embolization** decreases the amount of blood flow to the tumor. It is beneficial with highly vascularized tumors such as meningiomas or hemangiopericytomas.
- **Neuroendoscopes** are long, narrow, flexible tubes that the neurosurgeon uses to access areas of the brain through small openings. They are commonly used when a procedure is being performed on the ventricles.

19. How are stereotactic biopsy and stereotactically-guided craniotomy accomplished?

A spherical open frame (similar to a cervical stabilization device) is pinned to the skull, and the patient is taken for a CT or MRI scan. The films delineate the tumor and points of reference on the frame. With the aid of a computer program, the three-dimensional coordinates of the lesion are determined. During surgery, a special frame with degree markings is placed over the head and attached to the stereotactic halo. A needle is attached to the frame at a precise degree and trajectory and then passed to the target. If a biopsy is indicated, the target is usually the center of the lesion. Multiple samples are taken to ensure that representative tissue is obtained. If a craniotomy is indicated, the periphery of the lesion is targeted. During the craniotomy, the needle points to the edges of the lesion. A stereotactically guided craniotomy is indicated when the tumor is close to critical areas and the consistency of the tissue makes it difficult for the surgeon to differentiate between tumor and normal brain.

20. What is the role of radiation in the management of brain tumors?

Radiotherapy may be the treatment of choice, rather than surgery, if the tumor is deemed unresectable because it is located in an eloquent area of the brain or is too large and would cause extensive postsurgical deficits. Radiotherapy is beneficial as an adjunct to surgery (after optimal tumor removal), and increases the survival of patients with malignant gliomas.

21. What are the types of radiotherapy available for brain tumors?

- **Conventional radiation** can be initiated soon after surgery, when the surgical wound has healed. The radiation dose is limited by the risk of tissue necrosis and radiation injury. In general, the larger the treated area, the lower the tolerated radiation dose. Limitations of radiotherapy are cell resistance (hypoxia) and normal tissue tolerance. Radiosensitization with chemotherapy may help overcome this resistance.
- **Conformal radiation** therapy is external beam radiation shaped to the contour of the tumor in three dimensions, minimizing radiation exposure to surrounding tissue.
- **Brachytherapy** is often used for local disease control as a focal boost after conventional radiation. Sources of radiation are implanted directly into the tumor, minimizing radiation exposure to normal tissue.
- **Stereotactic radiosurgery** delivers high doses of radiation from an external source, either linear accelerator (LINAC), gamma knife, or heavy charged particle beams, (i.e., proton beam), to a targeted area and spares surrounding tissue. It can be used after conventional radiation therapy as a boost to the tumor site, at tumor recurrence, or for brain metastases. Despite its name, the procedure is noninvasive and requires no surgery. The benefit of stereotactic radiosurgery over brachytherapy is that it is less invasive.

22. What is the role of chemotherapy in the management of brain tumors?

Chemotherapy is used as adjuvant therapy to surgery and/or radiotherapy to kill remaining cancer cells, which should minimize tumor mass and the corresponding associated deficits. The success of chemotherapy depends on both the growth rate of the tumor and its inherent chemosensitivity. Slowly dividing tumor cells or benign tumors generally do not respond to chemotherapy; the rapidly dividing cells found in such diseases as CNS lymphoma or germ cell tumors are exquisitely sensitive. Unfortunately, most malignant brain tumors are relatively chemoresistant. However, because some tumors respond to chemotherapy, it is often offered to patients with malignant brain tumors. Attempts to identify patients that may benefit from chemotherapy before treatment have been of variable success. The response of oligodendroglial tumors to chemotherapy loosely correlates with the loss of heterozygosity of the 1p and 19q chromosomes. However, the absence of this genetic finding does not necessarily correlate with a negative treatment result. Additional factors, such as patient's age, functional status, and quality of life must also be considered in the decision to pursue chemotherapy.

23. What are the most commonly used chemotherapy regimens?

Until recently, intravenous carmustine (BCNU) as a single agent, and combination oral PCV (procarbazine, lomustine [CCNU], and vincristine) were standard therapies for high grade gliomas. Now Gliadel, biodegradable wafers impregnated with BCNU, can be implanted into the tumor resection site at the time of surgery. Temozolomide (Temodar) has been approved for treatment of anaplastic astrocytomas, recurrent glioblastomas (Grade IV astrocytomas). As of 2006 temozolomide is also FDA approved as first line therapy for glioblastomas. It is also used as a radiosensitizer with radiation therapy.

24. What is the blood-brain barrier and how does this affect chemotherapy treatment?

The blood-brain barrier (BBB) is a filter mechanism which protects the brain from toxic or foreign substances by blocking their passage from blood into the central nervous system. Although it is advantageous to healthy individuals, in brain tumor patients it prevents many chemotherapeutic agents from entering the brain. However, some chemotherapeutic agents adequately cross the BBB, including temozolomide, carmustine, lomustine, procarbazine, thiotepa, and high dose methotrexate. Approaches to bypass the BBB include the use of agents such as mannitol to temporarily disrupt the BBB in combination with intraarterial drug instillation, allowing chemotherapy agents to penetrate the brain.

25. How are recurrent brain tumors treated?

Most recurrences appear within 2 cm of the original resection site. The mass should be treated as a newly diagnosed tumor. Biopsy should be used to verify the pathologic diagnosis if there is a concern for treatment-related necrosis or infection versus tumor recurrence. Surgical resection may be offered depending on location (focal versus multifocal), extent of invasion, and size. Stereotactic radiotherapy may be an option. Chemotherapy is often provided. The choice of chemotherapeutic agent depends on the time of recurrence—during therapy, immediately after, or after an extended time. If the recurrence is found in the midst of treatment, changing the dosing schedule of the present therapy may be changed or it may be necessary to switch to another agent. If there is a significant time between the completion of chemotherapy and recurrence, reinitiation of a previous chemotherapeutic regimen is an option. If the time between treatment and recurrence is brief, generally the approach would be to select another chemotherapeutic agent or explore admission to clinical trials. Chemotherapeutic agents that may be used, individually or in combination, are carboplatin or cisplatin, high doses of tamoxifen, retinoic acid, etoposide, thalidomide, celecoxib (Celebrex), irinotecan, topotecan, and paclitaxel.

26. What novel treatment options are on the horizon?

Progress in the treatment of brain tumors has been slow; in the past decade, however, neurooncology has gained the attention of the health care community. New efforts focus on basic science as well as clinical research. Both local and systemic approaches are under evaluation:
- Tumor vaccines
- Biologic response modifiers
- High-dose chemotherapy with bone marrow rescue
- Gene therapy
- Steroid-sparing agents
- Antiangiogenic agents

27. What tumor-related symptoms might patients with a brain tumor experience?

Management of brain tumor–related symptoms

Tumor related symptoms	Time course	Management
Increased intracranial pressure (ICP) due to edema	At presentation or recurrence	Steroids Surgical tumor debulking or resection Mannitol
Increased ICP due to obstruction of cerebrospinal fluid (CSF) flow	At presentation or recurrence	Ventriculoperitoneal (VP) shunt placement Surgical tumor resection or debulking

Management of brain tumor-related symptoms—cont'd

Tumor related symptoms	Time course	Management
Seizures	At any time	Anticonvulsant medication therapies
		Surgical procedures
Focal neurological deficits	At presentation or tumor recurrence	Steroids
		Surgical tumor resection or debulking
		Radiation therapy
		Chemotherapy
		Physical therapy, occupational therapy, speech therapy

28. What side effects can occur in patients with brain tumors who are receiving radiation therapy?

Onset of radiation therapy side effects

Radiation therapy side effects	Acute reactions (during treatment)	Early delayed (2-4 months after therapy)	Late > 90 days after therapy
Alopecia	+		
Skin changes (dry desquamation, wet desquamation)	+		
Mucositis	+		
Fatigue	±	+	
Cognitive side effects			+
Radiation necrosis			+
Nausea/vomiting	+		
Encephalopathy	+		
Cerebral edema	+		
Myelosuppression	+		
Somnolence syndrome		+	
Transient focal neurologic symptoms		+	
White matter injury		±	+
Neurocognitive effects			+
Ophthalmic injury			+
Auditory injury			+
Radiation-induced tumors			+

29. Why are corticosteroids given to patients with brain tumors?

Patients with brain tumors may experience neurologic deficits or symptoms of increased intracranial pressure (headache, nausea, vomiting) caused by mass effect of the tumor plus surrounding edema. The edema is caused by abnormal blood vessels within the tumor, which allow fluid to leak from the intravascular space into surrounding brain tissue. Corticosteroids decrease the area of edema and improve symptoms, often dramatically. Corticosteroids are believed to improve the intercellular adherence of endothelial cells within the tumor blood vessels, thereby lessening leakage of fluid into the surrounding brain. This in turn decreases the abnormal mass effect responsible for symptoms.

30. Which corticosteroid is used and how is it dosed?

Effective management of peritumoral edema often requires steroids in doses that exceed standard recommendations. Dexamethasone (Decadron) is the steroid of choice because it has the most favorable side effect profile at the required doses compared to other available steroid medications (long half life, lower incidence of cognitive and behavioral side effects, and less peripheral edema). An average dose for patients who have neurologic symptoms is 2 to 4 mg of dexamethasone provided orally every 6 hours. There is rarely any benefit of exceeding a daily dose of 40 mg. For comparison, 1 mg of dexamethasone is equivalent to approximately 20 mg of prednisone.

31. What are the side effects of corticosteroids?

- **Acute side effects:** weight gain, fluid retention, increased appetite, sleep disturbance (insomnia), fatigue when the steroids are discontinued, gastric dyspepsia, and behavioral and personality changes (steroid psychosis)
- **Long-term side effects**: proximal myopathy; fragile skin; chemically induced diabetes; electrolyte imbalances, such as hypokalemia and hyponatremia; susceptibility to infection; hypertension; Cushingoid syndrome; osteoporosis; cataracts; and osteonecrosis.

32. How are seizures classified?

There are two main classifications of seizures— **Partial (focal)** and **Generalized:**

PARTIAL (FOCAL) SEIZURES

- **Simple partial seizure.** Loss of consciousness does not occur. Partial seizures are sometimes further subclassified as sensory or motor. Symptoms can start in one area of the body and spread to other areas. Psychic symptoms may occur, such as déjà vu, and imaginary sights, sounds, smells, or tastes.
- **Complex partial seizure.** Loss of consciousness does occur. A glazed look or inability to get the individual's attention with vigorous attempts can occur. Also lip smacking, eye blinking, and hand fumbling may be observed.

GENERALIZED SEIZURES

- **Generalized tonic-clonic (grand mal) seizure.** A recognizable or remembered focal onset may or may not be present. Loss of consciousness occurs and is followed by tonic (extending) and clonic (relaxing) muscle contractions. During the seizure, patients may bite their tongue, have a change in breathing pattern, and experience bowel or bladder incontinence. After seizure activity has resolved, the patient may experience lethargy, confusion, or sore muscles. This period is referred to as the postictal state.

33. When should patients be taken to the emergency room for seizures?

- If they injure themselves
- If they have difficulty breathing

- If a generalized tonic clonic seizure lasts longer than 10 minutes
- If a second seizure occurs immediately

34. Do all patients with a brain tumor require anticonvulsant therapy?

Anticonvulsants are often prescribed, depending on the physician's judgment and whether the patient has had a seizure. Seizures are caused by irritation to the brain cortex. The brain tumor functions as an irritant, as can normal scar formation after a craniotomy. Even if anticonvulsants are not prescribed for long-term use, most patients receive a bolus before surgery, which is continued for 3 to 4 weeks postoperatively. Patients who experience a seizure are likely to continue taking anticonvulsants for a longer period.

35. Do patients have to remain on anticonvulsants for life?

If a patient remains seizure-free, anticonvulsants may be stopped after 6 months or 1 year. Although anticonvulsants may be stopped abruptly, often they are tapered to reduce the risk of severe seizures. In patients with brain tumors, attention should be paid to all minor complaints, which in fact may represent unrecognized seizure activity. Seizures occur in various forms and degrees and often are not identified as seizures by the patient or family.

36. What should patients be told about taking anticonvulsants?

The anticonvulsants most commonly used by patients with brain tumor are phenytoin (Dilantin), carbamazepine (Tegretol), and levetiracetam (Keppra). These drugs must be taken for 5 to 10 days to reach a therapeutic blood level. The patient should take a missed dose if it is remembered on the same day. If a day has passed, the patient should not try to make up the dose and should *not* take a double dose! Taking anticonvulsants does not preclude a safe pregnancy. Discussion with the treating physician about pregnancy and the best anticonvulsants to use will help a patient with this decision. Anticonvulsants may limit the efficacy of oral contraceptive pills, underscoring the need for using two methods of contraception.

37. What are the side effects of anticonvulsants?

The most common side effects are slurred speech, gait imbalance, nausea, vomiting, and increased drowsiness. Major toxicities include nystagmus, dysarthria, hypotension, and coma (rare). If a patient develops a skin rash, the drug should be stopped immediately. Because the rash may become severe, even life-threatening (Stevens-Johnson syndrome), the patient should be told to call the physician immediately. Anticonvulsants are often metabolized by the liver; therefore, laboratory tests for liver function should be evaluated with reported symptoms, and at least annually. Often, combinations of drugs are used if a single agent is not effective. Other anticonvulsant agents that are available include clonazepam (Klonopin), gabapentin (Neurontin), valproic acid (Depakote), lamotrigine (Lamictal), zonisamide (Zonegran), and topiramate (Topomax).

38. Which cognitive impairments are most common?

- **Reasoning and judgment** may decline before patients are diagnosed. For example, a business owner may make poor decisions, not follow through with plans, or fail to meet deadlines. If there are no other overt symptoms of the brain tumor, the business may become bankrupt before someone challenges the owner's judgment or recognizes the problem.
- **Executive functioning** is the management of time, setting goals, planning, organizing, and "multi-tasking." These deficits make it difficult for a patient to function professionally.

- **Lack of initiative** is particularly common in patients with frontal lobe tumors. For example, the patient is aware that he or she needs to do something but cannot get started. The family may think that the patient is lazy or obstinate, and the supervisor at work knows only that the job is not getting done. Often relationships at work and home suffer, and the patient may be fired or divorced before the brain tumor is diagnosed. Activating agents such as methylphenidate (Ritalin) or modafinil (Provigil) may be prescribed to help alleviate symptoms related to this impairment.
- **Lack of awareness** is also a common neurologic deficit. If a family member tries to point out such deficits, the patient may refuse to believe that anything is wrong. Although the patient does not intend to be obstinate, this situation becomes exasperating for both patient and family member.
- **Short-term memory deficit** may complicate the lack of awareness. The patient asks the same question repeatedly and cannot follow through on tasks, because he or she does not remember. Many of these symptoms are similar to those of Alzheimer's disease.
- **Personality change** is particularly difficult for the family. Roles usually change because the patient cannot perform normal physical tasks or offer the usual emotional support and companionship. Antipsychotic medications may be prescribed in an attempt to minimize hostile or aggressive behavior that can occur with personality changes.

39. Should patients with brain tumors be allowed to drive?

Patients and families often ask when it is safe for the patient to drive. Reasons for restriction of driving privileges include seizures, cognitive deficits that affect processing information and judgment, impaired coordination, and visual field deficits. If a patient has had a seizure, many states have laws that restrict driving for 3 to 12 months. Although each state differs, most require a physician's approval for resumption of driving privileges. Rehabilitation programs often offer a safe driving evaluation. Removing the privilege to drive is one of the most difficult restrictions placed on a patient. It is a loss of autonomy that is met with passionate resistance. The patient who is not fit to drive but lacks awareness of deficits may resist the judgment of family and physician.

40. What are some common questions patients call about and what information is key to effective triage?

Telephone communication with the patient's caregiver is frequently necessary. Phone triage can be instrumental in helping patients and caregivers determine the best action to take: can the patient be managed at home, do they require evaluation at the physician's office, or does the patient need to report to the emergency room?

"I JUST FINISHED MY TREATMENT AND I FEEL AS BAD, IF NOT WORSE. WHY?"
The patient may feel worse for awhile after completion of therapy. Treatment itself may be responsible for this. Radiation therapy can cause swelling or edema that worsens symptoms. Reinitiating steroids, or if the patient is already taking steroids, increasing the dose for a brief time may minimize symptoms. Also, if steroid dosage is being tapered, symptoms may be exacerbated. Returning to a previously effective dose that controlled symptoms may be helpful before continuing the taper. Chemotherapy side effects, fatigue, nausea, vomiting, sleep disturbances, and dietary changes may also be contributing factors.

"I HAVEN'T HAD A SEIZURE IN A LONG TIME, BUT I DID TODAY. DO I NEED AN MRI?"
Not necessarily. Ask for explicit details about the event—length of time, body parts involved, loss of consciousness, incontinence, recent stress, long distance travel, and sleep disruption. Is this a random event or has this been occurring with some frequency? Determine if the patient missed any medication doses. If they have, taking the correct dose may be all that is necessary. If they assure you no doses have been missed, measuring the serum antiepileptic drug level may reveal that it is too low and a dose increase is needed. Approximately 5 days after changing a medication dose, a serum drug level should be drawn again to determine if the drug is at a therapeutic level. If questioning reveals worsening symptoms that are unexplained by these questions, an MRI may be the appropriate action.

"I TOOK MY FIRST DOSE OF TEMODAR AND EXPERIENCED A LOT OF VOMITING. WHAT SHOULD I DO?"
Determine if and when the patient took the prescribed antiemetics. If he/she took antiemetic medication before the chemotherapy, repeating a dose may be helpful. Explain that after the first few doses of chemotherapy, tolerance may occur and the side effects may resolve. Should symptoms continue, a combination of antiemetics may be helpful, such as ondansetron, lorazepam, and/or diphenhydramine.

"ALL OF A SUDDEN I HAVE A RASH. COULD THIS BE FROM ONE OF THE MEDICATIONS I'M TAKING?"
Think about the most simple explanation first, such as contact dermatitis. Has there been a change in detergents, soaps, or clothing? It could be a side effect of one or more drugs, such as steroids, antiseizure drugs (particularly phenytoin), and oral chemotherapy agents (temozolomide, gefitinib [Iressa], erlotinib [Tarceva]). Topical treatment may be all that is necessary. Drug-related rash may require discontinuation of the medication or treatment with steroids. Herpes zoster can occur with immunosuppression and can be treated with antiviral and pain medications.

"CAN I FLY WHILE I'M BEING TREATED FOR A BRAIN TUMOR?"
Yes. The cabin of the airplane is pressurized but not generally at the same level as ground pressure. A small dose of steroids immediately before and after flying can help with symptoms induced by pressure changes or neurologic symptoms such as headache.

 Key Points

- Some brain tumors arise from many different cell types (polyclonal); most tumors arise from one cell type (monoclonal).
- Brain tumor recurrence is generally within 2 cm of the original tumor.
- Brain tumor size does not correlate with prognosis.
- Brain tumors do not metastasize outside of the central nervous system.
- Symptoms depend on tumor size, location, and extent of ICP.
- The blood-brain barrier protects the brain, but it also prevents many treatment agents from entering the brain.
- Multimodal treatment includes: surgery, adjuvant radiation, and chemotherapy.
- Damaged tumor tissue (necrosis) may appear identical to a growing tumor on a radiograph.

Internet Resources

American Brain Tumor Association (ABTA):
   http://hope.abta.org/site/PageServer
   Services include a listing of support groups, pen-pal program, newsletter, and information
   about treatment facilities and research funding.
National Brain Tumor Foundation (NBTF):
   http://www.braintumor.org
   Provides free information; counseling and support services to patients with brain tumor,
   survivors, and families; newsletter; patient-to-patient telephone support line; free resource
   guide; and list of support groups.
National Comprehensive Cancer Network, Clinical Practice Guidelines in Oncology, Central
   Nervous System Cancers:
   http://www.nccn.org/professionals/physician_gls/PDF/cns.pdf
National Family Caregivers Association:
   http://www.nfcacares.org
   NFCA provides education, support, respite care, and advocacy for caregivers.

Acknowledgments

The authors wish to acknowledge Betty Owens, RN, MS, Kevin Lillehei MD, and Kim
Pollmiller, RN, MS, CNRN, for their contributions to the Brain Tumor chapter published in
the first and second editions of *Oncology Nursing Secrets*; a special acknowledgment to
Monica Robischon, RN, BSN, for her editing contributions.

Bibliography

Armstrong T, Hancock C: Temodar offers promise for treating astrocytomas. *Clin J Oncol Nurs* 4(4):
   159-160, 2000.
Armstrong TS, Kanusky JT, Gilbert MR: Seize the moment to learn about epilepsy in people with cancer.
   Clin J Oncol Nurs 7(2):163-169, 2003.
Ballonoff A, Kavanagh B: Complications of cranial irradiation. Available at: http://www.utdol.com/utd/
   content/topic.do?topicKey=rad_ther/2462&type=A&selectedTitle=1~49 Retrieved January 3, 2007.
Bauman G, Shaw EG: Low-grade glioma: Current management and controversies. *Clin Adv Hematol Oncol*
   1(9):546-553, 2003.
Birner A: Safe administration of oral chemotherapy. *Clin J Oncol Nurs* 7(2):158-162, 2003.
Brandes AA: State-of-the-art treatment of high-grade brain tumors. *Semin Oncol* 30(6), Suppl 19:4-9, 2003.
DeAngelis LM: Benefits of adjuvant chemotherapy in high-grade gliomas. *Semin Oncol* 30(6), Suppl
   19:15-18, 2003.
Fox SW, Mitchell SA, Booth-Jones M: Cognitive impairment in patients with brain tumors: Assessment and
   intervention in the clinic setting. *Clin J Oncol Nurs* 10:169-182, 2006.
Goetz C, Riva P, Poepperl G, et al: Locoregional radioimmunotherapy in selected patients with malignant
   glioma: Experiences, side effects and survival times. *J Neurooncol* 62(3):321-328, 2003.
Gordon BM, Myers JS: Leptomeningeal metastases. *Clin J Oncol Nurs* 7(2):151-155, 2003.
Jemal A, Siegel R, Ward E, et al: Cancer statistics, 2007. *CA Cancer J Clin* 57:43-66, 2007.
Kimmelman A, Liang B: Familial neurogenic tumor syndromes. *Hematol Oncol Clin North Am* 15(6):
   1073-84, 2001
Law E, Mangarin E: Nursing management of patients receiving stereotactic radiosurgery. *Clin J Oncol Nurs*
   7(4):387-392, 2003.
Moore D: Toxic leukoencephalopathy: A review and report of two chemotherapy-related cases. *Clin J Oncol
   Nurs* 7(4):413-417, 2003.
National Comprehensive Cancer Network, Clinical practice guidelines in oncology, central nervous system
   cancers, version 1, 2006. Available at: http://www.nccn.org/professionals/physician_gls/PDF/cns.pdf.
   Retrieved June 8, 2006.
Packer RJ, Mehta M: Neurocognitive sequelae of cancer treatment. *Neurology* 59:8-10, 2002.
Prados M: *Brain cancer*, BC Decker, Inc. 2002, Hamilton, Ontario, London.
Strickler R: Astrocytomas: The clinical picture. *Clin J Oncol Nurs* 4(4):153-158, 2000.

Breast Cancer

Kelly C. Mack and Dev Paul

Quick Facts

Incidence	180,510 newly diagnosed cases estimated in 2007 (2030 in men; 178,480 in women)	**Symptoms**	Firm, nontender mass, irregular without distinct borders, nonmovable, fixed to skin or deep fascia
Mortality	40,910 estimated deaths in 2007		Painless mass more common than painful mass
Risk factors	Increased age		Nipple discharge (serous or bloody), retraction, erosion
	Personal history of breast cancer		
	Early menarche, nulliparity, late menopause		Skin dimpling
	Increased age at birth of first child		Diffuse erythema of the breast
	Use of exogenous hormones		Peau d'orange (orange peel) skin
	History of atypical hyperplasia, lobular carcinoma in situ (LCIS)		Axillary or supraclavicular adenopathy
		Diagnosis and evaluation	History and physical examination (axillary and supraclavicular lymph node exam)
	Family history		
	Radiation exposure		Mammography
	Obesity		Ultrasound
	Higher socioeconomic status		Biopsy
			MRI/PET
	Increased parenchymal breast density on mammogram		Chest x-ray (PA and lateral)
			Computed tomography (CT) of chest and abdomen
Genetics	BRCA1 and BRCA2 mutation—5%-6% of all breast cancers		
Histopathology	Adenocarcinoma (infiltrating ductal) most common—80%		
	Lobular carcinoma— 5%-10%		
	Medullary, tubular, papillary, micropapillary, invasive cribriform—5%		

Continued

Quick Facts—cont'd

Staging and Stage Grouping

Stage	Description
Tumor, node, metastasis (TNM)	
Primary tumor (T)	
TX	Primary tumor cannot be assessed
T0	No evidence of primary tumor
Tis	Carcinoma in situ: intraductal carcinoma, lobular carcinoma in situ, or Paget's disease of the nipple with no tumor
T1	≤ 2 cm in greatest dimension
T2	> 2 cm up to 5 cm in greatest dimension
T3	> 5 cm in greatest dimension
T4	Tumors of any size with direct extension to chest wall or skin (e.g., peau d'orange, skin ulceration, satel-lite nodes, inflammatory carcinoma)
Regional lymph nodes (N)*	
pNX	Regional lymph nodes cannot be assessed
pN0	No regional lymph node metastasis
pN1	Metastasis in 1 to 3 ipsilateral axillary or internal mammary lymph node(s)
pN2	Metastasis in 4 to 9 ipsilateral axillary lymph nodes; or in clinically apparent internal mammary lymph nodes in the absence of axillary lymph node metastasis
pN3	Metastasis in 10 or more ipsilateral axillary lymph nodes; or infraclavicular lymph nodes, with or without axillary node involvement; or ipsilateral internal mammary lymph nodes in the presence of 1 or more positive axillary lymph nodes; or presence of ipsilateral supraclavicular lymph nodes
Distant metastasis (M)	
MX	Distant metastasis cannot be assessed
M0	No distant metastasis
M1	Distant metastasis

Stage	Primary Tumor	Regional Lymph Nodes	Distant Metastasis
0	Tis	N0	M0
I	T1	N0	M0
IIA	T0	N1	M0
	T1	N1	M0
	T2	N0	M0
IIB	T2	N1	M0
	T3	N0	M0
IIIA	T0	N2	M0
	T1	N2	M0
	T2	N2	M0
	T3	N1	M0
	T3	N2	M0
IIIB	T4	Any N	M0
IIIC	Any T	N3	M0
IV	Any T	Any N	M1

1. What is the incidence of breast cancer among American women?

Breast cancer is the most common cancer diagnosis and the second major cause of cancer-related deaths in women. With a life expectancy of 85 years, about 1 in 9 women will develop breast cancer at some time during their lives. Although the incidence has increased since 1980, the mortality rate has been decreasing since 1990. This is attributed to advances in early detection and in breast cancer treatment.

2. In which area of the breast are more cancers found?

The most common area is the upper outer quadrant, where approximately 50% of tumors are found. There is a 15% incidence in the upper inner quadrant, 11% in the lower outer quadrant, 6% in the lower inner quadrant, and 17% in the central region (near the areola).

3. Do all breast cancers grow at a steady rate?

No. Most breast cancers have a doubling time of approximately 60 to 90 days. On average, it takes 5 to 8 years for an invasive breast cancer to be detected by mammogram or physical examination; however, a small percentage of cancers double in size as quickly as every 15 days or as slowly as every 600 days. The latter are associated with late recurrences (> 10 years and sometimes > 20 years after the original diagnosis).

4. What is inflammatory breast cancer?

Inflammatory cancer (an aggressive form of breast cancer) is not a histologic subtype, but is a clinical diagnosis based on the presence of erythema and edema (peau d'orange) of the skin of the breast.

5. Which imaging modalities are used before biopsy is performed? Why?

- **Mammography**. Before biopsy of a dominant mass, a mammogram should be done to define the extent of the lesion and to identify other suspicious areas. Because mammograms can miss approximately 15% of cancers, a negative test should not dissuade a physician from performing a biopsy on a dominant, palpable mass.
- **Digital mammography** has been shown to be better in women with dense breasts under the age of 50 years. In other populations, digital mammography and traditional film mammography are equally effective in detecting abnormalities.
- **Breast ultrasound** is often used for highly dense breast tissue, because it can distinguish between fluid-filled and solid masses.
- **Bilateral dynamic magnetic resonance imaging (MRI)** is used to define extent of disease in the breast and can distinguish unifocal from multifocal disease. MRI results may influence the decision between having a mastectomy or a lumpectomy.
- **Positron emission tomography (PET)** scanning is used to stage breast cancer. It is not a screening tool to detect breast cancer.

6. What are the various biopsy methods for diagnosing breast cancer?

Most biopsies are performed in outpatient settings under local anesthesia.

- **Fine-needle aspiration (FNA)** is often performed on palpable nodules because it is quick, relatively painless, and inexpensive. It cannot distinguish between ductal carcinoma in situ (DCIS) and invasive cancers; its use is somewhat limited. A negative FNA does not rule out malignancy in a suspicious lesion.
- **Core-cutting needle biopsy** has advantages similar to those of FNA, and a larger sample is usually obtained, giving a higher degree of accuracy.
- **Stereotactic core biopsy** is performed with the patient lying face down with the breast suspended through an opening in the table. The breast is compressed, and multiple core samples can be obtained.

- **Mammotome** uses a vacuum-assisted system that yields a larger tissue sample with potentially less discomfort for the patient. A sterile probe is placed into the breast and rotated to obtain multiple samples.
- **Encor biopsy** is a fully automated form of obtaining a breast biopsy and is similar to a mammotome biopsy.
- **Needle localization.** If a suspicious, nonpalpable nodule is seen on mammogram, it may be localized with needles guided by mammography. The needle-localized lesion is excised.
- **Excisional biopsies** may be performed on any palpable nodule to provide the greatest diagnostic information, including size, receptor status, and margins.

7. How is noninvasive breast cancer (Stage 0) classified?

- Ductal carcinoma in situ (DCIS) is cancer confined within the lumen of the ducts.
- Lobular carcinoma in situ (LCIS) is cancer confined within the lobes of the breast, and is treated differently than DCIS is. It is a marker for increased risk of future cancer in either breast.

8. Discuss the significance and incidence of lymph node metastasis.

Axillary lymph node metastases are associated most closely with tumor size. Prognosis is related to the number of axillary lymph nodes involved; the greater the number, the poorer the overall survival rate. Medial tumors are more likely to metastasize to internal mammary and mediastinal lymph nodes than tumors located elsewhere in the breast. A complete axillary lymph node dissection has been the standard procedure for breast cancer staging and, based on studies from the 1990s, is associated with a 10% to 20% chance of developing lymphedema. The true incidence of lymphedema is difficult to ascertain because of the many years needed for follow-up, differences in reporting how lymphedema is measured, and the year in which the surgery was performed.

9. What is a sentinel lymph node biopsy and how is it performed?

The sentinel node is the first set of lymph nodes that drains a breast cancer. The principle of sentinel lymph node biopsy (SLNBx) rests on the theory that if metastatic spread has occurred, it involves the sentinel node first.

A blue dye and technetium-99m–labeled sulfur colloid are injected around the tumor. Alternatively, the dye and radioactive colloid may be injected around the nipple. Nodes that appear blue and are found to be "hot" by a hand-held gamma probe are sampled as the sentinel lymph nodes. Once the sentinel lymph node is identified, it can be removed through a small incision, with little disruption to the lymphatic system and low complication rates (lymphedema incidence is < 1%). On average, there are two sentinel lymph nodes that are removed. If SLNBx is positive, a complete axillary dissection is performed in most cases.

10. List the contraindications to SLNBx, according to the American College of Surgeons.

- Locally advanced disease
- Large biopsy cavity
- Palpable axillary lymph nodes
- Prior axillary surgery
- Pregnancy or lactation
- Prior radiation to the breast or axilla
- Known allergy to the dye

11. What are the cardinal prognostic factors in breast cancer staging?

The tumor-nodes-metastasis (TNM) staging system is used to predict the disease outcome by analysis of prognostic factors and survival rates. Approximately 98% of patients with localized disease are alive at 5 years after diagnosis. The 5-year survival rates for patients with regional disease (stages II and III) are approximately 81% and 65%, respectively. Less than 26% of patients with Stage IV metastatic disease are alive 5 years after diagnosis. Also important for prognosis, although not part of the staging system, are estrogen receptor (ER) and progesterone receptor (PR) status, HER-2/*neu* status, and S-phase status.

12. Define ER and PR status.

Receptor levels are measured in the primary tumor and provide valuable information for determining treatment. In general, tumors that are positive for estrogen and/or progesterone receptors have a better prognosis than tumors that are negative for ER and PR. Approximately 60% of breast cancers are ER positive. Postmenopausal women are more likely to be positive than premenopausal women. Receptor-positive tumors are generally responsive to endocrine therapies, such as selective estrogen receptor modulators (SERMs) and aromatase inhibitors.

13. What other prognostic criteria are helpful?

- **Elevated S-phase status or proliferative index (Ki67)** indicates a tumor that divides more rapidly and correlates with a more aggressive tumor.
- **HER-2/*neu*** (erbB2) oncogene, one of several epidermal growth factor receptors (EGFRs), is overexpressed in 25% of invasive breast tumors. Overexpression of HER-2/*neu* is associated with increased tumor growth, increased rate of metastases, ER negativity, and decreased overall survival.

14. What is the role of trastuzumab in the treatment of breast cancer?

Identification of HER-2/*neu* expression level has led to the development of the monoclonal antibody trastuzumab (Herceptin), which in combination with chemotherapy, has greater efficacy in patients with *metastatic* breast cancer. Three recent clinical trials combining trastuzumab with *adjuvant* chemotherapy in patients with positive lymph nodes have shown a 52% further decrease in recurrence when trastuzumab was given for 1 year in patients whose tumors were positive for HER-2/*neu*. Studies are currently underway evaluating the optimal duration of adjuvant therapy with trastuzumab. Many women with HER-2/*neu*-positive tumors (adjuvant or metastatic setting) will benefit from treatment with trastuzumab.

15. What is the OncotypeDX test?

OncotypeDX is a genomic study done on patients with ER-positive, stage I-II invasive breast cancers with no lymph node involvement. The test results have been shown to be correlated with disease outcome. This laboratory test analyzes 16 genes associated with breast cancer growth and metastasis and 5 regulatory/control genes to generate a recurrence score. Patients with low recurrence scores benefit from tamoxifen but not from adjuvant chemotherapy. Patients with high recurrence scores gain significant benefit from adjuvant chemotherapy. The role of adjuvant chemotherapy in patients with intermediate scores is undergoing additional study.

16. Is a lumpectomy as effective as a modified radical mastectomy?

Multiple randomized trials have demonstrated that the 10- to 20-year survival rate of patients with stage I or II breast cancer treated with lumpectomy (breast conservation with axillary lymph node dissection) and radiation therapy is equivalent to that of patients treated with modified radical mastectomy (removal of breast and lymph nodes) alone. Lumpectomy must be combined with radiation therapy for equivalent local control. Immediate or delayed reconstructive surgery is also an option for women who choose mastectomy. The decision is often difficult for women to make; it is based on personal preference, values, feelings about the body, priorities, and perceptions of risk.

17. What preoperative and postoperative teaching tips should the nurse include in the plan of care?

Because short-stay and outpatient procedures are becoming more common for both lumpectomy and mastectomy, patient education from the nurse is imperative. Individual coping is affected by exhaustion, anesthesia, change in body image, and emotional aspects of dealing with a new diagnosis.

- Remind patients to stop taking aspirin and nonsteroidal antiinflammatory agents before surgery, because they may decrease platelet function.
- Hormonal therapy (birth control or replacement) should be stopped as soon as a diagnosis of breast cancer is made. Discuss other appropriate birth control methods.
- Teach patients about signs and symptoms of infection, wound care, Jackson-Pratt drain management, prevention and management of lymphedema, pain control, and comfort measures at home.
- Recommend purchase of a postoperative bra.
- Initiate referral to the Reach to Recovery Program of the American Cancer Society (trained volunteers who have had breast cancer visit postoperatively, providing information about exercises, temporary prosthetic devices, bras, and available support services).
- Postoperatively, the patient should avoid lifting weights greater than 5 pounds for a few weeks.
- If adjuvant chemotherapy is indicated, there is usually a period of several weeks between surgery and start of chemotherapy. This is an ideal time to have a dental examination and cleaning, which should be avoided during chemotherapy treatments, when blood counts could be low.

18. What kind of bra, if any, should be worn in the postoperative period?

Women are most comfortable after biopsy or lumpectomy if the breast is well supported. A sports bra is ideal, especially one with frontal closure, which is easier to put on than the overhead type. Wearing a bra to bed for the first few nights helps some women, as does lying on the side opposite the surgical site, with a towel rolled under the breast for support. Women should avoid underwire support postoperatively and during radiation therapy, when the breast is tender and edematous.

19. What techniques are used for delivery of radiation therapy to the breast following lumpectomy? What are common side effects?

In general, 4500 to 5000 cGy are administered 5 days/week for 5 to 6 weeks after lumpectomy via tangential beam (through the breast instead of through the body to avoid the heart and lungs). Several other techniques are currently under investigation, including brachytherapy (short-term radiation implants), partial breast irradiation (radiating only the part of the breast where the tumor was) and more rapid fractionalization (more radiation in less time). The most common side effect is local skin irritation similar to a bad sunburn. This symptom varies among women and may cause pruritis, edema, and occasionally moist desquamation in severe cases.

20. Why do some women with a modified radical mastectomy receive radiation therapy?

Postmastectomy radiation therapy is recommended for women with a tumor at least 5 cm in diameter, skin or chest wall involvement, positive surgical margin, or at least 4 positive lymph nodes. Depending on institutional protocols, radiation therapy is administered at different times during treatment. Most commonly it is administered after completion of chemotherapy. Patients tend to have more severe side effects with concomitant chemotherapy (especially doxorubicin) and radiation therapy. Radiation therapy also is used to treat some spot bone or brain metastases.

21. Explain the role of neoadjuvant chemotherapy in breast cancer.

Neoadjuvant chemotherapy is administered before surgery in an effort to decrease the size of the primary tumor so that breast conservation is possible. Patients who have locally advanced or inflammatory breast cancers (stage IIIB) at initial diagnosis may benefit from neoadjuvant chemotherapy. Response rates appear to be 80% with a combination of doxorubicin, cyclophosphamide and docetaxel (Taxotere). The addition of neoadjuvant trastuzumab to chemotherapy, in HER-2/*neu*-positive patients results in an increase from 26% (chemotherapy alone) to 65% (chemotherapy + trastuzumab) complete pathologic response.

22. Why do some women receive adjuvant chemotherapy whereas others do not?

The potential increase in long-term survival weighed against the potential side effects determines whether a patient should be offered adjuvant chemotherapy. The general health of the patient is important in making this decision. According to the National Institutes of Health (NIH) Consensus Development Conference Statement on Adjuvant Therapy for Breast Cancer (2000), most women with primary invasive breast tumors that are greater than 1 cm in diameter (both node-negative and node-positive) should be offered cytotoxic chemotherapy. The decision to consider chemotherapy should be individualized for women with node-negative tumors that are less than 1 cm in diameter. OncotypeDX testing can help with this decision (see Question 15). For women with positive lymph nodes and any size tumor, adjuvant chemotherapy should be offered.

23. Summary of adjuvant treatment options (individualize for each patient).

- Surgical recommendations: mastectomy or lumpectomy plus radiation, with lymph node sampling for all patients; radiation therapy after surgery for any tumor greater than 5 cm or presence of more than 4 positive lymph nodes
- Any stage with positive estrogen or progesterone receptors: adjuvant hormonal therapy (tamoxifen in the premenopausal setting, tamoxifen or an aromatase inhibitor in the postmenopausal setting)
- HER-2/*neu*-positive tumors: consider 1 year adjuvant therapy with trastuzumab (Herceptin) plus chemotherapy
- Tumor larger than 1 cm (lymph node positive or negative): offer chemotherapy with or without adjuvant hormonal therapy, depending on estrogen and progesterone receptor status
- Positive lymph nodes: offer chemotherapy with or without adjuvant hormonal therapy, depending on estrogen and progesterone receptor status
- Consider OncotypeDX testing for stage I and II, ER-positive, lymph node-negative tumors to identify those patients who may not benefit from adjuvant chemotherapy

24. What are the most common chemotherapy drug combinations used to treat breast cancer?

Several hundred chemotherapy trials for breast cancer have provided data for the efficacious use of the following regimens:

- Combination of cyclophosphamide, methotrexate, and 5-fluorouracil (CMF) are administered on days 1 and 8, every 28 days for 6 cycles.
- Combination of 5-fluorouracil (5-FU), doxorubicin (Adriamycin), and cyclophosphamide (FAC) are administered on day 1, every 21 days.

Alternatively, 5-FU may be administered on days 1 and 8 of a 28-day cycle for 6 courses. A variation is oral cyclophosphamide for 14 days, with administration of doxorubicin and 5-FU on days 1 and 8 (CAF).

- Doxorubicin with cyclophosphamide (AC) are administered every 21 days for 4 cycles, followed by paclitaxel (Taxol) or docetaxel (Taxotere) every 21 days for 4 cycles. A recent study demonstrated equivalent response rates and survival between paclitaxel and docetaxel (see Question 25 on dose-dense chemotherapy).
- In Europe, regimens containing epirubicin instead of doxorubicin are commonly used.
- The NIH Consensus Development Statement states that inclusion of anthracyclines in adjuvant chemotherapy regimens produces a small but significant improvement in survival.
- In some women who are positive for the HER-2/*neu* receptor, adjuvant trastuzumab (Herceptin) should be offered for a period of 1 year.
- Other combinations, including TAC (Taxotere, Adriamycin, and Cytoxan), AT (Adriamycin and Taxotere), and THC (Taxotere, Herceptin, and Carboplatin), are under investigation.

25. What is dose-dense chemotherapy and how is it used to treat breast cancer?

Dose-dense chemotherapy is standard chemotherapy given on a more frequent schedule, such as every 14 days instead of every 21 days. The ECOG 9144 trial compared standard AC followed by Taxol every 21 days against the same drugs given every 14 days; additionally the same chemotherapy drugs were given as single agents in sequential fashion (Adriamycin × 4 cycles, followed by Cytoxan × 4 cycles, followed by Taxol × 4 cycles), also given in a cycle of 14 rather than 21 days. This study showed that chemotherapy given in a dose-dense fashion resulted in improved response rates. There was no difference in response rates if the chemotherapy was given in a dose-dense standard combination versus a dose-dense sequential single agent therapy. Dose-dense therapy requires support of hematopoeitic growth factors. Note that paclitaxel (Taxol) is used every 14 days instead of docetaxel (Taxotere); toxicity with docetaxel given every 14 days is too great.

26. When is stem cell transplant recommended for women with breast cancer?

Stem cell transplant is still investigational for patients with greater than 4 positive lymph nodes and no evidence of metastatic disease or inflammatory breast cancer. So far, no survival advantage has been noted for patients undergoing transplant versus conventional chemotherapy.

27. How does tamoxifen work? How long does treatment last?

Tamoxifen is considered a standard adjuvant therapy for women with ER-positive and/or PR-positive breast cancer. The current recommendation is 20 mg/day, orally for 5 years. The overall response rate is 60%. Formerly known as an antiestrogen, it is now classified as a SERM (selective estrogen receptor modifier). Tamoxifen binds to the estrogen or progesterone receptor on the breast cancer cell surface and activates a nuclear signaling pathway that results in cell death. It does not stop estrogen production in the body. Women taking tamoxifen generally are less likely to develop osteoporosis and usually have lower serum cholesterol levels. Postmenopausal women may take tamoxifen for 2 to 3 years and then switch to taking an aromatase inhibitor.

28. What are the side effects of tamoxifen?

The more common side effects are hot flashes and vaginal discharge. However, tamoxifen also may lead to a 2.5-fold increase in the incidence of endometrial cancer, a 2- to 4-fold increase in strokes and blood clots, and a slight increase in the incidence of posterior subcapsular cataracts.

29. Describe the role of aromatase inhibitors in management of breast cancer.

Because aromatase is important for the conversion of androgens into estrogens in postmenopausal women, drugs have been developed to inhibit this enzyme. Aminoglutethimide was the first aromatase inhibitor used with some effectiveness. Newer agents (anastrozole, letrozole, and exemestane) have been studied and have consistently shown to be superior to tamoxifen in preventing contralateral breast cancers, local recurrence, and metastatic disease. They are only effective in postmenopausal women with ER-positive or PR-positive tumor cells. They are currently being studied in the treatment of noninvasive breast cancer (DCIS) and for cancer prevention and risk reduction (in Europe).

30. Describe the current recommended regimens for aromatase inhibitors.

Anastrozole (Arimidex) is currently being used instead of tamoxifen in post-menopausal women, in the adjuvant setting for 5 years. Letrozole (Femara) is used in the "extended adjuvant" setting. In other words, following completion of 5 years of tamoxifen, women are offered 5 additional years of therapy with letrazole. Exemestane (Aromasin) has been used in cases of "switching" from tamoxifen after 2 to 3 years. The exemestane is continued for a total of 5 years including the time spent on tamoxifen. Recently the MA17 study has shown that letrozole therapy for 5 years after completing 5 years of tamoxifen is beneficial. There are also studies currently underway evaluating different aromatase inhibitors "head to head."

31. What are the side effects of aromatase inhibitors?

As a class, aromatase inhibitors may cause hot flashes and increase the risk for osteopenia and osteoporosis. There is no known associated risk for endometrial cancer. Women receiving aromatase inhibitor therapy should receive periodic DEXA (Dual Energy X-ray Absortiometry) to evaluate bone density, take calcium with vitamin D, and exercise.

32. How do aromatase inhibitors influence risk for heart disease?

Tamoxifen has been shown to reduce total cholesterol and increase high-density lipoprotein (HDL) cholesterol, yielding a favorable effect on the heart. Current studies are mixed in regard to the effect of aromatase inhibitors on the heart. Some studies suggest a neutral effect on the heart; other studies show a detrimental effect on blood lipid levels.

33. How are hot flashes treated?

- Hot flashes induced by treatment with SERMs or early menopause as a side effect of chemotherapy have been reported by 65% of women with breast cancer. Although many nonpharmacological and pharmacologic treatments have been tried or suggested, research is limited about the physiologic impact or mechanisms of action of these treatments.
- Nonpharmacological interventions: dressing in layers; relaxation training; exercise; homeopathic treatments; acupuncture; reflexology; avoidance of caffeine, alcohol, and spicy foods. Black cohosh; Vitamin E; Soy; acupuncture and magnets were found to be no more effective than placebo in reducing hot flashes.
- Pharmacologic treatments: venlafaxine and paroxetine (antidepressants); gabapentin (anticonvulsant); transdermal clonidine (antiadrenergic); Bellegral, a combination of

ergotiamine, belladonna alkaloid, and phenobarbital (anticholinergic); and megestrol acetate (progestin). Side effects and potential drug interactions need to be considered when choosing pharmacological interventions.

34. Which pharmacologic treatments are the most effective in treating hot flashes?

So far, the most effective drugs in reducing hot flashes are venlafaxine (Effexor) 37.5 to 150 mg daily (the 75 mg dose has been reported to be better than the 37.5-mg dose or placebo) and gabapentin (Neurontin) 200 to 900 mg daily (may be titrated up to 2400 mg daily). The selective serotonin reuptake inhibitor (SSRI) antidepressant, paroxetine 12.5 to 25 mg daily, fluoxetine 20 mg daily, and sertraline 50 mg daily, have also been reported to reduce hot flashes.

35. What is the concern about using SSRI antidepressants to treat hot flashes in women with breast cancer?

Recent research raises concern that the SSRI antidepressants, particularly paroxetine, fluoxetine, and sertraline inhibit the metabolism of tamoxifen through inhibition of the CYP2D6 enzyme. Venlafaxine, a SNRI (serotonin-norepinephrine reuptake inhibitor) is a weak inhibitor of the CYP2D6 enzyme. More research is needed on the effects of CYP2D6 inhibitors on tamoxifen metabolism. Until more is known about the clinical significance of the effects of SSRIs on tamoxifen metabolism, patients on tamoxifen should not receive paroxetine, fluoxetine, or sertraline to treat hot flashes.

36. How is vaginal dryness treated?

In addition to topical lubricants, such as Astroglide and Replens, it may be safe for women with breast cancer to use the Estring and Vagifem vaginal suppositories (low-dose, local estrogen treatments). Unlike estrogen creams (e.g., Premarin vaginal cream) which demonstrate detectable levels of circulating estradiol, these two products are related to minimal systemic absorption of estrogen. Research is pending to determine how much estrogen absorption is safe in women who have had breast cancer.

The vaginal estrogen ring (e.g., Femring) used for systemic estrogen replacement therapy should not be used by women with a history of breast cancer. The Estring and Vagifem should be avoided in women on aromatase inhibitors whose extremely low levels of circulating estrogen could enhance vaginal absorption of estrogen.

37. How often does breast cancer spread from one breast to the other?

It is rare for cancer to metastasize from one breast to the other. A woman who has had cancer in one breast, however, is at a higher risk of developing a new primary contralateral breast cancer. The risk in the opposite breast is 0.5% to 1.0% during each year of follow-up. Therefore most malignancies of the other breast are new cancers. It is also possible for one person to have one estrogen/progesterone receptor-positive tumor and a second receptor-negative tumor.

38. What are the most common sites of metastases?

Breast cancer may metastasize to several organs, including bone, liver, lung, brain, and skin, which are the tissues reported most frequently. Breast cancer in the ovaries, spleen, peritoneum, adrenal glands, stomach, leptomeninges, and retina of the eye is rare.

39. Discuss the prognosis of metastatic breast cancer.

Although metastatic disease is considered incurable, it does not always mean that death is imminent. One half of patients live more than 2 years, and 10% live a decade or more. Women with only bone metastases may live for a considerable time with the use of radiation, hormonal therapy, bisphosphonate treatment, and chemotherapy.

40. Discuss treatment options for metastatic breast cancer.

There are many options for treatment of metastatic disease. Multiple therapies are often used in sequence.

- If the tumor is positive for hormone receptors and disease is present in nonvisceral sites only, hormone therapy is first choice. Available hormones include: SERMS (tamoxifen), aromatase inhibitors, antiestrogen (Faslodex), megestrol acetate, fluoxymesterone (Halotestin), and high dose estrogen.
- If disease is in visceral sites and a rapid response is required, or if the tumor cells are hormone receptor-negative, the first line treatment is chemotherapy. Effective chemotherapy agents include: taxanes, cisplatin/carboplatin, gemcitabine, fluoropyrimidines (e.g., capecitabine [Xeloda]), and anthracyclines.
- Trastuzumab (Herceptin) is used in addition to chemotherapy if the tumor is positive for HER-2/*neu*.
- Bisphosphonates (zolendronate, pamidronate) are used to treat bone metastases.

41. What is the role of bisphosphonates in the treatment of metastatic bone disease?

Bisphosphonates have become a standard part of the treatment regimen. They interfere with tumor-mediated osteolysis by modulating the function and maturation of osteoclasts and can significantly reduce the risk of nonvertebral pathologic fractures. They also decrease the need for radiation therapy and surgery to treat bone complications, the incidence of hypercalcemia, and the degree of bone pain. Bisphosphonates are under study to see if they can prevent the incidence of bone metastasis in the adjuvant setting. The standard dose of zolendronate is 4 mg given intravenously over 15 minutes every 3 to 4 weeks. Alternatively, a dose of pamidronate, 90 mg, may be given intravenously over 2 hours every 3 to 4 weeks. Toxic effects of bisphosphonates include renal problems and risk of osteonecrosis of the jaw.

42. Should multiple regular screening tests be performed to monitor for metastatic disease or recurrence in women diagnosed with breast cancer?

The American Society of Clinical Oncology issued guidelines for the follow-up of patients with breast cancer. Routine screening for distant recurrences with laboratory tests, radiographs, computerized tomography, or bone scans in asymptomatic patients offers no survival advantage over performing the same tests when patients become symptomatic. Unlike distant metastasis, finding a new contralateral breast cancer or an ipsilateral recurrence is important because these are potentially still curable; therefore, mammograms are still important.

43. What is the ideal interval between mastectomy and breast reconstruction?

No interval can be considered ideal for all patients. Most mastectomy patients are candidates for reconstruction, which often may be performed at the same time that the breast is removed. For some women, delayed reconstruction may be best.

44. Discuss the options for breast reconstruction.

The options, which should be discussed with a plastic surgeon, depend on body type and breast size. Breast reconstruction may be accomplished as a prosthetic implant, tissue expansion, or flap procedure. After mastectomy, a balloon expander is inserted beneath the skin and chest muscle. Through a port mechanism, saline is injected periodically, stretching the skin until a more permanent saline or silicone implant may be inserted. An alternative approach involves creation of a skin flap using tissue from other parts of the body, such as the transverse rectus abdominis muscle (TRAM) or the latissimus dorsi muscle (LD). Although these alternatives do not require implants and generally result in a more natural contour, they involve more extensive surgical procedures and scarring. Additional surgical procedures are available to reconstruct the areola and nipple.

45. What critical psychological issues may confront partners and families of patients with breast cancer?

Breast cancer is a crisis for the entire family. It may result in depression among family members, impaired marital relationships, lowered self-esteem, developmental delays in children, and behavioral problems with adolescents. The oncology nurse is often the first observer of family dynamics in response to cancer. Identification of problems, provision of clear information, and referral to appropriate resources may help the family develop a successful coping style. Active listening is a valuable intervention, as is validation of concerns.

46. Women with a family history of breast cancer are often concerned about their increased risk of developing it. What can nurses say to these patients to decrease their fears?

Mutations in BRCA1 and BRCA2 genes account for approximately 5% to 10% of breast cancers, 45% of hereditary breast cancer, and the majority of heritable breast/ovarian cancer. Some women at high risk for developing breast cancer consider prophylactic mastectomies to reduce their risk; others may elect to take tamoxifen. However, taking tamoxifen to reduce the risk of breast cancer is not effective in women with a BRCA1 mutation; BRCA1 mutations are usually associated with the development of ER-negative tumors. Patients and family members should be referred to centers that offer genetic screening and counseling for women at risk. By emphasizing and facilitating breast cancer screening and detection through monthly breast self-examination, periodic clinical examination, and screening mammography (reduces the risk of dying from breast cancer by 33%-60% in women > 50 years old and by 17% in women age 40-49), the oncology nurse may reduce the fear of breast cancer.

47. Discuss the relationship between dietary fat intake and incidence of breast cancer, and the relationship between the role of exercise and the incidence of breast cancer.

Epidemiologists have long wondered whether a low-fat diet can prevent breast cancer. The incidence of breast cancer is clearly lower in countries where intake of animal fat is lower, but reproductive habits are also different in these countries. The ongoing Nurses' Health Study has not demonstrated an association between the two, but compliance has been a problem with participants in many studies to date. Diets high in raw fruits and vegetables are also under study. Although current data do not support specific dietary guidelines for reducing the risk of breast cancer, the American Cancer Society still recommends that women maintain a healthy weight and limit intake of high-fat foods, particularly those from animal sources, as part of a healthy lifestyle. Recent studies have confirmed that both diet and exercise can lower a women's risk for developing breast cancer. Furthermore, exercise has been shown to reduce the risk of breast cancer deaths in women with hormone responsive breast cancers (Holmes, 2005).

48. What is the modified Gail Model?

The modified Gail Model (for women age 35 years and older) is a computerized method of predicting a woman's 5-year and lifetime risk of developing invasive breast cancer. Risk factors include race, patient age, age at first menses, age at first live birth, number of first-degree relatives with breast cancer, number of previous breast biopsies, and biopsies showing atypical hyperplasia.

49. Does tamoxifen lower the risk of developing breast cancer?

The Breast Cancer Prevention Trial (BCPT) included 13,388 women at high risk for the development of breast cancer, based on the modified Gail Model. Patients were randomized to take either tamoxifen or placebo for 5 years. After a median follow-up of 54.6 months, the risk of invasive breast cancer was reduced by 49% in women receiving tamoxifen. Based on these results, tamoxifen has been approved in the United States for breast cancer prevention in high-risk women who meet criteria established by the National Cancer Institute. Women with LCIS or atypical hyperplasia who took tamoxifen had a 66% and 86% reduction respectively in developing invasive breast cancer on the P-1 trial.

50. What other preventive agents are under study?

Several trials are under way to evaluate the efficacy of newer agents that have fewer side effects than tamoxifen. The Multiple Outcomes of Raloxifene Evaluation (MORE) trial, designed to assess the value of raloxifene in prevention of osteoporosis, also evaluated as a secondary end point the incidence of newly diagnosed breast cancer. Although preliminary results show a reduction in new diagnoses of breast cancer, raloxifene currently is approved only for the treatment of osteoporosis. The first report of the Study of Tamoxifen and Raloxifene (STAR) trial was released in 2006 and showed approximately equal efficacy in reducing invasive breast cancer risk, with decreasing incidence of endometrial cancer, blood clots, and cataracts.

51. What issues related to breast cancer should we expect to hear about in the coming years?

Identification of additional oncogenes and genetic predisposition has scientific interest as well as ethical and legal implications. More research will be conducted on the selection of treatments based on molecular subtypes and the use of novel diagnostic tests or markers to predict treatment responses. A new screening/diagnostic tool currently under study is thermoscintigraphy. The more widespread use of lymphoscintigraphy or lymph node mapping (sentinel node procedure) will reduce the morbidity of lymph node dissections. New and improved treatments with less systemic toxicity are always of interest. Antiangiogenesis agents and other targeted therapies in the adjuvant and metastatic settings are being studied. Survivorship (e.g., quality of life, fatigue, exercise, diet, hormone use, pregnancy, financial impact, body image) is an area of increased interest.

52. What is the role for bevacizumab (Avastin) in breast cancer?

Bevacizumab is a humanized monoclonal antibody that targets the VEGF molecule. It is believed to act by inhibiting blood vessel growth and improve chemotherapy delivery to the tumor. A large trial conducted by ECOG (E2100) showed an increase in progression free survival in women with recurrent or metastatic breast cancer who received bevacizumab in addition to standard chemotherapy. It has not been shown to be effective as a single agent. Side effects include hypertension, proteinuria, bowel perforation, and hemorrhage. When given in combination with paclitaxel, there is worsening of neuropathy compared to paclitaxel alone. Adjuvant trials with chemotherapy plus bevacizumab are currently accruing patients.

53. What is the role of lapatinib (Tykerb) in the treatment of breast cancer?

Lapatinib is a dual kinase inhibitor targeting the EGFR-1 and EGFR-2 receptors. It has received FDA approval for use in combination with capecitabine for the treatment of women with HER-2/neu-positive metastatic breast cancer. Subjects included those who had disease progression after treatment with regimens containing trastuzumab (Herceptin), an anthracycline, and a taxane. Time to progression was significantly prolonged in the group who received lapatinib plus capecitabine compared to the group who received only capecitabine. Side effects were mild and included rash, fatigue, nausea, vomiting, diarrhea and anorexia. There was no significant increase in the risk of cardiotoxicity in the lapatinib arm of the study. There is a study evaluating lapatinib in the adjuvant setting; eligible patients must have HER-2/neu-positive tumors and not have received trastuzumab.

Key Points

- Breast cancer is the most common cancer diagnosis in women.
- New screening technology, including the use of digital mammography and dynamic breast MRI, is being used to screen for and detect breast cancer in high-risk women, including women carrying the BRCA1/2 gene mutations or women with dense breasts.
- Key prognostic indicators include: lymph node involvement, estrogen (ER) and progesterone receptor (PR) status, HER-2/*neu*, and S-phase status.
- Adjuvant chemotherapy should be offered to patients with lymph nodes positive for cancer and any size tumor.
- Aromatase inhibitors are effective only in postmenopausal women.
- The use of new agents, including aromatase inhibitors and trastuzumab, has made incremental advances in response rates. Newer targeted agents are under investigation.
- The mortality rate for women with breast cancer has been decreasing; advances in screening and treatment are credited with improved survival.
- In general, treatment of breast cancer in males is similar to that of breast cancer in females.

Internet Resources

National Comprehensive Cancer Network, Clinical Practice Guidelines in Oncology, Breast Cancer:
http://www.nccn.org/professionals/physician_gls/PDF/breast.pdf

San Antonio Breast Cancer Symposium, the largest conference devoted to reporting international research results on breast cancer:
http://www.sabcs.org

Myriad Genetic Laboratories:
http://www.myriadtests.com/provider/

National Cancer Institute, Breast Cancer Risk Assessment Tool. This site has the prevalence tables for BRCA1 and BRCA2 mutations, NCI clinical trials, and the interactive Gail Model breast cancer risk assessment tool:
http://bcra.nci.nih.gov/brc/

National Surgical Adjuvant Breast and Bowel Project (NSABP):
http://www.nsabp.pitt.edu

For Patients:

American Cancer Society, Reach to Recovery Program:
http://www.cancer.org/docroot/ESN/content/ESN_3_1x_Reach_to_Recovery_5.asp

Susan G. Komen Breast Cancer Foundation:
http://www.komen.org

Mothers Supporting Daughters with Breast Cancer (MSDBC):
http://www.mothersdaughters.org

National Alliance of Breast Cancer Organization (NABCO). Nonprofit agency representing over 300 organizations concerned about breast cancer; services range from physician referrals to job discrimination and professional education:
http://www.nabco.org

Y-ME National Breast Cancer Organization. This site provides information and support to anyone touched by breast cancer. They are also active in the political arena supporting research and the development of public policy for breast cancer:
http://www.y-me.org

Acknowledgment

The authors wish to acknowledge Patrice Y. Neese, MSN, RN, CS, ANP, for her contribution to the Breast Cancer chapter published in the first and second editions of *Oncology Nursing Secrets*.

Bibliography

Carpenter JS: State of the science: hot flashes and cancer, part 2: Management and future directions. *Oncol Nurs Forum,* 32(5):969-978, 2005.

Citron ML, Berry DA, Cirrincione C, et al: Randomized trial of dose-dense versus conventionally scheduled and sequential versus concurrent combination chemotherapy as postoperative adjuvant treatment of node-positive primary breast cancer: First report of Intergroup Trial C9741/Cancer and Leukemia Group B Trial 9741. *J Clin Oncol* 21(8):431-439, 2003.

Coombes RC, Hall E, Gibson LJ, et al: A randomized trial of exemestane after two to three years of tamoxifen therapy in postmenopausal women with primary breast cancer. *N Engl J Med* 350:1081-1092, 2004.

Fisher B, Costantino JP, Wickerham DL, et al: Tamoxifen for prevention of breast cancer: Report of the National Surgical Adjuvant Breast and Bowel Project P-1 study. *J Natl Cancer Instit* 90:1371-1388, 1998.

Fisher B, Montague E, Redmond C, et al: Comparison of radical mastectomy with alternative treatments for primary breast cancer. A first report results from a prospective randomized clinical trial. *Cancer* 39(suppl):2827-2839, 1977.

Goss PE, Ingle JN, Martino S, et al: Randomized trial of letrozole following tamoxifen in extended adjuvant therapy in receptor-positive breast cancer: Updated findings from NCIC CTG MA.17. *J Natl Cancer Instit* 97(17):1262-1271, 2005.

Greene FL, Page DL, Fleming ID, et al: *AJCC cancer staging manual,* ed 6, New York, 2002, Springer.

Gross R: Breast cancer: Risk factors, screening, and prevention. *Semin Oncol Nurs* 16:176-184, 2000.

Haber J, Noll Hoskins C: Meeting the challenges of adjuvant therapy: Strategies for partners and significant others. *Innov Br Cancer Care* 5:49-50, 2000.

Hilton BA: Issues, problems, and challenges for families coping with breast cancer. *Semin Oncol Nurs* 9:88-100, 1993.

Holmes MD, Chen WY, Feskanich D, et al: Physical activity after breast cancer diagnosis. *JAMA* 1293: 2479-2486, 2005.

Howell A, Cuzick J, Baum M, et al: Results of the ATAC (Arimidex, tamoxifen, alone or in combination) trial after completion of 5 years' adjuvant treatment for breast cancer. *Lancet* 365:60-62, 2005.

Jemal A, Siegel R, Ward E, et al: Cancer statistics, 2007. *CA Cancer J Clin* 57:43-66, 2007.

McMasters KM, Tuttle TM, Carlson DJ, et al: Sentinel lymph node biopsy for breast cancer: A suitable alternative to routine axillary dissection in multi-institutional practice when optimal technique is used. *J Clin Oncol* 18:2560-2566, 2000.

National Breast Cancer Coalition (NBCC): Bevacizumab (Avastin) in first-line treatment of metastatic breast cancer: The ECOG E2100 trial. Available at: http://www.natlbcc.org/bin/ index.asp?strid=745 &depid=9. Accessed January 15, 2007.

National Institutes of Health Consensus Development Conference Statement. Adjuvant therapy for breast cancer 2000. Available at: http://consensus.nih.gov/2000/2000AdjuvantTherapyBreastCancer114html.htm. Accessed January 14, 2007.

Paik S, Shak S, Tang G, et al: A multigene assay to predict recurrence of tamoxifen-treated, node-negative breast cancer. *N Engl J Med* 351:2817-2826, 2004.

Piccart-Gebhart MJ, Procter M, Leyland-Jones B, et al: Trastuzumab after adjuvant chemotherapy in HER2-positive breast cancer. *N Engl J Med* 353:1659-1672, 2005.

Pisano ED, Gatsonis C, Hendrick E, et al: Diagnostic performance of digital versus film mammography for breast cancer screening. *N Engl J Med* 353:1773-1383, 2005.

Romond E, Perez E, Bryant J, et al: Trastuzumab plus adjuvant chemotherapy for operable HER2-positive breast cancer. *N Engl J Med* 353:1673-1684, 2005.

Veronesi U, Paganelli G, Viale G, et al: A randomized comparison of sentinel-node biopsy with routine axillary dissection in breast cancer. *N Engl J Med* 349:546-553, 2003.

Winer EP, Hudis C, Burstein HJ, et al: American Society of Clinical Oncology technology assessment on the use of aromatase inhibitors as adjuvant therapy for post menopausal women with hormone receptor-positive breast cancer: status report 2004. *J Clin Oncol* 23: 619-629, 2005.

Yin Y, Desta Z, Stearns V, et al: CYP2D6 genotype, antidepressant use, and tamoxifen metabolism during adjuvant breast cancer treatment. *J Natl Cancer Inst* 97(1):30-39, 2005.

Colorectal Cancer (CRC)

Katherine Albert and Allen Cohn

Quick Facts

Incidence	112,340 newly diagnosed colon cancer (55,290 in men; 57,050 in women) cases; 41,420 rectal cancer (23,840 in men; 17,580 in women) cases estimated in 2007
Mortality	52,180 colorectal cancer deaths estimated in 2007
Risk factors	Personal history: adenomatous polyps; inflammatory bowel disease; ulcerative colitis, especially for > 10 years; Crohn's disease; breast, endometrial, ovarian cancers; pelvic irradiation for gynecologic cancers
	Diets rich in fat and cholesterol (high in red meat); obesity; alcohol consumption, especially beer; smoking; sedentary employment
Genetics	Familial adenomatous polyposis (FAP)
	Gardner's, Oldfield's, Turcot's, and Peutz-Jeghers syndromes
	Hereditary nonpolyposis colorectal carcinoma (HNPCC)
Histopathology	**Colon:** > 95% adenocarcinomas; remaining types: undifferentiated, squamous, carcinoid, leiomyosarcomas, hematopoietic, and lymphoid neoplasias
	Rectal: 98% adenocarcinomas; remaining types: carcinoid, lymphoma, and sarcoma
Symptoms	**Early:** usually asymptomatic; possible vague abdominal pain or flatulence
	Symptoms: vary according to location of tumor, but usually a change in bowel movements is the first symptom (i.e., change in shape of stool)
	Other signs and symptoms: pain, bleeding from the rectum, blood in stool or toilet, lower abdominal cramping, tenesmus, bowel obstruction, and weakness due to anemia
Diagnosis and evaluation	History and physical examination
	Digital rectal exam
	Fecal occult blood test (FOBT)
	Flexible sigmoidoscopy
	Double-contrast barium enema (DCBE)
	Colonoscopy with biopsy of any lesions; and/or air-contrast barium enema
	Other tests: endoscopic ultrasound, chest radiograph, computed tomography (CT) scan of abdomen and pelvis
	Laboratory data: complete blood count; complete metabolic panel, including liver and renal function tests; urinalysis; carcinoembryonic antigen (CEA)

Quick Facts—cont'd

Staging and Stage Grouping

Stage	Description
Tumor, nodes, metastasis (TNM)	
Primary tumor (T)	
TX	Primary tumor cannot be assessed
T0	No evidence of tumor
Tis	Carcinoma in situ
T1	Tumor invades submucosa
T2	Tumor invades muscularis propria
T3	Tumor invades through muscularis propria into submucosa
T4	Tumor perforates visceral peritoneum or invades other organs or structures
Regional lymph nodes (N)	
NX	Regional lymph nodes cannot be assessed
N0	No regional lymph nodes involved
N1	1-3 pericolic lymph nodes involved
N2	4 or more pericolic lymph nodes involved
N3	Regional nodes along major named vascular trunk
Distant metastasis (M)	
MX	Distant metastases cannot be assessed
M0	No distant metastasis
M1	Distant metastasis

Stage	Primary Tumor	Regional Lymph Nodes	Distant Metastasis
0	Tis	N0	M0
I	T1	N0	M0
	T2	N0	M0
IIA	T3	N0	M0
IIB	T4	N0	M0
IIIA	T1	N1	M0
	T2	N1	M0
IIIB	T3	N1	M0
	T4	N1	M0
IIIC	Any T	N2	M0
IV	Any T	Any N	M1

Used with permission of the American Joint Committee on Cancer (AJCC), Chicago, Illinois. The original source for this material is the AJCC Cancer Staging Handbook, Sixth Edition (2002) published by Springer New York, www.sprinfleronline.com.

1. What are some of the epidemiologic factors associated with colorectal cancer?

Colorectal cancer (CRC) is the third most common cancer and the second leading cause of cancer-related mortality in the United States for both genders; the incidence is higher in African Americans. The prevalence of colorectal cancer is nearly equal in men and women; rectal cancer is slightly more common in males. There is an increased risk of CRC incidence and death with age; 91% of new cases and 94% of deaths occur in individuals older than 50. Twenty to 25% of all CRC cases occur in individuals with a family history or predisposing illness. Overall CRC incidence rates have been declining since 1998 possibly reflecting increased screening and detection, and removal of precancerous polyps.

2. What is the most significant risk factor related to the development of CRC?

The presence of familial adenomatous polyps is the most common risk factor. The larger the polyps, the greater the likelihood of malignancy (up to 40% of patients with CRC had polyps > 2 cm).

3. What is the survival rate for CRC?

Prognosis is based on staging. The 5-year relative survival rates according to the stages of the American Joint Committee on Cancer (AJCC) are:

Stage I	93%
Stage II	85%
Stage IIIA	83%
Stage IIIB	64%
Stage IIIC	44%
Stage IV	8%

4. What are the most common signs and symptoms of CRC?

Symptoms are related to tumor location and include the following:

Right colon: vague, achy abdominal pain; bleeding (dark or mahogany red); anemia (common) and associated symptoms (weakness/fatigue, shortness of breath); obstruction (infrequent); palpable abdominal mass

Transverse colon: blood in stool; change in bowel pattern; potential bowel obstruction

Left colon: colicky pain, bleeding (red, mixed with stool), obstruction (common), weakness due to anemia (infrequent), nausea, vomiting, constipation alternating with diarrhea, change in bowel habits, decreased caliber of stool (pencil stools), tenesmus, fatigue, anorexia, failure to thrive, pain in the right upper quadrant of the abdomen (associated with liver metastases)

Rectum: steady, gnawing pain; bleeding (bright red, coating stool); change in bowel movements (constipation or diarrhea); pencil stools; rectal urgency or fecal incontinence; spasmodic contractions with pain; perineal and buttock pain

5. What percentage of CRC is accounted for by the different segments of the colon?

Descending and sigmoid colon: 52%
Ascending colon: 32%
Transverse colon: 16%

6. What is the value of carcinoembryonic antigen in monitoring patients with colorectal cancer?

Carcinoembryonic antigen (CEA) is a glycoprotein present in gastrointestinal mucosa. It is useful as a tumor marker for patients who have CEA-producing adenocarcinomas. CEA is most useful as a marker for tumor recurrence and in monitoring response to chemotherapy. An elevated, sustained postoperative level of CEA is correlated with tumor recurrence in most patients. Rising CEA levels (serial changes > 35% of baseline) may indicate progressive disease. Elevated CEA levels are found in patients with gastrointestinal, breast, and lung cancers; in smokers; and in patients with liver disease or cirrhosis, pancreatitis, inflammatory bowel disease, or rectal polyps.

7. What are common sites of colon and rectal metastases?

Common sites of metastasis for colon cancer are the liver, lungs, and peritoneum (with carcinomatosis). Colon cancer often metastasizes to the liver, because most of the colon's venous drainage is through the portal system. Uncommon sites are brain, bone, ovaries, and adrenal glands. Rectal cancer has a tendency to metastasize to the lungs, because its venous drainage is via the hemorrhoidal veins.

8. How is CRC detected if no symptoms are present?

Screening guidelines are controversial; however, the American Cancer Society recommends the following tests to screen for CRC in asymptomatic patients with no risk factors (approximate costs of each screening test are listed):

- Digital rectal examination plus fecal occult blood test (FOBT) for three specimens ($10) annually after age 50 years, in addition to one of the following screening tests:
  - Flexible sigmoidoscopy (examines up to 60 cm of rectum and distal colon; can detect about 50% of CRC; $200-$400) starting at age 50; repeat every 5 years if the results are normal
  - Double-contrast barium enema ($150-$200) (if results are normal, repeat every 5-10 years)
  - Colonoscopy with biopsy of any lesions (considered the gold standard of screening tests; $1500) after age 50 years; repeat every 10 years if results are normal

Follow-up colonoscopies should be obtained in individuals who have abnormal results from FOBTs, flexible sigmoidoscopies, and barium enemas. Screening examinations are recommended at more frequent intervals and should be started at a younger age in patients who have risk factors for developing CRC or have a family history of CRC.

9. Will a high-fiber diet protect against colon cancer?

The relationship between vegetable, fruit, and fiber consumption and colorectal cancer remains controversial. Recent studies have shown no risk reduction of colon cancer from high-fiber diets.

10. Have any studies provided evidence that the consumption of medications, vitamins, or other nutrients prevents colorectal cancer?

Some clinical trials have shown that calcium supplementation reduces the risk of colorectal adenomas, long-term use of aspirin reduces the incidence of colorectal polyps, and cyclooxygenase-2 (COX-2) inhibitors prevent colon polyps (see Chapter 2, Cancer Prevention and Detection). However, the American Cancer Society does not recommend any medications or supplements to prevent CRC because of uncertainties about their effectiveness, appropriate dose, and potential toxicity (e.g., risk of heart attacks associated with selective COX-2 inhibitors).

11. What is the treatment of choice for colorectal cancer?

Colon cancer: Surgical resection is the primary treatment of choice; more than one half of all patients can be cured by surgical resection of the involved intestinal segment and reanastomosis. Even if distant metastases are present, surgery is often performed to prevent complications from bleeding, perforation, or obstruction. Approximately 15% of all patients diagnosed with colorectal cancer require a permanent colostomy.

Rectal cancer: Abdominal-perineal resections may be indicated for low rectal lesions. Newer sphincter-sparing procedures are under study. Clinical trials are ongoing to compare laparoscopic surgery with traditional open surgery.

New advances in surgery for CRC include sentinel lymph node mapping and laparoscopy. Laparoscopic colectomies are being performed with increasing frequency, although their use for patients with CRC remains controversial. Shorter hospitalizations, earlier return of bowel function, and decreased need for opioid drugs have been documented in populations receiving this type of surgery.

Surgical treatment for colorectal cancer

Site	Procedure	Physical alteration
Appendix, cecum, ascending colon, hepatic flexure	Right hemicolectomy	Possible temporary or permanent cecostomy or ascending colostomy
Transverse colon	Transverse colectomy	Possible temporary or permanent transverse colostomy
Distal transverse colon	Left hemicolectomy	Possible temporary or permanent colostomy
Splenic flexure, descending colon	Left partial colectomy	Possible temporary or permanent colon descending colostomy
Sigmoid colon	Sigmoid colectomy	Possible temporary or permanent sigmoid colostomy
Rectum	Low anterior resection for tumors > 10 cm from anal verge (upper third of rectum)	Possible temporary or permanent sigmoid colostomy
	Abdominal perineal resection (APR)	Permanent sigmoid colostomy (APR) in distal 6 cm of rectum
	Low anterior resection or APR controversial (cancer in mid-rectum, 7-11 cm from anal verge)	Permanent sigmoid colostomy with APR

12. What instructions about lifestyle changes should be given to patients with a colostomy?

- **Hygiene**. Bathe with or without pouch; be aware that stool can pass while bathing. Hot tubs should be avoided or used with caution. Empty the pouch when it is one-third full of stool, flatus, or both. Change the pouch every 4 to 7 days if there is no leakage. Because pouches are now odor proof and waterproof, they should not be punctured, as recommended in the past.
- **Diet**. No restrictions. Continue to eat well-balanced meals with fluid intake of 6 to 8 glasses per day. Avoid or eat in moderation foods that may cause odor or gas.
- **Activity**. Avoid heavy lifting, pushing, and pulling during the first 3 postoperative months. Continue participation in sports, including swimming, but avoid contact sports.
- **Traveling**. No restrictions. Always hand-carry supplies and take along extras.
- **Sexual activity**. Empty the pouch or deodorize the pouch 6 to 12 hours before sexual activity and avoid foods that can cause gas, odor, or loose stools. Wear opaque pouch covers to conceal fecal material, or use lingerie or underwear made with pockets on the inside to hold the pouch. Experiment with sexual positions other

than the missionary position. For women, consider vaginal lubricants for dyspareunia; for men, consider prostheses or reconstructive surgery (high incidence of impotence in men after abdominal perineal resection).

13. Should colostomies be irrigated?

Patients are usually taught to irrigate the colostomy to maintain bowel regularity. Irrigation may also be necessary to cleanse the bowel for procedures. Colostomy irrigations can be done to regulate bowel activity in descending or sigmoid colostomies with formed stool. Irrigations are not recommended for the ascending or transverse colon because of the loose consistency of stool.

14. When is radiation therapy indicated?

- Preoperative radiation therapy is recommended to reduce bulky rectal cancers, increase the likelihood that the entire cancer can be resected, and eradicate microscopic disease. A decrease in local recurrence rate has been observed with neoadjuvant radiation, chemotherapy, or both.
- Postoperative radiation therapy is recommended for patients with stage II or III rectal cancers to prevent local recurrence, or eliminate remaining disease if surgical margins are positive.
- Postoperative radiation therapy is recommended for patients with colon cancer if disease invades other organs (e.g., bladder, abdominal wall).
- Palliative radiation therapy is recommended to decrease painful metastases or control bleeding in patients with inoperable cancers.

Note: No change in survival rate has been noted with radiation therapy.

15. What is the role of chemotherapy in treating colorectal cancer?

- Neoadjuvant treatment before surgery
- Adjuvant treatment after surgery (decreases the risk of recurrence by as much as 76%)
- Palliation of advanced or metastatic disease
- Radiation sensitizer

16. Which chemotherapeutic agents are used to treat CRC?

- **Fluorouracil** (5-FU) is the most widely used chemotherapy agent, with an overall response rate of 17% to 30%. Gastrointestinal effects (diarrhea and mucositis) or myelosuppression related to 5-FU vary according to total dose, timing, combination of drugs used, and method of administration. For example, continuous infusions commonly cause more gastrointestinal toxicity and hand-foot syndrome than bolus dosing, which causes more myelosuppression. A regimen of adjuvant postoperative radiation therapy plus 5-FU administration may have a detrimental effect on long-term bowel function. It may cause formation of liquid stools, frequent defecation, perineal skin irritation, and inability to differentiate stool from flatulence.
- **Capecitabine** (Xeloda), an oral 5-FU prodrug, is used for metastatic colorectal cancer.
- **Leucovorin** (a vitamin that enhances the effectiveness of 5-FU) is given with 5-FU postoperatively as adjuvant therapy in patients with Dukes' stage B and C colon cancer.
- **Irinotecan** (Camptosar) is used in patients with advanced disease refractory to 5-FU; it has a response rate of 23%. Irinotecan in combination with 5-FU and leucovorin (IFL or FOLFIRI regimen) has been shown to be superior to 5-FU and leucovorin alone in the metastatic setting. Studies are currently under way to explore the role of irinotecan in the adjuvant setting.

- **Bevacizumab** (Avastin) is currently approved for treatment of colon cancer in a metastatic setting. It is a humanized monoclonal antibody that targets and effectively neutralizes vascular endothelial growth factor (VEGF). Bevacizumab inhibits new blood vessel formation and tumor progression by decreasing or eliminating circulating VEGF levels. Whereas clinical trials have demonstrated increased survival when bevacizumab is added to IFL and FOLFOX (5-FU, leucovorin, oxaliplatin regimens, hypertension and grade 3 neurotoxicities are increased. There is some thought that bevacizumab may facilitate platinum entry into neurons.
- **Cetuximab** (Erbitux) is a monoclonal antibody that interferes with cancer cell growth by binding to an epidermal growth factor receptor (EGFR) so that the normal (natural) epidermal growth factors cannot bind and stimulate the cells to grow. Cetuximab is currently approved for use in combination with irinotecan for the treatment of EGFR-expressing, metastatic colorectal carcinoma in patients with cancer that is refractory to irinotecan-based chemotherapy. It is also used as a single agent for the treatment of EGFR-expressing, recurrent metastatic colorectal carcinoma in patients who are intolerant of irinotecan chemotherapy. Common toxicities are acne-like rash and diarrhea.
- **Oxaliplatin** (Eloxatin) is a platinum agent that is currently approved for first-line adjuvant treatment. Though it can be administered as a single agent, oxaliplatin alone is now known to be substantially inferior to FOLFOX in second line therapy. Common toxicities are oral-pharyngeal dysesthesias and peripheral neuropathies, which are typically exacerbated by cold exposure (see Chapter 6, Principles of Chemotherapy). Grade 3 neutropenia can also be observed when combined with a 5-FU regimen.
- **Panitumumab** (Vectibix) is a fully human monoclonal antibody. Like cetuximab, it binds to epidermal growth factor receptors (EGFR) on both normal and tumor cells. Panitumumab is currently indicated for EGFR expressing metastatic colorectal carcinoma with disease progression on or following treatment with 5-FU, oxaliplatin, or irinotecan containing chemotherapy regimens. Common toxicities include diarrhea and acne-form rash.

17. Compare the effectiveness of commonly used CRC chemotherapy regimens?

ADJUVANT
FOLFOX (fluorouracil [5-FU], leucovorin, oxaliplatin) has been proven to be more effective than the combination of 5-FU and leucovorin.
Xeloda as a single agent is equivalent to 5-FU and leucovorin combined.

METASTATIC
Currently, there is no one standard of care for metastatic colorectal cancer.
FOLFOX is equivalent to FOLFIRI (fluorouracil, leucovorin, irinotecan).

18. What newer agents show promise?

Experimental approaches include:
- Inhibitors of signal transduction, such as drugs that would inhibit an epidermal growth factor receptor and down-regulate cellular and molecular processes of malignant cells
- Monoclonal antibody therapy against the colon carcinoma-associated antigen, CO17-1A
- Vaccination against the tumor-associated antigen, CEA
- Folate-based specific inhibitors of thymidylate synthases, such as ICI D1694
- Inhibitors of tyrosine kinase vascular endothelial growth factor (VEGF) receptors
- UFT, another oral 5-FU prodrug; also in clinical trial

19. What rare adverse effects can occur from 5-FU therapy?

Severe reactions to standard doses of 5-FU are seen in 3% of patients who have a rare genetic enzyme deficiency called dihydropyrimidine dehydrogenase deficiency (DPD). This is an enzyme responsible for 5-FU catabolism. Adverse effects include diarrhea, stomatitis, mucositis, myelosuppression, neurotoxicity, hand-foot syndrome, nausea, vomiting, and mental status changes. Patients are not routinely tested for this enzyme deficiency before treatment with 5-FU.

20. Are other treatments available for metastatic disease?

Treatment depends on the symptoms and extent of metastatic disease. Metastatic disease in the liver can be treated with radiation, hepatic artery chemoinfusion, or surgical resection if disease is limited to one area of the liver.

 Key Points

- Surgical resection is the primary treatment for colorectal cancer.
- Chemotherapy is used as neoadjuvant therapy before surgery, adjuvant treatment after surgery, palliative treatment of advanced disease, and sensitizing agents for radiation therapy.
- Fluorouracil (5-FU), leucovorin, oxaliplatin, irinotecan, and oral capecitabine are chemotherapy agents commonly used to treat colorectal carcinomas.
- Currently, there is no one standard of care for metastatic colorectal cancer.
- Biologic agents, such as cetuximab, bevacizumab, and panitumumab have been shown to augment the effectiveness of chemotherapeutic agents commonly used in the metastatic setting.

 Internet Resources

American Cancer Society:
  http://www.cancer.org
Colon Cancer Network:
  http://www.colorectal-cancer.net/
United Ostomy Associations of America, Inc.:
  http://www.uoa.org
The Johns Hopkins Medical Institutions Gastroenterology and Hepatology Resource Center:
  http://hopkins-gi.nts.jhu.edu/pages/latin/templates/index.cfm
Myriad Genetics Laboratories (1-800-469-7423) provides information about genetic screening and counseling:
  http://www.myriad.com
National Cancer Institute:
  http://www.cancer.gov/
National Comprehensive Cancer Network (NCCN) Colon and Rectal Cancer Clinical Practice Guidelines, version 2:2006:
  http://www.nccn.org/professionals/physician_gls/PDF/colon.pdf
  http://www.nccn.org/professionals/physician_gls/PDF/rectal.pdf
Wound Ostomy & Continence Nurses Society:
  http://www.wocn.org/

Acknowledgments

The authors wish to acknowledge Diane K. Nakagaki, RN, BSN, ET, Brenda M. Hiromoto, RN, MS, CETN, OCN, and Kelly C. Mack, RN, MSN, AOCN, NP-C, for their contributions to the Colorectal Cancer chapter published in the first and second editions of *Oncology Nursing Secrets*.

Bibliography

American Gastroenterological Association Clinical Practice and Practice Economics Committee. AGA technical review: Impact of dietary fiber on colon cancer occurrence. *Gastroenterology* 118:1235-1257, 2000.

Bloomston M, Kaufman H, Winston J, et al: Surgical management of colorectal cancer in the laparoscopic era: A review of prospective randomized trials. *J Natl Compr Canc Netw* 3(4):517-524, 2005.

Ellis C, Saddler DAH: Colorectal cancer. In Yarbro CH, Frogge MH, Goodman M, et al, editors: *Cancer nursing: Principles and practice,* ed 6. Boston, 2005, Jones and Bartlett.

Govindan R: Colorectal malignancies. In *The Washington manual of oncology,* Philadelphia, 2002, Lippincott Williams & Wilkins.

Greene FL, Page DL, Fleming ID, et al: *AJCC cancer staging manual,* ed 6, New York, 2002, Springer.

Guthrie M: Alternative cancer treatments. Available at: http://www.alternative-cancer-treatments.com/colon-cancer-prognosis.htm. Accessed December 22, 2005.

Jemal A, Siegel R, Ward E, et al: Cancer statistics, 2007. *CA Cancer J Clin* 57:43-66, 2007.

Lorenz M, Muller HH: Randomized multicenter trial of fluorouracil plus leucovorin administered either via hepatic arterial or intravenous infusion versus flurordeoxyuridine administered via hepatic arterial infusion in patients with nonresectable liver metastases from colorectal carcinoma. *J Clin Oncol* 18: 243, 2000.

National Cancer Institute. A snapshot of colorectal cancer: Incidence and mortality trends. Available at: http://planning.cancer.gov/disease/Colorectal-Snapshot.pdf. Accessed December 22, 2005.

Saltz LB: Metastatic colorectal cancer: Is there one standard approach? *Oncology* 19(9):1147-1154, 2005.

Saltz LB, Cox JV, Blanke C, et al: Irinotecan plus fluorouracil and leucovorin for metastatic colorectal cancer. *N Engl J Med* 343:905-914, 2000.

Steinbach G, Lynch PM, Phillips RKS, et al: The effect of celecoxib, a cyclooxygenase-2 inhibitor, in familial adenomatous polyposis. *N Engl J Med* 342:1946-1952, 2000.

Endocrine Cancers

Michael T. McDermott

1. What are endocrine neoplasms?

Benign or malignant tumors may develop in endocrine glands and cause clinical disease by secreting excessive amounts of hormones, by compressing or invading surrounding structures, or by metastasizing to distant sites. An estimated 35,520 new cases of endocrine cancers will occur in 2007; 33,550 of these cases will be thyroid cancer. Only 2320 deaths are estimated for 2007, of which 1530 will be related to thyroid cancer.

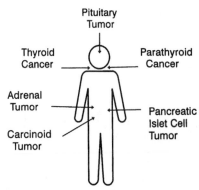

Location of endocrine neoplasms. Endocrine neoplasms arise from the hormone-secreting glands. The most common are tumors of the pituitary, thyroid, parathyroid, adrenal glands, and pancreatic islet cells. Carcinoid tumors, which may secrete large amounts of physiologic substances, are also often classified with the endocrine tumors, although they do not arise from an endocrine gland.

PITUITARY TUMORS

2. Name the different types of pituitary tumors.

Pituitary tumors may secrete prolactin (PRL), growth hormone (GH), adrenocorticotropic hormone (ACTH), thyrotropin (thyroid-stimulating hormone [TSH]), or gonadotropins (follicule-stimulating hormone [FSH] and luteinizing hormone [LH]). Some tumors secrete a mixture of hormones. Others do not secrete any hormones and are referred to as nonfunctioning pituitary tumors. The vast majority of pituitary tumors are benign neoplasms, with pituitary carcinoma being very rare. A pituitary tumor is considered a microadenoma if it is less than 10 mm in diameter, whereas macroadenomas are 10 mm or larger.

3. What syndromes are associated with pituitary tumors?

- Prolactin-secreting tumors cause galactorrhea (milk discharge from the breasts), amenorrhea (lack of menstrual periods), and infertility in women. They cause erectile dysfunction in men.
- Growth hormone-secreting tumors cause acromegaly in adults and gigantism in children.
- ACTH-producing tumors cause Cushing's disease.

- TSH-secreting tumors frequently cause hyperthyroidism, which can closely resemble Graves' disease.
- Gonadotropin-secreting tumors most often cause hypogonadism.

    If sufficiently large, any of these tumors may also cause symptoms through mass effects, similar to those seen in patients with large, nonfunctioning pituitary tumors. Mass effects include headaches, impaired vision, loss of peripheral vision, and cranial nerve palsies.

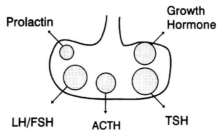

Functioning pituitary tumors. Pituitary tumors often secrete excessive amounts of one or more of the pituitary hormones: growth hormone, prolactin, thyrotropin, corticotropin, or gonadotropins (LH and FSH). Although the tumors are usually histologically benign, significant morbidity and mortality may result from the syndromes of hormone oversecretion or tumor mass compression of surrounding vascular or neural structures.

Clinical Features

ACROMEGALY

Enlargement of multiple organs

		Other features
Hands	Ears	Skin tags
Feet	Nose	Sleep apnea
Skull	Tongue	Osteoarthritis
Jaws	Heart	Hypertension
Sinuses	Liver	Diabetes mellitus

CUSHING'S SYNDROME

Central obesity	Purple striae	Emotional lability
Facial plethora	Easy bruising	Hypertension
Moon face	Muscle weakness	Diabetes mellitus
Buffalo hump		

4. How are benign pituitary tumors treated?

Many prolactin-secreting tumors can be treated with a dopamine agonist, such as bromocriptine (Parlodel) or cabergoline (Dostinex). Growth hormone-secreting tumors can be treated with either a somatostatin analog such as octreotide (Sandostatin), or a growth hormone receptor blocker such as pegvisomant (Somavert). Patients with tumors that don't respond adequately to these measures and the other hormone-secreting tumors are best treated by transphenoidal surgery. Radiation therapy, most commonly stereotactic radiosurgery, may be used if transphenoidal surgery is contraindicated or ineffective. Nonfunctioning asymptomatic microadenomas can be managed with observation by serial imaging studies, whereas macroadenomas usually require surgical removal.

5. What are the clinical features of pituitary carcinomas?

Pituitary carcinomas, which are extremely rare, expand rapidly and cause mass effects. Some secrete hormones causing endocrine syndromes similar to those seen with adenomas. Metastatic disease to the central nervous system, cervical lymph nodes, liver, and bone are commonly associated. Transphenoidal surgery is the primary therapy, followed by postoperative radiation. No significant use of chemotherapy has been reported for pituitary carcinoma. The mean survival is approximately 4 years.

6. Which cancers metastasize to the pituitary gland?

Metastatic disease to the pituitary gland occurs in approximately 3% to 5% of patients with widely disseminated carcinoma. The most commonly reported primary tumors that metastasize to the pituitary gland are breast, lung, kidney, prostate, liver, pancreas, nasopharynx, plasmacytoma, sarcoma, and adenocarcinoma of unknown primary site.

THYROID CANCER

7. Name the most common types of thyroid cancer.

The thyroid gland is composed of follicular cells, which synthesize thyroid hormones, and parafollicular C cells, which produce calcitonin. Three main histologic types of cancer arise from the follicular cells: papillary, follicular, and anaplastic carcinomas. Medullary carcinoma, in contrast, develops from the parafollicular C cells. The prognosis for papillary carcinoma is excellent. The cure rate exceeds 90%, and the 10-year mortality rate is only 5%. Similarly, follicular carcinoma has a cure rate of over 80% and a 10-year mortality rate of 10%. Patients with medullary carcinoma, however, have a 10-year mortality rate of approximately 30%, and most patients with anaplastic carcinoma die within 8 months of diagnosis.

8. How do thyroid cancers present clinically?

Patients with thyroid cancer usually develop a painless thyroid mass, much like a benign thyroid nodule. Features suggesting that such a mass is malignant include size greater than 3 cm, rock-hard consistency, lymphadenopathy, and hoarseness due to vocal cord paralysis. The diagnosis is most reliably made by fine-needle aspiration biopsy.

9. How are thyroid cancers treated?

- Papillary and follicular carcinomas are treated with near-total thyroidectomy, radioiodine (I-131) ablation, and levothyroxine (LT4) suppression therapy. I-131 is given after surgery, when appropriate, to destroy residual normal or neoplastic thyroid tissue. LT4 is then given in doses sufficient to suppress the serum TSH to below the reference range, since TSH is a growth factor for thyroid cancer.
- Medullary carcinoma requires a total thyroidectomy and LT4 replacement, keeping the TSH level within the reference range.
- Anaplastic carcinoma is treated by total thyroidectomy, LT4 suppression and, in some cases, external beam irradiation. Chemotherapy with paclitaxel or docetaxel, alone or with doxorubicin, may also be considered for aggressive or metastatic disease.

10. What are the features of parathyroid carcinoma?

The first symptoms of patients with parathyroid carcinoma may be a neck mass with associated lymphadenopathy or hypercalcemia discovered on serum testing. The most strongly suggestive finding is moderate to marked hypercalcemia with extremely elevated serum levels of parathyroid hormone (PTH). The diagnosis of parathyroid cancer, however, ultimately depends on tissue examination. The treatment of choice is removal of the tumor by an experienced surgeon. Chemotherapy and radiation therapies are rarely beneficial. The 5-year survival rate is less than 50%.

ADRENAL CANCER

11. What types of cancer occur in the adrenal glands?

Carcinomas may arise in the adrenal cortex (adrenocortical carcinomas) or the adrenal medulla (malignant pheochromocytomas). They also may metastasize to the adrenals from other primary sites. Approximately 50% to 70% secrete hormones, whereas 30% to 50% are nonfunctioning. The mean survival time is 15 months. The 5-year survival rate is about 20% to 35%. Prognosis is improved by young age, small tumor size, localized disease, complete tumor resection, and a nonfunctioning tumor.

12. What are the clinical features of adrenal carcinomas?

Functioning adrenal carcinomas secrete aldosterone, cortisol, androgens, or catecholamines. Excessive aldosterone (Conn's syndrome) causes hypertension and hypokalemia. Cortisol overproduction results in Cushing's syndrome. Excessive androgen secretion causes hirsutism and virilization in women and precocious puberty in children, but is often asymptomatic in men. Catecholamine excess causes severe hypertension, palpitations, headaches, and sweating. The first symptoms of nonfunctioning adrenocortical carcinomas are usually abdominal or flank pain, or an adrenal mass discovered incidentally during an imaging procedure.

13. What clues are most suggestive that an adrenocortical tumor is malignant?

Malignancy is suggested by tumor size larger than 6 cm, evidence of locally invasive or metastatic disease to the liver or lungs, and elevated urinary excretion of 17-ketosteroid. The diagnosis of malignancy is often not suspected, however, until histological examination after tumor removal.

14. What is the treatment for an adrenocortical carcinoma?

The treatment of choice is surgery. Mitotane, an adrenal cytotoxic agent, has produced partial or complete tumor regression, reduced production of adrenal hormones, and improved survival in nonrandomized, noncontrolled trials. The combination of mitotane with etoposide, cisplatin, and doxorubicin has shown some promise, but responses to chemotherapy have, in general, been disappointing. Radiation therapy has not been shown to be effective with these tumors.

15. What tumors metastasize to the adrenal glands?

The vascular adrenal glands are a frequent site of bilateral metastatic spread from cancers of the lung, breast, stomach, pancreas, colon, and kidney, and from melanomas and lymphomas.

ISLET CELL TUMORS

16. Name the most common pancreatic islet cell tumors.

The pancreatic islets normally secrete three major hormones: insulin, glucagon, and somatostatin. Nonetheless, the most common islet cell tumor is gastrinoma, a neoplasm that secretes gastrin, which is normally made only in the stomach. Insulinoma is the second most common islet cell tumor; glucagonomas and somatostatinomas are rare.

Occasionally islet cell tumors will also secrete pancreatic polypeptide. Insulinomas are usually benign (80%), whereas all other pancreatic islet cell tumors are most often (80% of cases) malignant.

17. What syndromes do pancreatic islet cell tumors produce?

Gastrinomas secrete excessive gastrin, which stimulates prolific gastric acid secretion, resulting in the development of multiple, recurrent peptic ulcers, and chronic watery diarrhea. This complex is also known as Zollinger-Ellison syndrome. Excessive insulin secretion by insulinomas causes episodes of severe hypoglycemia, manifested by confusion, convulsions, and coma.

18. Is there an effective treatment for islet cell tumors?

Surgery is the treatment of choice for islet cell tumors, whenever possible. For unresectable gastrinomas, symptom relief can be achieved with medications, such as omeprazole or octreotide. Hypoglycemia from a persistent insulinoma may be prevented by eating frequent small meals and taking diazoxide, propranolol, or verapamil. Chemotherapy is often required treatment for the malignant islet cell tumors. The most effective combinations include the following: streptozotocin, 5-fluorouracil, and leucovorin; lomustine and 5-fluorouracil; etoposide, doxorubicin, and 5-fluorouracil; and cisplatin, dacarbazine, and alpha interferon. Tumor embolization in conjunction with direct intraarterial infusions of chemotherapy agents has also shown promise as a palliative procedure.

CARCINOID

19. What is the difference between having a carcinoid tumor and having carcinoid syndrome?

Carcinoid tumors are neoplasms that arise from enterochromaffin cells, named because of their histologic staining characteristics. They occur most often in the lungs, the digestive tract (especially the appendix), and the gonads. Carcinoid syndrome is a symptom complex consisting of cutaneous flushing, diarrhea, and wheezing; it is associated with a tendency to develop progressive fibrosis of the valves on the right side of the heart, endocardium, pleura, peritoneum, and retroperitoneum.

20. Describe the pathophysiology of carcinoid syndrome.

Many carcinoid tumors produce substances, such as serotonin, bradykinin, tachykinin, histamine, prostaglandins, neurotensin, and substance P, all of which are readily metabolized by the liver. When carcinoid tumors metastasize to the liver, these humoral mediators gain access to the systemic circulation and cause the manifestations of carcinoid syndrome. The diagnosis is usually made by finding elevated serum levels of serotonin or increased urinary excretion of 5-hydroxyindoleacetic acid (5-HIAA), a breakdown product of serotonin.

21. Can carcinoid syndrome be treated or controlled?

Most patients with carcinoid syndrome have incurable metastatic disease; however, because of the slow growth rate of these tumors, prolonged survival is common, and control of the symptoms becomes necessary. Flushing may be treated with antihistamines (H_1 and H_2 antagonists), steroids, or octreotide injections, whereas diarrhea responds best to codeine, antidiarrheal agents, clonidine, or octreotide. Chemotherapy regimens with palliative effects include: streptozotocin, 5-fluorouracil, and leucovorin; lomustine and 5-fluorouracil; etoposide, doxorubicin, and 5-fluorouracil; and cisplatin, dacarbazine, and alpha interferon. Hepatic artery embolization along with direct intraarterial chemotherapy infusions are also sometimes useful.

ENDOCRINE PARANEOPLASTIC SYNDROMES

22. What are the endocrine paraneoplastic syndromes?

Endocrine paraneoplastic syndromes are associated with some tumors but are not due to tissue invasion or metastases. They result from secretion of hormones by the tumor into the circulation. The three best known examples are the syndrome of inappropriate antidiuretic hormone (SIADH), hypercalcemia of malignancy, and ectopic ACTH syndrome.

23. Explain the pathophysiology of SIADH.

Antidiuretic hormone (ADH) is normally secreted by the posterior pituitary gland and acts on the kidney to promote water retention. In doing so, it protects the body against dehydration. Tumors, particularly those of the lung and brain, sometimes secrete large amounts of ADH that result in excessive water retention and dilutional hyponatremia. Hyponatremia, when severe, may cause confusion, convulsions, and coma due to edema of the brain (refer to Chapter 50).

24. What are the mediators of hypercalcemia of malignancy?

Humoral hypercalcemia of malignancy (HHM) is usually caused by tumor production of parathyroid hormone-related peptide (PTHrp). Similar in some ways to parathyroid hormone (PTH), PTHrp normally controls the transfer of calcium across the placenta and from the maternal circulation into breast milk. When secreted in excessive quantities by tumors, such as those of the lung, it stimulates bone resorption and renal calcium retention, which combine to raise the serum calcium level.

25. Describe the pathophysiology of ectopic ACTH syndrome.

ACTH is normally secreted by the anterior pituitary gland and stimulates the adrenal glands to produce cortisol. Tumors of various organs, especially the lungs, occasionally produce enough ACTH to stimulate excessive secretion of adrenal cortisol. This causes Cushing's syndrome, the manifestations of which are partly masked by tumor cachexia.

 Key Points

- Treatment of thyroid cancer involves thyroidectomy, followed by treatment with radioactive iodine in appropriate cases, and levothyroxine suppression therapy in doses sufficient to maintain the serum TSH level just below the reference range.
- Papillary and follicular thyroid carcinomas have very low mortality rates, medullar carcinoma has an intermediate mortality rate, and anaplastic carcinoma has a very high mortality rate.
- The initial symptoms of adrenal carcinomas result from excess production of cortisol, aldosterone, androgen, or catecholamine. The patient may also experience abdominal or flank pain. In other patients, an adrenal mass is discovered incidentally. Adrenal carcinoma is best treated by surgical removal of the tumor.
- The treatment of pancreatic endocrine tumors is surgical removal when possible, but when the primary tumor is inoperable, symptomatic relief may be achieved with high-dose proton pump inhibitors or gastrectomy to reduce gastric acid production in patients with gastrinoma, and frequent small meals or medical therapy to reduce hypoglycemia in insulinoma patients.
- The treatment for carcinoid syndrome is surgery, when possible, but the treatment may be palliative, using medications that reduce secretion of the humoral mediators or antagonize their effects.

Internet Resources

American Cancer Society: Statistics for 2006:
http://www.cancer.org
National Comprehensive Cancer Network, Thyroid Carcinoma Practice Guidelines:
http://www.nccn.org
Clinical Trials:
http://www.clinicaltrials.gov

Bibliography

Ahlman H, Nilsson O, Olausson M: Interventional treatment of the carcinoid syndrome. *Neuroendocrinology* 80(suppl 1):67-73, 2004.

American Thyroid Association Guidelines Taskforce: Management guidelines for patients with thyroid nodules and differentiated thyroid cancer. *Thyroid* 16:109-139, 2006.

Beuschlein F, Looyenga BD, Reincke M, et al: Clinical impact of recent advances in the biology of adrenocortical cancer. *Endocrinologist* 13:470-478, 2003.

Bornstein SR, Stratakis CA, Chrousos GP: Adrenocortical tumors: Recent advances in basic concepts and clinical management. *Ann Intern Med* 130:759-771, 1999.

Busaidy NL, Jimenez C, Habra MA, et al: Parathyroid carcinoma: A 22 year experience. *Head Neck* 26(8):716-726, 2004.

Galanis E, Kvols LK, Rubin J: Carcinoid syndrome. *J Clin Oncol* 16:796-798, 1998.

Isidori AM, Kaltsas GA, Pozza C, et al: The ectopic adrenocorticotropin syndrome: Clinical features, diagnosis, management, and long-term follow-up. *J Clin Endocrinol Metab* 91:371-377, 2006.

Jemal A, Siegel R, Ward E, et al: Cancer statistics, 2007. *CA Cancer J Clin* 57:43-66, 2007.

Jensen RT: Pancreatic endocrine tumors: Recent advances. *Ann Oncol* 10(suppl 4):170-180, 1999.

Kaltsas GA, Mukherjee JJ, Plowman PN, et al: The role of cytotoxic chemotherapy in the management of aggressive and malignant pituitary tumors. *J Clin Endocrinol* Metab 83:4233-4238, 1998.

Kaltsas GA, Nomikos P, Kontogeorgos G, et al: Diagnosis and management of pituitary carcinomas. *J Clin Endocrinol Metab* 90:3089-3099, 2005.

Kebebew E, Clark OH: Differentiated thyroid cancer: "Complete" rational approach. *World J Surg* 24:942-951, 2000.

Kirschner LS: Emerging treatment strategies for adrenocortical carcinoma: A new hope. *J Clin Endocrinol Metab* 91:14-21, 2006.

Komninos J, Vlassopoulou V, Protopapa D, et al: Tumors metastatic to the pituitary gland: Case report and literature review. *J Clin Endocrinol Metab* 89:574-580, 2004.

Kulke MH, Mayer RJ: Carcinoid tumors. *N Engl J Med* 340:858-868, 1999.

Shane E: Parathyroid carcinoma. *J Clin Endocrinol Metab* 86:485-493, 2001.

Sherman SI: Thyroid carcinoma. *Lancet* 361(9356):501-511, 2003.

Soga J: Carcinoids and their variant endocrinomas: An analysis of 11,842 reported cases. *J Exp Clin Cancer Res* 22(4):517-30, 2003.

Stewart AF: Hypercalcemia associated with cancer. *N Engl J Med* 352:373-379, 2005.

Gastric, Pancreatic, Hepatocellular, and Gallbladder Cancers

Mary Kay Schultz and Michele Basche

GASTRIC CANCER
Quick Facts—Gastric Cancer

Incidence	21,260 newly diagnosed cases estimated in 2007 (13,000 in men; 8260 in women)
	Median age at diagnosis is 72 years
Mortality	11,210 deaths estimated in 2007
Risk factors	Male gender, advanced age
	Time postgastrectomy (> 15 years)
	Barrett's esophagus (proximal gastric cancer)
	Helicobacter pylori infection (distal gastric cancer)
	Chronic atrophic gastritis
	Ménétrier's disease (giant hypertophic gastritis)
	Pernicious anemia
	Gastric polyps
	Cigarette smoking
	Nutritional factors (diets low in fruits and vegetables; high in salted, smoked, or preserved foods)
Genetics	Family history of gastric cancer, blood type A, hereditary nonpolyposis colon cancer (HNPCC), and familial adenomatous polyposis
Histopathology	Adenocarcinoma, 90%-95%
	Lymphomas, sarcomas (including gastrointestinal stromal tumors [GIST]), and rarely carcinoid and squamous cell carcinomas, 5%-10%
Symptoms	Weight loss
	Abdominal pain (vague and mild in early disease; more severe and constant as the disease progresses)
	Dysphagia (gastric cardia or esophagogastric junction cancers)
	Postprandial emesis (distal gastric cancer due to pyloric obstruction)
	Other symptoms: nausea, bloating, early satiety, occult bleeding (common), melena or hematemesis (less common), anemia from chronic disease or iron deficiency, fatigue, and weakness
Diagnosis and evaluation	History and physical examination (palpable abdominal mass; nodal metastases in the supraclavicular fossa, axilla, or umbilical areas)
	Chest x-ray (PA and lateral)
	Computed tomography (CT) of chest, abdomen, pelvis
	Endoscopic ultrasonography (EUS)
	Capsule video endoscopy (useful in imaging the small intestine)
	PET scan

Quick Facts—cont'd

Staging and Stage Grouping

Stage	Description
Tumor, node, metastasis (TNM):	
Primary tumor (T)	
TX	Primary tumor cannot be assessed
T0	No evidence of primary tumor
Tis	Carcinoma in situ: intraepithelial tumor without invasion of lamina propria
T1	Tumor invades lamina propria or submucosa
T2	Tumor invades muscularis propria or subserosa
T2a	Tumor invades muscularis propria
T2b	Tumor invades subserosa
T3	Tumor penetrates serosa (visceral peritoneum) without invasion of adjacent structures
T4	Tumor invades adjacent structures
Regional lymph nodes (N)	
NX	Regional lymph node(s) cannot be assessed
N0	No regional lymph node metastasis
N1	Metastasis in 1-6 regional lymph node(s)
N2	Metastasis in 7-15 regional lymph nodes
N3	Metastasis in > 15 regional nodes
Distant metastasis (M)	
MX	Presence of distant metastasis cannot be assessed
M0	No distant metastasis
M1	Distant metastasis

Stage	Primary Tumor	Regional Lymph Nodes	Distant Metastasis
0	Tis	N0	M0
IA	T1	N0	M0
IB	T1	N1	M0
	T2a/b	N0	M0
II	T1	N	M0
	T2a/b	N1	M0
	T3	N0	M0
IIIA	T2a/b	N2	M0
	T3	N1	M0
	T4	N0	M0
IIIB	T3	N2	M0
IV	T4	N1-3	M0
	T1-3	N3	M0
	Any T	Any N	M1

1. In what part of the stomach does gastric cancer commonly occur?

Over recent decades, the site of cancer origin within the stomach has changed in frequency, with cancer of the distal half of the stomach decreasing. Cancer of the cardia and gastro-esophageal junction have been increasing in frequency, particularly in patients younger than 40 years.

2. What is the association between *Helicobacter pylori* infection and gastric cancer?

Gastric carcinoma is believed to evolve as a progression from atrophy to metaplasia, dysplasia, and then carcinoma. *Helicobacter pylori* infection, the most common cause of gastritis, is also associated with some types of lymphoma of the stomach, but the vast majority of people who carry this bacterium in their stomachs never develop gastric cancer. Therefore, gastric carcinogenesis cannot be explained by *H. pylori* infection alone.

3. Does treatment for gastric *H. pylori* infection reduce the risk of developing gastric cancer?

This is unknown. Data are insufficient to recommend mass screening programs of asymptomatic people for *H. pylori* infection for prevention of gastric cancer.

4. How does diet affect one's risk for developing gastric cancer?

Nitrates and nitrites, substances commonly found in cured meats, smoked foods, salted fish, pickled vegetables, and some drinking water, can be converted by certain bacteria, such as *H. pylori*, into compounds that have been found to cause stomach cancer in animals. Conversely, eating whole grain products and fresh fruits and vegetables containing vitamins A and C may lower the risk of stomach cancer. Some studies have linked alcohol use to stomach cancer; however, this association has never been clearly established.

5. What are the names of metastatic deposits associated with gastric cancer?

- Virchow's node: left supraclavicular lymph node enlargement
- Irish's node: left axillary lymph node enlargement
- Sister Mary Joseph's nodule: periumbilical nodule
- Krukenberg's tumor: metastatic disease to ovaries
- Blumer's shelf: mass in the cul-de-sac or rectal shelf

6. What role does surgery play in the treatment of gastric cancer?

Radical surgery is standard therapy for medically fit patients with potentially resectable (stages I-III) carcinoma, although it is curative in less than 40% of patients. The type of resection (subtotal vs. total gastrectomy) and extent of lymphadenectomy are subjects for debate. Survival rates are best improved in patients with stage I disease. Patients with T3, T4, or any nodal involvement have a significant risk for relapse after surgical resection.

7. Following gastrectomy, most patients develop some degree of "dumping syndrome." What is this?

Dumping syndrome is a postoperative complication of gastric resection. Clinical manifestations include nausea, vomiting, diarrhea, epigastric fullness, tachycardia, diaphoresis, and weakness. Dumping syndrome most likely is due to removal of the reservoir function (antrum) of the stomach. Hypertonic foodstuffs empty directly into the small bowel, resulting in a major fluid shift out of the intravascular space and into the bowel. To improve symptoms, patients should decrease the osmotic load presented to the small bowel by eating small, frequent meals that are low in carbohydrate and high in protein.

8. Why are monthly injections of Vitamin B$_{12}$ necessary after subtotal or total gastrectomy?

Intrinsic factor, a glycoprotein produced by the parietal cells of the gastric mucosa, is necessary for the absorption of Vitamin B$_{12}$. Following gastrectomy, there is inadequate production of intrinsic factor, eventually resulting in vitamin B$_{12}$ deficiency and pernicious anemia. Because of the liver's ability to store vitamin B_{12}, deficiency usually does not develop for 2 to 10 years after surgery. Once these stores are exhausted, the deficiency becomes evident and monthly administration of vitamin B_{12} becomes necessary.

9. What adjuvant therapy protocols are used to treat gastric cancer?

- Recently a multicenter phase III randomized controlled trial, INT-0116, demonstrated that adjuvant chemoradiotherapy with fluorouracil (5-FU), administered to patients who have undergone curative-intent resection of adenocarcinoma of the stomach or gastroesophageal junction conferred a significant survival advantage compared to observation alone. This regimen has become a standard of care in the United States.
- Only 5-FU/leucovorin has been studied in conjunction with radiation therapy in the phase III setting. Other chemotherapy regimens currently being evaluated in combination with radiation in clinical trials include cisplatin, taxanes, and irinotecan-based combinations, and ECF (epirubicin, cisplatin, and 5-FU).
- Neoadjuvant treatment (chemotherapy or chemoradiotherapy) may be performed to convert an initially unresectable cancer to resectable status.

10. How should patients with advanced gastric cancer be treated?

Patients with advanced gastric carcinoma are incurable. Palliative treatment options include:

- **External beam radiation therapy or endoscopic techniques** may be used in patients with locally advanced tumors that are unresectable to reduce pain, relieve obstruction, and/or control bleeding.
- **Chemotherapy** may improve quality of life and overall survival. Outside of clinical trials, the recommended chemotherapy for patients with advanced gastric carcinoma and good performance status is either cisplatin-based or 5-FU–based combination therapy.
- **Palliative resection** should be reserved for patients with uncontrolled bleeding or obstruction.
- Participation in **clinical trials** should be offered to medically fit patients with stage III-IV disease.

11. How does the survival rate vary by stage for the patient with gastric cancer?

Five-year survival rates vary greatly depending on stage at diagnosis:

Stage 0	> 90%
Stage IA	60%-80%
Stage IB	50%-60%
Stage II	30%-50%
Stage III	10%-20%
Stage IV	< 5%

PANCREATIC CANCER

Quick Facts—Pancreatic Cancer

Incidence	37,170 newly diagnosed cases estimated in 2007 (18,830 in men; 18,340 in women)	Cigarette smoking Occupational chemical exposure (beta-naphthylamine, benzidine [used in textile dyes])
Mortality	33,370 deaths estimated in 2007	High dietary fat intake
Risk factors	Advanced age (80% of cases in persons aged 60-80 years)	Chronic high alcohol use in smokers

Continued

Quick Facts—cont'd

Genetics	Genetic predisposition in approximately 5% of patients		Nausea, vomiting, bloating, dyspepsia
	Germline mutations in genes causing familial cancer syndromes		Diarrhea, steatorrhea, or floating stools
			New-onset diabetes
Histopathology	Adenocarcinoma arising from the exocrine gland ductal system (95%)	**Diagnosis and evaluation**	History and physical examination
			Multiphase spiral computed tomography (CT)
	Islet cell and carcinoid tumors are considered endocrine tumors and are not included in this chapter (see Chapter 24)		Transabdominal ultrasound; endoscopic ultrasound (EUS)
			CT of abdomen and pelvis
Symptoms	Abdominal pain (advanced disease)		Endoscopic retrograde cholangiopancreatography (ERCP)
	Anorexia, weight loss, early satiety		CT/PET (positron emission tomography)
	Jaundice		

Staging and Stage Grouping

Stage   Description

Tumor, node, metastasis (TNM)

Primary tumor (T)

TX   Primary tumor cannot be assessed
T0   No evidence of primary tumor
Tis   Carcinoma in situ
T1   Tumor limited to the pancreas, 2 cm or less in greatest dimension
T2   Tumor limited to the pancreas, more than 2 cm in greatest dimension
T3   Tumor extends beyond the pancreas but without involvement of the celiac axis or the superior mesenteric artery
T4   Tumor involves the celiac axis or the superior mesenteric artery (unresectable primary tumor)

Regional lymph nodes (N)

NX   Regional lymph nodes cannot be assessed
N0   No regional lymph node metastasis
N1   Regional lymph node metastasis

Distant metastasis (M)

MX   Distant metastasis cannot be assessed
M0   No distant metastasis
M1   Distant metastasis

Stage	Primary Tumor	Regional Lymph Nodes	Distant Metastasis
0	Tis	N0	M0
IA	T1	N0	M0
IB	T2	N0	M0
IIA	T3	N0	M0
IIB	T1-3	N1	M0
III	T4	Any N	M0
IV	Any T	Any N	M1

12. Isn't chronic pancreatitis a risk factor for pancreatic cancer?

Chronic pancreatitis has long been thought to be a risk factor; however, recent studies suggest that the increased risk may be due to smoking, alcohol consumption, and selection bias.

13. What are the 5-year survival rates for pancreatic cancer and why are they so low?

The median survival of patients with pancreatic cancer is 9 to 12 months, and the overall 5-year survival rate is only 3%. The prognosis is poor because at the time of diagnosis, more than half of patients have distant metastatic disease, and 40% of patients have locally advanced but unresectable disease.

Resectable disease is defined by absence of extrapancreatic disease, absence of tumor extension to the superior mesenteric artery and celiac axis, and a patent superior mesenteric-portal vein confluence. Median survival of resected patients ranges from 15 to 19 months, with the 5-year survival rate at approximately 20%. Among patients whose disease is considered to be resectable, 50% will die of recurrent tumor within 2 years. Local recurrence occurs in 50% to 80% of patients, peritoneal recurrence in 25%, and liver metastases in 50%.

The average survival rate for patients with unresectable, locally advanced, non-metastatic pancreatic cancer treated without surgery is 9 to 10 months, and the median survival for metastatic disease is 6 months.

14. What surgical procedures are used to treat pancreatic cancer?

The approach to therapy differs according to stage of disease when diagnosed. Complete surgical resection remains the only effective treatment (possible in only 15%-20% of patients). Procedures include pancreaticoduodenectomy (Whipple procedure) for tumors in the head of the pancreas, distal pancreatectomy for lesions in the tail, and total pancreatectomy for large or diffuse lesions. Since there are no universally accepted criteria for resection, the National Comprehensive Cancer Network (NCCN) Guidelines Panel recommends that decisions about diagnostic management and resectability require multidisciplinary consultation.

15. What is a Whipple procedure?

The standard operation for pancreatic cancer within the head of the pancreas is a pancreaticoduodenectomy, or Whipple procedure. It is the only potentially curative approach to cancer in the head of the pancreas. The standard Whipple procedure involves removal of the pancreatic head, duodenum, common bile duct, gallbladder, and the first 15 cm of the jejunum. A vagotomy and partial gastrectomy are also performed. Unfortunately, resection is feasible in only 10% to 20% of cases, because most patients have advanced disease. Factors that predict long-term survival after resection include clear surgical margins, negative lymph nodes, and reduced perioperative mortality. Because Whipple procedures are associated with significant morbidity and mortality, the NCCN recommends that this procedure be performed at high volume centers. Mortality rate following pancreaticoduodenectomy is less than 2% when surgery is performed at a major medical center by experienced surgeons.

16. Is adjuvant therapy indicated in patients with pancreatic cancer?

Adjuvant therapy for resected pancreatic cancer is controversial.

- In the United States many patients are offered chemotherapy with 5-FU and radiotherapy after recovery from surgery. This approach is based on the results of a small randomized controlled trial (stopped early because of poor accrual) that was conducted by the Gastrointestinal Tumor Study Group (GITSG). However, a larger randomized study conducted by the European Study Group for Pancreatic Cancer (ESPAC-1) reported greater improvement in median survival in patients with resected pancreatic cancer who received adjuvant 5-FU versus no chemotherapy, and a decrease in median survival in patients who received radiotherapy versus no radiotherapy.

- Chemoradiotherapy is an option for managing unresectable, locally advanced pancreatic cancer. It confers a modest improvement in survival when compared to best supportive care alone.
- Gemcitabine is clinically beneficial and slightly increases survival time for patients with locally advanced or metastatic pancreatic cancer. Clinical benefits include decreased pain, increased appetite, weight gain, and improved functional status. Other gemcitabine combination regimens have shown no statistically significant trend toward improved survival time.
- There is no consensus on second-line therapy for pancreatic cancer. Capecitabine and 5-FU have been used to treat patients not enrolled in clinical trials.
- Because of poor response to conventional chemotherapy, radiation therapy, and surgery, medically fit patients with pancreatic cancer should be offered enrollment in clinical trials.

17. What is Courvoisier's sign?

A palpable gallbladder is called Courvoisier's sign. Carcinoma of the head of the pancreas may cause biliary obstruction, resulting in a distended gallbladder, which can be palpated on physical exam. The distended gallbladder is typically not tender, and is present in approximately 25% of all patients with pancreatic cancer.

18. Which serologic tumor-associated antigen is followed in the patient with pancreatic cancer?

CA 19-9 is commonly expressed and shed in patients with pancreatic and hepatobiliary disease as well as many other malignancies. A decrease in serial CA 19-9 levels is correlated with survival of patients with pancreatic cancer after surgical resection or chemotherapy. Therefore, in some patients, CA 19-9 levels are monitored to evaluate response to treatment.

19. How is advanced pancreatic cancer treated?

The primary goals for treatment of advanced pancreatic cancer are palliation and improved quality of life.

- Patients are often malnourished from anorexia, nausea, tumor cachexia, biliary or gastric obstruction, and pancreatic insufficiency. Treatment with pancreatic enzyme tablets can aid absorption and decrease symptoms of dyspepsia, nausea, and bloating. Nutritional consultation with an oncology dietician can help relieve effects of anorexia and decreased calorie and protein intake.
- Biliary obstruction may cause jaundice, nausea, pruritus, malaise and impaired liver function. Placement of a biliary stent, either endoscopically or percutaneously, may relieve obstruction and diminish symptoms.
- Gastric outlet obstruction causes nausea, vomiting, early satiety, and pain. These symptoms may be palliated by the endoscopic placement of stents by experienced gastroenterologists. Alternatively, surgery to relieve or bypass an obstruction may be considered, depending on the patient's disease, anticipated life expectancy, and symptoms. Feeding tube placement might be considered as a less invasive alternative.

20. What can be done for pain associated with pancreatic cancer?

Pancreatic cancers may invade the celiac plexus, causing significant neuropathic pain, which is often the worst symptom experienced by patients with advanced pancreatic cancer. The pain is usually described as severe, gnawing, and radiating to the back. If the bile duct is obstructed, pain may also occur outside the stomach or in the right upper quadrant (RUQ) of the abdomen. Opioids are usually employed at first symptoms of pain; however, the sedative effects of the large doses required to control pain may interfere with quality of life. Chemical neurolysis (celiac block) by injection of 50% alcohol directly into the region of the celiac plexus, either endoscopically, intraoperatively, or percutaneously, is very effective for alleviating pain. Surgical neurotomy and radiation therapy may also be used to control pain from pancreatic cancer.

21. What new treatments are in development for pancreatic cancer?

- Trials investigating the effectiveness of gemcitabine combined with new targeted drugs are ongoing. When compared to gemcitabine alone, erlotinib plus gemcitabine was shown to have a nominal but statistically significant improvement in median and 1-year survival.
- Additional current research will evaluate pancreatic cancer vaccines, which are intended to stimulate the patient's immune system and prevent recurrence of pancreatic cancer following surgical resection.

HEPATOCELLULAR CANCER

Quick Facts—Hepatocellular Cancer

Incidence	19,160 newly diagnosed cases estimated in 2007 (13,650 in men; 5510 in women) Incidence increases with age; median age at diagnosis is 66 years	**Histopathology**	Primarily adenocarcinomas, with two major cell types: hepatocellular and cholangiocarcinoma (intrahepatic bile duct carcinoma)
Mortality	16,780 deaths estimated in 2007	**Symptoms**	Abdominal or RUQ pain Fatigue Anorexia, nausea, weight loss Jaundice
Risk factors	Hepatitis B (HBV) and Hepatitis C (HCV) Excessive alcohol consumption Cirrhosis Oral contraceptive and androgenic steroid use Ingestion of foods contaminated with the fungal toxin, aflatoxin Tobacco smoking Hemochromatosis or alpha$_1$-antitrypsin deficiency	**Diagnosis and evaluation**	History and physical examination (abdominal mass is noted on physical exam in ⅓ of patients) Elevated alpha fetoprotein (AFP) Ultrasonography High resolution CT of abdomen CT/PET Contrast-enhanced MRI

Continued

Quick Facts—cont'd

Staging and Stage Grouping

Stage	Description
Tumor, node, metastasis (TNM)	
Primary tumor (T)	
TX	Primary tumor cannot be assessed
T0	No evidence of primary tumor
T1	Solitary tumor without vascular invasion
T2	Solitary tumor with vascular invasion, or multiple tumors with none > 5 cm
T3	Multiple tumors > 5 cm, or tumor involving a major branch of the portal or hepatic vein(s)
T4	Tumors with direct invasion of adjacent organs other than the gallbladder, or with perforation of visceral peritoneum
Regional lymph nodes (N)	
NX	Regional lymph nodes cannot be assessed
N0	No regional lymph node metastasis
N1	Regional lymph node metastasis
Distant metastasis (M)	
MX	Distant metastasis cannot be assessed
M0	No distant metastasis
M1	Distant metastasis

Stage	Primary Tumor	Regional Lymph Nodes	Distant Metastasis
I	T1	N0	M0
II	T2	N0	M0
IIIA	T3	N0	M0
IIIB	T4	N0	M0
IIIC	Any T	N1	M0
IV	Any T	Any N	M1

Used with permission of the American Joint Committee on Cancer (AJCC), Chicago, Illinois. The original source for this material is the AJCC Cancer Staging Handbook, Sixth Edition (2002) published by Springer New York, www.sprinfleronline.com.

22. Is the incidence of hepatocellular carcinoma increasing in the United States?

The presence of hepatitis C virus (HCV) has been positively correlated with the development of hepatocellular carcinoma (HCC). With the current epidemic of HCV in the United States, incidence of HCC will likely increase in the next 20 years.

23. What role does alcohol consumption have in the development of HCC?

Excessive alcohol consumption is a definite risk factor for developing hepatocellular carcinoma. Additionally, alcohol consumption by persons with hepatitis B virus (HBV) or HCV increases the risk of developing cancer when compared to infected persons who abstain from alcohol. Cirrhosis is a risk factor for HCC irrespective of etiology; the majority (50%-80%) of patients with HCC have underlying liver cirrhosis.

24. What is the Okuda staging system and how does it impact staging and treatment?

Because the degree of cirrhosis affects treatment options for HCC and the patient's response, the Okuda staging system may be more practical and relevant to the treatment outcome than the TNM staging. The Okuda staging system assigns weight to the percentage of liver that is replaced by tumor, to biochemical indicators of the severity of cirrhosis (serum albumin and bilirubin levels, prothrombin time), and to the presence of ascites.

25. Can HCC be cured?

Surgery provides the only potential cure for hepatocellular carcinoma, but its use depends on tumor size, location, and condition of the uninvolved liver. Only 10% of patients with hepatocellular carcinoma have resectable disease at the time of diagnosis. Liver transplant is an option for the patient with HCC and cirrhosis who meets the United Network for Organ Sharing criteria (single tumor < 5 cm, or 2-3 tumors < 3 cm; no macrovascular invasion; no extrahepatic spread).

26. What is the 5-year survival rate for HCC?

The overall 5-year survival rate is approximately 9%. Most patients have unresectable disease when it is first diagnosed, but in those patients who undergo curative resections, the 5-year survival rate is 20%. (Resectable disease is defined as noncirrhotic liver with solitary or unilobar hepatic lesions). Following resection, recurrence is common, with metastases arising in the remaining liver, lungs, bone, kidneys, and heart.

27. What treatment options are available for patients with unresectable disease?

Other treatment options for those with unresectable disease, or who are not candidates for surgery include: ablative surgery (alcohol, cryotherapy, radiofrequency, microwave), hepatic intraarterial infusion of chemotherapy, chemoembolization, radiation therapy, radiotherapeutic microspheres, and chemotherapy combined with radiation or targeted therapies.

28. Does chemotherapy improve survival?

Systemic chemotherapy has shown no survival benefit for patients with hepatocellular cancer. Durable remissions have rarely been reported, but a few agents that have shown partial response rates above 10% include doxorubicin, 5-FU, and cisplatin. At present there is no indication for adjuvant systemic chemotherapy. The National Cancer Institute (NCI) recommends that patients without surgically resectable disease be offered treatment through a clinical trial.

29. What is transarterial chemoembolization?

Transarterial chemoembolization (TACE) is a treatment used in some patients with hepatocellular carcinoma. If the cancer is in the region of the liver served by the hepatic artery, it can be treated in isolation from the remaining liver, which depends on the portal system for its blood supply. The goal is to eliminate the blood supply to the cancer by occluding the hepatic artery with gelfoam, alcohol, iodized oil, or other substance, and at the same time administering cytotoxic chemotherapy directly to the tumor to cause necrosis (cell death). TACE is frequently complicated by abdominal pain and fever (postembolization syndrome) and is usually self-limiting. TACE has been used to treat patients with large unresectable hepatocellular carcinoma before resection and before transplant. Careful patient selection is important and depends on several patient characteristics (e.g., alpha-fetoprotein [AFP], tumor volume). The effect of TACE on survival remains controversial.

30. What tumor marker can be used for screening and/or to follow hepatocellular carcinoma?

Serum AFP is a fetal protein that is not normally detectable in healthy adults but is elevated in most persons (approximately 70%) with HCC. Unfortunately, AFP is not specific for hepatocellular carcinoma and modest elevations may be seen in patients with benign liver disease, germ cell tumors, gastric cancer, and pancreatic cancer. Although a normal AFP level does not exclude the diagnosis of HCC, an AFP level greater than 500 ng/ml is considered indicative of HCC and warrants further investigation. Even in cases where no identifiable lesion is found on imaging, elevated and rising serum AFP may indicate the early presence of HCC, and these patients should be followed closely. AFP level can also be used to follow response to therapy, and it is prognostically important, with the median survival of patients with no detectable AFP significantly longer than those with elevated AFP.

GALLBLADDER CANCER

31. How common is gallbladder cancer?

Gallbladder cancer is an uncommon but usually fatal malignancy. In the United States approximately 9250 cases (4380 in men; 4870 in women) and 3250 deaths are estimated in 2007.

32. Who gets gallbladder cancer?

The incidence of gallbladder cancer increases with age and peaks in the sixth to seventh decades of life; it is rare before the age of 40 years. Women are affected more frequently than men (ratio of 1.7:1). The incidence of gallbladder cancer is 5 to 6 times higher in Hispanics, Native Americans, and Alaska Natives.

33. What risk factors are associated with the development of gallbladder cancer?

The greatest risk factor is the presence of gallstones, particularly when associated with chronic cholecystitis. People who have calcified "porcelain" gallbladder or gallbladder polyps, are carriers of *Salmonella typhi*, or have been exposed to carcinogens (e.g., azotoluene, nitrosamines) also have a higher risk of developing gallbladder cancer.

34. Why is the prognosis for gallbladder cancer so poor?

Gallbladder cancer is typically asymptomatic in its early resectable stages. By the time symptoms develop, the disease is often advanced and unresectable. When symptoms develop, they are typically similar to benign gallbladder disease. Up to 20% of gallbladder cancers are diagnosed incidentally at the time of gallbladder surgery. The cancer usually grows into the liver, stomach, and duodenum by direct extension, making resection impossible. At the time of attempted surgical resection, 25% of patients have lymphatic involvement, and 70% have direct extension of disease into the liver. The overall 5-year survival rate is 5% to 12%. The few patients who are incidentally found to have stage I or II tumors during a cholecystectomy have an improved survival rate and may be cured.

35. What is the role of chemotherapy in the treatment of gallbladder cancer?

- Resected gallbladder cancer: adjuvant treatment with 5-FU and mitomycin-C has improved survival time.
- Unresectable gallbladder cancer: treatment with 5-FU, mitomycin-C, capecitabine, gemcitabine, cisplatin, docetaxel, doxorubicin, and the nitrosureas alone or in combination, have produced responses in patients with unresectable gallbladder cancer. There is no evidence that combination chemotherapy improves quality of life or survival in this patient population.

36. Klatskin's tumor refers to a cancer in what location?

Klatskin's tumor is a primary extrahepatic bile duct cancer (cholangiocarcinoma) near the confluence of the left and right hepatic bile ducts.

Key Points

- Upper GI cancers, such as pancreatic, gastric, and gallbladder cancers, often have progressed to advanced stages at the time of diagnosis.
- The symptoms of gastric, pancreatic, hepatocellular, and gallbladder cancers often correlate with obstruction of an intestinal or biliary lumen. For example, gastric outlet obstruction will cause bloating, early satiety, nausea, and vomiting in patients with gastric or pancreatic cancer. Obstruction of the bile ducts by pancreatic or hepatocellular cancer will cause jaundice, nausea, and elevated bilirubin level.
- The major therapeutic goal for advanced pancreatic cancer is palliation, which often requires a multidisciplinary approach to best manage pain and nutritional needs.
- The symptoms that accompany advanced liver disease severely limit treatment options.

Internet Resources

American Cancer Society:
   http://www.cancer.org
Memorial Sloan-Kettering Cancer Center:
   http://www.mskcc.org
National Cancer Institute (NCI):
   http://www.cancer.gov
National Cancer Institute, Surveillance Epidemiology and End Results (SEER), Cancer Stat Fact Sheets:
   http://www.seer.cancer.gov/statfacts

Bibliography

Abdella E, Pisters P, Evans D: Clinical aspects and management of pancreatic adenocarcinoma, management options: Potentially resectable pancreatic cancer. In Abbruzzese J, Evans D, Willett C, et al editors: *Gastrointestinal oncology,* Oxford, 2005, Oxford University Press.

American Cancer Society: What are the risk factors for stomach cancer? Available at: http://www.cancer.org/docroot/CRI/content/CRI_2_4_2X_What_are_the_risk_factors_for_stomach_cancer_40.asp?sitearea. Accessed January 3, 2006.

Benson A, Myerson J, Hoffman J: Pancreatic, neuroendocrine, GI and adrenal cancers. In Pazdur R, Coia L, Hoskins J, et al, editors: *Cancer management: A multidisciplinary approach,* ed 9, Lawrence, KS, 2005, CMP Healthcare Media.

Blanke C, Coia L, Schwarz R, et al: Gastric cancer. In Pazdur R, Coia L, Hoskins J, et al editors: *Cancer management: A multidisciplinary approach,* ed 9, Lawrence, KS, 2005, CMP Healthcare Media.

Choti M: Clinical aspects and management of hepatocellular cancer: Diagnostic and staging procedures. In Abbruzzese J, Evans D, Willett C, et al, editors: *Gastrointestinal oncology,* Oxford, 2005, Oxford University Press.

Greene FL, Page DL, Fleming ID, et al, editors: *AJCC cancer staging manual,* ed 6, New York, 2002, Springer.

Hassan M, Patt Y: Epidemiology and molecular epidemiology of hepatocellular cancer. In Abbruzzese J, Evans D, Willett C, et al, editors: *Gastrointestinal oncology,* Oxford, 2005, Oxford University Press.

Jemal A, Siegel R, Ward E, et al: Cancer statistics, 2007. *CA Cancer J Clin* 57:43-66, 2007.

Ko AH, Tempero MA: Treatment of metastatic pancreatic cancer. *J Natl Compr Canc Netw* 3:627-636, 2005.

Macdonald J, Smalley S, Benedetti J, et al: Chemoradiotherapy after surgery compared with surgery alone for adenocarcinoma of the stomach or gastroesophageal junction. *N Engl J Med* 345(10):725-730, 2001.

Mansfield P: Clinical aspects and management of gastric carcinoma, management options: Potentially resectable gastric cancer. In Abbruzzese J, Evans D, Willett C, et al, editors: *Gastrointestinal oncology,* Oxford, 2005, Oxford University Press.

Marshall J: Novel vaccines for the treatment of gastrointestinal cancers. *Oncology* 19:1557-1565, 2005.

McBride G: Researchers optimistic about targeted drugs for pancreatic cancer. *J Natl Cancer Inst* 96: 1570-1572, 2004.

Moss S, Shirin H: Epidemiology and molecular epidemiology of gastric cancer. In Abbruzzese J, Evans D, Willett C, et al, editors: *Gastrointestinal oncology,* Oxford, 2005, Oxford University Press.

Mulcahy MF, Wahl AO, Small W: The current status of combined radiotherapy and chemotherapy for locally advanced or resected pancreas cancer. *J Natl Compr Canc Netw* 3:637-642, 2005.

National Comprehensive Cancer Network: Clinical practice guidelines in oncology: Gastric cancer. Available at: http://www.nccn.org/professional/physician_gls/PDF/gastric.pdf. Accessed January 14, 2007.

National Comprehensive Cancer Network: Clinical practice guidelines in oncology: Hepatobiliary cancers. Available at: http://www.nccn.org/professional/physician_gls/PDF/hepatobiliary.pdf. Accessed January 14, 2007.

National Comprehensive Cancer Network: Clinical practice guidelines in oncology: Pancreatic adenocarcinoma. Available at: http://www.nccn.org/professional/physician_gls/PDF/pancreatic.pdf. Accessed January 14, 2007.

National Cancer Institute: Adult primary liver cancer: Treatment. Available at: http://cancer.gov/cancertopics/pdq/treatment/adult-primary-liver/healthprofessionals. Accessed January 3, 2006.

National Cancer Institute: Cancer topics: Gastric cancer screening. Available at: http://nci.nih.gov/cancertopics/pdq/screening/gastric/healthprofessional/page2. Accessed January 14, 2007.

National Cancer Institute: General information about gastric cancer. Available at: http://cancer.gov/cancertopics/pdq/treatment/gastric/Patient. Accessed January 3, 2006.

National Cancer Institute: Surveillance Epidemiology and End Results (SEER) cancer statistics review. Available at: http://seer.cancer.gov/csr/1975_2003/. Accessed January 3, 2006.

Neoptolemos JP, Stocken DD, Friess H, et al: A randomized trial of chemoradiotherapy and chemotherapy after resection of pancreatic cancer. *N Engl J Med* 350(12):1200-1210, 2004.

Shinchi H, Takao S, Noma H et al: Length and quality of survival after external-beam radiotherapy with concurrent continuous 5-fluorouracil infusion for locally unresectable pancreatic cancer. *Int J Radiat Oncol Biol Phys* 53(1):146-150, 2002.

Tempero M, Termuhlen P, Brand R, et al. Clinical aspects and management of pancreatic adenocarcinoma, management options: Locally advanced unresectable pancreatic cancer. In Abbruzzese J, Evans D, Willett C, et al, editors: *Gastrointestinal oncology,* Oxford, 2005, Oxford University Press.

Wagman L, Robertson J, O'Neil B: Liver, gallbladder, and biliary tract cancers. In Pazdur R, Coia L, Hoskins J, et al, editors: *Cancer management: A multidisciplinary approach,* ed 9, Lawrence, KS, 2005, CMP Healthcare Media.

Wanebo H, Savarese D: Gallbladder cancer. Available at: http://www.patients.uptodate.com/topic.asp?file=gicancer/17390. Accessed January 14, 2007.

Yang GY, Wagner TD, Fuss M, et al: Multimodality approaches for pancreatic cancer. *CA Cancer J Clin* 55:352-367, 2005.

Gynecologic Cancers

Susan Adnan-Koch and Susan A. Davidson

1. What are the primary sites of gynecologic cancer?

Gynecologic cancers are associated with the female reproductive organs. The principal sites include the ovaries, fallopian tubes, uterus, cervix, vagina, and vulva. Additional rare cancers that are classified as gynecologic include gestational trophoblastic neoplasias (GTN), a group of pregnancy-related tumors that may persist and metastasize (e.g., hydatidiform mole, choriocarcinoma), and primary peritoneal carcinoma, a tumor that originates on the peritoneal surfaces but demonstrates behavior similar to epithelial ovarian cancers. The three most commonly diagnosed gynecologic cancers are the focus of this chapter: cervical, ovarian, and endometrial (epithelial surface of the uterus).

2. How are gynecologic cancers staged?

Gynecologic cancers are staged according to guidelines established by the International Federation of Gynecology and Obstetrics (FIGO), which adapted the traditional primary tumor-regional lymph nodes-distant metastasis (TNM) system to ensure consistency on the international level. The primary features that distinguish this system from other staging systems are: (1) reliance on clinical staging for cervical and vaginal cancer, which includes but is not limited to physical examination, chest radiograph, and intravenous pyelogram; (2) use of specific surgical staging for all other gynecologic cancers; and (3) adherence to the original staging designation for all disease sites, despite later findings of persistence, metastasis, or recurrence.

Quick Facts—Cervical Cancer

Incidence	11,150 newly diagnosed cases estimated in 2007		cervical secretions, are thought to favor development of precancerous changes of the cervix)
Mortality	3670 deaths estimated in 2007		
Risk factors	Early coitus	**Genetics**	No genetic risk factors
	Multiple sexual partners	**Histopathology**	Squamous cell carcinomas (most common)
	Human papillomavirus (HPV), especially types 16 and 18		Other cell types: adenocarcinoma, adenosquamous carcinoma, small cell, and glassy cell
	Human immunodeficiency virus (HIV)	**Symptoms**	Most common: thin, watery vaginal discharge; heavier menses; postcoital spotting
	Low socioeconomic status (decreases access to routine Pap test screening)		
	Smoking (nicotine by-products, measured in		Spontaneous, intermittent, painless uterine bleeding (menometrorrhagia)

Continued

Quick Facts—cont'd

	Back, flank, or leg pain	CT or MRI of abdomen and pelvis to detect hydronephrosis and occult metastases
	Lower extremity edema	
	Dysuria	
	Hematuria or rectal bleeding	Chest x-ray (PA and lateral) to detect metastatic disease
	Cough	
Diagnosis and evaluation	History and physical examination	PET to identify foci of abnormal uptake in anatomically normal structures
	Pap test and pelvic examination	
	Intravenous pyelogram (IVP)	

Staging and Stage Grouping

Stage	Description
I	Confined to cervix
IA$_1$	Invasion of stroma ≤ 3 mm deep and ≤ 7 mm wide
IA$_2$	Invasion of stroma > 3 mm to ≤ 5 mm deep and ≤ 7 mm wide
IB$_1$	Invasion of stroma > 5 mm deep or > 7 mm wide, and clinical lesions ≤ 4 cm
IB$_2$	Clinical lesions > 4 cm
II	Extension beyond cervix and/or upper ⅔ of vagina
IIA	No parametrial involvement
IIB	Parametrial involvement
III	Extension to lower third of vagina
IIIA	No extension to pelvic side wall
IIIB	Extension to pelvic side wall and/or hydronephrosis
IV	Extension beyond true pelvis
IVA	Involvement of adjacent organs (bladder, rectum)
IVB	Distant metastasis

3. Why is cervical cancer considered preventable?

It is characterized by a lengthy premalignant, preinvasive state that can be detected early through routine Papanicolaou (Pap) tests. These premalignant conditions may not be visible to the naked eye, and with colposcopic examination and detection, may be eradicated completely before malignant transformation occurs. All premalignant lesions may regress, persist, or become invasive. It may take up to 7 years for early changes to progress to an invasive cancer.

4. What about the new cervical cancer vaccine? When is it used?

The FDA recently approved Gardasil (quadrivalent human papillomavirus [HPV] recombinant vaccine) to protect females aged 9 to 26 years against cervical cancer, cervical adenocarcinoma in situ, cervical intraepithelial neoplasia, and genital warts caused by HPV types 6, 11, 16, and 18. This vaccine, which is administered three times (every 2 months) over a 6-month period, is not intended to substitute for routine cervical cancer screening and should not be used to treat cervical cancer. The most common toxicities associated with the vaccination are pain, swelling, and erythema at the injection site and possible fever and nausea.

5. What terms are used to explain an abnormal Pap test?

- **Atypia** refers to cells with abnormal features that are not diagnostic and have undetermined significance.
- **Dysplasia** indicates a distinct abnormality of cellular development and is associated with premalignant disease of the cervix. It is reported as mild, moderate, or severe, depending on the degree of deviation from the normal cells found on the cervix.
- **Cervical intraepithelial neoplasia** (CIN) includes three categories of dysplasia: (1) mild dysplasia/CIN 1; (2) moderate dysplasia/CIN 2; and (3) severe dysplasia/ carcinoma in situ (CIS)/CIN 3.
- **Squamous intraepithelial lesions** (SIL) were introduced in the current Bethesda classification system to include the emergence of human papillomavirus (HPV) as a deviation from normal cervical cytology and its association as a risk factor in the development of cervical cancer. Low-grade SIL (LSIL) encompasses changes due to HPV as well as CIN 1 or mild dysplasia. High-grade SIL (HSIL) includes CIN 2 or moderate dysplasia, CIN 3 or severe dysplasia, and CIS.

6. How should the nurse explain abnormal Pap test findings to the patient?

Stress that the classification is used to identify degrees of abnormality that are universally understood and to direct appropriate treatment and follow-up. The Pap test is only a screening test; the actual cervical abnormality may be better or worse than the screening test indicates. To determine why the findings of the Pap test are abnormal, the cervix must be examined with a colposcope, and diagnostic biopsies may be required.

7. How should the nurse explain treatment for abnormal Pap test findings?

Treatment recommendations for an abnormal Pap test depend on colposcopy findings and, if necessary, biopsy results. A colposcope enhances visual inspection and allows thorough examination of the cervical surface. The procedure is comparable to the Pap test, although it takes longer to complete. After the speculum is inserted, the cervix is examined through the magnification of the colposcope. A 3% to 5% acetic acid (household vinegar) or other staining solution, such as Lugol's iodine stain, may be used to demarcate cervical abnormalities. These solutions may cause a stinging or burning sensation, but they are not harmful to cervical mucosa. Biopsies of abnormal areas, as well as curettage (scraping) of the endocervical canal above the external opening of the cervix, are then performed. These procedures may produce mild discomfort, such as pinching or cramping sensations, and light vaginal bleeding or spotting. If precancerous changes are detected, further treatment is necessary. Treatment options that may be discussed with the patient include laser ablation, cryotherapy (freezing of abnormal tissue), loop excision, cold knife cone biopsy, and hysterectomy.

8. What should the nurse tell a patient who asks about the use of Pap test screening for gynecologic cancers?

Patients often believe that Pap tests are used as screening tests for all gynecologic cancers. In reality, the Pap test is specifically intended to detect abnormalities in the cells on the surface of the cervix, particularly preinvasive CIN (see Question 5). On occasion, cellular abnormality of vaginal, endometrial, or ovarian origin may be detected. In these situations, additional tests are required to determine the origin and significance of the abnormality. Patients should be informed that the Pap test does not screen for either invasive cervical cancer or other gynecologic malignancies. Despite this limited application, the Pap test provides valuable information to the practitioner. Before insertion of the speculum, inspection of the external genitalia under bright light facilitates identification of abnormal or suspicious lesions on the vulva. Direct visualization of the cervix and vaginal tissue may reveal a gross lesion in an asymptomatic woman. After the speculum examination, palpation during bimanual examination assesses the ovaries for enlargement, a possible symptom of ovarian pathology.

9. When should women begin annual Pap test screening?

Women should begin annual Pap test screening and pelvic examination with the initiation of sexual activity or by age 21 years. After three or more consecutive normal annual screening tests and examinations, the Pap test may be done less frequently as suggested by the clinician. A lifelong habit of annual testing as part of a well-woman examination increases the likelihood of detecting abnormalities early. Both the American Cancer Society and the American College of Obstetricians and Gynecologists recommend annual examinations. After hysterectomy, Pap test recommendations vary according to patient history.

10. Why is a pelvic examination often performed under anesthesia in patients with cervical cancer?

Cervical cancer spreads primarily by direct extension to surrounding tissues and organs and involvement of regional lymph node chains. In the presence of visible, measurable tumor, the surrounding parametrial tissue should be examined for evidence of tumor infiltration. Although a pelvic examination is performed in the office, full assessment is not always possible because of patient discomfort during the examination, presence of stool in the bowel, and anxiety about the findings. Therefore, patients are usually anesthetized so that a thorough pelvic examination may be performed with the patient completely relaxed. Under these conditions, the clinical stage of disease can be more accurately assessed. In addition, cystoscopic and sigmoidoscopic examinations may be carried out at the same time to rule out bladder and bowel involvement.

11. What is meant by parametrial spread in cervical cancer?

The parametrium is the space between the lateral portion of the cervix and the bony structure of the pelvic sidewall. It contains the supporting structures, such as the uterosacral and transverse cervical ligaments, that maintain the cervix in its relatively immobile position. The ureters pass through this area rather close to the uterus before insertion into the urinary bladder. Invasion of this space is common when a cervical tumor expands laterally. It may extend and adhere to the bony structure of the pelvic side wall. Patients with parametrial spread have an increased incidence of hydronephrosis, which requires ureteral stent placement because of compression by tumor growth. In addition, such patients commonly complain of radiating hip or back pain secondary to mass effect, nerve infiltration, and possible bony metastasis. Spread of tumor to this location is an indication for primary treatment with radiation therapy.

Chemotherapy is used as a radiation sensitizer. Surgical excision after radiation therapy is generally not undertaken because irradiated tissue heals poorly and fistulas often develop. When parametrial spread is documented on bimanual pelvic examination, the patient has a more advanced stage of disease, which, as described above, affects treatment recommendations.

12. How is cervical cancer treated?

Stage I: cone biopsy up to radical hysterectomy
Stages IB, IIA: radical hysterectomy with lymph node dissection or radiation with chemotherapy; combination therapy (radiation and surgery) for some IB tumors

Stages IIB, III, IVA: radiation therapy with chemotherapy used as radiation sensitizer
Stage IVB: palliative radiation, chemotherapy, or both

13. When is hysterectomy indicated in patients with cervical cancer?

The decision is based on the stage of the cancer, age and health status of the patient, treatment plan, and patient preference. Proper treatment of cervical cancer and potential sites of spread with surgery alone requires a radical hysterectomy with lymph node dissection. Patients with early cancers, characterized by tumors confined to the cervix that are smaller than 4 cm, may be the most appropriate candidates for this procedure if surgery does not expose them to increased morbidity. Patients with tumors that are larger than 4 cm but still confined to the cervix usually receive radiation therapy and weekly sensitizing chemotherapy first. This may be followed by a simple hysterectomy to remove any residual cervical tumor.

When the cancer extends beyond the cervix to the parametrium and other surrounding tissue, radiation therapy without hysterectomy is the most effective treatment. Cervical cancer may be effectively treated with radiation therapy. If the patient has an early-stage cervical cancer in the presence of comorbid factors that significantly increase operative risks, treatment with definitive radiation therapy offers survival rates comparable to those of the surgical procedure.

14. Distinguish among an extrafascial, modified radical, and radical hysterectomy.

- **Extrafascial hysterectomy** (simple hysterectomy) includes removal of the entire uterus and cervix through either the vagina or abdomen; adjacent supporting ligaments and vagina remain intact. This procedure may be used for benign conditions, such as fibroids. It is also the procedure of choice after pelvic irradiation, because it allows removal of the uterus and cervix with minimal cutting damage to irradiated tissue. The associated complications are low and include common surgical risks, such as bleeding and infection.
- **Modified radical hysterectomy** involves removal of a small portion of the upper vagina and the inner third of the parametrium (the space containing the uterosacral and cardinal ligaments), along with the entire uterus and cervix. The ureters, bladder, and rectum are partially dissected out of the uterosacral ligaments. The higher complication rate for this surgery is due to the increased potential for blood loss, ureteral injury, and postoperative bladder dysfunction. Patients have a longer postoperative recovery period and usually need either an indwelling Foley or suprapubic catheter until normal voiding patterns are reestablished. Some patients may need to perform self-catheterization as a result of continued bladder dysfunction.
- **Radical hysterectomy** includes removal of the upper 3 cm of the vagina and most of the parametrium, along with the entire uterus and cervix. The ureters are completely dissected out of the uterosacral ligaments. The bladder and rectum must be dissected further from the supporting tissue than for the modified radical hysterectomy. The serious complication rate is approximately 5% and includes infection, blood loss, ureteral injury, chronic bladder or rectal dysfunction, fistula formation (from ureter, bladder, or rectum), small bowel obstruction, and nerve injury. Patients should expect to have an indwelling Foley or suprapubic catheter for 1 to 4 weeks after surgery. Chronic problems, such as urinary frequency or incontinence, change in bowel elimination patterns, and pain or hypersensation associated with femoral-genital nerve disruption, may occur.

15. Why is lymph node dissection often performed during hysterectomy?

Regional pelvic lymph node dissection is usually combined with the more radical hysterectomy procedures to assess for metastasis. The complications associated with this procedure include lymphocyst formation, lower extremity edema, and nerve injury.

16. What is salpingo-oophorectomy? Why is it performed?

The decision to perform a salpingo-oophorectomy (removal of the fallopian tubes and ovaries) at the time of hysterectomy depends on the age of the patient and prior treatments. Women over the age of 45 years, who are approaching menopause, may choose to have the ovaries removed at the time of hysterectomy. For women with non-functioning ovaries, such as those who are postmenopausal or have received prior pelvic radiation therapy, removal of the ovaries is often recommended to reduce future risk of ovarian cancer. Surgical induction of menopause in premenopausal or perimenopausal patients reduces circulating estrogen and thus causes an acute vasomotor response. Depending on the diagnosis, estrogen replacement may be recommended for such patients.

17. What is a pelvic exenteration?

Pelvic exenteration is a radical surgical procedure that involves the removal of the uterus, vagina, parametrium, bladder (in a total or anterior exenteration), and rectum (in a total or posterior exenteration). The type of exenterative procedure—anterior, posterior, or total—is determined by the location of the cancer in the pelvis. The exenteration is followed by reconstructive procedures that include formation of a neovagina (with skin grafts or flaps), a urinary drainage system (either a conduit or continent pouch) fashioned from bowel, and either a colostomy or reanastomosis of the lower rectum to the sigmoid colon.

18. When is pelvic exenteration used?

Pelvic exenteration is used most commonly for cervical cancer that recurs in the central pelvis after radiation therapy. It also may be used for recurrent vaginal or endometrial cancer and for primary treatment of some extensive pelvic cancers. The rationale for complete and radical removal of tissues and organs in the pelvis after radiation therapy, as opposed to simple local excision, is based on the circulatory compromise and poor healing properties of irradiated tissue and the need to achieve free margins around the tumor. Tissue that has been irradiated is less likely to heal normally. This compromise further increases the risk of infection, abscess, and fistula formation, requiring ongoing intervention and corrective procedures. The intent of an exenterative procedure is curative. It should not be performed for palliation because of the high morbidity rate. For this reason, evidence of disease outside the central pelvis is a contraindication for exenteration.

19. Why are radiation implants used in the treatment of cervical cancer?

Successful radiation therapy depends, in part, on the ability to deliver an adequate dose of radiation to the source of the cancer. Tissue tolerance of the effects of radiation varies throughout the body. Irradiation beyond the known level of tolerance may cause permanent tissue damage. The vagina and cervix are relatively radiation-resistant compared with the surrounding bowel and bladder. Therefore, higher doses of radiation therapy may be used to deliver a curative dose to the cervix. The usual radiation treatment plan for cervical cancer is biphasic. Approximately 5 weeks of external beam radiation therapy along with weekly sensitizing chemotherapy is administered to the pelvis to shrink the tumor and treat regional lymph nodes. This is followed by brachytherapy, which is the placement of an intracavitary radiation source, kept in place by a holder, such as a tandem and ovoid device, vaginal cylinder, or interstitial template. When loaded with the radioactive source, these devices deliver additional high doses of radiation to the vagina, cervix, and adjacent parametrial tissue. While the radiation source is implanted, the uterus insulates the small bowel from higher doses of radiation. In addition, packing placed into the vagina pushes the bladder and rectum further away from the radiation source. Thus, the cervix and vagina receive at least twice the dose of radiation that could be delivered by external radiation alone.

20. What nursing care should be provided to patients receiving a radiation implant?

Nursing care should focus on safe delivery of the treatment and recognition and prevention of complications. The most common devices used to deliver intracavitary radiation in gynecologic cancer are tandem and ovoid devices, vaginal cylinders, and interstitial afterload needles. This may be an outpatient or an inpatient procedure, depending on radiation dosing. If inpatient treatment is planned, the nurse should have adequate time to perform a thorough postoperative assessment of the patient, review the postoperative orders, inform the patient of restrictions on activity, and prepare the patient for the loading procedure. The following should be included in the patient's care plan:

- Vital sign assessment every 4 hours to monitor for sepsis from the introduction of a foreign object (tandem or interstitial needle) through the necrotic tumor mass
- Strict bed rest with minimal side-to-side turning to prevent hardware dislodgment
- Elevation of the head of the bed to no more than 30° to prevent perforation from the tandem or interstitial afterload needles
- Foley catheter placement to eliminate bedpan use
- Complete bowel rest to prevent hardware dislodgement; use of a low-residue diet along with Lomotil and/or opioid pain medications around the clock to promote constipation and discourage defecation
- Administration of intravenous fluids until the patient has recovered from nausea due to anesthesia
- Prevention of deep vein thrombosis (DVT) through the use of antiembolism or intermittent inflation stockings, and treatment with subcutaneous heparin
- Hourly incentive spirometry
- Use of a patient-controlled analgesia (PCA) pump or epidural analgesia catheter to prevent discomfort from hardware placement

21. How are staff members protected from radiation exposure?

Because minimal time should be spent at the bedside after the radiation source has been placed, routine care activities, such as bathing, maintaining oral hygiene, and changing linens, are severely restricted. Lead shields may be placed around the patient's bed, just inside the entrance to the room, or both, to absorb emitted radiation. Staff should position themselves behind a shield when inside the room to minimize radiation exposure. Shields may be impractical, however, when the patient requires direct care. Lead aprons do not afford additional protection from the gamma rays of this type of radiation; therefore, their use is not advocated. A coordinated team effort is required to ensure that the principles of time, distance, and shielding are followed without compromising the patient's physical and emotional care needs.

22. What is high dose rate brachytherapy?

In some institutions, high dose rate brachytherapy is used to deliver radiation directly to the tumor source. This method follows the principles of conventional implant devices through the insertion of an applicator or holder into the tumor (cervix) or cavity (vagina, uterus). The radiation source emits a much higher hourly rate of radiation. Thus, the time that the implant needs to stay in place is reduced dramatically. In addition, the procedure can be done on an outpatient basis. The major disadvantages are the requirements for specialized equipment and a highly trained staff.

23. Does chemotherapy have a role in the treatment of cervical cancer?

Because patients are traditionally treated with surgery and radiation therapy with good response, the role of chemotherapy is limited. Chemotherapy has been generally reserved for patients with recurrent or advanced disease, not amenable to surgery or radiation therapy. However, there are factors that may preclude the use of chemotherapy in this patient population: decreased bone marrow reserves and cellular resistance due to previous radiation, and impaired renal function due to disease spread. Chemotherapeutic agents include:

- Cisplatin and fluorouracil (5-FU), used as radiation sensitizers in the treatment of Stage IIB-IV disease
- Various combinations of cisplatin, ifosfamide, paclitaxel, gemcitabine, topotecan, and vinorelbine (Navelbine) used to treat Stage IVB or recurrent disease

Quick Facts—Ovarian Cancer

Incidence	22,430 newly diagnosed cases estimated in 2007	**Genetics**	Familial cancer syndromes are autosomal dominant conditions accounting for 10% of ovarian cancers.
Mortality	15,280 deaths estimated in 2007		
Risk factors	Age: risk increases with age until 70 years old	**Histopathology**	Adenocarcinoma of mucinous or serous papillary origin (most common)
	Family history of ovarian cancer, breast-ovarian cancer, or breast-ovarian-endometrial-colon cancer (ovarian cancer in two 1st-degree relatives [mother, sister] may increase the risk to as much as 50%).		Other cell types include: endometrial, clear cell, Brenner, undifferentiated, sarcomas
	Incessant ovulation, and such conditions as nulliparity or infertility	**Symptoms**	Most common: abdominal distention and bloating
	Northern European ancestry		Increased abdominal girth, nonspecific changes in GI function, increased flatus, weight gain, vaginal bleeding, and pain
	Industrialization/higher socioeconomic class	**Diagnosis and evaluation**	History and physical examination
	Association with perineal talc use, high dietary fat, and excessive coffee and alcohol consumption have been suggested but are considered weak.		Pelvic examination
			CA-125 marker
			CT/MRI of abdomen and pelvis
			Ultrasound

Quick Facts—cont'd

Staging and Stage Grouping

Stage	Description
I	Limited to ovaries
IA	1 ovary; capsule intact; no tumor on ovarian surface
IB	2 ovaries; capsules intact; no tumor on ovarian surface
IC	Tumor limited to 1 or both ovaries with any of the following: ruptured capsule, surface tumor, positive peritoneal cytology
II	Pelvic extension
IIA	Uterus or tubes
IIB	Other tissues
IIC	Ruptured capsule, surface tumor, positive cytology
III	Abdominal or nodal metastasis
IIIA	Microscopic seeding of abdominal-peritoneal surfaces
IIIB	Abdominal peritoneal implants $\leq$ 2 cm, no metastasis to nodes
IIIC	Abdominal peritoneal implants > 2 cm and/or metastasis to nodes
IV	Distant metastasis; includes pleural effusion with positive cytology, parenchymal liver metastases

24. Are there any screening studies that can detect ovarian cancer?

Unfortunately, no reliable tests are available for screening asymptomatic women for ovarian cancer. Although a combination of bimanual pelvic examination, transvaginal ultrasound, and assay of serum tumor marker CA-125 has been suggested, little evidence supports the effectiveness of this triad in an asymptomatic population. Bimanual pelvic examination may not alert the practitioner to the presence of an abnormality, particularly if the cancer is in an early stage or if the body habitus of the patient prevents optimal examination. Transvaginal ultrasound may define the characteristics of an enlarged ovary, but, like many radiographic studies, it has limited diagnostic value. Although CA-125 level is useful for monitoring treatment response, it lacks specificity for distinguishing ovarian cancer from various benign and malignant conditions. CA-125 tumor marker is elevated in 80% of patients with advanced ovarian cancer, but is normal in 50% to 75% of patients with Stage I ovarian cancer. The degree of elevation varies, and the actual CA-125 level may not directly reflect the amount of tumor present.

25. When is the CA-125 assay useful?

If CA-125 level is elevated when ovarian cancer is diagnosed, the assay is useful for monitoring response to treatment and detecting cancer recurrence. The CA-125 level may be obtained monthly during treatment and every few months during follow-up after remission. Although the return of the CA-125 to normal levels early in the course of chemotherapy treatment may be considered a favorable prognostic indicator, it is not an indication of cure. Approximately one half of women with ovarian cancer who have a normal CA-125 level after initial debulking surgery and chemotherapy have residual cancer if a second-look operation is performed. Residual cancer is frequently microscopic or of small volume; it may not be visible on radiographic studies or palpable on bimanual pelvic examination.

26. Can anything protect women from developing ovarian cancer?

Oral contraceptive pills (OCPs) significantly reduce the risk of ovarian cancer by up to 50% in women who use them consistently for 5 years. This reduction is attributed to the ovulatory suppression of OCPs; the progesterone component of OCPs may also play a role. Protection is also obtained from breastfeeding and having one or more full-term pregnancies, because both situations suppress ovulation. Tubal ligation also gives some protection, although the reasons are unclear. A prophylactic bilateral salpingo-oophorectomy should be considered in women with a gene mutation associated with breast-ovarian syndrome or a strong family history suggestive of hereditary syndrome, because removal of the ovaries and fallopian tubes reduces cancer risk by 90%.

27. How is ovarian cancer treated?

For ovarian cancers of all stages except IA and IB with well-differentiated or moderately well-differentiated tumors, a staging laparotomy with tumor debulking (< 1 cm residual disease is optimal) is performed and followed by chemotherapy (6 cycles of paclitaxel or platinum-based chemotherapy preferred).

28. A patient with ovarian cancer is told by her gynecologic oncologist that all visible cancer was removed at the time of debulking surgery, but she still needs chemotherapy. Why?

Although the removal of all visible tumor markedly improves prognosis, microscopic tumor is most likely still present because of the spread patterns of ovarian cancer. Epithelial ovarian cancer, the most common type, arises from the surface of the ovary. The cancer cells can exfoliate and spread throughout the abdominal cavity early in the course of disease. This often results in peritoneal seeding of tumor, which may form microscopic implants of tumor on the peritoneal surfaces. Without chemotherapy, these implants may potentially grow and reform bulky tumor. Chemotherapy (paclitaxel plus carboplatin or cisplatin) is needed to treat the microscopic tumor and may be administered intravenously, intraperitoneally (chemotherapy delivered directly into the abdomen through a subcutaneous port and catheter), or both. The FDA recently approved gemcitabine in combination with carboplatin for advanced ovarian cancer patients who have relapsed 6 months after platinum-based therapy.

29. Intraperitoneal chemotherapy seems to be making a comeback. Why is this so?

Results of a 7-year clinical trial have confirmed that intraperitoneal (IP) chemotherapy improves survival in women with optimally debulked stage III ovarian cancer compared to women of the same stage who receive intravenous (IV) chemotherapy. The drugs typically used in combination are IP cisplatin, IP paclitaxel, and IV paclitaxel. However, IP therapy may cause increased toxicities for some patients, causing nausea, vomiting, abdominal pain, and peripheral neuropathies.

30. What is a second-look laparotomy? When should a nurse expect a patient to undergo this procedure?

A second-look laparotomy is an exploratory procedure performed after completion of the initial chemotherapy regimen for ovarian cancer. It is initiated when there is no evidence of cancer on physical examination or computed tomography (CT) scan. The purpose is to determine whether residual cancer is present, which is possible despite the lack of physical evidence of disease in 50% of women who have undergone debulking surgery and chemotherapy. During the procedure, the abdominal and pelvic cavities are thoroughly explored. Visible tumor is removed when possible, and multiple biopsies of the peritoneal surfaces are obtained.

Although it was considered standard practice for many years, second-look laparotomy has limited value. Gynecologic oncologists moved to abandon the procedure when it became apparent that as many as 50% of women with negative second-look surgeries developed recurrent disease at a future time. Thus, survival was not positively affected, and patients were exposed to the increased morbidity and mortality of additional surgery. The procedure may be used on some individuals or when a patient is enrolled in a study that examines the efficacy of existing or new treatments.

31. What is borderline ovarian cancer?

Borderline ovarian cancer is also known as ovarian adenocarcinoma of low malignant potential. Pathologically, the cells resemble those of an ovarian carcinoma, but they are not invasive. Patients generally develop symptoms similar to those of ovarian carcinoma, such as increased abdominal girth, ascites, and enlarged ovaries. Tumors usually occur in the fourth and fifth decades of life, are more commonly confined to the ovary at diagnosis, and are associated with a good prognosis. When they have spread beyond the ovary, which is uncommon, the primary treatment is surgical debulking. In the event that they recur, surgical debulking may be repeated. Chemotherapy is rarely used because there is little data to indicate that it improves survival. Whereas borderline ovarian cancer can be extensive and recurrent, it is treated primarily with surgical excision and has a much more favorable prognosis than epithelial ovarian cancers.

Quick Facts—Endometrial Cancer

Incidence	39,080 newly diagnosed cases estimated in 2007	**Histopathology**	Endometrial adenocarcinoma (most common)
Mortality	7400 deaths estimated in 2007		Adenosquamous, squamous, mucinous, serous papillary, clear cell, and undifferentiated
Risk factors	Unopposed exogenous estrogen (progesterone is protective)	**Symptoms**	Abnormal uterine bleeding in postmenopausal women (80% of patients)
	Nulliparity, infertility, anovulation		Pap test abnormality, presence of endometrial cells suspicious; symptoms of uterine enlargement or pelvic pressure may be signs of advanced disease
	Late menopause (after age 52 years)		
	Obesity (increased levels of endogenous estrogen)		
	Diabetes mellitus, hypertension	**Diagnosis and evaluation**	History and physical examination
	Family history (ovarian-endometrial-colon cancer)		Pelvic examination
	Complex atypical hyperplasia (thickened endometrium with cytologic atypia of glands)		Dilation and curettage
			Endometrial biopsy
			Intravenous pyelogram
	Prolonged adjuvant tamoxifen therapy for breast cancer		CT or MRI of abdomen or pelvis
Genetics	Hereditary nonpolyposis colorectal cancer (HNPCC) genetic abnormality increases risk (10-fold)		Chest x-ray (PA and lateral)

Continued

Quick Facts—cont'd

Staging and Stage Grouping

Stage	Description
I	Confined to corpus
IA	Limited to endometrium
IB	Invades < half of myometrium
IC	Invades > half of myometrium
II	Extends to cervix
IIA	Involves endocervical glands
IIB	Invades cervical stroma
III	Involves adjacent structures
IIIA	Invades uterine serosa, adnexae, or peritoneal cytology positive
IIB	Vaginal extension
IIIC	Metastasis to pelvic or para-aortic lymph nodes
IV	Distant metastasis, including intraabdominal or inguinal lymph nodes, lungs

32. How are estrogen levels and estrogen replacement therapy related to endometrial cancer?

Endometrial cancer depends on the unopposed supply of estrogen from endogenous (within the body) and exogenous (outside the body) sources. During the reproductive years, neuroendocrine changes occur each month to promote a regular menstrual cycle. Cyclical estrogen production in the form of estradiol from the ovary promotes proliferation of the lining of the uterus in anticipation of implantation of a fertilized ovum. After ovulation, secretion of estradiol continues, and progesterone is produced to maintain the endometrial lining. In the absence of pregnancy and the associated release of human chorionic gonadotropin (HCG) from the developing placenta, the level of progesterone falls dramatically. The drop in progesterone causes the endometrial lining to be shed within 1 to 2 days.

Estrogen production that is not challenged or opposed by progesterone causes ongoing proliferation of the endometrial lining. Continued growth of the endometrial lining favors the development of atypical cells and cancer. When a woman has either increased endogenous sources of estrogen (e.g., with anovulation and obesity) or increased exogenous sources of estrogen (e.g., estrogen replacement without progesterone), the risk of developing endometrial cancer is greater. Any woman with an intact uterus who takes estrogen replacement also should receive progesterone either cyclically or daily to counteract the proliferative effects of estrogen on the lining of the uterus. Women who have had the uterus removed do not require progesterone therapy when estrogen replacement is initiated.

33. How should the nurse respond to the woman who asks if obesity increases the risk for endometrial cancer?

Associations among obesity, excessive estrogen levels, and endometrial cancer have been documented. Obese women typically have higher levels of endogenous estrogen because of two mechanisms. First, the adrenal cortex produces androstenedione, which is converted to estrogen by adipose tissue. Consequently, excessive fat tissue leads to excessive production of estrogen. Second, obesity depresses the level of sex hormone-binding globulin (SHBG) and thus, leads to higher free (unbound) levels of estrogen. Unbound estrogen is the hormonally active form. The nurse should explain that obese women face a higher risk for the development of endometrial cancer because increased levels of endogenous estrogen promote proliferation of the uterine lining.

34. How is endometrial cancer treated?

Total abdominal hysterectomy with bilateral salpingo-oophorectomy and lymph node dissection is considered the gold standard. For Stage IC cancer and above, a poorly differentiated tumor, or cancer with histologic signs (e.g., clear cell, serous papillary) of an aggressive form, the recommended treatment is adjuvant radiation therapy, chemotherapy (doxorubicin, cisplatin, carboplatin, paclitaxel), or both.

35. After hysterectomy for endometrial cancer, a patient is told by her physician that the final surgical pathology report will determine the need for additional radiation or chemotherapy. How may the nurse clarify this statement?

Several pathologic determinations are required to ascertain the need for adjunctive treatment. These results include histology, tumor grade, extent of myometrial invasion, findings from cytologic washings, extent of spread to other organs, and lymph node status.

- Adenocarcinomas are the most common histologic types of endometrial cancer. Additional cell types, such as clear cell or papillary serous carcinomas, are considered more aggressive and require adjuvant treatment.
- Tumor grade is applied to all histologic types and is stated in degree of differentiation: well, moderately, or poorly differentiated cells. A less favorable prognosis is associated with moderately to poorly differentiated tumors; thus, adjuvant treatment is desirable.
- Myometrial invasion refers to the depth of cancer cell penetration into the wall of the uterus. Myometrial invasion that is less than one half the thickness of the uterine wall is less likely to have spread beyond the uterus than tumors that invade the outer half. Such patients frequently require treatment with radiation and/or chemotherapy.
- Cytologic washings from the abdominal-peritoneal cavity collected at the beginning of the surgery are checked for malignant cells that may have disseminated through either the fallopian tubes or the uterine wall before removal of the uterus.
- Lymph nodes sampled at the time of the surgery are also examined microscopically for evidence of disease.

Positive findings in cytologic washings or lymph nodes require additional treatment, usually chemotherapy or radiation, for disease that has spread outside the uterus. Despite the appearance of "normal" tissue at the time of gross visual inspection, any of these pathologic findings may alter the treatment recommendations. The nurse should know that the treatment plan cannot be determined until the final pathology report has been received, so that he or she can offer emotional support to the patient during this time of uncertainty.

 ## Key Points

- Cervical cancer is considered preventable. It is characterized by a lengthy premalignant, preinvasive state that can be detected early through routine Papanicolaou (Pap) tests.
- Cervical cancer spreads primarily by direct extension to surrounding tissues and organs, and by flowing through the lymphatic system to regional lymph node chains.
- If CA-125 is elevated when ovarian cancer is diagnosed, the assay is useful for monitoring response to treatment and to detect cancer recurrence.
- Several pathologic traits, including histologic findings, tumor grade, myometrial invasion, cytologic washings, spread to other organs and lymph nodes, determine whether adjunctive treatment is recommended for a patient.

Continued

Key Points—cont'd

- Treatment of gynecologic malignancies includes a multimodal approach, usually involving hysterectomy and other procedures that may change organ function, body image, and sexuality. Treatment decisions are based on the stage of the cancer, age and health status of the patient, and preferences of the patient.

Internet Resources

National Ovarian Cancer Coalition:
  http://www.ovarian.org
Gilda Radner Familial Ovarian Cancer Registry:
  http://www.ovariancancer.com
Gynecologic Cancer Foundation:
  http://www.wcn.org/gcf
National Comprehensive Cancer Network, Clinical Practice Guidelines:
  http://www.nccn.org/professionals/physician_gls/PDF/cervical.pdf

Acknowledgment

The authors wish to acknowledge Patricia Novak-Smith, RN, MSN, AOCN, for her contributions to the Gynecologic Cancers chapter published in the first and second editions of *Oncology Nursing Secrets*.

Bibliography

Armstrong DK, Bundy B, Wenzel L, et al: Intraperitoneal cisplatin and paclitaxel in ovarian cancer. *N Engl J Med* 354:34-43, 2006.

Ault KA: Vaccines for the prevention of human papillomavirus and associated gynecologic disease: A review. *Obstet Gynecol Surv* 61(6):S26-S31, 2006.

Berek JS, Hacker NF, editors: *Practical gynecologic oncology,* ed 4, Philadelphia, 2005, Lippincott Williams & Wilkins.

Greene FL, Page DL, Fleming ID, et al, editors: *AJCC cancer staging manual,* ed 6, New York, 2002, Springer.

Jemal A, Siegel R, Ward E, et al: Cancer statistics, 2007. *CA Cancer J Clin* 57:43-66, 2007.

Moore-Higgs GJ, Almadrones LA, Colvin-Huff B, et al, editors: *Women and cancer: A gynecologic oncology nursing perspective,* ed 2, Boston, 2000, Jones & Bartlett.

Thomas GM: Improved treatment for cervical cancer: Concurrent chemotherapy and radiotherapy. *N Engl J Med* 340:1198-1200, 2000.

Villa LL, Costa RLR, Petta CA, et al: Prophylactic quadrivalent human papillomavirus double-blind placebo-controlled multicentre phase II efficacy trial. *Lancet Oncol* 6(5):271-278, 2005.

Head and Neck Cancers

R. Lee Jennings and Lenore L. Harris

Quick Facts

Incidence	34,360 newly diagnosed oral cavity and pharynx cancer cases estimated in 2007 (24,180 in men; 10,180 in women) 11,300 newly diagnosed larynx cancer cases estimated in 2007 (8960 in men; 2340 in women)	**Nasopharyngeal cancer** Epstein-Barr virus (EBV) Frequent ingestion of smoked foods beginning in childhood
Mortality	7550 oral cavity and pharynx deaths estimated in 2007 3660 larynx cancer deaths estimated in 2007	**Genetics** Mutations of the p53 tumor suppressor gene may be related to head and neck cancer development
Risk factors	**Squamous cell cancer of the upper aerodigestive tract** Habitual use of tobacco in any form (greatest risk factor in 90% of cases): cigarettes, cigars, pipes, bidis, kreteks, smokeless tobacco/snuff	**Histopathology** Squamous cell carcinomas (approximately 95% of all head and neck cancers) Salivary gland primary cancers Sarcomas (rare)
	Marijuana use	**Symptoms** Pain, tenderness
	Chronic irritation to mucosa, leukoplakia	Unilateral sinusitis or nasal obstruction
	Advancing age (more common after age 50)	Persistent scaly or ulcerated lesion
	Male gender (male-female ratio = 3:1)	Neck or submucosal mass Persistent hoarseness or change in voice
	Excessive use of alcohol (synergistic effect with tobacco)	Unilateral ear pain, not explained by infection Chronic dysphagia
	Industrial exposure to wood dust, leather, metal (nickel), asbestos, chemical inhalants (woodworking)	**Diagnosis and evaluation** History and physical examination (comorbid conditions, tobacco and alcohol use, nutritional assessment)
	Daily skin exposure to sun (outdoor workers)	Complete blood count, chemistry screen (albumin and magnesium) Chest x-ray (PA and lateral)
	Radiation exposure (salivary gland and thyroid cancers)	Biopsy, fine-needle aspiration cytology, biopsy with direct laryngoscopy CT/MRI of primary site

Continued

293

Quick Facts—cont'd

	PET evaluation of tumor extent; residual or recurrent cancer	More extensive imaging if distant metastases found

Staging and Stage Grouping

Stage	Description
Tumor, node, metastasis (TNM)	
Primary tumor (T) for lip and oral cavity	
T1	Greatest diameter of primary tumor ≤ 2 cm
T2	Greatest diameter of primary tumor > 2-4 cm
T3	Greatest diameter of primary tumor > 4 cm
T4	Lip: invades adjacent structure, such as bone, tongue, skin
	Oral cavity: invades adjacent structures, such as deep muscles of tongue, bone (deep invasion), maxillary sinus, skin
Primary tumor (T) for salivary glands	
T1	Greatest dimension of tumor ≤ 2 cm (no local extension)
T2	Greatest dimension of tumor > 2-4 cm (no local extension)
T3	Greatest dimension of tumor > 4-6 cm (with local extension but no cranial nerve (CN) VII involvement)
T4	Invades base of skull, CN VII, and/or greatest dimension of tumor < 6 cm; local extension is defined as clinical or macroscopic; evidence of spread to skin, nerve, or bone
Cervical node involvement (N), oral cavity and salivary glands	
NX	Regional nodes cannot be assessed
N0	No nodal involvement
N1	Single clinically positive ipsilateral node = 3 cm
N2a	Single clinically positive ipsilateral node > 3-6 cm
N2b	Multiple clinically positive ipsilateral nodes, none > 6 cm
N2c	Bilateral or contralateral positive nodes, none > 6 cm
N3	One clinically positive lymph node > 6 cm
Distant metastasis (M)	
MX	Distant metastasis cannot be assessed
M0	No known distant metastasis
M1	Distant metastasis present (common sites of metastasis include: lung, bone, liver)

Stage	Primary Tumor	Cervical Node Involvement	Distant Metastasis
Cancer of lip, oral cavity, and pharynx			
I	T1	N0	M0
II	T2	N0	M0
III	T3	N0	M0
	T1	N1	M0
	T2	N1	M0
	T3	N1	M0
IVA	T4	N0	M0
	T4	N1	M0
	Any T	N2	M0
IVB	Any T	N3	M0
IVC	Any T	Any N	M1

Quick Facts—cont'd

Stage	Primary Tumor	Cervical Node Involvement	Distant Metastasis
Salivary glands:			
I	T1	N0	M0
II	T2	N0	M0
III	T3	N0	M0
	T1	N1	M0
	T2	N1	M0
	T3	N1	M0
IVA	T4	N0	M0
	T4	N1	M0
	Any T	N2	M0
IVB	Any T	N3	M0
	T4 (invades skull)	Any N	M0
IVC	Any T	Any N	M1

1. Describe the types and sites of head and neck cancer.

All cancers arising in the upper food and airway passages (upper aerodigestive tract) are included: lips, oral cavity, pharynx (oropharynx, nasopharynx, hypopharynx), nasal cavity, and paranasal sinuses. Also included are the major and minor salivary glands and the thyroid gland (see Chapter 24 on endocrine tumors).

Subdivisions of the major sites include buccal mucosa, gingivae, palate, tongue, tonsils, pyriform sinus, and larynx. Subsite designation is important because prognosis, treatment, and morbidity of treatment may change dramatically for each one. Cancers arising in the skin (melanoma, basal cell and squamous cell carcinoma, skin adnexal tumors) and lymphomas are excluded for reporting purposes, but are important in any discussion of malignancies of the head and neck (see Chapter 17, Non-Hodgkin Lymphoma, and Chapter 29, Malignant Melanoma).

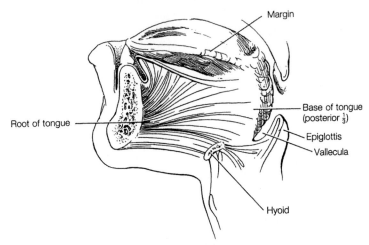

Posterior oral anatomy. *(From Jennings RL: Tumors of the head and neck. In Ritchie WP Jr, Steele G Jr, Dean RH, editors: General surgery, Philadelphia, 1995, Lippincott-Raven. By permission.)*

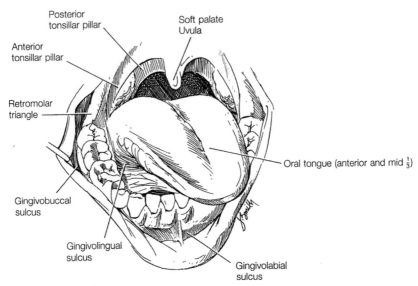

Anterior oral anatomy. *(From Jennings RL: Tumors of the head and neck. In Ritchie WP Jr, Steele G Jr, Dean RH, editors: General surgery, Philadelphia, 1995, Lippincott-Raven. By permission.)*

2. How do patients with head and neck cancers differ from patients with other types of cancer?

The head and neck region is unique among the sites requiring cancer treatment. The complex interaction of the face, oral cavity, voice, and air passages in personal presentation, food intake, and comfort makes treatment planning highly demanding. Even a microscopic cosmetic or functional defect is viewed with concern. The importance of maintaining acceptable cosmetic and functional results must be balanced with the necessity of adequately treating the patient's primary cancer. Primary tumors of the head and neck create functional and cosmetic problems if the malignancy is not adequately treated and controlled. Good palliation is seldom achieved without cure of the primary tumor.

3. Describe the role of chemoprevention.

Chemoprevention using retinoids, including natural vitamin A and synthetic analogs, beta carotene, and vitamin E, has shown some promise in reversing premalignant lesions and preventing second primary tumors. Other studies have employed vitamin C or zinc.

4. What are the presenting symptoms of head and neck cancer?

Presenting complaints vary because of the complex anatomy of the region and the variety of functions performed by the head and neck. Significant changes in facial appearance, sight, smell, swallowing, and/or voice may be early symptoms of cancer. Nonhealing ulceration, pain at the primary site, and referred pain also may be early symptoms. Often the patient visits the dentist first because of changes in the oral cavity, including loosening teeth, or ill-fitting dentures. Pharyngeal primary tumors are the most subtle and varied in presentation. Changes are less noticeable to the patient because these areas are

Symptoms according to primary tumor site

Site	Presenting symptoms	Late symptoms
Lip	Sore that does not heal	Large ulceration, mass, pain, foul breath, loss of lip function
Buccal mucosa	Ulceration or mass; acidic drinks may cause burning	Pain, mass in cheek
Gingiva	Ulceration; dentures do not fit	Pain, loose teeth, trismus (lockjaw)
Tongue	Ulceration, mild pain, mass	Decreased range of motion, pain, dysphagia, malnutrition
Hard palate	Ulcer or mass	Ulceration, loose teeth
Floor of mouth ± tongue invasion	Ulceration	Pain, mass
Nasopharynx	Nasal stuffiness, nosebleeds	Bleeding, nasal obstruction, cranial nerve paralysis, pain, vision changes
Oropharynx, base of tongue	Sore throat, usually unilateral and persistent	Dysphagia, pain, malnutrition, muffled voice
Tonsil, soft palate	Ulceration or mass	Mass or large ulceration, dysphagia
Pharyngoesophageal junction	Possible dysphagia	Mass or large ulceration, dysphagia
Hypopharynx (pyriform sinus)	Possible dysphagia	Dysphagia, pain, aspiration, voice change
Larynx	Hoarseness	Severe hoarseness, airway obstruction, aspiration
Salivary gland (major and minor)	Preauricular or submandibular mass Mucosa-covered mass in oral cavity (no ulceration)	Enlarged neck masses, ulceration in oral cavity (minor salivary gland), facial nerve paralysis with parotid gland cancer, mandibular invasion with submandibular gland cancers
Thyroid gland	Thyroid mass	Enlarged neck masses, vocal cord paralysis, dysphagia

not visible. Hoarseness and persistent unilateral throat irritation should be assessed, because these symptoms can lead to an early diagnosis.

5. When does treatment planning begin?

Planning for treatment and rehabilitation starts with the initial visit. Plan to monitor the patient's nutritional status to prevent weight loss, so that nutritional repair is supported as the diagnostic workup continues.

6. What does the practitioner need to perform a head and neck examination?

Instruments required for clinical head and neck examination are simple, fairly inexpensive, and easily available in the head and neck surgeon's office but often absent from the hospital unit or outpatient clinic. Needed equipment includes a high-backed chair for the patient and a stool for the examiner. A flashlight is inadequate; a headlight is needed to free both hands. Also needed are laryngeal mirrors, a heat source to warm the mirror to prevent fogging, tongue blades, finger cots, local and topical anesthetics, and biopsy forceps. A fiberoptic laryngoscope is used to examine the nasopharynx of patients with a severe gag reflex. Physical examination of the oral cavity, pharynx, and larynx requires visualization of all mucosal surfaces. The oral cavity, base of tongue, and tonsils are palpated with a gloved finger. The nasopharynx, hypopharynx, and larynx are visualized with a mirror or fiberoptic laryngoscope.

7. What histologic types of cancer occur on skin surfaces of the head and neck, including the lip?

Skin malignancies are the most common head and neck cancers that require surgical treatment. Over 800,000 skin malignancies are reported each year, along with 2,300 deaths. Basal cell and squamous cell carcinomas are by far the most numerous, with 85% occurring in the head and neck region. Ninety-four percent of recurrent basal cell cancers occur in the head and neck region, with 75% occurring in the central face. Melanoma is a more common malignancy of the head and neck skin surface, whereas Merkel cell carcinoma is rare.

8. How are skin cancers of the head and neck treated?

Most basal cell malignancies are small and can be treated adequately with desiccation and curettage by the patient's dermatologist or primary care physician. Biopsy for pathology examination is mandatory. Larger skin cancers, multicentric basal cell cancers, or recurrent skin cancers should be treated with wide excision and pathology confirmation that margins are free of tumor. Wide elliptical excision is usually adequate, but flap reconstruction is considered when the pathologist reports close or positive margins. Lymph node metastasis is unusual except with large squamous cell skin cancers. Merkel cell cancer and skin appendage cancers are rare but important, because nodal metastasis and distant spread are more likely. Sentinel lymph node biopsy should be considered for melanoma and Merkel cell carcinoma. Wide surgical removal with flap or skin graft reconstruction is necessary, and lymph node dissection may be required, depending on the location of the primary tumor. Melanoma may occur on any skin surface in the head and neck and on mucosal surfaces, such as the oral cavity and nasal cavity (see Chapter 29 for more information on melanomas).

9. What are salivary gland malignancies?

Malignancies may occur in the major (parotid, submandibular, sublingual) and minor salivary glands. Minor salivary glands are present in all mucosal surfaces of the upper food and airway passages. A mass in one of the major salivary glands has a 20% to 50% chance of being malignant. A mass covered by intact mucosa in the oral cavity may be a minor salivary tumor, and the risk of malignancy is as high as 50%.

10. How are salivary gland malignancies treated?

Complete surgical excision is the treatment of choice, and may be accomplished when the biopsy is obtained. Most benign tumors of the salivary glands are pleomorphic adenomas (mixed tumors); when excision is incomplete, the recurrence rate is 70%.

Treatment of major salivary neoplasms

Tumor	Parotid	Submandibular
Benign mixed, Warthin's tumor, nonneoplastic benign masses	Superficial parotidectomy Facial nerve preservation	Digastric triangle dissection Preservation of facial nerve marginal branch
T1 or T2 low grade tumor, mucoepidermoid or acinic cell cancer	Total parotidectomy Facial nerve preservation No radiation therapy	Digastric triangle dissection Preservation of facial nerve marginal branch No radiation therapy
T1 or T2 high-grade tumor*	Total parotidectomy Facial nerve preservation (unless involved) No postoperative radiation therapy	Digastric triangle dissection Preservation of facial nerve marginal branch (unless involved) Neck dissection if N+ Postoperative radiation therapy
T3, N0, or N+ recurrent salivary cancers	Radical parotidectomy Facial nerve resection Neck dissection if N+ Postoperative radiation therapy	Radical neck dissection Removal of facial nerve marginal branch and lingual nerve as necessary Postoperative radiation therapy
T4	Radical parotidectomy Resection of ear canal, including muscle Sacrifice of facial nerve Neck dissection if N+ Postoperative radiation therapy	Resection of involved structures Radical neck dissection Postoperative radiation therapy

*Includes malignant mixed, squamous, and poorly differentiated adenocarcinomas, and anaplastic and adenoid cysts. *From Jennings RL, Nelson WR: Tumors of the head and neck. In Ritchie WP Jr, Steele G Jr, Dean RH, editors:* General surgery, *Philadelphia, 1995, Lippincott-Raven, p 35. By permission.*

11. When the patient has a thyroid nodule and cancer is suspected, what type of thyroidectomy is advised?

It is unusual to have a definitive diagnosis of cancer before a thyroidectomy is performed. Total thyroid lobectomy on the side of the nodule is the preferred procedure. An attempt to excise the nodule for biopsy is not advised because of: (1) the risk of contaminating the surgical field if the diagnosis is cancer, (2) the greater risk of injury to the recurrent nerve, and (3) the greater difficulty in making a definitive diagnosis from frozen sections of the tumor. A delayed cancer diagnosis requires a return to surgery for completion of the thyroidectomy, again placing the patient's recurrent nerve and parathyroid glands at greater risk for injury. When cancer is identified on frozen section, many surgeons favor performing a total thyroidectomy to allow for total thyroid ablation with iodine-131 and later radioactive iodine scanning in the event of metastasis. Small (< 2 cm), well-differentiated cancers contained within the thyroid capsule require only total lobectomy. Lymph node dissection for the patient with well-differentiated thyroid cancer is necessary only if nodes are clinically involved (see Chapter 24 for more information on endocrine cancers).

12. What are the types of lip cancer?

Most lip malignancies involve the lower lip and are squamous in type. Basal cell carcinoma is the usual histologic type for lesions of the upper lip. Other lip malignancies are minor salivary gland cancers that arise on mucosal surfaces of the lips.

13. How are the various types of lip cancer treated?

Malignancies of the lip are treated with a wide excision, including removal of the mucosal surface. Postoperative radiation therapy is used to treat advanced or high-grade malignancies. Basal cell and squamous cell cancers are best treated with surgery. Radiation therapy may be used alone to achieve an equal cure rate, but may further damage surrounding skin already injured from sun exposure. The damage usually makes later surgical excision difficult, should the primary tumor recur or new skin cancers develop in the same area. Locally advanced cancers or node-positive cancers may require a combination of radiation and surgery. Surgical procedures are usually performed in one stage. Tumors requiring removal of up to one third of the lip width are treated with a V excision and primary repair. Cosmetic and functional results are excellent with this procedure. Upper neck dissection is necessary for a node-positive neck cancer as well as advanced malignancy directly invading skin and bone. Basal cell cancers of the upper lip require special attention. This tumor is more likely to recur locally, perhaps because it is more difficult to obtain clear margins with wide excision and cosmetic repair.

14. What are other histologic types of oral and pharyngeal cancer?

Well over 90% of malignancies involving the mucosal surfaces are squamous cell tumors. The remainder are minor salivary gland tumors (see Question 9).

15. How are T1 squamous cell cancers treated?

Small (T1) squamous cell cancers in the anterior oral cavity may be treated with radiation therapy alone or surgery alone; the cure rates are the same for the two treatments. Many believe that a malignancy that is diagnosed early and has minimal risk of nodal spread is better treated with surgery alone, because treatment is generally completed in one day, morbidity should be minimal, and the risks of xerostomia (hyposalivation), dental caries, and bone loss (osteoradionecrosis) are decreased.

16. How are T2 and more advanced squamous carcinomas best treated?

Treatment generally includes a combination of surgery and radiation therapy. Both the radiation therapist and the surgeon should examine the patient to plan the treatment before it begins. When combined treatment is recommended, most surgeons prefer that the surgical procedure be done first, if the primary tumor is well defined and a complete excision with free margins is possible. Otherwise, surgery may be scheduled between 3 and 7 weeks after completion of radiation therapy. Surgery earlier than 3 weeks after radiation therapy may result in excessive bleeding due to inflammation, and after 7 to 8 weeks, excessive fibrosis may prevent proper wound healing.

Nasopharyngeal primary tumors are most frequently treated with radiation therapy alone; skull base surgical techniques are reserved for tumors that have not responded to radiation therapy and for primary tumors with local extension that are not treatable with radiation therapy for cure. Hypopharyngeal and laryngeal cancers are usually treated with radiation therapy alone when diagnosed early, before the tumor has spread. A combination of surgery and radiation therapy is reserved for advanced-stage primary tumors. Surgical salvage is necessary when radiation therapy fails to eliminate the malignancy and a partial or total laryngectomy is needed.

17. What repair techniques are used for advanced cancer?

Removal of advanced cancers of the posterior oral cavity and oropharynx by surgery requires specialized repair techniques, usually involving myocutaneous flaps, to replace the large amount of functional tissue removed. Repair techniques improve functional and cosmetic results. Microvascular free flap procedures can be used to repair mandible, tonsil, and tongue defects with bone and soft tissue from distant sites.

18. What is a carotid rupture? How common is it?

The carotid artery ruptures when it becomes exposed because of flap necrosis, fistula formation and associated infection, or recurrent tumor around the artery. The first hint of this complication may be a trickle of blood that occurs hours or days before rupture. Carotid rupture is rare because of improved techniques in both radiation therapy and surgery.

19. How is a carotid rupture managed?

Preparations are made in advance when the potential for rupture exists. The patient must be moved to a bed near the nurse's station. Blood is typed and cross-matched, intravenous access ensured, tracheotomy established, and a hemostat placed in the room. If a rupture occurs, the nurse applies firm pressure over the artery with a towel, immediately calls for help, initiates oxygen and intravenous fluids, and calls for blood. When a rupture occurs in a palliative setting, comfort measures, reassurance, and supportive care are provided in place of surgery. The rupture is not painful but may be terrifying to the patient and those with the patient.

20. What is important in the postoperative nursing care of patients with head and neck cancer?

Major areas of nursing care include the following:
- **Assurance of an adequate airway**. Often the patient will have a tracheotomy, which should be sutured in place or secured at all times. A dislodged tracheotomy may result in hypoxia or death. Attention to secretion clearance is mandatory for airway maintenance, patient comfort, and wound healing.
- **Self-care**. Patients should be taught self-care techniques for airway clearance, wound care, and possible complications, as soon as possible after surgery. The confidence that results from airway assurance, secretion clearance, and wound care gives the patient control of what could otherwise be a terrifying situation.
- **Speech and swallowing rehabilitation**. Techniques taught by a speech pathologist or dysphagia therapist should be reinforced by nursing staff. Patients need to be taught proper head and body posture, food texture and portions, ways to prevent aspiration, and use of assistive devices for speaking and swallowing.
- **Repair of nutritional defects**. A dietary consult is indicated to optimize caloric intake. Teaching includes the importance of meeting the nutritional requirements for adequate calories and protein essential for wound healing. Total parenteral nutrition provides excellent short-term support, but it is not the optimal method of feeding for patients with head and neck cancer. Enteral feeding should start as

soon as possible. Oral feedings usually start as soon as suture lines have sufficiently healed. Nasogastric or percutaneous endoscopic gastrostomy (PEG) tubes allow patients with long-term swallowing problems to be discharged while outpatient rehabilitation continues. A PEG tube can be placed preoperatively so that nutritional repair may begin preoperatively and continue immediately after surgery.

21. Outline patient education needs according to tumor site.

Patient education needs

Organ site	Treatment	Patient teaching
Nasal fossa/paranasal sinus	Surgery alone or combination therapy	Elevate head of bed Wound care/irrigating graft Oral hygiene Technique for removing, cleaning, and replacing oral obturator Care of prosthesis
Nasopharynx	Radiation therapy Chemoradiotherapy ± surgery	Wound care Management of xerostomia, pain, otitis media
Oral cavity/oropharynx	Stage I-II: surgery or radiation therapy Stage III-IV: surgery + radiation therapy	Wound care Oral hygiene Speech and swallowing therapy reinforcement Management of pain, xerostomia Tracheostomy care and suctioning Gastric tube care
Salivary gland	Stage I-II: surgery ± radiation therapy Stage III-IV: surgery + chemoradiotherapy	Wound care Oral hygiene If cranial nerve VIII is involved, protect and moisten affected cornea (eye drops/ointment), tape eyelids Protect skin from elements (because of facial numbness)
Larynx/hypopharynx/neck	Stage I-II: surgery or radiation therapy Stage III-IV: surgery + chemoradiotherapy OR Chemoradiotherapy + neck dissection (laryngeal preservation)	Prevent aspiration Provide humidification Wound care Management of fistula drainage Oral hygiene Tracheostomy care and suctioning Gastric tube care Speech and swallowing therapy reinforcement With insufficient tissue coverage of carotid artery: carotid artery rupture precautions

22. What are the choices for speech production after total laryngectomy?

Vocalization requires the movement of air through the larynx and vocal tract, so it is not possible when the larynx has been removed. The referral to the speech pathologist should include the surgeon's description of the patient's postoperative physiologic status. The speech pathologist teaches the patient to use at least one of the following voice alternatives:

- Artificial larynx
  - Handheld, electronic, battery-powered device with robot-like sound
  - Either neck-type (diaphragm causes vibration of neck tissue with resonance into oral cavity) or mouth-type (directs sound into oral cavity through small tube placed in mouth)
  - Easy to use; minimal training is required
- Esophageal speech
  - Air swallowed into and momentarily held in the esophagus and released as words are articulated (called "burping speech")
  - May require up to 6 months of speech therapy to become proficient
- Tracheoesophageal puncture (TEP) speech
  - Surgical procedure to create a tracheoesophageal fistula and placement of a one-way valve (silicone tube) prosthesis
  - Speech is produced by inhaling air and covering the tracheostoma with the thumb; valve may be fitted in place to allow hands-free speech (husky voice results)
  - Cleaning and maintenance of the prosthesis by the patient (as often as necessary) or practitioner (usually every 6 months)
  - Requires awareness and reporting of possible symptoms of fungal colonization on valve

23. When may radiation therapy alone be the treatment of choice?

Patients with small (T1 or T2) tumors may receive radiation therapy alone, which achieves better function and cosmesis than can be obtained with surgery alone. If the patient has a stage III or IV unresectable malignancy, radiation therapy may be prescribed to maintain or improve swallowing and/or speech, but treatment is not expected to be curative.

24. What assessments are needed for the patient receiving radiation therapy?

If radiation therapy precedes surgery, the patient's nutritional status should be monitored to prevent malnutrition. Prophylactic dental care is necessary before treatment begins because of the risk of radionecrosis and mandibular bone loss. With preoperative radiation therapy, treatment is usually stopped at around a total dose of 5500 cGy because most patients develop mucositis with a higher dose. Redness and dysphagia usually disappear by 3 weeks after the last treatment. When radiation therapy is the only treatment, additional dosage to the primary site is necessary. This boost may be given with external beam or implant techniques. Implants usually are performed under general anesthesia and require hospitalization and often a tracheotomy until the implants are removed.

25. When is chemotherapy used to treat patients with head and neck cancer?

Chemotherapy has an increasing role in the treatment of oral, pharyngeal, and laryngeal carcinoma and is usually given in conjunction with radiation therapy for organ (larynx) preservation. After chemotherapy, surgery may be performed for salvage in case of recurrence or persistent tumor, or as a planned treatment with a lesser surgical procedure to preserve function. The role of chemotherapy is palliative with metastatic or recurrent head and neck cancer. The chemotherapy agents showing response are carboplatin, cisplatin, 5-fluorouracil with leucovorin, paclitaxel, doxorubicin, and methotrexate.

26. What are the 5-year survival rates for head and neck cancers?

Trends in relative 5-year survival rates vary according to stage and site. Stage I-II cancers are small; 5-year survival rates are approximately 80%. Because stage III-IV tumors involve surrounding tissue and have lymph node involvement, 5-year survival rates are 40% or less. The survival rate of patients with tumors in the oral cavity has shown a statistically significant increase, whereas the 5-year survival rate for patients with cancer of the larynx has not shown statistically significant improvement during the past 25 years.

27. Describe the management of xerostomia.

- Thin the saliva with sodium bicarbonate.
- Pilocarpine is usually prescribed at the start of radiation therapy to stimulate salivary glands.
- Promote frequent hydration (carry a water bottle).
- Use artificial saliva products or oral lubricants (e.g., Numoisyn™ [liquid or lozenges])

28. How are skin problems managed?

- Protect patient's skin from irritation (e.g., abrasion from folds of shirt [neck or collar] or tracheostomy tube).
- Dry desquamation (flaky or itchy skin) is treated with meticulous skin care, topical cream as prescribed by the radiation therapist, and diphenhydramine as needed.
- Wet desquamation (oozing or dripping wound) is treated with moist dressings, which promote healing. Hydrogel dressings may not need changing for up to 12 hours.

29. What strategies are appropriate for tube feeding problems?

- Monitor weight and tolerance.
- A nasogastric tube should be inserted only by a surgical team member familiar with the patient's altered anatomy.
- Percutaneous endoscopic gastrostomy (PEG) tube placement for feeding during radiation therapy and chemotherapy and after surgery has replaced nasogastric tube feeding in many centers because of increased patient comfort and improved safety from aspiration.

 Key Points

- Ninety percent of patients with primary tumors of the oral cavity, pharynx, or larynx have a smoking history. Excessive alcohol intake is also a risk factor; it has a synergistic effect with tobacco use and further increases incidence.
- Primary tumors of the head and neck create functional and cosmetic problems if the malignancy is not adequately treated and controlled.
- Effective palliation is seldom achieved without cure of the primary tumor.
- The patient's nutritional status must be monitored to prevent weight loss, so that nutritional repair is supported through diagnostic workup and treatment.
- Early cancer diagnosis with minimal risk of nodal spread is better treated with surgery alone. Treatment is generally completed in one day, morbidity should be minimal, and the risk of xerostomia (hyposalivation) is avoided, along with the risk of dental caries and bone loss (osteoradionecrosis).

Internet Resources

Patient and Caregivers

Cancer Information Service provides booklets on head and neck, larynx, and skin cancer:
https://cissecure.nci.nih.gov/ncipubs/searchResults.asp?subject1=Oral+Cancers

American Cancer Society, All About Laryngeal and Hypopharyngeal Cancer:
http://www.cancer.org/docroot/CRI/CRI_2x.asp?sitearea=&dt=23

International Association of Laryngectomies:
http://www.larynxlink.com

Support for People with Oral and Head and Neck Cancer (SPOHNC):
http://www.spohnc.org

Let's Face It (LFI):
http://www.faceit.org

National Foundation for Facial Reconstruction:
http://www.nffr.org

Health Care Professional

National Comprehensive Cancer Network, Clinical Practice Guidelines in Oncology, Head
and Neck Cancers:
http://www.nccn.org/professionals/physician_gls/PDF/head-and-neck.pdf

American Cancer Society:
http://www.cancer.org

Oncology Nursing Society:
http://www.ons.org

National Cancer Institute Clinical Trials:
http://www.cancer.gov/clinicaltrials

Bibliography

Blom ED: Current status of voice restoration following total laryngectomy. *Oncology* 14(6):915-922, 2000.

Centers for Disease Control and Prevention: Tobacco use, access, and exposure to tobacco in media among middle and high school students—United States, 2004. *MMWR Morb Mortal Wkly Rep* 54(12):297-301, 2005. Available at: http://www.cdc.gov/mmwr/PDF/wk/mm5412.pdf. Accessed December 2005.

Cox J, Ang KK: *Radiation oncology: Rationale, techniques, results,* ed 8, St Louis, 2003, Elsevier Mosby.

Greene FL, Page DL, Fleming ID, et al, editors: *AJCC cancer staging manual,* ed 6, Head and Neck Sites, New York, 2002, Springer.

Harris LL: Head and neck malignancies. In Yarbro CH, Frogge MH, Goodman M, editors: *Cancer nursing Principles and practice,* ed 5, Boston, 2000, Jones and Bartlett.

Harris LL, Huntoon MB, editors: *Core curriculum for otorhinolaryngology and head-neck nursing,* ed 2, New Smyrna Beach, FL, 2007, Society of Otorhinolaryngology and Head-Neck Nurses.

Harrison LR, Sessions RB, Hong WK, editors: *Head and neck cancer: A multidisciplinary approach,* ed 2, Philadelphia, 2003, Lippincott Williams & Wilkins.

Jemal A, Siegel R, Ward E, et al: Cancer statistics, 2007. *CA Cancer J Clin* 57:43-66, 2007.

Jennings RL, Nelson, WR: Tumors of the head and neck. In Ritchie WP Jr, Steele G Jr, Dean RH, editors: *General surgery,* Philadelphia, 1995, JB Lippincott.

Lee KJ: *Essential otolaryngology,* ed 8, Columbus, OH, 2003, McGraw-Hill.

Myers EN, Suen J, Myers JN, et al, editors: *Cancer of the head and neck,* ed 4, Philadelphia, 2003, Elsevier Saunders.

Nelson WR, Jennings RL: Pre- and postoperative care. In Loré JM, Medina JE, editors: *An atlas of head and neck surgery,* ed 4, Philadelphia, 2005, Elsevier Saunders.

Shah JP, Patel SG: *Head and neck surgery and oncology,* ed 3, Edinburgh, 2004, Elsevier Mosby.

Tsottles ND, Reedy AM: Head and neck cancer. In Shelton BK, Ziegfield CR, Olsen MM, editors: *Manual of cancer nursing,* Philadelphia, 2004, Lippincott Williams & Wilkins.

Lung Cancer

Tina Russell and Karen Kelly

Quick Facts

Incidence	213,380 newly diagnosed cases estimated in 2007 (114,760 in men; 98,620 in women)
Mortality	160,390 deaths estimated in 2007
Risk factors	Cigarette smoking and tobacco use
	Exposure to environmental tobacco smoke, radon gas, asbestos, occupational respiratory carcinogens
Genetics	Genetic predisposition
Histopathology	Non–small cell lung cancers (NSCLC): 84%
	Adenocarcinoma (most common): 30%-50% (includes bronchoalveolar)
	Squamous cell (epidermoid): 30%
	Large cell lung cancers: 10%-15%
	Small cell lung cancers (SCLC): 16%

Symptoms	Cough, hemoptysis
	Dyspnea, wheezing
	Hoarseness
	Weight loss, anorexia
	Recurring pneumonia or bronchitis
	Chest, shoulder, arm, or back pain
Diagnosis and evaluation	History and physical examination (supraclavicular lymph node exam)
	Chest x-ray (PA and lateral)
	Biopsy (bronchoscopy, transthoracic fine-needle aspiration, mediastinoscopy, thoracoscopy, thoracotomy)
	Computed tomography (CT) of chest and abdomen
	Whole body CT/PET scan
	Brain MRI

Staging and Stage Grouping

Stage	Description
Tumor, node, metastasis (TNM)	
Primary tumor (T)	
TX	Primary tumor cannot be assessed, or tumor proven by the presence of malignant cells in sputum or bronchial washings, but not visualized by imaging or bronchoscopy
T1	Tumor ≤ 3 cm in greatest dimension, surrounded by lung or visceral pleura, without bronchoscopic evidence of invasion more proximal than the lobar bronchus
T2	Tumor with any of the following features of size or extent: > 3 cm in greatest dimension; involves main bronchus, 2 cm or more distal to carina; invades visceral pleura; associated with atelectasis or obstructive pneumonitis that extends to the hilar region but does not involve the entire lung

Used with permission of the American Joint Committee on Cancer (AJCC), Chicago, Illinois. The original source for this material is the AJCC Cancer Staging Handbook, Sixth Edition (2002) published by Springer New York, www.sprinfleronline.com.

Quick Facts—cont'd

Stage	Description
T3	Tumor of any size that directly invades any of the following: chest wall (including superior sulcus tumors), diaphragm, mediastinal pleura, parietal pericardium; tumor in main bronchus < 2 cm distal to the carina but without involvement of carina; associated atelectasis or obstructive pneumonitis of entire lung
T4	Tumor of any size that invades any of the following: mediastinum, heart, great vessels, trachea, esophagus, vertebral body, carina; separate tumor nodules in same lobe; tumor with a malignant pleural effusion; satellite tumor nodules within primary tumor of the lung

Regional lymph nodes (N)

NX	Regional lymph nodes cannot be assessed
N0	No regional lymph node metastasis
N1	Metastasis to ipsilateral peribronchial and/or ipsilateral hilar lymph nodes, and intrapulmonary nodes, including involvement by direct extension of primary tumor
N2	Metastasis to ipsilateral mediastinal and/or subcarinal lymph node(s)
N3	Metastasis to contralateral mediastinal, contralateral hilar, ipsilateral or contralateral scalene, or supraclavicular lymph node(s)

Distant metastasis (M)

MX	Distant metastasis cannot be assessed
M0	No distant metastasis
M1	Distant metastasis present; tumor nodules in more than 1 lobe (common sites of metastasis include brain, liver, bone, adrenal gland)

Stage	Primary Tumor	Regional Lymph nodes	Distant Metastasis
NSCLC			
IA	T1	N0	M0
IB	T2	N0	M0
IIA	T1	N1	M0
IIB	T2	N1	M0
	T3	N0	M0
IIIA	T3	N1	M0
	T1-3	N2	M0
IIIB	Any T4	Any N3	M0
IV	Any T	Any N	M1 (distant metastasis present)
SCLC			
Limited	Tumor confined to one hemithorax and regional lymph nodes		
Extensive	Tumor that has spread beyond the boundaries of limited disease; malignant pleural effusion		

Used with permission of the American Joint Committee on Cancer (AJCC), Chicago, Illinois. The original source for this material is the AJCC Cancer Staging Handbook, Sixth Edition (2002) published by Springer New York, www.sprinfleronline.com.

1. How common is lung cancer?

Lung cancer is the second most common cancer in men and women, closely following breast cancer in women and prostate cancer in men. The median age of diagnosis is 70 years. The marked increase in lung cancer in women began in the late 1960s, but more recently, the rate is decreasing.

2. What is the 5-year survival rate?

Unfortunately, lung cancer is the leading cause of death in both men and women; only 14% of patients with lung cancer live more than 5 years after diagnosis.

5-year survival rates	
Stage IA-IIB	57%-67%
Stage IIIA	13%-25%
Stage IIIB	5%
Stage IV	1%

3. What role does cigarette smoking play in the development of lung cancer?

Cigarette smoking is the chief preventable cause of lung cancer worldwide. Death rates from cancer would decrease by approximately 25% if people stopped or never started smoking. About 30% of all cancer deaths and 85% of all lung cancer deaths are directly attributable to smoking. The rate for developing lung cancer in nonsmokers ranges from 12 to 15 people per 100,000 population. For people who smoke less than 1 pack per day, the risk is 10 times greater than for nonsmokers; for those who smoke more than 1 pack per day, the risk is 21 times greater than for nonsmokers.

Tobacco smoke is considered a group A (known human) carcinogen and is both an initiator and promoter of carcinogenesis. Although a causal link has been established between smoking cigarettes and lung cancer, only 10% to 13% of people who smoke eventually develop lung cancer. The risk for developing lung cancer increases with the number of cigarettes smoked per day and the number of years of smoking. A risk model (Bach model) to determine an adult's risk for getting lung cancer has been developed and is based on age (50 to 75 years), the number of cigarettes smoked, and smoking status. It is available at: http://www.mskcc.org/mskcc/html/12463.cfm.

4. How has the pattern of tobacco use changed over the past 15 years?

Although the percentage of Americans who smoke has decreased (approximately 30% of the adult population smoked in 1985, including 10% to 15% of physicians and 20% to 30% of nurses), about 20% of men and 22% of women were smokers in the year 2000. In general, women have a shorter smoking history than men at diagnosis of lung cancer, but may be more vulnerable to smoking-related risks than men. However, lung cancer mortality rates remain 23 times higher for men who continue to smoke versus men who quit smoking; whereas for women mortality rates are 13 times higher than lifetime nonsmokers. The marked increase in tobacco use by teenagers is a serious health care concern, because the risk of developing lung cancer is higher for people who begin to smoke before age 15 years than for people who begin to smoke after age 25 years.

5. When do the benefits of smoking cessation become apparent?

The lung cancer risk for a one pack per day smoker (who has ceased smoking) compared to a nonsmoker with a risk of 1 is:

- 20 times at 3 to 5 years after quitting
- 11 times at 6 to 10 years after quitting
- 4.1 times at 10 to 15 years after quitting
- 4.0 times at more than 15 years after quitting

Former smokers will always have a greater risk for lung cancer than "never smokers" (lifelong nonsmokers). Former smokers constitute about 50% of patients diagnosed with lung cancer. Lifelong abstinence from smoking is the key to eradicating this disease.

6. Does passive smoke play a role in the development of lung cancer?

Passive smoking or environmental tobacco smoke (ETS) is the involuntary exposure of nonsmokers to tobacco smoke. ETS is believed to be qualitatively similar to smoke inhaled by smokers and has been labeled by the Environmental Protection Agency as a group A carcinogen (known to cause cancer in humans). Although significantly fewer cases of lung cancer have been directly attributed to ETS than to smoking, 20% of all lung cancers and 3,000 lung cancer deaths per year are estimated to be related to ETS exposure. This number may well increase when the amount of smoke exposure in ETS can be measured.

7. What are the symptoms of lung cancer?

The **most common** symptoms of lung cancer include cough, hemoptysis, dyspnea, wheezing, and pain (chest, shoulder, arm or back). **Systemic** symptoms include anorexia, weight loss, fatigue, and paraneoplastic syndromes, such as syndrome of inappropriate secretion of antidiuretic hormone (SIADH), Cushing's syndrome, and hypercalcemia. Other symptoms include facial swelling (from superior vena cava syndrome), headache or seizures (from brain metastases), pleural effusions, bone pain, recurrent bronchitis, and hoarseness (due to tumor impinging on the laryngeal nerve). Pneumonia that is unresolved after 2 months of treatment should be investigated as a symptom of lung cancer. Yet at time of diagnosis, 10% of patients are asymptomatic.

8. How is lung cancer diagnosed and staged?

Adults with a mass on a chest x-ray have lung cancer until proven otherwise. A biopsy of the mass is required by either bronchoscopy with washings, brushings, and biopsies; transthoracic fine-needle aspirations; or core biopsies. Additional diagnostic measures include lymph node biopsy, mediastinoscopy, thoracoscopy, and thoracotomy. Once the diagnosis is made, staging is performed. Patients should have a CT/PET fusion or a PET scan if possible. If these studies are not available, a CT of the chest with images through the upper abdomen including the adrenal glands is the minimal requirement. Brain MRI scans are very sensitive for detecting small metastatic lesions and are usually done only if clinically indicated. However, their use is increasing, particularly if surgery is planned.

9. What are the differences among the types of lung cancer?

Lung cancer is divided into two histologic classes: non–small cell lung cancer (NSCLC) and small cell lung cancer (SCLC).

- NSCLC accounts for approximately 84% of all lung cancers and has three major subtypes:
  - Adenocarcinomas (including bronchoalveolar) are the most common type of lung cancer and are found more frequently in women and younger people.
  - Squamous cell lung cancer usually arises centrally, grows more slowly, and tends to remain localized.
  - Large cell lung cancers are associated with a poor prognosis.
- SCLC or oat cell carcinoma accounts for the remaining 16% of lung cancers. Incidence of SCLC is strongly correlated with smoking habits. SCLC multiplies rapidly and is generally a systemic disease at diagnosis. More than 50% of patients have extensive (widespread) disease at diagnosis; approximately 25% have regional involvement, and less than 10% have only local disease at diagnosis. SCLC metastasizes early and is associated with a poor prognosis.

10. What are the most significant prognostic indicators for patients with lung cancer?

For both SCLC and NSCLC, the single most common prognostic indicator for overall survival and response to treatment is weight loss. Patients who have lost more than

5% of total body weight within the previous 6 months have a worse prognosis than patients who have not lost weight. Other indicators include tumor stage, tumor bulk, presence and site(s) of metastases, gender (women usually fare better than men), and performance status (ambulatory patients have a longer survival rate than nonambulatory patients). In addition, increased serum levels of lactate dehydrogenase (LDH) or alkaline phosphatase and a decreased level of serum sodium are associated with a poorer prognosis in patients with SCLC.

11. How is NSCLC treated?

- Surgery is the mainstay for NSCLC treatment. However, only 20% to 25% of patients have localized disease that is amenable to surgery. It is the only modality that offers a chance for cure, and it is used to treat patients with stage I-III disease deemed to be resectable. The treatment of choice is lobectomy, video-assisted thoracoscopic surgery (VATS), or rarely pneumonectomy.
- Radiation therapy (RT) is recommended for patients with stage I and stage II disease who are not surgical candidates or for patients who refuse surgery.
- A major advance in the treatment of localized lung cancer was recently demonstrated in five randomized clinical trials that compared the efficacy of adjuvant chemotherapy versus observation only. The results showed a statistically significant reduction in the 5-year mortality rate of 5% to 15% in patients who received chemotherapy. Adjuvant chemotherapy is now the standard of care after definitive resection. However, the likelihood of cure is much lower than with surgery combined with RT.

12. How are patients with Stage III NSCLC treated?

Patients with stage III NSCLC pose a treatment challenge. The standard treatment for all patients with stage IIIA disease is concurrent chemotherapy and radiotherapy. However, selected patients with minimal N2 disease (microscopic lymph node involvement) deemed eligible for a lobectomy (not a pneumonectomy) by the thoracic surgeon may benefit from a neoadjuvant approach of chemotherapy or chemoradiotherapy followed by surgery. Patients with stage IIIB disease are treated with concurrent chemotherapy and radiotherapy. Patients with T4 N0 disease may also be candidates for the neoadjuvant approach with chemoradiotherapy followed by surgery. Patients with stage III disease should be encouraged to participate in the international trial of prophylactic brain radiation because recent studies have demonstrated an isolated brain recurrence rate at 18%.

13. Should chemotherapy be used in patients with stage IV NSCLC?

Chemotherapy (3-6 cycles) is the treatment of choice for patients with stage IV disease. For these patients, chemotherapy has been shown to increase survival, improve quality of life, decrease symptoms, and be more cost-effective than the best supportive care alone. Patients with nonsquamous cell cancer, no brain metastases, and no evidence of hemoptysis are eligible to receive a triple drug combination of paclitaxel, carboplatin and bevacizumab (Avastin). Results from a recent randomized controlled clinical trial showed that patients who received this regimen had a survival advantage over patients who received the standard regimen of paclitaxel plus carboplatin. Patients who relapse after first line therapy should be considered for second line therapy. The FDA has three approved agents in this setting: docetaxel, pemetrexed, and erlotinib (Tarceva). Erlotinib, which is an oral epidermal growth factor receptor (EGFR) tyrosine kinase inhibitor, is also approved in third line settings. Treatment with these new agents has extended patient survival periods.

14. How is SCLC treated?

SCLC is considered to be a systemic disease at time of diagnosis; thus surgical resection alone is not appropriate. Chemotherapy is the mainstay of treatment, which includes either cisplatin or carboplatin plus etoposide. Another option would be irinotecan and cisplatin. Topotecan has been used to treat patients who have relapsed. Patients with limited stage disease usually receive 4 cycles of cisplatin plus etoposide, with concurrent radiation starting at cycle 1 or 2 of chemotherapy. The average survival for patients with SCLC is 9 to 11 months; approximately 40% of patients with limited stage disease survive 2 years. Patients who continue to smoke during their concurrent treatment have decreased survival due to their inability to tolerate treatment.

15. What is the role of radiation therapy in the treatment of lung cancer?

- RT in doses of 61 to 66 Gy is used with the intent to cure (in combination with other treatment modalities) some patients with NSCLC who are not candidates for surgery. RT is also used to shrink the primary tumor and regional lymph nodes.
- External beam radiation therapy (30 Gy in 10 fractions or less) has been commonly used to palliate symptoms of cough, dyspnea, hemoptysis, and postobstructive pneumonia due to bronchial obstruction, with effectiveness ranging from 50% to 90%.
- Three-dimensional conformal radiation therapy, which pinpoints the tumor in three rather than the usual two dimensions, is considered standard.
- Radiostereotactic radiation (RSR or gamma knife) is frequently used to treat 1 to 3 brain metastases.
- Stereotactic body radiation therapy (SBRT) is being evaluated in patients with stage I inoperable NSCLC and liver metastasis. The development of body frames in combination with stereotactic localization of the tumor allows ultrahigh dose RT to be delivered to discrete tumor nodules in a hypofractionated regimen, typically 1 to 5 treatments, while minimizing the damage to nontumor tissues.

16. What paraneoplastic syndromes are commonly associated with lung cancer?

SIADH, Cushing's syndrome (ectopic production of adrenocorticotropic hormone [ACTH]), peripheral neuropathies, Eaton-Lambert syndrome (myasthenia-like transverse myelitis, polymyositis, and weakness), and carcinoid syndrome are commonly associated with SCLC. Squamous cell lung cancer is associated with hypercalcemia and peripheral neuropathies, whereas adenocarcinoma of the lung is associated with hypercoagulable states and hypertrophic pulmonary osteoarthropathy. Hypercalcemia (rare), hypertrophic pulmonary osteoarthropathy, and peripheral neuropathies are also seen in patients with large cell lung cancers.

17. What oncologic emergencies most commonly occur with lung cancer?

The most common oncologic emergencies seen in patients with lung cancer are superior vena cava syndrome (SVCS) and airway obstruction. Of all instances of SVCS, 75% are related to obstruction by either squamous cell or small cell lung cancers. Partial or complete airway obstruction is seen in 53% of patients with squamous cell carcinoma, 38% with SCLC, and 33% with large cell carcinoma. In 70% of all patients with lung cancer, endobrachial lesions are found during thoracotomy. Pericardial effusions, neoplastic cardiac tamponade (direct extension into the pericardium), and spinal cord compression may occur, and metabolic emergencies, including hypercalcemia and hyponatremia (due to SIADH), are not uncommon.

18. What is Pancoast tumor syndrome?

Named after Henry Pancoast (who described the tumor that bears his name) in 1924, it is a lung tumor usually found after a lengthy investigation associated with severe shoulder and arm pain. Ipsilateral Horner's syndrome, which is characterized by a small pupil, ptosis of the eyelid, and lack of facial sweating, may also may be present. The tumor may cause rib destruction and involve spinal nerve roots (C8 or T1). It is located near the brachial plexus, major thoracic vessels, and vertebral bodies. The staging workup is the same as any other patient with lung cancer. Patients without mediastinal disease (stages I-IIIA) are treated with combined modality chemotherapy plus RT followed by surgery. Patients with mediastinal involvement (stages IIIA/B) are treated with definitive chemotherapy and radiation therapy. Neuropathic pain medications are the mainstay of symptomatic treatment for shoulder and arm pain.

19. What new treatments are in development for lung cancer?

The integration of molecularly targeted therapies into the treatment of all stages of lung cancer is ongoing with the two agents that have shown a survival advantage, bevacizumab (Avastin) and erlotinib (Tarceva). Meanwhile, a host of novel targeted agents are being evaluated alone, with cytotoxic agents, and in combination with bevacizumab and erlotinib.

Tailored therapy based on tumor profiling and/or clinical characteristic is emerging. For example, a patient whose tumor displays EGFR mutations or fluorescence in situ hybridization (FISH) amplification are highly responsive to EGFR inhibitors. Never smokers have the longest survival times when treated with these agents. Clinical trials selecting patients based on these criteria have begun. Molecular profiling for response to cytotoxic chemotherapy is also under study.

20. How does mesothelioma differ from lung cancer?

Mesothelioma, a rare neoplasm commonly involving the pleura or peritoneum, is directly linked to asbestos exposure; people with occupational exposure to asbestos (e.g., ship builders, pipe fitters, brake repairers, insulation installers) have a 6- to 7-fold greater risk of death from any cancer than an unexposed population. Short-term exposure (< 1 month) carries a continued risk for the development of cancer 25 years later. More than 8 million people are believed to be at risk for developing mesothelioma, and it is estimated that 4720 new cases will be diagnosed in 2007 in the United States. The most common symptom of mesothelioma is pleural effusion. The three subtypes are epithelial, fibrosarcomatous, and mixed. Disease spreads locally in the mediastinum and chest wall through direct tumor extension. Mesotheliomas rarely metastasize distally.

21. Describe the current treatment for mesothelioma.

Mesothelioma is unresponsive to most cytotoxic agents. Administration of single agent cisplatin or doxorubicin (Adriamycin) was commonly used until recently, when a randomized phase III trial of pemetrexed plus cisplatin produced a median survival of 12 months compared to 9 months for cisplatin alone. Other newer cytotoxic agents that are used include paclitaxel and gemcitabine. In the rare patient (less than 5%) who does not have mediastinal lymph node involvement or diaphragm invasion, extrapleural pneumonectomy (EPP) should be considered. However, patients who are candidates for an EPP should be told that surgery is only one part of the treatment. These patients should have chemotherapy (neoadjuvant, adjuvant, or both) and hemithoracic radiation therapy; their survival is 20 to 24 months.

22. Why should smokers with lung cancer quit smoking?

According to Sarna (1998), reasons for smokers with lung cancer to quit smoking include:

- Decreasing symptoms, such as cough and shortness of breath
- Decreasing the risk of recurrence or a second primary lung tumor and the risk of worsening tobacco-related diseases
- Decreasing the risk of household members developing lung cancer or heart disease related to inhaling secondhand smoke
- Increasing feelings of control and overall well-being
- Being a role model for friends and family

 Key Points

- Lung cancer is the leading cause of death among men and women.
- Incidence of lung cancer is strongly linked to smoking.
- Cough is one of the most common symptoms of disease.
- Lung cancer classification is based on histopathology: NSCLC and SCLC.
- Staging, weight loss, and performance status are the most common prognostic indicators.
- Treatment is based on histopathology, stage, and symptoms.

 Internet Resources

American Cancer Society (ACS):
   http://www.cancer.org
American Lung Association:
   http://www.lungusa.org
American Society of Clinical Oncology (ASCO):
   http://www.asco.org
Agency for Healthcare Research and Quality (AHRQ):
   http://www.ahrq.gov
Association of Cancer Online Resources (ACOR):
   http://www.acor.org
Lung Cancer:
   http://www.lungcancer.org
Lung Cancer Alliance:
   http://www.alcase.org
National Cancer Institute (NCI):
   http://www.cancer.gov
National Lung Cancer Partnership:
   http://www.nationallungcancerpartnership.org/main.cfm

Acknowledgment

The authors wish to acknowledge the previous work of Linda Krebs, RN, PhD, FAAN, AOCN, for her contribution to the Lung Cancer chapter published in the first and second editions of *Oncology Nursing Secrets*.

Bibliography

Bressler TR: Small cell lung cancer. In Miaskowski C, Buchsel P, editors: *Oncology nursing assessment and clinical care,* St Louis, 2000, Mosby.

Greene FL, Page DL, Fleming ID, et al, editors: AJCC *cancer staging manual,* ed 6, New York, 2002, Springer.

Hoffman PC, Mauer AM, Vokes EE: Lung cancer. *Lancet* 355:479-485, 2000.

Iwamoto R: Lung cancer. In Nevidjon BM, Sowers KW, editors: *A nurse's guide to cancer care.* Philadelphia, 2000, Lippincott.

Jemal A, Siegel R, Ward E, et al: Cancer statistics, 2007. *CA Cancer J Clin* 57:43-66, 2007.

Kemp CS: Lung cancers. In Yarbro CH, Frogge MH, Goodman M, et al, editors: *Cancer nursing: Principles and practice,* ed 6, Boston, 2005, Jones & Bartlett.

Mountain, CF: Revisions in the international system for staging lung cancer. *Chest* 111:1710-1717, 1997.

Sandler AB, Gray R, Brahmer J, et al: Randomized phase II/III Trial of paclitaxel plus carboplatin in patients with advanced non-squamous non-small cell lung cancer: An Eastern Cooperative Oncology Group Trial-E4599. *Proc Am Soc Clin Oncol* 23:2s, abstract LBA4, 2005.

Sarna L: Smoking cessation after the diagnosis of lung cancer. *Develop Support Care* 2:45-49, 1998.

Van Cleave JH: Nursing perspectives on the diagnosis and management of stage III NSCLC. *Clin Oncol Updates Oncol Nurse* 1(3):1A-6A, 2000.

Visbal AL, Leighl NB, Feld R, et al: Adjuvant chemotherapy for early-stage non-small cell lung cancer. *Chest* 128(4):2933-2943, 2005.

Vogelzang NJ: Multimodality therapy in mesothelioma: Role of chemotherapy. *Thorac Surg Clin* 14:531-542, 2004.

White EJ: Lung cancer. In Varrichio C, editor: *A cancer source book for nurses,* ed 8, Atlanta, 2004, American Cancer Society.

Malignant Melanoma

Maude Becker and Rene Gonzalez

Quick Facts

Incidence	59,940 newly diagnosed estimated cases in 2007 (33,910 in men; 26,030 in women)
Mortality	8110 deaths estimated in 2007
Risk factors	Large number of moles
	Family history of melanoma
	History of severe sunburns in childhood and adolescence
	Light skin type, blue or green eyes, blond or red hair
	Clinically atypical moles, dysplastic nevus syndrome
	History of acute and intermittent exposure to sun or ultraviolet radiation

Genetics	Genetic predisposition
Histopathology	Superficial spreading is the most common, followed by nodular melanomas
	Other forms: acral lentiginous melanoma, lentigo maligna melanoma, desmoplastic melanoma, and uveal melanoma (rare)
Symptoms	Mole that changes in size, elevation, color, surface, surroundings, and sensation
Diagnosis and evaluation	History and physical examination
	Biopsy
	Chemistry panel
	Chest x-ray (PA and lateral)

Microstaging

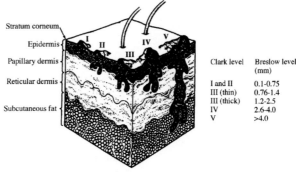

Clark level	Breslow level (mm)
I and II	0.1-0.75
III (thin)	0.76-1.4
III (thick)	1.2-2.5
IV	2.6-4.0
V	>4.0

Both level of invasion and maximal thickness determine the T (primary tumor) classification: **Breslow's thickness** = thickness of tumor tissue; **Clark's level** = anatomic level of invasion. *(From Gronewald S, Frogge M, Goodman M, Yarbo C: Comprehensive cancer nursing review, ed 2, Research Triangle Park, NC, 1995, Glaxo Wellcome. By permission.)*

Continued

Quick Facts—cont'd

Computed tomography (CT) of abdomen and pelvis Brain MRI PET/CT	Sentinel lymph node biopsy should be considered before wide excision in patients with tumors > 1 mm

Staging and Stage Grouping

Stage	Description

Tumor, node, metastasis (TNM)
Primary tumor (T)

TX	Primary tumor cannot be assessed
T0	No evidence of primary tumor
Tis	Melanoma in situ
T1	≤1.0 mm
T2	1.01-2.0 mm
T3	2.01-4.0 mm
T4	> 4.0 mm

a. without ulceration

b. with ulceration

Regional lymph nodes (N)

NX	Regional lymph nodes cannot be assessed
N0	No regional lymph node metastasis

N1	1 lymph node
	   a. microscopic
	   b. macroscopic

N2	2-3 lymph nodes
	   a. microscopic
	   b. macroscopic
	   c. satellite or in-transit metastasis without nodal metastasis

N3	4 or more nodes, matted lymph nodes, combination of in-transit metastasis/satellite, or ulcerated melanoma and lymph node(s)

Distant metastasis (M)

MX	Distant metastasis cannot be assessed
M0	No distant metastasis
M1	Distant skin, subcutaneous, or lymph nodes with normal lactate dehydrogenase (LDH)
M2	Lung metastases with normal LDH
M3	All other visceral or any distant metastases with elevated LDH

Stage	Primary Tumor	Regional Lymph Nodes	Distant Metastasis
0	Melanoma in situ		
IA	T1a	N0	M0
IB	T1b, T2a	N0	M0
IIA	T2b, T3a	N0	M0
IIB	T3b, T4a	N0	M0

Quick Facts—cont'd

Stage	Primary Tumor	Regional Lymph Nodes	Distant Metastasis
IIC	T4b	N0	M0
IIIA	Any T	N1a	M0
IIIB	Any T	N1b, N2a	M0
IIIC	Any T	N2b, N3	M0
IV	Any T	Any N	M1-3

Used with permission of the American Joint Committee on Cancer (AJCC), Chicago, Illinois. The original source for this material is the AJCC Cancer Staging Handbook, Sixth Edition (2002) published by Springer New York, www.sprinfleronline.com.

1. What is melanoma and how often does it occur?

Melanoma is a malignant tumor originating from melanocytes, the pigment (melanin)-producing cells in the skin. Melanocytes are found throughout the skin but are most common in the basal layers of the epidermis. Melanoma may arise from a preexisting nevus or occur spontaneously.

The lifetime risk of developing melanoma is increasing: 1991, 1 in 105; 2000, 1 in 75. It is a tumor that strikes fear because of its unpredictable behavior. For example, a melanoma can be completely excised, recur years later in another site, and cause rapid progression and death in less than 1 year.

2. What is dysplastic nevus syndrome?

A dysplastic nevus is a distinct melanocytic lesion that may be a precursor to melanoma. People with dysplastic nevus syndrome (DNS) develop many of these lesions. They may occur sporadically or be associated with a personal or family history of melanoma (familial DNS). Regardless of family history, persons with DNS have a higher risk of developing melanoma. Clinically, dysplastic nevi tend to be larger than commonly acquired nevi, often measuring greater than 5 mm. The lesions may have fuzzy or irregular borders, and the pigmentation pattern is often irregular. Another distinctive feature is the "fried-egg" appearance, created when the central nevus component is one color and the peripheral component is another shade. Patients often have dozens or even hundreds of lesions.

3. Where do melanomas commonly occur?

Melanomas can be located anywhere on the body but occur most commonly on the lower extremities in women and on the trunk in men, especially on the back.

4. What type of biopsy should be done if melanoma is suspected?

Because tumor thickness is the most important factor in determining prognosis and treatment, the biopsy should be excisional through the underlying fat, using a punch-type biopsy when possible. After the diagnosis is established, lesions less than 1 mm thick should be excised with a 1-cm margin, whereas primary lesions that are 1 to 4 mm thick require a 2-cm margin. Studies have shown that large and disfiguring surgical excisions are unnecessary because they do not improve outcome or decrease local recurrence rates.

5. What are the warning signs of malignant melanoma?

The warning signs of malignant melanoma can be summarized as the **ABCDs**:
Asymmetry in shape, color, or appearance of mole; **a**ppearance of new pigmented lesion
Borders that are notched, irregular in shape, or both; **b**leeding moles
Color of mole is variable or contains blue, gray, white, pink, or red
Diameter greater than 6 mm in any direction

6. What preventive measures should be taken to reduce the risk of developing melanoma?

- Avoid peak times of intense ultraviolet (UV) radiation exposure from the sun (10 AM to 4 PM).
- Use sunscreen with a sun protection factor (SPF) of at least 15; reapply if swimming, perspiring, or outdoors longer than 2 hours.
- Apply 1 ounce of sunscreen evenly over the body at least 30 minutes before sun exposure.
- Wear protective clothing while outdoors.
- Do not use artificial sun tanning lamps.
- Do regular self-examinations of skin, and evaluate suspicious lesions using the ABCDs.

7. What is the relationship between melanoma and sunlight?

Sunlight is composed of UV radiation that damages the DNA of skin cells. This damage may cause mutations that lead to the development of all forms of skin cancer, including melanoma. The same process occurs with the use of tanning booths. There is no such thing as a safe tan. The damaging effects of sunlight may occur many years before tumors appear; therefore, sun protection during childhood and youth is particularly important.

8. What does SPF mean?

Minimal erythematous dose (MED) is the minimal dose of UV that causes erythema. SPF is the relative protection offered by a sunscreen versus no sunscreen protection. For example, a person who can be exposed to the sun for only 20 minutes without developing erythema can apply sunscreen with an SPF of 8 and stay outside for 160 (20×8) minutes without burning. More sun protection is offered by sunscreens with higher SPF numbers. A sunscreen with a SPF of 15 offers complete protection in most cases; it is recommended that patients use sunscreen with an SPF of at least 15 for protecting skin after chemotherapy and radiation therapy.

9. What type of sunscreen is recommended?

Newer generations of sunscreens provide UVA and UVB protection. When choosing a sunscreen, check the label to see if it contains both UVA and UVB protection. The SPF refers only to UVB coverage. Research suggests that brief intense exposure to UVA is a risk factor for the development of melanoma.

10. What role do sentinel lymph node mapping and biopsy play in melanoma?

Sentinel lymph node mapping and biopsy have evolved as a means of accurately staging the regional lymph nodes. The draining lymphatic vessels from a high-risk primary melanoma (i.e., T1b or greater) are identified by injecting a vital blue dye, a radioisotope, or both. The first ("sentinel") lymph node that takes up the dye is surgically removed and analyzed histologically. If this node is not involved with melanoma, there is a less than 5% chance that any lymph node in that drainage site is pathologically involved. Sentinel lymph node biopsy is the current standard of care at many centers for surgical staging of melanoma when there is no clinical evidence of regional or distant metastases. Likewise, patients at high risk for recurrence (i.e., positive sentinel lymph node) can be identified and targeted for aggressive systemic therapy.

11. Is there a benefit to prophylactic lymph node dissection?

An elective or prophylactic lymph node dissection is generally performed in patients with deep primary tumors, under the assumption that they have a higher risk of regional node involvement, and that early surgical treatment of the regional nodal basin will

Malignant melanoma: Histologic subtypes

Type (%)	Demographics/ male:female ratio	Color and characteristics	Growth	Location
Superficial spreading (70%-75%)	5th decade 1:1	Tan, brown, flat, crusty, irregular borders; red, blue, ulcerated lesion—vertical phase	Radial growth (1-5 years); vertical rapid growth (color change)	Women: legs Men: upper back
Nodular (10-15%)	5th decade 2:1	Blue-black, blue-gray, red-blue Raised, possible bleeding	No radial growth All vertical growth (< 1 year) Aggressive	Head, neck, trunk
Acral lentiginous (5-10%)	Occurs equally in all races	Tan, brown, black	Radial growth (months-years)	Palms, soles, subungual
Lentigo maligna (5%) (best prognosis of all melanomas)	7th decade 1:3	Tan, brown; mottled irregular borders	Slow radial growth (decades)	Head, neck, cheek, temple

improve prognosis. Although this approach seems intuitively reasonable, two large randomized studies failed to demonstrate benefit from this treatment; thus its use remains controversial. Most experts do not recommend prophylactic lymph node dissection. In contrast, a therapeutic lymph node dissection is one in which the involved lymph nodes are removed. This technique remains a cornerstone of treatment for patients with stage III melanoma.

12. What are the histologic subtypes of melanoma?

Malignant melanoma has four major subtypes, each with unique clinical features. (Refer to table on p. 319).

13. What are the most common sites of metastases?

Malignant melanoma can metastasize to most body organs. The most frequent sites for metastases are the regional lymph nodes, followed by the lungs. Other sites include skin, subcutaneous tissue, liver, brain, and bone.

14. What is the prognosis of a patient who develops brain metastases?

Melanoma ranks with small cell lung cancer as the most common tumor that metastasizes to the brain. Headaches, seizures, and neurologic deficits are the most common symptoms. The median survival once a patient develops brain metastases is less than 6 months.

15. Does melanoma always occur on the skin?

No. Melanoma may originate in any area of the body that contains pigment cells. Unusual variants of melanoma include ocular melanoma (originating in the pigment cells of the retina or iris); conjunctival melanoma; and mucosal melanomas, such as nasopharyngeal, oral, vulvar, and anorectal melanomas. At diagnosis, 1% to 12% of patients have metastatic disease originating from an unknown primary site.

16. Where do ocular melanomas commonly spread?

Ocular melanomas usually spread to the liver.

17. How is melanoma usually treated?

Current treatment is based on stage of disease.
  Stage IA: Surgical excision of primary tumor
  Stages IB-II: Consider sentinel lymph node (SLN) biopsy before wide excision
  Stage III: Surgical excision of primary tumor with radical lymphadenectomy, possibly with interferon therapy
  Stage IV: No standard treatment; all patients encouraged to participate in clinical trials

18. What is the role of interferon in the treatment of melanoma?

Alpha interferon is currently indicated for postsurgical adjuvant therapy in patients with tumors greater than 4 mm thick and after therapeutic lymph node dissection. Interferon is also commonly used alone or in combination for treatment of metastatic disease. As a single agent, it produces a 15–20% response rate. Interferon is being evaluated for treatment of earlier-stage melanoma. The Food and Drug Administration (FDA) has approved a regimen of high-dose interferon for 1 year, based on a large randomized study that showed improved disease-free and overall survival in treated patients. However, side effects, such as fatigue, were substantial.

19. What is the role of chemotherapy in treatment of melanoma?

Chemotherapy has generally been considered ineffective in the treatment of melanoma. Studies have shown no benefit in the adjuvant setting in patients at high risk for relapse.

The only FDA-approved chemotherapy agent for treating the advanced stages of melanoma is dacarbazine (DTIC), which in many parts of the country remains the standard treatment. The response rate to DTIC is not high, at 15% to 20% with a median duration of response of 5 to 6 months. Complete responses were observed in only 5% of 580 patients entered into phase III trials. Only 3% of patients who achieved a complete response remained disease-free at 6 years after treatment. Several multidrug regimens have been evaluated but have shown no benefit over DTIC in randomized trials.

20. What are the latest treatment options for melanoma?

High-dose bolus interleukin-2 (IL-2) was approved by the FDA for treating patients with stage IV melanoma, based on a small but definite proportion of patients who achieved durable complete responses. Newer modalities of diagnosis and treatment are currently under investigation, including: (1) sentinel node biopsy with molecular evaluation of lymph nodes, (2) stereotactic radiation with either a gamma knife or linear accelerator for brain metastases, (3) hyperthermic limb perfusion, and (4) chemoembolization for liver metastases. Several new systemic agents and regimens are in various stages of development, including combinations of biologic agents and chemotherapy, gene therapy, agents that inhibit angiogenesis, and melanoma vaccines.

21. Who is at risk for recurrent melanoma?

Patients who have had one melanoma are at greater risk for developing a second melanoma. The lifetime risk of developing a second primary tumor ranges from 3% to 6%. Patients who have multiple dysplastic nevi or a familial form have an even greater risk of developing multiple primary melanomas. Persons with familial melanoma account for approximately 10% of all patients with melanoma.

22. Is melanoma radioresistant?

Traditionally, melanoma has been described as radioresistant. However, an increasing number of clinical studies have questioned this concept. More recent studies have supported hypofractionated radiotherapy (larger doses over a shorter interval) as potentially beneficial in the treatment of melanoma. Stereotactic radiation may be effective in selected cases with CNS involvement.

23. What follow-up care should a patient have after a diagnosis of melanoma?

Lifetime follow-up is indicated because local recurrences and metastases are always possible. All follow-up visits should include a thorough skin and lymph node examination. The following schedule is recommended: for the first 3 years, every 3 to 4 months; for years 4 and 5, every 6 months; and annually thereafter.

24. What are the 10-year survival rates for the various stages of melanoma?

Stage*	10-year survival rate
I	85%
II	60%
III	20%
IV	< 5%

* According to the American Joint Committee on Cancer

Key Points

- There is no "safe" tan.
- Melanoma can be cured when it is diagnosed early.
- Sentinel node involvement is the best predictor of survival.
- Any suspicious lesion should be checked by a doctor.

Internet Resources

The Melanoma Research Foundation:
  http://www.melanoma.org
Medline Plus, Melanoma:
  http://www.nlm.nih.gov/medlineplus/melanoma.html
National Cancer Institute:
  http://www.cancer.gov
Skin Cancer Foundation, Melanoma:
  http://www.skincancer.org/melanoma/index.php
American Cancer Society:
  http://www.cancer.org

Bibliography

Atallah E, Flaherty L: Treatment of metastatic malignant melanoma. *Curr Treat Options Oncol* 6(3):185-193, 2005.

Atkins MB: Interleukin-2 in metastatic melanoma: What is the current role? *Cancer J Sci Am* 6(suppl 1):S8-S10, 2000.

Atkins MB, Kunkel L, Sznol M, et al: High-dose recombinant interleukin-2 therapy in patients with metastatic melanoma: Long-term survival update. *Cancer J Sci Am* 6(suppl 1):S11-S14, 2000.

Balch CM, Soong SJ, Atkins MB, et al: An evidence-based staging system for cutaneous melanoma. *CA Cancer J Clin* 54(3):131-149, 182-184, 2004.

Groenwald S, Frogge M, Goodman M, et al: *Comprehensive cancer nursing review,* ed 2, Research Triangle Park, NC, 1995, Glaxo Wellcome.

Hurley KE, Chapman PB: Helping melanoma patients decide whether to choose adjuvant high-dose interferon-alpha2b. *Oncologist* 10(9):739-742, 2005.

Jemal A, Siegel R, Ward E, et al: Cancer statistics, 2007. *CA Cancer J Clin* 57:43-66, 2007.

Kirkwood JM: Adjuvant interferon in the treatment of melanoma. *Br J Cancer* 82:1755-1756, 2000.

Li W, Stall A, Shivers SC, et al: Clinical relevance of molecular staging for melanoma: Comparison of RT-PCR and immunohistochemistry staining in sentinel lymph nodes of patients with melanoma. *Ann Surg* 231:795-803, 2000.

Reintgen D, Li W, Stall A, et al: Metastatic melanoma to regional lymph nodes. *In Vivo* 14:213-220, 2000.

Thompson JF, Uren RF, Scolyer RA, et al: Selective sentinel lymphadenectomy: Progress to date and prospects for the future. *Cancer Treat Res* 127:269-287, 2005.

Walsh P, Gibbs P, Gonzalez R: Newer strategies for effective evaluation of primary melanoma and treatment of stage III and IV disease. *J Am Acad Dermatol* 42:480-490, 2000.

Prostate Cancer

Thomas W. Flaig and Frances Crighton

Quick Facts

Incidence	218,890 newly diagnosed cases estimated in 2007	**Diagnosis and evaluation**	History and physical examination
Mortality	27,050 deaths estimated in 2007		Digital rectal examination
			Prostate-specific antigen
Risk factors	Increased risk with increasing age		Transrectal ultrasound (TRUS) guided biopsy
	African American		Core biopsy
	Family history		Pelvic CT
	Dietary fat		Bone scan
Genetics	Genetic predisposition		CBC, acid phosphatase level, blood chemistry
Histopathology	95% adenocarcinoma		

Gleason score

2-4	Well differentiated
5-7	Moderately differentiated
8-10	Poorly differentiated

Symptoms Early: none

Late: May be asymptomatic, urinary symptoms (frequency, dysuria, nocturia, hematuria, obstructive symptoms, slow urine stream, retention, hydronephrosis), pedal edema, painful defecation, bone pain, weight loss

Staging and Stage Grouping

Stage	Description
Tumor, node, metastasis (TNM) and American Urological Association (AUA) systems	
Primary tumor (T)	
TX	Primary tumor cannot be assessed
T0	No evidence of primary tumor
T1	Clinically inapparent tumor not palpable or visible by imaging
T1a	Tumor incidental histologic finding in 5% or less of tissue resected
T1b	Tumor incidental histologic finding in greater than 5% of tissue resected
T1c	Tumor identified by needle biopsy (e.g., because of elevated PSA)
T2	Tumor confined within prostate

Used with permission of the American Joint Committee on Cancer (AJCC), Chicago, Illinois. The original source for this material is the AJCC Cancer Staging Handbook, Sixth Edition (2002) published by Springer New York, www.sprinfleronline.com.

Continued

Quick Facts—cont'd

Stage	Description
T2a	Tumor involves half of one lobe or less
T2b	Tumor involves more than half of one lobe but not both lobes
T2c	Tumor involves both lobes
T3	Tumor extends through the prostatic capsule
T3a	Extracapsular extension (unilateral or bilateral)
T3b	Tumor invades the seminal vesicle(s)
T4	Tumor is fixed or invades adjacent structures other than seminal vesicles: bladder neck, external sphincter, rectum, levator muscles, and/or pelvic wall

Regional lymph nodes (N)

NX	Regional lymph nodes cannot be assessed
N0	No regional lymph node metastasis
N1	Metastasis in regional lymph node(s)

Distant metastasis (M)

MX	Distant metastasis cannot be assessed
M0	No distant metastasis
M1	Distant metastasis

Histopathologic grade (G)

GX	Grade cannot be assessed
G1	Well differentiated (slight anaplasia)
G2	Moderately differentiated (moderate anaplasia)
G3-4	Poorly differentiated or undifferentiated (marked anaplasia)

Stage	Primary Tumor	Regional Lymph Nodes	Distant Metastasis	Histopathologic Grade
I	T1a	N0	M0	G1
II	T1	N0	M0	Any G
	T2	N0	M0	Any G
III	T3	N0	M0	Any G
IV	T4	N0	M0	Any G
	Any T	N1	M0	Any G
	Any T	Any N	M1	Any G

Used with permission of the American Joint Committee on Cancer (AJCC), Chicago, Illinois. The original source for this material is the AJCC Cancer Staging Handbook, Sixth Edition (2002) published by Springer New York, www.sprinfleronline.com.

1. How common is prostate cancer?

Rates of prostate cancer, which is the most common cancer in men, peaked among white men in 1992 and among African American men in 1993. This apparent spike in the incidence of prostate cancer was likely from the widespread application of prostate specific antigen (PSA) screening in the late 1980s. Approximately 90% of new prostate cancer cases are expected to be diagnosed as locally confined disease, for which the 5-year survival rate approaches 100%.

2. Can we predict who is at risk for developing prostate cancer?

The strongest predictors for prostate cancer are age, race, and family history. Eighty percent of men are 65 years or older when initially diagnosed. In comparison with white men, African American men have a 50% higher chance of being diagnosed with prostate cancer, develop it at an earlier age, have a greater extent of disease at time of diagnosis, and have a mortality rate two times higher. Availability of health care services and beliefs about the health care system may be contributing factors to these disparities.

Many putative risk factors, including androgens, diet, physical activity, sexual factors, inflammation, and obesity, have been implicated, but their roles in prostate cancer etiology remain unclear. War veterans of the Asian theaters who were exposed to Agent Orange are at increased risk for prostate cancer. Obesity may increase the risk of dying from prostate cancer. Men with a body mass index of over 32.5 are 33% more likely to die from prostate cancer.

3. How do family history and hereditary risks affect the incidence of prostate cancer?

As much as 42% of the risk of developing prostate cancer may be accounted for by genetic influences, including individual and combined effects of both highly or weakly penetrant genes and genes acting in concert with each other. Familial aggregation (at least 2 cases in a family) is observed in about 20% of the cases with a hereditary form of prostate cancer. This proportion increases with younger age at diagnosis. Aggregation of prostate cancer and other cancers in some families suggest the involvement of common susceptibility genes. A man whose father or brother has been diagnosed with prostate cancer has a 3-fold risk of developing the disease. Men with two affected first-degree relatives are at a 9-fold increased risk.

4. Do hormones play a role in prostate cancer?

The important role of hormones in prostate cancer has been appreciated for over 50 years, because of the pioneering work of Huggins and Hodges in the 1940s. They specifically showed the beneficial effects of androgen deprivation in prostate cancer. Over the last 50 years, the method of androgen deprivation has shifted from surgical to pharmacological castration. Recent studies indicate that hormone receptors may play a role in targeted therapies for prostate cancer. In addition, both epidemiologic and laboratory studies indicate that another endogenous substance, insulin-like growth factor 1 (IGF1), may contribute to prostate cancer development. IGF1 is similar to insulin, but its function is to control cell growth, not insulin metabolism.

5. Can dietary habits and lifestyle changes affect prostate cancer progression?

Research has shown that diets high in fat or calcium may increase risk. Possible risk-reducers of prostate cancer include decreased fat consumption and increased consumption of soybeans (legumes), because of their high concentration of isoflavones; cruciferous vegetables; and foods that contain a high concentration of lycopenes (e.g., tomatoes, grapefruit, and watermelon). One small study reports that intensive lifestyle changes may affect prostate cancer progression. Patients with low risk for developing prostate cancer had low Gleason scores (refer to Question 14) and decreased PSA levels and were randomly assigned to standard care or an intensive lifestyle modification arm. The active therapy intervention included adopting a vegan diet; moderate aerobic exercise; gentle yoga; weekly support group; and diet supplementation with soy, fish oil, selenium, and vitamin C. The PSA level of those in the experimental group showed a small decrease, whereas the PSA level of those in the control group had a small increase.

6. Can pharmacologic intervention help prevent prostate cancer?

Results from the large NCI-funded Prostate Cancer Prevention Trial (PCPT) were reported in 2003. This trial examined the ability of finasteride (Proscar), which inhibits the conversion of testosterone into dihydrotestosterone (DHT), to prevent prostate cancer. Men between 55 and 75 years of age, with no evidence of prostate cancer were eligible to participate; 18,882 men were randomly assigned to two treatment groups, one of which received 5 mg of finasteride daily, and the other a placebo. The results of this important study are mixed; although there was a 25% relative reduction in total cases of prostate cancer with finasteride treatment, high grade cancers (Gleason score ≥ 7) were more common in the group receiving finasteride. Concern over these high-grade cancers, which are likely to be more lethal, has limited finasteride's use in a prevention setting.

7. What are the current recommendations or guidelines for prostate cancer screening?

American Cancer Society Guidelines: Men 50 years old with a 10-year life expectancy, and men at high risk (African Americans, men with family history) at 45 years of age should have both a digital rectal exam (DRE) and prostate-specific antigen (PSA) test annually.

American Urological Association (AUA) Guidelines: All men 50 years and older should be offered an annual DRE and PSA test.

The **National Cancer Institute** is currently conducting a large prospective, randomized trial to study whether early detection increases survival and decreases disease-related mortality. Results will not be available for several years.

8. Discuss the role of PSA in detection of prostate cancer.

Increased ability to diagnose prostate cancer by PSA level and transrectal ultrasound (TRUS) have greatly increased the number of men diagnosed with prostate cancer over the past decade. Whether survival rates are increased by early detection is still controversial. PSA is a glycoprotein enzyme that liquefies semen. Synthesized in the prostate, PSA level is considered to be elevated when it is > 4.0 ng/ml (normal range: 0-4.0 ng/ml). PSA blood screening was first available in 1987 and has led to an increase in the number of men diagnosed with prostate cancer. Even though PSA is specific to the prostate, it lacks both sensitivity and specificity for predicting the presence of prostate cancer. In other words, men with a PSA less than 4 ng/ml may have prostate cancer, and those with mild to moderate elevations may not. False positive PSA readings are associated with presence of other conditions, such as benign prostatic hypertrophy and prostatitis, and with recent medical procedures, such as cystoscopy, transurethral resection of the prostate (TURP), and needle biopsy. However, performing a routine DRE before measuring PSA level does not appear to cause significant PSA elevation.

9. How is PSA evaluated?

Prostatic specific antigen (PSA) is a protein produced by the cells of the prostate gland. The PSA test measures the level of PSA in the blood. Several approaches are available to increase the specificity of total PSA:

- **PSA velocity** is based on the rate of increase in PSA levels over time. A sharp rise in PSA raises the suspicion of cancer.
- **PSA density** considers the relationship of PSA level to the prostate gland size. For example, an elevated PSA might not arouse suspicion if a man has a very enlarged prostate.
- **Age-specific PSA** (refer to question 10)
- **Free versus total PSA** is a ratio, expressed as a percent. PSA circulates in the blood in two forms: free or total (attached to a protein molecule). There is more free PSA in benign prostate disease; cancer produces more of the total PSA form.

In men with an increased PSA of 4 to 10 ng/ml, the **free-to-total PSA ratio** is lower in men with prostate cancer than in men with benign disease. The appropriate free-to-total PSA cut-off level remains controversial. Studies suggest that a cut-off level of 25% would enable negative biopsies to be avoided in 20% of patients. A PSA increase of 2 ng/ml or greater in the year before prostatectomy for prostate cancer is associated with reduced survival.

10. What is meant by age-specific PSA reference ranges?

Because normal PSA levels increase as men become older, many researchers suggest that age-specific reference ranges should be used to increase the sensitivity of the PSA test among younger men and increase the specificity for older men. These ranges have not been approved or accepted by all urologists and clinicians.

Age-specific PSA reference ranges	
Age (yr)	PSA reference range (ng/ml)
40-49	0-2.5
50-59	0-3.5
60-69	0-4.5
70-79	0-6.5

11. Should prostate cancer be treated aggressively in all patients?

Because most men diagnosed with prostate cancer will not die from it, treatment decisions need to be individualized based on a patient's prognostic factors and overall health. For patients with localized disease, initial treatment options include radical prostatectomy, radiation therapy (external beam or brachytherapy), or watchful waiting. A Scandinavian study that started in the late 1980s and included patients with early-stage prostate cancer randomized participants to two groups; members of one group were treated with radical prostatectomy, and the other group was subjected to watchful waiting. While both overall survival and the prostate-specific survival were better in the prostatectomy group, some have argued that many of the patients included in this study would be considered at least intermediate risk by current standards and not good candidates for surveillance. Another approach, active surveillance, will be studied in the START (standard treatment against restricted treatment) trial. In this study, low-risk patients (Gleason score < 7, PSA < 10 ng/ml, localized disease), will be randomized between definitive local therapy and active surveillance. The surveillance group will have close PSA monitoring and repeated prostate biopsies, with significant changes in these measures triggering definitive therapy.

12. What are the signs and symptoms of prostate cancer?

Generally, **early-stage prostate cancer** is asymptomatic. However, as the tumor progresses, the patient may complain of symptoms consistent with urinary obstruction, such as nocturia, hesitancy, and straining to void; or irritative symptoms, such as urgency, dysuria, feeling of incomplete voiding, or hematuria.

Symptoms of **late-stage prostate cancer** are often associated with bone metastasis; consequently, pain is the most common complaint. Pain is often located in the pelvis and femur. The quality of the pain is commonly described as migratory (pain that radiates from one site to another). Complaints of back pain require thorough assessment for possible spinal cord compression. Liver involvement is manifested by elevated liver function tests, tenderness on palpation, anorexia, and nausea. Rarely, coagulopathies, such as thrombophlebitis and disseminated intravascular coagulation, may occur in the late stages. Lung metastasis is rare, but may be manifested by shortness of breath.

13. What are the survival rates for prostate cancer?

Prostate cancer survival rates

TNM	AUA stage	5-year survival rate
T1-T1c	A	90%-94%
T2-T2c	B	74%-90%
T3-T3c	C	55%-72%
T4-M+	D	1-4 year survival

14. What is the significance of the Gleason score and its impact on prognosis?

The Gleason score is based on the pathologic evaluation of the tumor's histology and correlates very well with the clinical behavior of prostate cancer. It is composed of two grade assessments, each on a 1 to 5 scale, which are added together to derive the final score. For example, if the most prevalent histologic grade is 4, but the pathologist also notes a secondary area of grade 5, the patient's Gleason score is 9. The higher the Gleason score, the worse the prognosis, with a score of 7 or higher commonly used as a crude dividing line between more and less aggressive prostate cancers.

15. What questions should the patient ask about proposed treatments?

- What is the chance of cure?
- What is the survival rate with each proposed treatment?
- Is the cancer confined to the prostate? How can you tell?
- What are the complication rates of each treatment?

16. What is a radical prostatectomy?

Radical prostatectomy involves removal of the entire prostate, including the true prostatic capsule, seminal vesicles, and a portion of the bladder neck. It can be performed by the perineal or retropubic approach. Recently, laparoscopy and the minimally invasive robot-assisted laparoscopy provide an alternative to the traditional surgical approach. Laparoscopy procedures require a longer learning curve for the surgeon and oncological control is not yet clearly validated. New surgical techniques do provide options for patients, including shorter hospital stay, faster recovery, decreased bleeding and transfusion rate, and enhanced visualization by the surgeon.

17. Discuss the surgical complications of radical prostatectomy.

Surgical complications are rare but may include atelectasis, wound infection, pulmonary emboli, bleeding, deep vein thrombosis, and urinary incontinence. Some complications (other organ perforation) are slightly higher with laparoscopic techniques than with open techniques. Advances in surgical techniques, anesthesia, pain control, and early ambulation have shortened the hospital stay to 1 to 2 days. Patients are taught catheter care and are sent home with a Foley catheter in place, which is removed at 2 weeks after surgery.

18. What are the complications of lymph node dissection?

Deep vein thrombosis or edema of the penis, scrotum, or lower extremities may result.

19. What are the side effects of radical prostatectomy?

- Incontinence incidence ranges from 0% to 57%, depending on the definition and type of incontinence, patient age, and skill of the surgeon. The most frequently reported incidence for stress incontinence (leakage of urine when coughing, straining, or lifting) is approximately 10% for all procedures; the incidence of total incontinence (no control over urination) is 5%.
- Loss of potency after radical prostatectomy depends on patient age, potency before surgery, and use of nerve-sparing techniques. In potent patients whose surgeon uses bilateral nerve-sparing techniques, the reported postsurgical potency is approximately 68%. Previously potent men whose surgeon uses unilateral nerve-sparing techniques have a reported potency of 47% postoperatively. The use of cavernous nerve mapping and stimulation to identify the nerve may improve nerve sparing.

20. How is incontinence managed?

Surgical techniques to preserve the urethral sphincter and muscle help to improve urinary continence. Treatments such as injection of collagen around the urethra and implantation of an artificial urinary sphincter are used to correct incontinence when it persists after other methods, such as pelvic floor (Kegel) exercises and biofeedback, do not work.

21. What treatments are available for erectile dysfunction?

The most common treatments, in order of patient preference, are oral medication, vacuum devices, urethral suppository, injectable drugs, and implants.

- Oral medications, such as sildenafil, tadalafil, and vardenafil, are patients' treatment of choice; however, they are generally not effective until the patient begins to experience some erectile function. As suggested by recent studies, sildenafil should be started soon after radical prostatectomy to maintain and promote blood vessel integrity and improve efficacy.
- Vacuum devices are the least invasive and help the penis become erect by suction. The vacuum device may be used daily. Its use is encouraged after radical prostatectomy to maintain normal erectile function.
- Urethral suppositories are easy to use but have poor efficacy (< 20%).
- A combination of drugs can be injected subcutaneously into the corpus cavernosum by the patient or significant other. Patients must be counseled about potential priapism.
- Penile implants require surgical intervention. Hollow tubes are placed in the corpus cavernosum and erection results from pumping a reservoir that inflates the tubes with normal saline. In addition, rods may be surgically placed into the corpus cavernosum to maintain a permanent erection. Patients should be told that infection is a potential complication of penile implants.

22. What forms of radiation therapy are used in the treatment of prostate cancer?

Radiation therapy may be used as initial definitive therapy, as a salvage treatment for local recurrence after a prostatectomy, and for palliation of bone pain. Radiation may be delivered via an external beam or by directly inserting the radioactive source into the prostate (brachytherapy). Studies comparing radiation therapy to surgical prostatectomies are largely retrospective, making a definitive assessment of each modality's relative efficacy and toxicity problematic.

23. Discuss the role of brachytherapy in prostate cancer.

Recent advances in ultrasound equipment and computer planning techniques have increased the popularity of brachytherapy. Low dose rate brachytherapy involves the insertion of "radioactive seeds" in the prostate, uniformly placed in the prostate tissue. This approach is used most commonly for lower risk patients (PSA < 10 ng/ml; Gleason score < 7) with a prostate volume of less than 40 grams.

24. What are the advantages of brachytherapy?

Radioactive seeds have the advantages of reduced side effects and a single outpatient administration. Retrospective data from observational series report similar outcomes with brachytherapy, external beam radiation, and surgical prostatectomy in low-risk patients.

25. What is high dose rate brachytherapy and in what setting is it used for prostate cancer?

High-dose-rate brachytherapy (HDRBT) is the administration of high dose radiation via needles placed temporarily in the prostate. HDRBT is used in combination with external beam radiation in some high-risk patients (Gleason score ≥ 7; PSA ≥ 10 ng/ml or a lesion rated T2c or greater). This combination increases radiation delivery to the prostate, while attempting to minimize the toxicity to surrounding tissues. Available data indicates that probability of urethral stricture may be increased with HDRBT, especially if transurethral resection of the prostate (TURP) was previously performed.

26. Discuss the advantages of conformal and intensity modulated radiation therapy.

Modern radiation therapy uses several innovations to maximize radiation delivery to the target, while minimizing the radiation exposure of the surrounding tissue. With 3-D conformal therapy, advanced imaging techniques and specialized computer software are used to create a 3-D representation of the anatomy in the treatment area. Improved planning results from defining the tumor volume and surrounding organs at risk. Intensity modulated radiation therapy (IMRT) adds further refinement by modulating the dose intensity of radiation to further maximize radiation delivery to the prostate, while minimizing toxicity.

27. What is the role of particle beam proton therapy in prostate cancer?

Particle beam proton therapy is currently under study in patients with prostate cancer. Protons have different physical and biologic properties than conventional x-ray beams, potentially increasing radiation delivery without increasing toxicity. Because proton beam therapy requires specialized facilities, its general availability is limited. Researchers in California at Loma Linda University reported good outcomes in prostate cancer patients with minimal morbidity, but the results of larger investigations using this approach are needed.

28. What are the side effects of radiation therapy for prostate cancer?

Modern radiation therapy is generally well tolerated. Minimal fatigue, mild dysuria, and urinary frequency have been reported during therapy. The long-term incidence of impotence is similar to that associated with radical prostatectomy. Brachytherapy has a higher incidence of urinary irritation and obstructive symptoms. Although these side effects resolve over weeks to several months, they may be uncomfortable and require self-catheterization. The incidence of side effects is greater for patients receiving high dose combination radiation therapy. Approximately 17% of patients experience proctitis and 5% report irritative urinary symptoms lasting longer than 1 year. Only 0.5% experience urinary retention. The incidence of proctitis is similar for proton beam therapy.

29. What is the significance of the PSA level after primary treatment?

Patients in whom PSA returns to an undetectable level (< 0.1 ng/ml) after radical prostatectomy are less likely to have a subsequent relapse than patients with higher levels (> 1.0 ng/ml). PSA levels should decrease rapidly after prostate removal in patients with organ-confined disease. Close attention to postoperative PSA level is important, since salvage radiation therapy to treat a local relapse is more successful if performed when PSA level is less than 2 ng/ml. In contrast to surgery, the PSA level may take over 18 months to reach the nadir after primary radiation therapy, and may additionally fluctuate rather than decline linearly.

30. What is cryosurgery? When is it used?

Cryosurgery is controlled freezing of the prostate with liquid nitrogen or other agents used for rapid freezing. This procedure consists of implanting ultrasound-guided percutaneous perineal wire trocars into the prostate. Cryoprobes are placed through cannulas or dilators and positioned over each wire. Urethral freezing is prevented by perfusing a urethral catheter with warm saline. The freezing process begins anteriorly and stops before the freezing agent reaches the rectal serosa. Cryosurgery was popular in the late 1980s and early 1990s but lost its popularity because of poor treatment outcomes and side effects. Recently cryosurgery has gained popularity among patients with both low and high risk disease and with cancer that has not responded to radiation therapy. The incidence of cryosurgery morbidity is reduced with newer equipment. Five-year follow-up from cryosurgical ablation shows a PSA less than 1 ng/ml in 83.3% of patients with early-stage prostate cancer. Currently, clinical trials are available for focal cryosurgery in patients with early-stage prostate disease.

31. What are the side effects of cryosurgery?

Patient-reported side effects from cryosurgery compare favorably with the side effects reported after radical prostatectomy. Immediate side effects include urinary leakage (4.3%), erectile dysfunction (85%), urethrorectal fistula (0.4%), bladder outlet obstruction (10%), scrotal swelling (18%), penile tingling and burning (15%), and pelvic pain (12%). These side effects usually resolve within 1 year of surgery, except for erectile dysfunction, which may take longer. Some men, however, do not regain potency.

32. What hormonal therapy is available for prostate cancer?

Luteinizing hormone-releasing hormone (LHRH) agonists, antiandrogens, and, less commonly, newer LHRH antagonists are used to treat patients with prostate cancer. Hormonal therapy is used in a variety of settings, including biochemical failure (rising PSA level) after localized therapy, in patients with advanced disease at diagnosis, and in the metastatic setting. Because of an initial surge in testosterone caused by treatment with LHRH agonists (before an eventual down-regulation of the LHRH receptors), antiandrogens are often prescribed during the start of LHRH agonist therapy. Hormonal ablation is also used with radiation therapy and after a radical prostatectomy in selected patients. Surgical bilateral orchiectomy is another effective method for quickly decreasing testosterone levels; however, bilateral orchiectomy is not commonly performed because of available pharmacologic alternatives and the psychological impact of the procedure.

33. What are the side effects of hormonal therapy?

Men who are potent when therapy is initiated should be told that the risk of losing potency and libido is almost 100%. In addition, hot flashes, weight gain, loss of bone density, and gynecomastia may occur.

34. How does hormonal therapy work?

Approximately 95% of testosterone comes from the testicles; the other 5% is produced by the adrenal glands. The goal of endocrine manipulation is to inhibit the formation or activity of testosterone. This goal can be achieved either surgically by orchiectomy or pharmacologically with oral hormones or injections that inhibit testosterone formation. Response rates are equal. Therapy can be aimed at one or both testosterone-producing systems. Single-agent androgen blockade can be achieved by: (1) surgical orchiectomy, (2) injections of analogs of LHRH agonists, such as leuprolide (Lupron), or (3) goserelin acetate (Zoladex) implant. LHRH analogs can be given as a depot injection monthly or every 3 or 4 months. The hormone injections "trick" the pituitary into thinking that testosterone production does not need to be initiated. In contrast, flutamide (Eulexin) and bicalutamide (Casodex) are oral antiandrogens that inhibit testosterone effects at the target tissue.

35. What is combined androgen blockade?

Combined androgen blockade (CAB) refers to the use of combination therapy (e.g., LHRH agonist plus an antiandrogen) to achieve maximal reduction of testosterone level and activity. The results of large, prospective trials examining CAB versus androgen deprivation monotherapy are mixed. Some clinicians use CAB only after progression on monotherapy with LHRH agonists. A paradoxical decline in PSA may be seen after stopping the antiandrogen treatment and continuing with the LHRH agonist in men whose cancer does not respond to CAB (termed antiandrogen withdrawal syndrome).

36. Can prostate cancer cells become hormone-refractory over time?

Yes. Relapse typically occurs 18 to 36 months after treatment. Studies are under way to determine whether an androgen-independent state can be delayed by the intermittent administration of an LHRH agonist. This therapy may decrease the likelihood that prostate cancer will become hormone refractory by returning cells to their normal pathways of differentiation and apoptosis.

37. How are hot flashes controlled?

Hot flashes are the most frequently reported side effect of hormonal ablative therapy for prostate cancer. Controlling hot flashes is a challenge. The severity may be diminished, but total eradication is rare. A combination of medications and complementary therapies may be offered. Commonly prescribed medications are vitamin E, clonidine, megestrol acetate (Megace), transdermal estrogen patches, and venlafaxine (Effexor). Venlafaxine, a serotonin and norepinephrine reuptake inhibitor used to treat depression, has been shown to reduce hot flashes in patients with prostate cancer (12.5 mg twice daily). Hot flashes may also be reduced by taking a related medication, paroxetine (Paxil).

38. What can be done about gynecomastia?

Gynecomastia is seen with all forms of androgen deprivation, but has a high incidence with antiandrogen therapy. Radiation therapy to the breasts is partially effective in reducing breast pain from gynecomastia, but is less effective in reducing breast size after the development of gynecomastia. Some clinicians recommend prophylactic breast irradiation for this reason. More recent investigations suggest that tamoxifen, a selective estrogen receptor modulator, may also be an effective treatment for gynecomastia from taking antiandrogens, but long-term safety data in patients with prostate cancer is not yet available.

39. What is the role of bisphosphonates in prostate cancer?

Bisphosphonates inhibit bone resorption and are helpful in the treatment of osteoporosis and hypercalcemia. Both oral (alendronate) and intravenous (zoledronic acid, pamidronate) formulations of bisphosphonates are available. Patients with prostate cancer who are treated with zoledronic acid had fewer skeletal-related events (bone fracture, worsening bone pain) compared to those treated with a placebo. Two serious adverse events from zoledronic acid are renal insufficiency and osteonecrosis of the jaw. There has been no clear survival benefit with bisphosphonate therapy in prostate cancer to date.

40. When is chemotherapy indicated?

Historically, the efficacy of chemotherapy in prostate cancer has been limited. However, two prospective, randomized clinical trials of chemotherapy from 2004 showed a small survival benefit in patients with metastatic, hormone-refractory prostate cancer. Although the absolute improvement in survival was approximately 2 months, many clinicians now use the combination of docetaxel every 3 weeks with twice daily dosing of prednisone as first-line therapy for advanced prostate cancer. Mitoxantrone is also approved by the FDA for use in prostate cancer, based on improved quality of life measures. Adjuvant chemotherapy in high-risk patients after a radical prostatectomy is being studied in several ongoing or planned trials.

41. Discuss the role of radionuclides in the treatment of bone metastases.

Strontium-89 and samarium-153 are radioisotopes that are administered intravenously to patients with far-advanced prostate cancer who have failed all other therapy and have a life expectancy of less than 2 months. These isotopes travel to areas of bone with metastatic disease, follow the biochemical pathways of calcium in the body, and are taken into the mineral structure of the bone. Initially they may cause a flaring of pain and myelosuppression. They also may cause prolonged anemia and thrombocytopenia. Patients should be instructed to continue taking prescribed pain medication for 2 to 3 weeks after receiving either radionuclide because of the delayed response before pain relief occurs. Pain relief can be maintained for 4 to 15 months. Response rates to radionuclide treatment are 40% to 80%. Patients also may benefit from a second injection; however, caution must be used because of the prolonged side effects. Use of radionuclides may compromise further chemotherapy, because of prolonged myelosuppression.

42. Are newer, targeted therapies being used to treat prostate cancer?

Targeted agents are likely to play a more important role in treating prostate cancer in the future. Although preliminary data for the use of single agents (e.g., trastuzumab) has been disappointing, combination trials of targeted agents with traditional chemotherapy are underway. Immunotherapy, enhancing the body's immune response to cancer, has received much attention in prostate cancer. Vaccines against prostate antigens have been developed and are being examined in clinical trials. For example, the Provenge vaccine uses the patient's own dendritic cells, which are removed, exposed to specific prostate antigens, and then reintroduced into the patient. In one early study, this vaccine appears to slow the time to progressive disease, and larger phase III studies, examining its effect on survival, are underway.

 Key Points

- Prostate cancer is the most common noncutaneous cancer in men and the second leading cause of cancer deaths in men.
- Treatments for localized disease include surgery, radiation therapy, and cryosurgery.
- LHRH, antiandrogen therapy, or both are the most effective systemic treatments.
- Chemotherapy is used for palliative therapy and may slightly increase survival.
- New targeted therapies to treat prostate cancer are being studied.

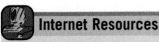

Internet Resources

American Cancer Society:
  http://www.cancer.org
American Prostate Society:
  http://www.americanprostatesociety.com/
American Urological Association and Urology Health:
  http://afud.org
National Cancer Institute:
  http://www.cancer.gov
Prostate Cancer Education Council:
  http://www.pcaw.com
Prostate Cancer Foundation:
  http://www.prostatecancerfoundation.org
US TOO International, Inc., Prostate Cancer Education and Support:
  http://www.ustoo.com

Acknowledgment

The authors wish to acknowledge Susanne Cook, RN, BSN, for her contributions to the Prostate Cancer chapter published in the first and second editions of *Oncology Nursing Secrets.*

Bibliography

Abeloff MD, Armitage JO, Lichter AS, et al, editors: *Clinical oncology,* ed 3, New York, 2004, Churchill Livingstone.
Bill-Axelman A, Holmberg L, Ruutu M, et al: Radical prostatectomy versus watchful waiting in early prostate cancer. *N Engl J Med* 352:1977-1984, 2005.
Boccardo F, Rubagotti A, Battaglia M, et al: Evaluation of tamoxifen and anastrozole in the prevention of gynecomastia and breast pain induced by bicalutamide monotherapy of prostate cancer. *J Clin Oncol* 23:808-815, 2005.
DiAmico A, Ming-Hui C, Roehl K, et al: Preoperative PSA velocity and risk of death from prostate cancer after radical prostatectomy. *N Engl J Med* 351:125-135, 2004.
Greene FL, Page DL, Fleming ID, et al, editors: *AJCC cancer staging manual,* ed 6, New York, 2002, Springer.
Hsing AW, Chokkalingam AP: Prostate cancer epidemiology. *Front Biosci* 1:1388-1413, 2006.
Jemal A, Siegel R, Ward E, et al: Cancer statistics, 2007. *CA Cancer J Clin* 57:43-66, 2007.
Klotz L: Active surveillance for prostate cancer: For whom. *J Clin Oncol* 23:8165-8169, 2005.
McGlynn B, Al-Saffar N, Begg H: Management of urinary incontinence following radical prostatectomy. *Urol Nurs* 24:475-482, 2004.
Moul JW, Pienta KJ, Hollenbeck BK, et al: Prostate cancer. In Pazdur R, Coia LR, Hoskins WJ, et al: *Cancer management: A multidisciplinary approach,* ed 9, Lawrence, KS, 2005, CMP Health Care Media.
Ornish D, Weidner G, Fair W, et al: Intensive lifestyle changes may affect the progression of prostate cancer. *J Urol* 174:1065-1070, 2005.
Pienta KJ, Smith DC: Advances in prostate cancer chemotherapy: A new era begins, *CA Cancer J Clin* 55:300-318, 2005.
Raina R, Agarwal A, Zippe CD: Management of erectile dysfunction after radical prostatectomy. *Urology* 66:923-929, 2005.
Slater JD, Rossi CJ, Yonemoto LT, et al: Proton therapy for prostate cancer: The initial Loma Linda University experience. *Int J Radiat Oncol Biol Phys* 59:348-352, 2004.
Smith RA, Cokkinides V, Eyre HJ: American Cancer Society guidelines for the early detection of cancer, 2005. *CA Cancer J Clin* 55:31-44, 2005.
Stephenson AJ, Shariat SF, Zelefsky MJ, et al: Salvage radiotherapy for recurrent prostate cancer after radical prostatectomy. *JAMA* 291:1325-1332, 2004.
Tannock IF, de Wit R, Berry WR, et al: Docetaxel plus prednisone or mitoxantrone plus prednisone for advanced prostate cancer. *N Engl J Med* 351:1502-1512, 2004.

Tewari A, El-Hakim A, Leung RA: Robotic prostatectomy: A pooled analysis of published literature. *Expert Rev Anticancer Ther* 6:11-20, 2006.

Thompson IM, Goodman PJ, Tangen CM, et al: The influence of finasteride on the development of prostate cancer. *N Engl J Med* 349:215-224, 2003.

Willener R, Hantikainen V: Individual quality of life following radical prostatectomy in men with prostate cancer. *Urol Nurs* 25:88-100, 2005.

Chapter 31

Renal Cell Carcinoma

Patrick H. Judson and Carolyn Phillips

Quick Facts

Incidence	51,190 newly diagnosed cases estimated in 2007 (31,590 in men; 19,600 in women)
Mortality	12,890 deaths estimated in 2007
Risk factors	Cigarette smoking
	Exposure to asbestos
	Family history of kidney cancer
	Development of renal cystic disease on hemodialysis
	Obesity
	Hypertension (diastolic)
	Advancing age (median age at diagnosis is 55 years)
Genetics	von Hippel-Lindau syndrome
Histopathology	Clear cell or conventional (75%-85% of tumors)
	Papillary (10%-15%)
	Chromophobe (3%-5%)
	Oncocytoma (uncommon)
	Collecting duct (very rare)
	Each subtype may feature high-grade sarcomatoid characteristics
Symptoms	Hematuria
	Flank pain
Diagnosis and evaluation	History and physical examination
	CBC and chemistry screen
	Cystoscopy (if hematuria is present)
	Ultrasound
	Computed tomography (CT) of chest and abdomen
	Venogram of inferior vena cava (IVC), or magnetic resonance imaging (MRI) to evaluate IVC involvement

Staging and Stage Grouping

Stage	Description
I	Tumor is confined to the kidney
II	Tumor invades through perinephric fat but is confined within Gerota's fascia
III	Tumor has invaded the renal vein (A), regional lymph nodes (B), or both (C)
IV	Contiguous organ involvement (A) or distant metastases (B)

1. Is renal cell carcinoma associated with genetic predispositions?

Some families have an inherited autosomal dominant predisposition to develop renal cell carcinoma. Affected family members have a balanced translocation involving chromosome 3p, whereas family members without the disease do not have this translocation. Another form of hereditary renal cell carcinoma is seen with Von Hippel-Lindau (VHL) disease, which is characterized by development of multiple, bilateral renal cysts and carcinomas; pheochromocytomas; retinal hemangiomas; hemangioblastomas of the central nervous system (CNS); pancreatic cysts and tumors; and epididymal cystadenomas.

Affected families have a germ line mutation of the VHL gene on chromosome 3p. Roughly 50% of sporadic renal cell carcinomas have mutations affecting the VHL gene on the short arm of chromosome 3.

2. Summarize the histopathologic findings in renal cell carcinoma.

- 2% to 4% are bilateral.
- 4% to 10% have extension into the renal vein or the inferior vena cava.
- The histologic types are clear cell or conventional (75%-85% of tumors), papillary (10%-15%), chromophobe (3%-5%), oncocytoma (uncommon), and collecting duct (very rare). Each subtype may feature high-grade sarcomatoid characteristics.
- The most common grading system is the nuclear grading system by Fuhrman, ranging from 1 to 4 with higher grades having poorer prognoses.
- The Heidelberg classification of renal tumors was introduced in 1997 to increase the correlation between the histopathologic features of the tumor with the identified genetic defects.

3. List unusual biological characteristics of renal cell carcinoma.

- De novo drug resistance
- Complete or partial spontaneous regression (which has led to research on biologic therapy)

4. What are the signs and symptoms of renal cell carcinoma?

The most common symptom is hematuria. Approximately 50% of renal cell carcinomas are found serendipitously on imaging studies obtained for unrelated reasons. The classic triad of symptoms (flank pain, flank mass, and hematuria) is unusual today (10%-15% of cases) and indicates advanced disease. In addition, only 40% of patients have disease confined to the kidney upon diagnosis; at initial diagnosis 25% have metastatic disease. Therefore, a patient's primary symptoms at diagnosis may be caused by metastases.

5. Describe the distant effects of renal cell carcinoma.

Paraneoplastic syndromes are relatively common. Examples include an increased erythrocyte sedimentation rate, hypertension, anemia, cachexia and weight loss, fever, abnormal liver functions (e.g., Stauffer's syndrome), hypercalcemia, erythrocytosis, neuromyopathies, and amyloidosis.

6. What are the usual sites of metastases?

The primary sites of metastatic disease are the lungs, liver, bones, lymph nodes, and CNS.

7. Describe the staging system for renal cell carcinoma.

The TNM system is unwieldy for everyday use in renal cell carcinoma. A staging system modified by Robson is in general use (see Quick Facts).

8. What determines prognosis and treatment?

Prognosis depends on the size, stage, and grade of the tumor. Sarcomatoid variants are more aggressive and have a poorer prognosis. Resectable, early-stage disease is curable only with surgery. Patients with stage I or stage II disease have a 5-year survival of 50% to 80%. Selected patients with stage I disease may be treated with a radical, simple, or partial nephrectomy. Radical resection involves removal of the kidney, adrenal gland, perirenal fat, and Gerota's fascia, with or without dissection of regional lymph nodes. Surgical excision of solitary or multiple metastatic lesions may also benefit the patient.

9. What is the role of adjuvant therapy outside of clinical trials?

There is no proven benefit for adjuvant systemic therapy or radiation therapy. Patient participation in clinical trials is encouraged.

10. Summarize the prognosis for metastatic disease.

A 5-year survival rate of 35% to 50% has been reported for tumors extending beyond the renal capsule. Patients with stage IV or metastatic disease have a median survival of only 18 months, and approximately 2% survive 5 years.

11. How is metastatic disease treated?

Chemotherapy regimens do not have a significant benefit (< 10% response rate) for renal cell carcinoma. Patients should be encouraged to participate in clinical trials. For almost twenty years, the standard first line therapy has been interferon alpha or interleukin-2 (IL-2). IL-2 has a response rate of approximately 15% and some complete responders have been disease-free for 5 years. So far, long-lasting remissions have been seen only with high doses of IL-2. This therapy can be quite toxic and should be given only to patients with adequate cardiac function and good performance status. Interferon-alpha has a response rate of 15% to 20%, with median durations of response of 6 months. External-beam radiation can be used to palliate metastatic renal cell carcinoma (bone and CNS lesions).

New targeted therapies are rapidly becoming the new standard of care for renal cell carcinoma. Evidence has been presented for the use of the tyrosine kinase inhibitors (TKI). Sunitinib malate recently received U.S. Food and Drug Administration (FDA) approval as first-line therapy for metastatic renal cell carcinoma. In addition, sorafenib tosylate, which inhibits the vascular endothelial growth factor (VEGF) pathway and c-Raf kinase isoforms, was approved by the FDA based on substantial improvement in progression-free survival.

12. What investigational treatments for metastatic renal cell carcinoma are available?

- Nonmyeloablative allogeneic stem cell transplantation
- Tumor vaccines
- Targeted therapies
  - Bevacizumab is a recombinant human monoclonal antibody against VEGF
  - Erlotinib is an endothelial growth factor receptor inhibitor. Treatment with a combination of bevacizumab and erlotinib is showing great promise in early studies
  - In clinical trials, temsirolimus, an inhibitor of the protein mTOR, is showing a significant survival advantage for poor-risk renal cell carcinoma.

Patients are encouraged to participate in clinical trials involving these agents.

 Key Points

- Approximately 50% of renal cell carcinomas are found serendipitously on imaging studies obtained for unrelated reasons.
- 25% of renal cell carcinomas are metastatic upon initial diagnosis.
- Most renal cell carcinoma is unresponsive to chemotherapy.
- Biologic therapy is an exciting possibility for future treatments.

Internet Resources

American Cancer Society, Kidney Cancer:
   http://www.cancer.org/docroot/cri/content/cri_2_4_1x_what_is_kidney_cancer_22.asp
National Cancer Institute:
   http://cancer.gov/kidney
American Kidney Fund:
   http://www.kidneyfund.org
Kidney Cancer Association:
   http://www.kidneycancerassociation.org

Bibliography

Atkins MB: Clinical manifestations, evaluation, and staging of renal cell carcinoma. Available at:
   http://www.utdol.com/utd/content/topic.do?topicKey=gucancer/4484&type=A&selectedTitle=2~51
   Accessed January 7, 2007.
Atkins MB: Epidemiology, pathology, and pathogenesis of renal cell carcinoma, Available at:
   http://www.utdol.com/utd/content/topic.do?topicKey=gucancer/2829&type=A&selectedTitle=3~51
   Accessed January 7, 2007.
Atkins MB: Medical management of renal cell carcinoma Available at:
   http://www.utdol.com/utd/content/topic.do?topicKey=gucancer/14296&type=A&selectedTitle=1~51
   Accessed January 7, 2007.
Atkins MB: Molecularly targeted therapy for renal cell carcinoma. Available at:
   http://www.utdol.com/utd/content/topic.do?topicKey=gucancer/14941&type=A&selectedTitle=5~51
   Accessed January 7, 2007.
Atkins MB, Richie JP: Surgical management of renal cell carcinoma. Available at:
   http://www.utdol.com/utd/content/topic.do?topicKey=gucancer/5071&type=A&selectedTitle=6~51
   Accessed January 7, 2007.
Cohen HT, McGovern FJ: Renal cell carcinoma. *N Engl J Med* 353:2477-2490, 2005.
Hainsworth JD, Sosman JA, Spigel DR, et al: Treatment of metastatic renal cell carcinoma with combination
   of bevacizumab and erlotinib. *J Clin Oncol* 23:7889-7896, 2005.
Hudes G, Carducci M, Tomczak P, et al: 2006 ASCO Annual Meeting Proceedings Part I. *J Clin Oncol* 24:18,
   2006: LBA4
Jemal A, Siegel R, Ward E, et al: Cancer statistics, 2007. *CA Cancer J Clin* 57:43-66, 2007.
Motzer RJ, Michaelson MD, Redman BG, et al: Activity of SU11248, a multitargeted inhibitor of vascular
   endothelial growth factor receptor and platelet-derived growth factor receptor in patients with metastatic
   renal cell carcinoma, *J Clin Oncol* 24:16-24, 2006.
Rini BI, Small EJ: Biology and clinical development of vascular endothelial growth factor-targeted therapy
   in renal cell carcinoma, *J Clin Oncol* 23:1028-1043, 2005.
Simmons J, Marshall F: Kidney and ureter. In Abeloff M, Armitage J, Niederhuber J, et al, editors: *Clinical
   oncology,* ed 3, New York, 2000, Churchill Livingstone.
Stadler WM: New targets, therapies, and toxicities: Lessons to be learned (editorial), *J Clin Oncol* 24:4-5, 2006.
Vogelzang NJ: Treatment options in metastatic renal carcinoma: An embarrassment of riches (editorial),
   J Clin Oncol 24:1-3, 2006.
Vogelzang NJ, Scardino P, Shipley W, et al, editors: *Comprehensive textbook of genitourinary oncology,* ed 2,
   Philadelphia, 2000, Lippincott Williams & Wilkins.

Chapter 32

Testicular Cancer

Jeffrey L. Berenberg

Quick Facts

Incidence	7920 newly diagnosed cases estimated in 2007 (accounts for 1% of all cancers in men); most common tumor in men aged 15-35 years
Mortality	380 deaths estimated in 2007
Etiology	Unknown; testicular germ cell tumors probably start in utero
Risk factors	History of cryptorchid testis (several-fold increased risk); orchiopexy performed before 6 years of age slightly reduces the risk
	Klinefelter's syndrome and extragonadal germ cell tumors
	Personal or family history of testis tumor
	Carcinoma in situ
Genetics	Isochrome of short arm of chromosome 12 [i(12p)] (80% of germ cell cases); increased copy number in 100%
Histopathology	Germ cell neoplasms make up more than 94% of primary tumors; the remaining 5% are non-germ cell types (e.g., Sertoli cell, Leydig cell, and gonadoblastomas)
	Two categories of germ cell tumors: Seminoma (60%) Nonseminoma (40%)

- Embryonal
- Teratoma
- Yolk sac (endodermal sinus; most common in children)
- Choriocarcinoma (rare; 1%)
- 40% of tumors are mixed (seminoma + nonseminoma)

Symptoms	Painless mass
	Swelling has often been present for > 3 months
	Low back pain (secondary to retroperitoneal lymph node involvement) and gynecomastia are less common as initial symptoms
	Advanced disease: cough, dyspnea, headache, seizures
Diagnosis and evaluation	History and physical examination
	Testicular examination: tumor is unlikely if the mass clearly separates from the body of the testis
	Ultrasound examination
	Radical inguinal orchiectomy (removal of testis, epididymis, part of vas deferens, and parts of gonadal lymph nodes and blood vessels)
	Tumor markers: beta human chorionic gonadotropin (βHCG), alpha-fetoprotein (AFP), and lactate dehydrogenase (LDH)
	Chest x-ray (PA and lateral)
	Computed tomography (CT) of chest, abdomen, and pelvis

Quick Facts—cont'd

Staging and Stage Grouping

MRI for identification of brain metastases

Stage	Description

Tumor, node, metastasis (TNM)

Primary tumor (T)

The extent of primary tumor is classified after radical orchiectomy.

T	Primary tumor cannot be assessed (if no radical orchiectomy has been performed, TX is used)
T0	No evidence of primary tumor (e.g., histologic scar in testis)
Tis	Intratubular germ cell tumor (carcinoma in situ)
T1	Tumor limited to testis and epididymis without vascular/lymphatic invasion; tumor may invade tunica albuginea but not tunica vaginalis
T2	Tumor limited to testis and epididymis with vascular/lymphatic invasion; or tumor extends through tunica albuginea with involvement of tunica vaginalis
T3	Tumor invades spermatic cord with or without vascular/lymphatic invasion
T4	Tumor invades scrotum with or without vascular/lymphatic invasion

Regional lymph nodes (N)

NX	Regional lymph nodes cannot be assessed
N0	No regional lymph node metastasis
N1	Metastasis with lymph node mass ≤ 2 cm in greatest dimension; or multiple lymph nodes, none > 2 cm in greatest dimension
N2	Metastasis with a lymph node mass > 2 cm but not > 5 cm in greatest dimension; or multiple lymph nodes, none > 5 cm in greatest dimension
N3	Metastasis with a lymph node mass > 5 cm in greatest dimension

Distant metastasis (M)

MX	Distant metastasis cannot be assessed
M0	No distant metastasis
M1	Distant metastasis
M1a	Nonregional nodal or pulmonary metastasis
M1b	Nonpulmonary visceral metastasis

Serum tumor markers (S)

SX	Marker studies not available or not performed
SO	Marker study levels within normal limits
S1	LDH $< 1.5 \times$ N; HCG (mIU/ml) < 5000; and AFP (ng/ml) < 1000
S2	LDH 1.5-$10 \times$ N; or HCG (mIU/ml) $= 5000$-$50,000$; or AFP(ng/ml) $= 1000$-$10,000$
S3	LDH $> 10 \times$ N; or HCG (mIU/ml) $< 50,000$; or AFP (ng/ml) $> 10,000$
	N = upper limit of normal for LDH assay

Stage	Description
0	Tis, N0, M0
I (40%*)	Any T, N0, M0 Tumor limited to testis and adjacent structures

*Incidence at presentation

Used with permission of the American Joint Committee on Cancer (AJCC), Chicago, Illinois. The original source for this material is the AJCC Cancer Staging Handbook, Sixth Edition (2002) published by Springer New York, www.sprinfleronline.com.

Continued

Quick Facts—cont'd

Stage	Description
IS	Any T, N0, M0, S1-3 Tumor limited to testis and adjacent structures with marker positive
II (40%*)	Any T, N1-3, M0, S0-1 Tumor beyond testis but not beyond regional retroperitoneal lymph nodes
III (20%*)	Any T, Any N, M0, S2-3; or Any T, Any N, M1 Any S Disseminated metastasis beyond lymphatic drainage or above diaphragm or regional nodes with S3

*Incidence at presentation
Used with permission of the American Joint Committee on Cancer (AJCC), Chicago, Illinois. The original source for this material is the AJCC Cancer Staging Handbook, Sixth Edition (2002) published by Springer New York, www.sprinfleronline.com.

1. What is unique about testicular cancer?

Testicular carcinoma is the most curable solid tumor in adults (> 95% cure rate in patients with stage I or II disease). It is unique because even 72% of patients with advanced stage disease are cured.

2. How often are patients with testicular cancer diagnosed correctly on presentation?

In one series, only 33% of cases were correctly diagnosed. Delay in diagnosis from 1 to 3 months is not unusual because signs or symptoms are mistaken for benign abnormalities (varicocele, spermatocele, epididymitis, hydrocele, and torsion) and patients delay seeking medical attention.

3. Is screening for testicular cancer of proven value?

The American Cancer Society recommends monthly testicular self-examination (TSE) starting at puberty; this approach has not been validated and continues to be controversial. Some researchers believe that the potential yield from TSE is outweighed by increased anxiety in an already body conscious age group. Others believe that testicular examination provides an opportunity to initiate education and discussion about male sexuality and sexually transmitted diseases.

4. What raises the suspicion of cancer when a patient develops a testicular mass?

A patient who has the combination of gynecomastia, a swollen left supraclavicular lymph node, and testicular mass almost always has testicular cancer.

5. How is an intrascrotal mass evaluated?

Trauma and infection should be ruled out as a cause of intrascrotal pain or swelling.
- Examine the patient for the following:
  - Varicocele (vein engorgement within scrotum)
  - Spermatocele (irregular grapelike sac)
  - Hydrocele (accumulation of scrotal fluid)
  - Torsion (swelling)
- Transilluminate the scrotum with a flashlight. Cysts, such as hydroceles, often appear transparent, whereas tumors appear dense.
- Scrotal ultrasound is highly accurate in identifying intratesticular masses.

6. How often does testicular cancer occur in both testes?

Only 1% to 2% of all germ cell tumors are bilateral. Both tumors may occur synchronously, or the second tumor may occur years later.

7. Why are needle biopsy and transscrotal orchiectomy contraindicated?

These procedures can cause both scrotal recurrence from implantation of tumor cells and inguinal spread of disease from a change in lymphatic drainage.

8. Where does testicular cancer spread?

Retroperitoneal nodes are usually the first area of spread; hematogenous metastases occur later to the lungs, liver, and brain. Brain metastases may occur earlier in patients with choriocarcinoma.

9. Discuss the value of tumor markers.

AFP (alpha-fetoprotein), βHCG (beta subunit-human chorionic gonadotropin) and LDH (lactate dehydrogenase) help to identify nonseminomatous elements, predict prognosis (very high levels), determine residual disease after orchiectomy or retroperitoneal lymph node dissection (RPLND), confirm response to treatment, and detect recurrence. At least one abnormal marker is found in 80% to 85% of nonseminomatous tumors. Patients with pure seminoma usually do not have elevated tumor marker levels. Occasionally βHCG is mildly elevated in seminoma (< 10% of patients). AFP elevations in seminoma indicate other nonseminomatous elements, whether or not the pathologist can confirm their presence. False-positive results are extremely rare except in patients with hypogonadism in whom βHCG level may be falsely elevated when leuteinizing hormone (LH) levels are high. AFP level may be elevated in cases of hepatoma or liver inflammation due to cirrhosis or hepatitis. Increased LDH levels may correlate with widespread disease.

10. How reliable is the CT scan in staging retroperitoneal disease in patients with nonseminomatous tumors?

About 20% to 25% of patients with clinical stage II disease are found to have a higher stage after RPLND. A similar percentage of patients with clinical stage I disease are found to have a lower stage.

11. What prognostic factors are useful in patients with stage I nonseminoma?

Vascular or lymphatic invasion, embryonal histology, and tunica invasion predict a higher relapse rate when patients are observed without RPLND after orchiectomy.

12. When is observation after orchiectomy a reasonable treatment choice?

Orchiectomy followed by RPLND yields an anticipated disease free survival of 81% to 94% in patients with nonseminomatous disease. However, the morbidity associated with RPLND includes injury to nerves supplying the prostate, seminal vesicles, vasa deferentia, and bladder neck. Even if erectile potency is preserved, there may be reduction or loss of ejaculate. A nerve-sparing lymphadenectomy may be done to preserve ejaculation.

Observation with assessment of tumor markers every month and chest radiographs and CT scans every 2 months for 2 years yields an overall relapse rate of 27%; the salvage rate is greater than 90% with 3 or 4 cycles of platinum-based chemotherapy. However, this approach requires examination of risks and benefits, patient commitment, and personal involvement of both nurses and physicians during follow-up care.

13. What prognostic classifications are commonly used for advanced testicular cancer?

An International Germ Cell Cancer Collaborative Group (IGCC-CG) used tumor extent and marker levels to classify prognosis. This system, which has been incorporated into AJCC (American Joint Committee on Cancer) staging, is based on a combination of location of primary site (testis/retroperitoneal vs. mediastinal), elevation of tumor marker levels, histologic analysis, and location of metastatic sites (pulmonary or nonpulmonary). Patients with good risk (low serum marker elevations and pulmonary metastases) may need only three courses of chemotherapy. High-risk patients have disseminated visceral metastases, primary tumor in the mediastinum, or very high tumor marker levels. All patients with seminoma have good prognoses.

14. What is the standard treatment for seminoma?

The tumor is usually localized and especially radiosensitive. All stages of seminoma require removal of the testicle by radical inguinal orchiectomy. Patients with stage I and stage II disease have radiation therapy to the ipsilateral iliac and retroperitoneal lymph nodes. This treatment is curative in more than 95% of patients with stage I disease. Stage II nonbulky tumors (< 5 cm) are eliminated in more than 90% of patients by irradiation. Usually patients with bulky stage II and stage III disease receive combination cisplatin-based chemotherapy or radiation to the abdominal and pelvic lymph nodes.

15. Do all Stage I seminoma patients require radiation therapy?

Prolonged intensive surveillance similar to that outlined in Question 12 leads to cure rates similar to that of radiation; 15% to 20% of patients relapse but respond to either radiation therapy or chemotherapy. At 3 years after treatment in a recent European trial, patients who received a single course of adjuvant carboplatin experienced disease-free periods that were equivalent to those patients treated with radiation. Phase II trials suggest two cycles of carboplatin may be more effective.

16. What is the impact of testicular cancer and its treatment on fertility?

Sterility due to chemotherapy, radiation therapy, and surgery is a major concern to young men diagnosed with testicular cancer. For unknown reasons, oligospermia, azoospermia, and Leydig cell dysfunction are often seen before treatment is initiated. At the time of diagnosis, approximately 80% to 90% of men have oligospermia or azoospermia. Sperm banking may not always be an option because of the urgency of chemotherapy and rapid tumor growth. Chemotherapy may affect spermatogenesis. Patients remain azoospermic for almost 1 year after therapy. Approximately 50% of patients regain both spermatogenesis and Leydig cell function within 2 years. About 33% of patients are able to father children. Oligospermia after radiation is usually reversible. Congenital malformations are not increased.

The size and location of the tumor may preclude the use of nerve-sparing RPLND. Fertility may be affected by retrograde "dry" ejaculation (ejaculate enters the bladder upon orgasm) due to the severing of the sympathetic plexus, which occurs in many patients undergoing RPLND.

17. When should chemotherapy be the initial treatment?

Patients with bulky seminoma and patients with stage III or bulky stage II (> 5 cm or palpable mass) nonseminomatous disease should receive treatment with 3 to 4 cycles of bleomycin, etoposide, and cisplatin (BEP). Three cycles should result in a long-term disease-free survival rate in more than 85% of patients if minimal metastatic disease is present. A recent update of a trial comparing treatment with etoposide and cisplatin with either bleomycin or ifosfamide showed that high-risk patients should receive four cycles of treatment, which yields a disease-free survival rate of greater than 50%. Modern radiotherapy may be curative for patients with bulky stage II seminoma, but many oncologists prefer cisplatin-based chemotherapy.

18. What is the role of RPLND in nonseminomatous patients?

If serum marker levels do not return to normal after orchiectomy or rise after an initial decrease, chemotherapy should be instituted immediately even without objective disease.

RPLND is indicated after chemotherapy when discernible residual disease is found even with normal markers. Fibrosis, necrosis, cancer, and/or teratoma may be found during this surgical procedure. Unresected teratoma may transform into malignancy or grow and cause symptoms. If no teratoma was present initially and the residual masses are small, residual cancer or teratoma are less likely to be found.

19. **What acute and long-term toxicities are associated with chemotherapy for testicular cancer?**

Acute toxicities:
- Gastrointestinal effects (nausea and vomiting)
- Renal effects (decreased creatinine clearance and tubular loss of sodium, potassium, and magnesium)
- Bone marrow depression

Long-term toxicities:
- Bleomycin pneumonitis (rarely fatal if < 400 U are given)
- Sterility
- Secondary acute myelogenous leukemia (related to treatment with etoposide; typically shows 11q23 translocation; incidence < 5% at 5 years after treatment)
- Peripheral neuropathies
- Cisplatin-induced renal tubular wasting and hearing loss

20. **If a patient develops progressive disease after therapy with BEP, what are the options for salvage treatment?**

Patients who have progressive disease following primary chemotherapy may be salvaged with vinblastine, cisplatin, and ifosfamide (30%). Surgery also may have a role. High dose chemotherapy using etoposide/carboplatin with or without cyclophosphamide or ifosfamide offers a limited potential for cure when combined with peripheral stem cell transplant.

21. **What are the significant nursing implications in caring for patients with testicular cancer?**

Because all types of testicular cancer require that patients undergo radical inguinal orchiectomy for diagnostic and therapeutic purposes and possibly RPLND for nonseminoma, nurses need to address concerns about body image and fear of sexual dysfunction. Patients are likely to be worried about the surgical consequences and toxicities of radiation or chemotherapy. Their fears should be explored and unfounded concerns should be corrected and explained. They should be reassured about positive outcomes. Patients may

 Key Points

- Testicular cancer is the most common cancer in men between the ages of 15 and 35 years.
- Testicular cancer is unique because even in advanced stages 72% of patients are cured.
- Retroperitoneal nodes are usually the first area of spread; hematogenous metastases occur later to lungs, liver, and brain.
- Serum tumor markers (AFP, βHCG and LDH) predict prognosis, determine residual disease after orchiectomy or retroperitoneal lymph node dissection (RPLND), confirm response to treatment, and detect recurrence.
- Treatment is determined by stage of disease and histological factors.
- Radiation is still used in the treatment of patients with early stage seminoma.
- Chemotherapy is often curative, even in patients with advanced stage disease.

be so afraid of sexual dysfunction that they refuse potentially curative therapies. Patients should be prepared about the effect of the orchiectomy on genital appearance and about the possibility of retrograde ejaculation after RPLND. Inform patients about testicular prostheses, and, if indicated, make appropriate referrals. (See Chapter 44 for information about sexual counseling, retrograde ejaculation, and sperm banking.)

 Internet Resources

National Comprehensive Cancer Network (NCCN) Clinical Practice Guidelines in Oncology, Testicular Cancer:
   http://www.nccn.org/professionals/physician_gls/PDF/testicular.pdf
National Cancer Institute, Testicular Cancer:
   http://www.cancer.gov/cancertopics/types/testicular
National Cancer Institute, Testicular Cancer (PDQ): Treatment (guide for health care professionals):
   http://www.cancer.gov/cancertopics/pdq/treatment/testicular/healthprofessional
National Cancer Institute, Testicular Cancer (PDQ): Treatment (guide for patients):
   http://www.cancer.gov/cancertopics/pdq/treatment/testicular/Patient
Testicular Cancer Resource Center (guide for patients):
   http://tcrc.acor.org/index.html
American Cancer Society, All About Testicular Cancer (guide for patients):
   http://www.cancer.org/docroot/CRI/CRI_2x.asp?sitearea−LRN&dt−41
Lance Armstrong Foundation (supports managing and surviving cancer):
   http://www.livestrong.org
National Action Plan for Cancer Survivorship:
   http://www.cdc.gov/cancer/survivorship/survivorpdf/plan.pdf

Bibliography

Bosl GJ, Bajorin DF, Sheinfeld J, et al: Cancer of the testis. In: DeVita VT Jr, Hellman S, Rosenberg SA, editors: *Cancer: Principles and practice of oncology,* ed 7. Philadelphia, PA, 2005, Lippincott Williams & Wilkins.

Choo R, Thomas G, Woo T, et al: Long-term outcome of postorchiectomy surveillance for stage I testicular seminoma. *Int J Radiat Oncol Biol Phys* 61(3):736-740, 2005.

Einhorn L: Curing metastatic testicular cancer. *Proc Natl Acad Sci USA* 99:4592-4595, 2002.

Greene FL, Page DL, Fleming ID, et al, editors: *AJCC cancer staging manual,* ed 6, New York, 2002, Springer.

Hinton S, Catalano PJ, Einhorn LH, et al: Cisplatin, etoposide with either bleomycin or ifosfamide in the treatment of disseminated germ cell tumors: Final analysis of an intergroup trial. *Cancer* 15:1869-1875, 2003.

International Germ Cell Cancer Collaborative Group: International Germ Cell Consensus Classification: A prognostic factor-based staging system for metastatic germ cell cancers. *J Clin Oncol* 15:594-603, 1997.

Jemal A, Siegel R, Ward E, et al: Cancer statistics, 2007. *CA Cancer J Clin* 57:43-66, 2007.

Loehrer PJ, Ahlering TE, Pollack A: Testicular cancer. In Pazdur R, Coia LR, Hoskins WJ, et al, editors: *Cancer management: A multidisciplinary approach,* ed 9, New York, 2005, Oncology Publishing Group.

Oliver RT, Mason MD, Mead GM, et al: Radiotherapy versus single-dose carboplatin in adjuvant treatment of stage I seminoma: A randomized trial. *Lancet* 366(9482):293-300, 2005.

Williams SD, Birch R, Einhorn LH, et al: Treatment of disseminated germ-cell tumors with cisplatin, bleomycin, and either vinblastine or etoposide. *N Engl J Med* 316:1435-1440, 1987.

Zack E: Testicular germ call cancer. In Yarbro CH, Frogge MH, Goodman M, et al, editors: *Cancer nursing: Principles and practice,* ed 6, Boston, 2005, Jones and Bartlett.

Disclaimer: The views contained in this chapter are solely those of the author and do not reflect the views or policies of Tripler Army Medical Command, the Department of Defense, or the U.S. Government.

Cancer of Unknown Primary Sites (CUPs)

Jamie S. Myers and Kelly Pendergrass

1. What are cancers of unknown primary sites, and how often do they occur?

Cancers of unknown primary sites (CUPs) or occult primary malignancies are metastatic malignancies for which the primary malignancy cannot be identified. Estimates of the incidence of CUPs vary from 3% to 10% of cancer diagnoses. Incidence is equal between men and women and is on the decline because of increased use of enhanced evaluation techniques, including magnetic resonance imaging (MRI), positron emission tomography (PET), and serum and tissue immunohistochemical tests. CUP is the seventh most common cause of cancer death. For certain categories of CUPs it is estimated that the primary site becomes obvious during the patient's lifetime in 15% to 20% of cases. Even at autopsy, the primary site cannot be identified in 20% to 30% of patients with CUP. CUPs may occur in metastatic sites not expected for the site of origin.

2. How are CUPs categorized?

There are four major categories of CUPs:
- Poorly differentiated neoplasm
- Well-differentiated and moderately well-differentiated adenocarcinoma
- Squamous cell carcinoma
- Poorly differentiated carcinoma (with or without features of adenocarcinoma)

3. How do the clinical evaluations differ for the various categories of CUPs?

The categories are important to the clinical evaluation and management of the disease, and may be predictive of treatment response.

Poorly differentiated neoplasm: About 5% of oncology patients will have an initial diagnosis of poorly differentiated neoplasm by initial light microscopy. Most patients' diagnoses can be further defined into a general histologic category of neoplasm (e.g., carcinoma, lymphoma, melanoma, and sarcoma) by conducting further specialized pathologic studies, such as immunoperoxidase staining, electron microscopy, and/or genetic analysis. Because of the need for preservation of the histologic pattern and the necessary volume of tissue to conduct special studies, a generous biopsy is preferred over a fine needle aspiration. Until a general category of neoplasm can be determined, it is very difficult to make treatment decisions. Accurate histologic analysis leads to a rational and potentially effective treatment plan.

Well differentiated and moderately well differentiated adenocarcinoma (also referred to as ACUP): This is the most common category of CUP and represents about 60% of the cases. The most common types of cancer in this category are lung and pancreas (40%). Gastrointestinal cancers (stomach, colon, liver) also occur relatively frequently. Cancers of the breast, prostate, and ovary are more rare. Patients tend to be older adults with metastatic tumors at multiple sites (e.g., lymph nodes, liver, lung, and bone). These patients typically have a poor prognosis with a median survival of 3 to 4 months. Clinical evaluation should include a thorough history and physical (H&P), including patterns of tobacco use, complete blood count (CBC), liver function tests, serum creatinine, prostatic acid phosphatase, prostate-specific antigen (PSA), urinalysis, chest radiograph, mammogram, and computed tomography (CT) of the abdomen and pelvis. Positron emission tomography (PET) scanning may also be used to attempt determination of the primary site.

Women with a malignancy in an axillary node may have a primary breast cancer. Lymph node biopsy, HER-2/neu, and estrogen/progesterone receptor (ER/PR) status should be performed even when mammography is negative.

Elevated PSA levels, presence of osteoblastic bone metastases, or both may indicate a primary prostate cancer in men (about 3% of cases), in spite of an unusual metastatic pattern. Radiolabeled imaging such as the ProstaScint scan (Indium-111 labeled capromab pendetide) targets specific proteins on the surface of prostate cancer cells and may be a valuable tool for recognizing primary prostate cancers. Breast and prostate cancers may respond to hormonal therapy and be more amenable to treatment than tumors of gastrointestinal origin.

Squamous cell carcinoma: This category represents about 5% of cases of CUP.

Cervical lymph nodes are the most common metastatic site for middle-aged or older patients. Most patients have a history of alcohol and/or tobacco use. Malignant lesions in upper or middle cervical nodes may indicate that the primary site is in the head or neck. Evaluation should include panendoscopy with biopsies of any suspicious lesions. PET scanning has been shown to be a valuable tool for the identification of primary tumors, as well as occult metastatic disease.

Lung cancer should be suspected when lower or supraclavicular nodes are involved. Evaluation should include chest CT and examination of the head and neck. If no evidence of malignancy is found, fiberoptic bronchoscopy is indicated.

Malignant lesions in inguinal lymph nodes may indicate a genital or anorectal primary. Evaluation should include digital rectal exam and anoscopy.

Poorly differentiated carcinoma: About 30% of CUP cases fall into this category. The malignancies in approximately one third of these cases have some features of adenocarcinoma. The patients are typically younger than those in the other categories and demonstrate a rapid progression of symptoms and tumor growth. Predominant sites of involvement are the lymph nodes, particularly in the retroperitoneum and mediastinum. As with poorly differentiated neoplasms, these cases should be assessed with immunoperoxidase staining. Electron microscopy may be helpful when immunoperoxidase staining is not definitive. Clinical evaluation should include H&P, CT of chest and abdomen, CBC, liver function tests, and serum levels of creatinine, beta subunit-human chorionic gonadotropin (βHCG), and alpha-fetoprotein (AFP). Elevations of βHCG and AFP levels with a mediastinal or retroperitoneal lesion suggest the presence of a germ cell tumor. It is hypothesized that some highly chemotherapy responsive tumors are marker-negative germ cell tumors that are not identifiable by current pathologic methods. Genetic analysis of the i(12p) marker chromosome may be a useful diagnostic method for patients suspected of having midline germ cell tumors. These are neuroendocrine tumors that may respond favorably to treatment with chemotherapy. NeoTect (technetium-99m depreotide) scanning may be used to identify primary small cell and non–small cell-lung cancers that overexpress somatostatin. PET scanning has proven valuable in detecting primary tumors in 20% to 60% of patients with these lesions.

Clinical evaluation for carcinoma of unknown primary site (CUP)

CUP category	Radiographic tests/exams	Lab tests	Pathologic studies
Adenocarcinoma (Well/moderately differentiated)	CT abdomen	AFP CEA CA 19-9	Mucin stain
	Women: mammography	CA 15-3 CA 125 CA 27-29	ER/PR receptors HER-2/neu expression
	Men: ProstaScint scan	PSA	PSA stain
Squamous carcinoma			
Cervical nodes	Panendoscopy PET scan		Genetic analysis Keratin
Supraclavicular nodes	Bronchoscopy		
Inguinal nodes	Pelvic/rectal exam Anoscopy		
Poorly differentiated carcinoma			
(with or without adenocarcinoma)	CT of chest/abdomen NeoTect scan	βHCG AFP	Immunoperoxidase stains Electron microscopy Genetic analysis

4. How are treatment decisions made for CUPs?

Treatment decisions are based on the most likely primary site for the CUP as indicated by the cell type (e.g., adenocarcinoma vs. squamous cell carcinoma), location of CUP (e.g., axilla vs. cervical lymph nodes), risk factors (such as use of alcohol or tobacco), and tumor markers (i.e., elevated levels of PSA, Cancer Antigen 15-3[CA 15-3], or βHCG/AFP). The patient's performance status and any comorbidities are also considered before deciding whether the patient should receive aggressive treatment or supportive care.

5. Are some subsets of CUPs more responsive to treatment than others?

Yes. There are subgroups within the categories that have a greater chance of treatment response. About 10% of patients with well differentiated or moderately well differentiated adenocarcinomas may respond. For example, a woman with peritoneal carcinomatosis may have an ovarian or endometrial cancer. These women may benefit from platinum-based or taxane-based chemotherapy after aggressive surgical cytoreduction. An axillary lymph node lesion that is ER/PR positive with no other sites of metastases may respond to treatment like a stage II breast cancer. These women may be successfully treated with locoregional radiation therapy. Women with positive axillary lymph nodes will most likely benefit from systemic treatment with chemotherapy, hormonal manipulation, or both. Presence of elevated PSA level, osteoblastic bone metastases, or both in men may indicate prostate cancer that will respond to an empirical trial of hormonal therapy.

Poorly differentiated carcinomas are most responsive to treatment. Within this category, patients with elevated βHCG or AFP levels and a mediastinal or retroperitoneal mass typically have a germ cell tumor and can be successfully treated, and even cured, with a chemotherapy regimen of paclitaxel, carboplatin, and etoposide. Favorable prognostic factors include tumor location, limitation to one or two metastatic sites, younger age, and no smoking history. Electron microscopy will detect neurosecretory granules in 10% of patients. These patients can be treated for neuroendocrine carcinoma of unknown primary site. The response rate to a platinum agent and etoposide ranges as high as 77%. Neuroendocrine carcinomas have now been divided into three categories: well differentiated or low grade; poorly differentiated by light microscopy with neuroendocrine features; and high grade biology with no distinctive neuroendocrine features by light microscopy. The well differentiated variety may be treated with somatostatin analogues, streptozocin, doxorubicin, and fluorouracil (5-FU) based chemotherapy. A combination regimen of paclitaxel, carboplatin, and etoposide has been used for the poorly differentiated type. Cisplatin-based regimens are used for the high-grade variety. Thymomas (primary tumors of the thymus gland) may also be the primary site for CUPs that are poorly differentiated carcinomas. These too respond to platinum-based chemotherapy. Many clinicians believe that all patients with poorly differentiated carcinomas should be considered for treatment with platinum-based chemotherapy.

Patients diagnosed with metastatic melanoma of unknown primary site to a single nodal site are treated as stage II disease. These patients have slightly better survival rates than patients with stage II disease and a documented primary site. Patients with more advanced disease may still be managed with curative intent and be offered adjuvant therapy protocols.

Patients with squamous cell carcinoma and a head and neck presentation may be treated with radiation therapy, combination chemotherapy, or both. Although radical neck dissection yields the primary tumor in 20% to 40% of patients, it is avoided when possible because of the devastating cosmetic and functional effects on a patient's quality of life. Patients with N1 and N2 involvement fare better than those with N3 or massive nodal disease. Local regional management yields 5-year survival rates of 35% to 50%.

6. What treatment is recommended for patients who do not have a CUP that falls into the favorable subsets?

Up until recently, for 90% of patients who have well differentiated or moderately well differentiated adenocarcinomas, chemotherapy has not been highly successful. However, a variety of recent trials has evaluated combination chemotherapy regimens with the taxanes, gemcitabine, vinorelbine, irinotecan, and topotecan. Results have shown response rates of 30% and median survival of 9 months. Combination regimens have now become the standard of care for patients with good performance status.

Patients with squamous cell carcinoma that are suspected lung cancer primaries may be candidates for chemotherapy.

7. How do I discuss this diagnosis with my patients and their families?

Discussing a cancer diagnosis can be difficult enough without having to deal with not knowing where the cancer started. Educating patients and families that the treatment recommendation is based on the most likely primary site requires patience and the development of trust. Ideally the topic of CUP is brought up during the clinical evaluation, as the work-up proceeds without identification of a definitive primary site. Once all the test results are in, an important function of the oncology nurse is participation in the physician/patient/family conference as the diagnosis and treatment options are discussed. The nurse will hear what treatment options are presented and can observe the patient/family reactions to the diagnosis of CUP. It will then be a little easier to answer questions and provide emotional support and education about the treatments, expected side effects, and possible toxicities.

8. Has progress been made for reimbursement for treatment of CUP?

Yes. After years without an ICD-9 code for carcinoma of unknown primary, the diagnosis code is now listed in both the American Hospital Formulary Drug Information and the United States Pharmacopeia Drug Information. The three drugs that are listed as indicated for this diagnosis code are paclitaxel, carboplatin, and etoposide. Drugs currently being considered include docetaxel, gemcitabine, and irinotecan.

 Key Points

- Cancers of unknown primary sites (CUPs) are malignancies that are diagnosed as a metastatic lesion for which the primary malignancy cannot be identified.
- The four major categories of CUPs are: (1) poorly differentiated neoplasm, (2) well differentiated and moderately well differentiated adenocarcinoma, (3) squamous cell carcinoma, and (4) poorly differentiated carcinoma (with or without features of adenocarcinoma).
- Some subsets of CUPs are more responsive to treatment:
  - Axillary lymph node lesions that are positive for hormone receptor markers in women
  - Lesions accompanied by elevation of PSA level and/or osteoblastic bone metastases in men
  - Mediastinal or retroperitoneal lesions accompanied by elevations of βHCG or AFP levels
  - Lesions with neurosecretory granules present
- The American Hospital Formulary Drug Information and United States Pharmacopeia Drug Information compendia now list an ICD-9 code for carcinoma of unknown primary. Indicated drugs include paclitaxel, carboplatin, and etoposide.

 Internet Resources

National Cancer Institute, Carcinoma of Unknown Primary:
   http://www.nci.nih.gov/cancertopics/types/unknownprimary
   Includes information on treatment, clinical trials, current literature, and links to: What You Need to Know About Cancer, CUP Origin Fact Sheet, Coping With Cancer, Taking Time, and When Someone in your Family is Facing Cancer

Bibliography

Ghosh L, Dahut W, Kakar S, et al: Management of patients with metastatic cancer of unknown primary. *Curr Probl Surg* 2:12-66, 2005.

Greco FA, Hainsworth JD: Cancer of unknown primary site. In DeVita VT, Hellman S, Rosenberg SA, editors: *Cancer: Principles & practice of oncology,* ed 7, Philadelphia, 2005, Lippincott-Raven.

Greco FA, Litchy S, Dannaher C, et al: Carcinoma of unknown primary site with unfavorable characteristics: Survival of 396 patients after treatment with five consecutive phase II trials by the Minnie Pearl Cancer Research Network. *J Clin Oncol* 22(14S):4186, 2004.

Miller FR, Hussey D, Beeram M, et al: Positron emission tomography in the management of unknown primary head and neck carcinoma, *Arch Otolaryngol Head Neck Surg* 7:626-629, 2005.

National Cancer Institute: Carcinoma of unknown primary (PDQ): Treatment. Last modified March 21, 2005. Available at: http://cancernet.nci.nih.gov/cancertopics/pdq/treatment/unknownprimary/ healthprofessional. Accessed May 6, 2006.

Pavlidis N, Fizazi K: Cancer of unknown primary (CUP), *Crit Rev Oncol Hematol* 3:243-250, 2005.

Ross MI, Cormier JN, Xing Y, et al: Prognosis and survival outcomes in melanoma patients with unknown primary (MUP), *J Clin Oncol* 22(14S):7544, 2004.

Veach SR, Saeed M, Beschloss J, et al: Survival prediction in carcinoma of unknown primary (CUP) based on the metastatic site, *Proc Am Soc Clin Oncol* 22:4159, 2004.

Unit V

Symptom Management

Depression, Distress, and Anxiety

Barbara I. Damron and Rose A. Gates

1. Define depression.

Depression is a mood or feeling related to disappointment or loss. In cancer patients, depression refers to "the entire range of depressive symptoms, including normal sadness in response to loss, as well as chronic depressed emotional affect and clinical depression meeting specific criteria for psychiatric disorder" (Barsevick, Sweeney, Haney, Chung, 2002, p. 74). Major depression is a clinical syndrome lasting at least 2 weeks with at least five of the following symptoms:

- Depressed mood most of the day, almost every day
- Markedly decreased interest or pleasure in most activities most of the day
- Significant weight loss/gain or appetite disorder
- Insomnia or too much sleeping
- Psychomotor agitation or retardation
- Inappropriate guilt
- Indecisiveness or difficulty in concentrating
- Recurring thoughts of death, including suicidal ideation

2. How does depression compare to distress in cancer patients?

Distress, as defined in the National Comprehensive Cancer Network (NCCN) Practice Guidelines, is a "multifactorial, unpleasant experience of an emotional, psychological (cognitive, behavioral, emotional), social, and/or spiritual nature that may interfere with the ability to cope effectively with cancer, its physical symptoms, and its treatment. Distress extends along a continuum, ranging from common normal feelings of vulnerability, sadness, and fears to problems that can become disabling, such as depression, anxiety, panic, social isolation, and existential or spiritual crisis." Thus, depression is one aspect of distress. The term *distress* was selected by the NCCN to describe psychosocial aspects of the patient's experiences because it is less stigmatizing, may be seen as a more normal or natural response to a cancer diagnosis, and can be defined by self-report. Using the word *distress* may facilitate health care providers in obtaining information about patients' emotions, as well as depression. It may also be easier or less embarrassing for patients to talk about their distress rather than depression. Depression and "distress should be recognized, monitored, documented, and treated promptly at all stages of disease" (NCCN, 2007).

3. What is the prevalence of depression among cancer patients?

Depression is the most common psychiatric problem in the United States (15% prevalence rate). However, it is an under-recognized problem in cancer patients that affects treatment outcomes, patients' quality of life, and satisfaction with care. The reported prevalence of depression in cancer patients varies widely from 1% to 50%; depression is more frequent among hospitalized and advanced cancer patients. About 25% of patients with cancer continue to have high levels of depression and anxiety that persist for weeks to months. These disorders are called adjustment disorders with depressed, anxious, or mixed moods, depending on the major symptoms.

4. Describe how symptoms of depression differ in cancer patients.

The biologic correlates or somatic symptoms, typically used for diagnosing depression in physically healthy adults, are frequently unreliable in patients with cancer. These symptoms (e.g., decreased appetite, insomnia, fatigue, loss of energy, loss of libido, psychomotor slowing) are similar to symptoms caused by many cancer treatments or cancer itself. Patients with cancer frequently have no appetite because of chemotherapy or radiotherapy, sleep poorly because of pain or hospitalization, and are fatigued by cancer or its treatments.

More reliable indicators of depression in cancer are the psychological symptoms expressed by the patient: a depressed mood that is persistent or worsens, hopelessness, helplessness, worthlessness, despondency, guilt feelings, and suicidal ideation. Other signs of depression in cancer patients include depressed appearance, social withdrawal or decreased talkativeness, pessimism, and lack of response to situations that are normally enjoyable. Depression is treatable and should not be considered normal in most patients with cancer.

5. How is depression diagnosed in patients with cancer?

Depression is best diagnosed with a thorough interview and by simply asking patients whether they are depressed. Many tools are also available to screen for depression (e.g., Patient Questionnaire PHQ-9, visual analogue scale for depressed mood). In terminally ill patients, it is often difficult to differentiate depression from sadness or the normal grieving that is part of the dying process. Some patients can tell you that they are depressed, whereas others may not be aware of their own depression. The nurse needs to assess for risk factors (see Question 6) and constantly assess the patient's psychological status (mood, severity of depression, and suicide risk), paying attention to such cues as an unexpected decision to discontinue treatment.

The nurse should carefully determine whether certain symptoms (e.g., fatigue, insomnia, confusion, decreased libido) are caused by depression, cancer, treatment, drugs, or other medical conditions. For example, mental disorders mimicking depression may be due to metastatic disease or a paraneoplastic syndrome.

6. What are some risk factors for depression in cancer patients?

- Psychiatric factors: personal or family history of depression or other psychiatric diagnoses (e.g., bipolar disorder), history of substance abuse
- Social factors: multiple stressors or losses, lack of perceived social support
- Cancer-related factors: diagnosis of lung, pancreatic, brain, oropharyngeal, or breast cancer; high symptom distress; advanced illness; neurological disorders; and chemotherapy/medications
- Age younger than 30 or older than 80 years
- History of medical nonadherence

7. What are the common causes of psychological distress in cancer patients and their families?

- Learning of the diagnosis of cancer or discovery of a suspicious symptom
- Painful medical procedures
- Fear of dying from the illness
- Beginning new treatment (surgery, radiation therapy, chemotherapy)
- Difficulty of treatments related to new demands on time and side effects of treatment (e.g., fatigue, appetite and weight loss, pain)
- Managing side effects and symptoms related to treatment and cancer (e.g., pain, fatigue, loss of appetite and weight, loss of intimacy or sexuality)
- Threats of disfigurement

- Learning that treatment efforts have failed or that disease has progressed or recurred
- Loss of job
- Additional financial expenses
- Social isolation
- End of treatment and stresses related to survivorship
- Advanced cancer and end of life

8. **Describe a normal response to the stressors related to the diagnosis and treatment of cancer.**

Normal responses are highly individualized and are affected by many factors, including extent of the disease, presence of side effects, prognosis, past experiences, coping skills, support systems, culture, and religious and spiritual beliefs. The normal response to the diagnosis and treatment of cancer can include brief periods of denial or despair, followed by distress and a mixture of symptoms, such as depressed mood, anxiety, insomnia, anorexia, and irritability. Patients may have difficulty in performing activities of daily living and may experience recurring thoughts about an uncertain future. These symptoms can last for days to several weeks, after which usual patterns of adaptation and coping return. Distress is recurrent during frequent crisis points experienced by patients along the cancer trajectory.

Normal coping is an active, conscious response to stress, with or without unconscious behaviors. Coping efforts are aimed not only at reducing or eliminating stressful conditions but also at minimizing the inherent emotional distress.

9. **What are the medical causes of depression that patients with cancer may experience?**

- Surgeries (e.g., mastectomy, head and neck surgery)
- Radiation therapy and its side effects (e.g., whole brain radiation)
- Chemotherapy (e.g., asparaginase, procarbazine, vincristine, vinblastine) and its side effects
- Treatment with cytokines: interferon-alfa, interleukin-2
- Uncontrolled pain
- Hormonal abnormalities (e.g., hyperthyroidism or hypothyroidism, adrenal insufficiency)
- Metabolic abnormalities (e.g., anemia, vitamin B_{12} or folate deficiency, hypercalcemia, sodium or potassium imbalances)
- Medications: beta-blockers, antihypertensives, opioids, barbiturates, benzodiazepines, methyldopa, reserpine, amphotericin B, corticosteroids, antiestrogens (tamoxifen), cyproterone acetate

10. **What is a major risk factor for depression among patients with cancer?**

Uncontrolled pain is a major risk factor for depression and suicide among cancer patients. The presence of clinically significant pain nearly doubles the likelihood of a major psychiatric complication of cancer, particularly depressive disorders and confusional states. Any patient experiencing overwhelming physical symptoms and functional limitations should be considered at risk for developing psychologic distress.

11. **When should a patient be referred to a psychologist or a psychiatrist?**

A consultation is warranted whenever the nurse or physician is uncomfortable addressing the patient's psychologic needs. Early consultations can be extremely helpful in facilitating the establishment of a supportive relationship for the patient. The following signs are indications for a psychologic or psychiatric consultation:

- The patient requests the consultation
- The patient is suicidal or requests suicide or euthanasia
- The patient and/or family is experiencing multiple stressors, or the family is dysfunctional

- The patient exhibits signs and symptoms of a depressive disorder, extreme anxiety, or psychosis
- The patient is not responding to current treatment for depression or anxiety
- The patient's psychological symptoms interfere with medical treatment
- The patient is in need of specific psychologic therapy, such as biofeedback, hypnosis, or relaxation

12. How is depression managed in patients with cancer?

Although, psychopharmacologic interventions are the mainstay of depression treatment, depression in cancer patients is optimally managed within the context of an interdisciplinary team (psychologist, psychiatrist, social worker, advanced practice nurse, staff nurses, oncologist, chaplain) by a combination of supportive psychotherapy or counseling (individual or group), cognitive-behavioral techniques (CBT), and antidepressant medications. Additional treatments may include exercise, family support/counseling, relaxation, meditation, art, dance, and music. Treatment is directed toward helping patients adapt to stresses and strengthen their coping abilities.

13. How do cognitive behavioral techniques help patients with cancer?

Cognitive-behavioral interventions focus on inaccurate perceptions and assessments that lead to anxious and depressed feelings. These techniques can help patients develop an adaptive perspective and have been shown to decrease depressive symptoms in patients with mild to moderate levels of depression. By using CBTs, nurses can help patients reframe their situation, using realistically positive perspectives, and therefore alter negative perceptions that impair quality of life.

14. When should antidepressants be considered in patients with cancer?

The use of psychotropic medication should be determined by the patient's level of distress, inability to carry out daily activities, and response to psychotherapeutic interventions. A patient does not need a psychiatric diagnosis to receive treatment for psychological distress. According to the American College of Physicians–American Society of Internal Medicine (ACP-ASIM) End-of-Life Care Consensus Panel, clinicians should have a low threshold for prescribing antidepressants. Effective psychotherapeutic and pharmacologic therapy can reduce distress, improve quality of life, and even increase survival. A trial of antidepressants is warranted when both depression and debilitation are observed in patients with advanced cancer because it may be difficult to determine which condition is primary.

15. Which antidepressants are most useful for patients with cancer?

Clinicians have a wide array of antidepressants from which to choose: first- and second-generation tricyclic antidepressants (TCAs), heterocyclic antidepressants, monoamine oxidase inhibitors (MAOIs), selective serotonin reuptake inhibitors (SSRIs), serotonin and noradrenaline reuptake inhibitors, and dopamine antagonists. In addition, drugs such as alprazolam (Xanax), a benzodiazepine, can be used for antidepressant effects in patients with anxiety. Lithium carbonate, an antipsychotic drug, is useful for treating depression in bipolar illness; however, it must be used cautiously in patients receiving cisplatin because of the potential for nephrotoxicity.

16. How is the appropriate antidepressant chosen for individual patients?

Antidepressants should be selected according to their mechanism of action, side-effect profile, and secondary actions. The patient's existing medical problems, nature of the depressive symptoms, and past response to specific antidepressants should also be considered. (Refer to table on opposite page).

Characteristics of antidepressants used during cancer treatment

Medication	Oral dose (mg/day)	Primary side effects	Comments
First-generation tricyclics (TCAs)			
Amitriptyline (Elavil)	25-125	Sedation, anticholinergic effects (dry mouth, delirium, constipation), orthostasis	Onset of action: 2-4 weeks Administer at bedtime. All first-generation TCAs: start at low doses (10-25 mg) at bedtime; slowly increase by 10-24 mg every 1-2 days until effective.
Doxepin (Sinequan)	25-125	Highly sedating; orthostatic hypotension, intermediate anticholinergic effects; potent antihistamine	Useful for neuropathic pain and as an adjunct to opioids Alternate routes: parenteral or rectal
Imipramine (Tofranil)	50-200	Intermediate sedation; anticholinergic effects; orthostasis	Not tolerated well in terminally ill patients because of anticholinergic effects. Monitor plasma levels to establish therapeutic dosage.
Desipramine (Norpramin)	12.5-200	Little sedation or orthostasis; moderate anticholinergic effects	
Nortriptyline (Pamelor)	10-150	Little anticholinergic or orthostatic effects; intermediate sedation	
Trazodone (Desyrel)	150-300	Sedating; not anticholinergic; risk of priapism	Second-generation TCA Generally less cardiotoxic than first-generation TCAs Highly serotonergic; adjuvant analgesic effect
Monoamine oxidase inhibitors (MAOIs)			
Isocarboxazid (Marplan)	20-40		Use with caution. Avoid tyramine-containing foods.
Phenelzine (Nardil)	30-60		
Tranylcypromine (Parnate)	20-40	Myoclonus and delirium have been reported.	Use of meperidine while taking MAOIs absolutely contraindicated because of potential for hyperpyrexia and cardiovascular collapse

Continued

Characteristics of antidepressants used during cancer treatment—cont'd

Medication	Oral dose (mg/day)	Primary side effects	Comments
Selective serotonin reuptake inhibitors (SSRIs)			
SSRIs		Few anticholinergic or cardiovascular side effects; can cause sexual dysfunction; rare side effects: bradycardia, increased risk of bleeding, hyponatremia, serotonin syndrome, and mania	Onset of action: 2-4 weeks Drug of choice in medically ill patients because of favorable side-effect profile Beware of possible drug interactions because of metabolism by cytochrome P450 isoenzyme 2D6. Because SSRIs are strongly protein-bound, consider possibility of increased levels of other drugs (e.g., warfarin, digoxin, cisplatin, some anticonvulsants).
Citalopram (Celexa)	20-60	Less gastrointestinal side effects; low potential for drug interactions	Good choice for elderly patients
Escitalopram (Lexapro)	10-20	Low potential for drug interactions	No dosage adjustment required for hepatic or mild to moderate renal impairment Available as elixir
Fluoxetine (Prozac/Sarafem)	20-40	Sexual dysfunction, including anorgasmia; anticholinergic effects; headache; nausea; anxiety; insomnia	Increased half-life in elderly patients Available as elixir
Paroxetine (Paxil)	10-50	Nausea, somnolence, asthenia; may cause anticholinergic symptoms	No active metabolites; excreted relatively quickly on discontinuation Available as elixir Also available as Paxil CR to decrease gastrointestinal side effects
Sertraline (Zoloft)	25-200	Nausea; insomnia	Useful in medically ill: shorter half-life than fluoxetine and more rapid hepatic and renal clearance

Characteristics of antidepressants used during cancer treatment—cont'd

Medication	Oral dose (mg/day)	Primary side effects	Comments
Heterocyclic antidepressants			
Maprotiline (Ludiomil)	50-75	Side-effect profile similar to TCAs; increase in seizure incidence	
Amoxapine (Asendin)	100-150	Side-effect profile similar to TCAs; mild dopamine-blocking activity	Patients taking dopamine blockers (e.g., antiemetics) have increased risk of developing extrapyramidal symptoms and dyskinesias.
Mixed-action			
Bupropion (Wellbutrin)	75-450	May cause seizures in those with low seizure threshold/brain tumors; initially activating: tremor anxiety and insomnia; low risk of sexual side effects	Norepinephrine/dopamine reuptake inhibitor Limited role in oncology Energizing effects may have role for psychomotor retardation in depressed, terminally ill patients Useful for smoking cessation Sustained-release formulation is better tolerated.
Duloxetine (Cymbalta)	40-60	Nausea; dry mouth; constipation	Selective norepinephrine reuptake inhibitor (SNRI) Approved for diabetic peripheral neuropathic pain and may be useful for other types of chronic pain
Mirtazapine (Remeron)	15-45	Sedating at lower doses; dry mouth; constipation; neutropenia (rare); weight gain; fewer reported GI problems; sexual side effects are unlikely	Stimulates release of norepinephrine and serotonin Useful for agitated depression and insomnia Good for cancer patients who have anorexia or who want to gain weight Available as oral disintegrating tablets
Nefazodone (Serzone)	200-500	Sedating; nausea; dizziness; less cardiotoxicity; low risk of sexual dysfunction	Serotonin-2 antagonist/ reuptake inhibitor: affects serotonin and norepinephrine. Metabolized by cytochrome P450 3A4 isoenzyme.

Continued

Characteristics of antidepressants used during cancer treatment—cont'd

Medication	Oral dose (mg/day)	Primary side effects	Comments
Venlafaxine (Effexor, Effexor XR)	225-375; XR: 37.5-225	May increase blood pressure; fewer sexual side effects; achieves steady state in 3 days	SNRI, also inhibits dopamine reuptake Avoid abrupt discontinuation Effective in treatment of hot flashes related to chemotherapy and hormonal therapy Available as extended release

17. How do antidepressants work?

Most antidepressants work by restoring balance between receptors that control neurotransmitter release. For example, amitriptyline inhibits the membrane pump mechanism responsible for uptake of norepinephrine and serotonin in adrenergic and serotonergic neurons, thereby potentiating serotonin and norepinephrine activity. SSRIs selectively inhibit the reuptake of serotonin ($5HT_3$) at the presynaptic neuronal membrane.

18. Are the newer antidepressants more effective than the older TCAs?

Clinicians often believe that the newer antidepressants (e.g., SSRIs) are more effective with fewer side effects (e.g., less sedating and autonomic side effects). However, evidence-based guidelines commissioned by the Agency for Healthcare Research and Quality recommend that clinicians should consider TCAs and newer antidepressants as equally effective in the treatment of primary care patients with acute major depression or dysthymia. The side-effect profiles of both old and new antidepressants should be reviewed jointly by clinician and patient to accommodate the patient's clinical needs.

19. Do patients with cancer require lower doses of TCAs?

Although the reason is not clear, depressed patients with cancer often have a therapeutic response at much lower doses (10-125 mg/day) than other populations (150-300 mg/day). Plasma levels should be monitored to ensure adequate dosing, because medically ill patients and those with advanced cancer often have therapeutic plasma levels at modest dosages.

20. Can antidepressants be administered by alternatative routes?

- For patients who cannot take medications orally, most TCAs are available as rectal suppositories. However, absorption by this route has not been studied in patients with cancer.
- Some antidepressants are also available in an elixir (amitriptyline, nortriptyline, doxepin, fluoxetine, or paroxetine).
- Parenteral administration of TCAs should be considered for patients who are unable to tolerate oral administration because of absence of the swallowing reflex, presence of gastric or jejunal drainage tubes, or intestinal obstruction.
  - Although intravenous (IV) clomipramine (Anafranil), imipramine (Tofranil), maprotiline (Ludiomil) have been widely used abroad, only amitriptyline (Elavil)

and citalopram (Celexa) are approved and available for parenteral administration in the United States.

○ Amitriptyline, imipramine, and doxepin can be given intramuscularly (IM). However, the IM route may cause excessive bleeding in patients with low platelet levels as well as discomfort due to the volume of the diluent. The maximal dose that can be delivered by IM injection is usually 50 mg.

● Emsam (selegiline transdermal system), an MAOI, is the first transdermal patch for the treatment of major depressive disorder (MDD) in adults.

21. How effective are psychostimulants in treating depression in patients with cancer?

The psychostimulants (e.g., dextroamphetamine, methylphenidate, and pemoline) offer an alternative and effective pharmacologic approach to the treatment of depression in patients with cancer. They have a more rapid onset of action than TCAs, and relatively low doses are useful for patients with depressed mood, apathy, decreased energy, poor concentration, weakness, psychomotor slowing, and mild cognitive impairment. These agents stimulate appetite, promote a sense of well-being, improve attention and concentration, and improve feelings of weakness and fatigue in patients with cancer. Psychostimulants also help to counter the sedating effects of opioids.

22. Describe the dosing of psychostimulants in patients with cancer.

Treatment with dextroamphetamine or methylphenidate typically begins with a dose of 2.5 mg at 8:00 AM and at noon. The dosage is slowly increased over several days until a desired effect is achieved or until side effects intervene. Usually a dose greater than 30 mg/day is not necessary, although occasionally a patient may require up to 60 mg/day. Patients usually are maintained on methylphenidate for 1 to 2 months; in approximately two thirds of patients, methylphenidate can be withdrawn without recurrence of depressive symptoms. Patients with recurring symptoms can be maintained on a psychostimulant for up to 1 year without significant abuse problems. Pemoline has the advantage of less abuse potential, mild sympathomimetic effects, and lack of federal regulation through special triplicate prescriptions.

Dosing of psychostimulants in patients with cancer

Medication	Daily oral dose (mg)	Primary side effects	Comments
All psychostimulants		May cause nightmares	Onset of action < 24 hours. Administer in morning and at noon. Advantages in patients with cancer: rapid onset, analgesic adjuvant, counter sedation of opiates

Continued

Dosing of psychostimulants in patients with cancer—cont'd

Medication	Daily oral dose (mg)	Primary side effects	Comments
Dextroamphetamine (Dexedrine)	2.5-3.0	Insomnia, anxiety, agitation, restlessness	Energizes, stimulates appetite, promotes sense of well-being, improves feelings of weakness and fatigue
Methylphendidate (Ritalin)	2.5-3.0	Mild increase in blood pressure and pulse Confusion in elderly Possible cardiac complications in elderly or those with heart disease Rare: dyskinesias or motor tics, mood liability, paranoid psychosis	Particularly useful in patients with advanced cancer, psychomotor slowing, and mild cognitive impairment
Pemoline (Cylert)	37.5-150	Liver injury (monitor liver function tests) Use with caution in renal failure	Onset of action: 1-2 days Unrelated to amphetamine Advantages for patients with cancer: mild sympathomimetic effects, lack of abuse potential, available as a chewable tablet

23. How frequently does anxiety occur in patients with cancer?

About 4% to 5% of patients with cancer have preexisting anxiety disorders. More than two thirds of patients with cancer who have a psychiatric disorder also have reactive depression or anxiety, which is an adjustment disorder with depressed or anxious mood.

24. List the different types of anxiety.

- Reactive anxiety
- Organic anxiety disorders
- Phobias, panic disorders, chronic anxiety disorders

25. What causes reactive anxiety?

Reactive anxiety usually is related to the stresses of cancer and its treatment. It is an exaggerated form of the normal anxious response and is the most common type of anxiety in patients with cancer. Many, if not all, patients experience some anxiety at critical moments during evaluation, diagnosis, and treatment (e.g., various tests, surgery, chemotherapy, awaiting test results). Reactive anxiety is distinguished from typical fears of cancer by the duration and intensity of symptoms and the degree of functional impairment.

Such anxiety may disrupt the ability to function normally, interfere with interpersonal relationships, and even affect the ability to understand and comply with cancer treatments.

26. What are organic anxiety disorders?

Organic anxiety disorders are anxiety disorders of medical origin. Patients with pain are exposed to multiple potential organic causes of anxiety: medications that produce withdrawal states, uncontrolled pain, infection, some hormone-producing tumors, and abnormal metabolic states. Patients in acute pain and those with acute or chronic respiratory distress often appear anxious.

27. Describe the relationship between cancer and chronic anxiety disorders.

Phobias, panic, and chronic anxiety disorders may predate the cancer diagnosis but can be exacerbated during illness. Occasionally, patients have their first episode of panic or phobia in the cancer setting. A number of variants of anxiety disorders (e.g., panic attack, needle phobia, claustrophobia) can prevent cancer diagnostic work-ups and complicate or halt treatment.

28. What are the common symptoms of anxiety?

Common symptoms of anxiety include nervousness, fidgeting, palpitations, tremulousness, diaphoresis, shortness of breath, diarrhea, intestinal cramping, numbness and tingling of extremities, feelings of imminent death, derealization or depersonalization, phobias, and fearfulness.

29. What types of psychological treatments are used for anxiety in patients with cancer?

Several psychological approaches—cognitive-behavioral therapy, brief supportive therapy, crisis intervention, insight-oriented psychotherapy, and behavioral interventions—can be used alone or in combination to treat anxiety in patients with cancer. Biofeedback, guided imagery, meditation, progressive relaxation, and hypnosis are behavioral approaches that can be used to treat anxiety symptoms associated with adverse side effects to cancer and its treatment, pain syndromes, anxiety while awaiting test results, and anticipatory fears.

30. What pharmacologic agents are useful in treating anxiety?

Usually an anxiolytic medication is combined with a psychologic approach. Pharmacotherapy for anxiety in patients with cancer involves the judicious use of the following classes of drugs: benzodiazepines, neuroleptics, antihistamines, antidepressants, and opioid analgesics.

31. List the commonly used benzodiazepine anxiolytics, along with dosage, duration of action, half-life, and route of administration.

Commonly used benzodiazepine anxiolytics

Medication	Dosage range (mg)	Duration of action	Half-life (hr)	Route	Comments
Midazolam (Versed)	10-60/day	Very short	2-7	IV, SC	Used to decrease anxiety in patients undergoing procedures

Continued

Commonly used benzodiazepine anxiolytics—cont'd

Medication	Dosage range (mg)	Duration of action	Half-life (hr)	Route	Comments
Alprazolam (Xanax)	0.25-2.0 tid-qid	Short	10-15	PO, SL	Metabolized through oxidative pathways in liver, making it more vulnerable to cause hepatic damage. Can be absorbed SL in patients with dysphagia
Oxazepam (Serax)	10-15 tid-qid	Short	5-15	PO	Metabolized by liver and excreted by kidney. Safest in patients with hepatic disease
Lorazepam (Ativan)	0.5-2.0 tid-qid	Short	10-20	PO, SL, IV, IM	Metabolized by liver and excreted by kidney. Safest in patients with hepatic disease. Lacks active metabolites
Chlordiazep-oxide (Librium)	10-50 tid-qid	Intermediate	5-30	PO, IM	
Diazepam (Valium)	5-10 bid-qid	Long	20-70	PO, IM, IV, PR	Can be administered rectally and parenterally to dying patients
Clorazepate (Tranxene)	7.5-15 bid-qid	Long	30-200	PO	
Clonazepam (Klonopin)	0.5-2 bid-qid	Long	30-40	PO	Useful for painful symptoms, insomnia, neuropathic pain, depersonalization in patients with seizure disorders, brain tumors, and mild organic mental disorders

tid = 3 times/day; qid = 4 times/day; bid = 2 times/day; IV = intravenously; SC = subcutaneously; PO = orally; SL = sublingually; IM = intramuscularly; PR = rectally

32. How are the benzodiazepines used in the oncology setting?

Benzodiazepines are the most commonly used pharmacologic treatment of anxiety in patients with cancer. They not only decrease daytime anxiety but also reduce insomnia. The dosing schedule depends on tolerance and requires individual titration. The most common side effects are dose-dependent and controlled by titration: drowsiness, confusion, lack of motor coordination, and sedation. All benzodiazepines can cause respiratory depression and must be used cautiously, if at all, in patients with respiratory impairment. The depressant effects are additive or even synergistic in the presence of other drugs, such as antidepressants, antiemetics, and opioids.

The shorter-acting benzodiazepines (lorazepam, alprazolam, and oxazepam) are the safest to prescribe for patients with cancer. However, their disadvantage is that patients often experience breakthrough anxiety or end-of-dose failure. If either occurs, patients should be switched to longer-acting benzodiazepines, such as diazepam or clonazepam. Diazepam can be administered rectally or parenterally to dying patients with dosages equivalent to oral regimens. Rectal diazepam has been used widely in palliative care to control anxiety, restlessness, and agitation associated with the final days of life. Drugs with rapid onset of effect (e.g., lorazepam, diazepam) are most effective for high levels of distress.

33. Besides the benzodiazepines, what other agents can be used to treat anxiety?

- **Neuroleptics,** such as thioridazine and haloperidol, are useful in the treatment of anxiety when benzodiazepines are not sufficient and when anxiety is accompanied by psychotic symptoms (e.g., delusions, hallucinations).
- **Hydroxyzine,** an antihistamine, can be quite useful in treating anxious, terminally ill patients who are in pain, because it may potentiate the analgesic effects of opioids.
- **Buspirone** is a useful adjunct to psychotherapy in patients with chronic anxiety or anxiety related to adjustment disorders. The onset of anxiolytic action is delayed compared to the benzodiazepines (5-10 days). Because buspirone is not a benzodiazepine, it does not block benzodiazepine withdrawal; thus the clinician must be cautious when switching from a benzodiazepine to buspirone. It is best used for older adult patients, patients who have not previously been treated with a benzodiazepine, and patients at risk of habituation with benzodiazepines.
- **Tricyclic and heterocyclic antidepressants** are the most effective treatment for anxiety accompanying depression and are helpful in treating panic disorder. In dying patients, however, their usefulness is often limited by anticholinergic and sedative side effects and slower onset of action (5-10 days).

34. List the dosage range and route of administration for nonbenzodiazepine anxiolytics.

Commonly used nonbenzodiazepine anxiolytics

Medication	Dosage range (mg)	Route	Comments
Buspirone (BuSpar)	5-20 tid	PO	Useful adjunct to psychotherapy in patients with chronic anxiety or anxiety related to adjustment disorders Onset of anxiolytic action is delayed

Continued

Commonly used nonbenzodiazepine anxiolytics—cont'd

Medication	Dosage range (mg)	Route	Comments
Neuroleptics			
Haloperidol (Haldol)	0.5-5 every 2-12 hr	PO, IV, SC, IM	Indicated when an organic cause is suspected, or psychotic symptoms, such as delusions or hallucinations, accompany anxiety
Trifluoperazine (Stelazine)	1-6 once a day	PO, IM	
Chlorpromazine (Thorazine)	12.5-50 every 4-12 hr	PO, IM, IV	Low doses are safe and relatively effective when respiratory distress is a concern
Antihistamine			
Hydroxyzine (Atarax, Vistaril)	25-50 every 4-6 hr	PO, IV, SC	Mild anxiolytic, mild antiemetic, sedative, and analgesic properties. Low doses are safe and relatively effective when respiratory distress is a concern
Tricyclic antidepressants			
Imipramine (Tofranil)	12.5-150 q HS	PO, IM	Indicated in anxiety accompanying depression, helpful in treating panic disorder. Limited use in dying patients because of anticholinergic and sedative side effects
Clomipramine (Anafranil)	10-150 q HS	PO	Same as for imipramine

35. Are patients with cancer who take drugs for depression or anxiety at risk for addiction?

Concerns about addiction in patients with no history of drug abuse are exaggerated. Fear of addiction is a factor in the under treatment of depression, anxiety, and pain. Patients, physicians, and nurses share this fear. Although tolerance and physical dependence commonly occur, addiction (psychologic dependence) is rare in patients with no history of substance abuse.

36. Should cancer patients with a history of substance abuse receive any pharmacologic treatment for depression or anxiety?

Treatment of depression and anxiety should not be neglected in patients with a history of substance abuse. They should be assessed carefully and given the opportunity for treatment with psychological techniques in conjunction with cautious medication use and observation for signs of drug dependence.

37. How common is suicide in patients with cancer?

Patients with cancer have a 2- to 3-fold greater risk of committing suicide compared to the general population, and a 2.5- to 10-fold increase in suicide rates compared with the general population. The greatest risk is immediately after diagnosis (within 6 months). Published studies report a 0% to 17% incidence of suicidal ideation, which is limited to significantly depressed patients. Clinically, however, many health care providers report that thoughts of suicide probably occur quite frequently, particularly in patients with advanced cancer. Suicidal thoughts are often fleeting and may act as an outlet for feelings related to an overwhelming situation. They may be a last attempt at control by the patient who views suicide as a way out. Within the context of a trusting, safe relationship with the nurse, patients may reveal that they have had occasional or even persisting thoughts of suicide as a means of escaping the threat of overwhelming pain or cancer itself.

38. When does suicide most frequently occur in cancer patients?

Patients with advanced illness are at highest risk, perhaps because they have the highest incidence of cancer complications, such as pain, depression, and debilitating side effects. Depression is a factor in 50% of all suicides. Patients suffering from depression are at 25-fold greater risk of suicide than the general population. The role of depression in cancer-related suicide is equally significant. Many patients with cancer experience hopelessness, which is a key variable that links depression and suicide in the general population.

39. What are the risk factors for suicide in patients with advanced cancer?

- Psychiatric factors: personal history of suicide attempts, family history of suicide, preexisting psychopathology, delirium, history of substance /alcohol abuse, depression, feelings of hopelessness
- Social factors: few or no social supports (not married, fewer than 6 friends or relatives, no membership in church or community groups), history of recent death of friends or spouse
- Cancer-related factors: diagnosis of head and neck or pancreatic cancers, uncontrolled pain or suffering associated with cancer, overwhelming fatigue, advanced illness or poor prognosis
- Advanced age

40. How can the nurse assess suicidal risk in patients with cancer?

Nurses must be willing to talk openly about suicide. To do so does *not* mean that the patient is going to commit suicide. No evidence supports the belief that suicidal thoughts are exacerbated by exploration. Warning signs that a patient is considering suicide include such actions as saying goodbye, giving away a treasured object, and wishing to be dead. The following strategies provide the nurse with a way to initiate a conversation about suicide (Roth & Brietbart, 1996). Open with a statement: "Most patients with cancer have passing thoughts about suicide, such as 'I might do something if things get bad enough.'"

- Acknowledge: "Have you ever had thoughts like that? Any thoughts of not wanting to go on or that it would be easier to die?"
- Plan: "Do you ever think about suicide? Have you ever thought about how you would do it?"
- Personal history: "Have you ever been depressed or treated for depression?"
- Substance abuse: "Have you ever had any drug or alcohol problems?"
- Bereavement: "Have you recently lost someone close to you?"

41. How can the nurse form a supportive relationship with the patient?

Nurses must be aware of their own emotional abilities and limitations to provide the best communication to patients. Ways for nurses to form a supportive relationship with the patient include the following:

- Listening
- Projecting an empathetic and welcoming attitude to the patient's concerns
- Reinforcing the patient's strengths
- Facilitating dialogue with family members
- Assuring the patient that what is said in confidence will not be shared unless permission is obtained
- Offering hope that something can be done to make the situation more tolerable

42. Give examples of unsupportive comments to cancer patients.

Usually it is not helpful for the nurse to tell the patient that he or she "knows" what the patient is feeling. Although a sympathetic approach is helpful, for the health professional to assume that he or she can know what the patient is feeling is dismissive of the patient's concerns. Each person's pain, emotional or physical, is unique and highly individualized. It is also not helpful to tell the patient that "this is God's will," or to minimize the patient's emotional pain.

Key Points

- Depression is an under-recognized problem in cancer patients that affects treatment outcomes and patients' quality of life and satisfaction with care.
- Distress extends along a continuum, ranging from normal feelings of vulnerability, sadness and fear, to disabling conditions, such as clinical depression, anxiety, panic, isolation, and existential or spiritual crisis.
- The biologic correlates, typically used for diagnosing depression in physically healthy adults, are frequently unreliable in patients with cancer.
- Depression is best diagnosed with a thorough interview and by simply asking patients whether they are depressed.
- A patient does not have to have a psychiatric diagnosis to receive treatment for psychological distress.
- Uncontrolled pain is a major risk factor for depression and suicide among cancer patients.
- Benzodiazepines are the most commonly used pharmacologic treatment of anxiety in patients with cancer.

Internet Resources

Agency for Health Care Research and Quality (AHRQ) Evidence Report, Management of Cancer Symptoms: Pain, Depression, Fatigue:
   http://www.ncbi.nlm.nih.gov/books/bv.fcgi?rid=hstat1a.chapter.5.
Antidepressant comparison table:
   http://www.CommunityOncology.net/journal/articles/0206528t.pdf
National Cancer Institute, Cancer Topics, Depression:
   http://www.cancer.gov/cancertopics/pdq/supportivecare/depression/HealthProfessional

Bibliography

Ables AZ, Baughman OL: Antidepressants: Update on new agents and indications. *Am Fam Physician* 67(3):547-554, 2003.

Adkins B, Titus-Howard T, Massey V, et al: Recognizing depression in cancer outpatients. *Community Oncology*, 528-533, 2005.

Barsevick AM, Sweeney C, Haney E, et al: A systematic qualitative analysis of psychoeducational interventions for depression in patients with cancer. *Oncol Nurs Forum* 29: 73-84, 2002.

Block SD: Assessing and managing depression in the terminally ill patient. *Ann Intern Med* 132:209-218, 2000.

Camp-Sorrell D, Hawkins RA, editors: *Clinical manual for the oncology advanced practice nurse,* ed 2, Pittsburgh, PA, 2006, Oncology Nursing Society.

Fulcher CD: Clinical challenges: Depression management during cancer treatment. *Oncol Nurs Forum* 33(1): 33-35, 2006.

Haight RJ: Choosing an antidepressant part 1: The selective serotonin reuptake inhibitors. *Hem/Onc Today,* 6-7, August 2005. Available at: http://www.hemonctoday.com/200508/frameset.asp?article= antidepressant.asp/. Accessed January 14, 2007.

Haight RJ: Choosing an antidepressant part 2: Mixed reuptake inhibitors. *Hem/Onc Today,* 16-17, September 2005. Available at: http://www.hemonctoday.com/200509/frameset.asp?article= antidepressant.asp. Accessed January 14, 2007.

Kroenke K, Spitzer RL, Williams JBW: The PHQ-9: Validity of a brief depression severity measure. *J Gen Intern Med* 16:606-613, 2001.

Lovejoy N, Tabor D, Deloney P: Cancer-related depression. Part II: Neurological alterations and evolving approaches to psychopharmacology. *Oncol Nurs Forum* 27:795-810, 2000.

Lovejoy N, Tabor D, Mattels M, et al: Cancer-related depression. Part I: Neurological alterations and cognitive-behavior therapy. *Oncol Nurs Forum* 27:667-680, 2000.

National Comprehensive Cancer Network: Distress management, clinical practice guidelines in oncology, Version.1. 2007. Available at: http://www.nccn.org/professionals/physician_gls/PDF/distress.pdf. Accessed January 16, 2007.

Massie MJ: Prevalence of depression in cancer. *J Natl Cancer Inst Monogr* 32:105-111, 2004.

Patrick DL, Ferketich SL, Frame PS, et al: National Institutes of Health State-of-the-Science Conference Statement, Symptom Management in Cancer: Pain, Depression, and Fatigue, July 15-17, 2002. *J Natl Cancer Inst*, 95, 1110-1117, 2003.

Roth A, Brietbart W: Psychiatric emergencies in terminally ill cancer patients. *Hematol Oncol Clin North Am* 10:235-259, 1996.

Roth A, Massie MJ, Redd WH: Consultation for the cancer patient. In Jacobson JL, Jacobson AJ, editors: *Psychiatric secrets,* ed 2, Philadelphia, 2001, Hanley & Belfus.

Snow V, Lascher S, Mottur-Pilson D: Clinical guideline. Part 1: Pharmacologic treatment of acute major depression and dysthymia. *Ann Intern Med* 132:738-742, 2000.

Valentine A: Depression, anxiety, and delirium. In R Padzur, LR Coia, WJ Hoskins, et al, editors: *Cancer management: Multidisciplinary approach,* ed 9, Lawrence, KS, 2005, CMP Healthcare Media.

Williams JW, Mulrow CD, Chiquette E, et al: Clinical guideline. Part 2: A systematic review of newer pharmacotherapies for depression in adults: Evidence report summary. *Ann Intern Med* 132:743-756, 2000.

Zabora J, Brintzenofeszoc K, Curbow B, et al: The prevalence of psychological distress by cancer site. *Psychooncology,* 10:19-28, 2001.

Chapter 35

Diarrhea and Constipation

Constance Engelking

1. Distinguish between diarrhea and constipation.

Although diarrhea and constipation are relatively high incidence problems in cancer patients, both are underreported and often mismanaged. Both gastrointestinal abnormalities are multicausal and associated with degree of stool consistency and defecation frequency. Because bowel patterns vary from patient to patient, it is important to determine whether changes in frequency and consistency are of sufficient magnitude to constitute an abnormal change in the patient's established bowel pattern. Using standardized definitions or objective measurements can help to make that determination.

- Diarrhea is an increase in stool liquidity and frequency. It is defined as more than 3 stools and/or 300 ml per day, or stool that conforms to the shape of its container.
- Constipation is a decrease in stools that are smaller, harder, and drier than the patient's normal stool consistency. According to the Rome II Criteria, constipation is characterized by two or more of the following symptoms occurring at least 25% of the time: straining to evacuate stool, passing lumpy or hard stools, having a sensation of incomplete bowel evacuation, needing manual evacuation of stool, and having two or fewer bowel movements per week.

2. What symptoms may be associated with both diarrhea and constipation?

- Abdominal cramping
- Pain
- Flatulence
- Bloating or distension of abdomen
- Anorexia, nausea and/or vomiting, according to severity

3. What are the consequences of untreated or inadequately managed diarrhea and constipation?

- **Undertreated or untreated diarrhea and constipation** may affect quality of life, causing irregular sleep patterns, fatigue and discomfort, reduction in performance, disturbance in interpersonal relationships and socialization, altered self-image, travel restrictions, absenteeism from work, hospitalization, and increased family/caregiver burden.
- **Uncontrolled diarrhea** can result in volume depletion, significant losses of potassium and bicarbonate, perianal irritation and denuding with secondary infection. It may also affect tumor response by producing treatment dose reductions and delays, thus limiting the total dose patients are able to receive.
- **Undertreated or untreated constipation** can lead to obstipation (fecal impaction) severe enough to require surgical intervention. Reluctance or refusal to take opioids because of their constipating effects can result in poor pain control.

4. What pathophysiologic mechanisms produce diarrhea and constipation?

The pathophysiologic changes are related to the movement of fluid and fecal matter through the bowel and the rate of water absorption and/or secretion. Balanced transport of intestinal fluid and electrolytes in the bowel are the result of two principal processes: (1) secretion, believed to take place in the crypt cells, and (2) absorption, which occurs in the enterocytes lining the wall of the gastrointestinal (GI) villi. These physiologic processes are mediated by neural, endocrine, and luminal physiologic mechanisms. Normally, the intestines handle about 8.5 L of fluid per day (7 L secreted through the gut wall plus 1.5 L ingested). All but approximately 1 L is reabsorbed in the jejunum. That liter of fluid enters the colon, where another 800 ml is absorbed, leaving about 200 ml to be excreted in the stool. Interestingly, there is only about a 100 ml difference between constipation and diarrhea in relation to fluid excretion.

5. What are key assessment parameters for diarrhea and constipation?

Key parameters in comprehensive bowel evaluation include:

HISTORY

- **Usual bowel pattern:** Determine the consistency and number of stools per day or week.
- **Tumor type, location, and extent of disease.** Determine whether the patient's cancer can produce bowel dysfunction. Some malignant diseases, such as carcinoid and VIPoma, are specifically associated with diarrhea. Others, such as colorectal and pancreatic cancers, can produce diarrhea as secondary effects. Obstructing bowel tumors or neurologic tumors involving the nerves responsible for producing peristalsis can cause constipation.
- **Coexisting conditions and treatments.** Abdominopelvic radiation, bowel resection (with or without diversion), irritable or inflammatory bowel syndrome, or other conditions (e.g., neurologic disorder, malnutrition) can cause or intensify diarrhea. Constipation can accompany vinca alkaloid or opioid therapy, tumors that produce bowel obstruction, or spinal cord compression that interfere with bowel innervation.
- **Medications.** Obtain the patient's medications list because drugs are often responsible for bowel dysfunction (see Questions 10, 11, and 19). The temporal relationship between onset/duration and initiation or discontinuation of chemotherapy, radiotherapy, or other medication helps to distinguish whether bowel dysfunction is a response to treatment or due to some other cause.
- **Dietary pattern.** Assess current diet, daily fluid intake, and changes in diet habits or pattern. Food allergies, lactose intolerance, consumption of alcohol and sorbitol-based products can all produce diarrhea. Patients whose oral intake of food and fluids has decreased are at risk for developing constipation. Also query the patient about weight trends during the previous few weeks to a month.
- **Other factors.** Patients who have traveled outside the country during the past year or live with family members who have diarrhea could be at risk for developing diarrhea related to infectious etiologies. Patients who are unable to move their bowels because they lack privacy or need to use unfamiliar or uncomfortable facilities (e.g., public bathrooms, bedpans) are at risk for developing constipation.

PHYSICAL EXAMINATION

- **Presenting signs and symptoms.** Ask patients to describe recent changes and current bowel pattern, including stool character (consistency, color, odor), volume, frequency, and associated symptoms (e.g., pain, cramping, flatulence). Visually inspect stool for consistency and evidence of blood, pus, or mucus. Patient weight is particularly important when quantification of diarrheal stool volume is difficult. The presence of fever and bloody diarrhea may point to an infectious cause.
- **Abdominorectal evaluation.** Auscultate for hyperactive or absent bowel sounds, and perform abdominal palpation for tenderness or presence of masses (stool-filled colon). A rectal examination also may be indicated to rule out fecal impaction in patients who are constipated. In patients with stool incontinence or

severe diarrhea, inspect anal and peristomal areas for impaired skin integrity, hemorrhoids, evidence of fecal impaction, or rectal malignancy.

- **Hydration status**. Assess objective measures of hydration, including thirst level, vein filling and emptying times, skin turgor and resiliency, degree of mucosal moisture (conjunctiva, lips, tongue, oral mucosa), vital signs, fluid intake and output, and osmolality and specific gravity of urine. Note indicators of dehydration and electrolyte imbalances (e.g. poor skin turgor, dry mucosal surfaces, periorbital edema, highly concentrated urine, changes in mentation, weight loss exceeding 2 lbs/day, tachycardia, and orthostatic blood pressure changes with accompanying vertigo and weakness).

LABORATORY AND DIAGNOSTIC ANALYSES
- Laboratory studies are done to detect electrolyte/metabolic abnormalities (hypokalemia, hypercalcemia) and evidence of protein/calorie malnutrition (e.g., hypoalbuminemia).
- Complete blood count; an elevated white blood cell count may indicate an infection.
- Positive findings of a Hemoccult test may signal an intraluminal lesion is causing the constipation.
- To rule out infection in cases of diarrhea, obtain stool cultures to test for the presence of enteric pathogens, including *Shigella, Campylobacter*, and *Salmonella spp.* Stool samples should also be tested for the presence of *Clostridium difficile* toxin, and ova/parasites (ova and parasite testing are not necessary for patients who develop diarrhea while hospitalized). Obtain tests for viral agents (adeno-viruses, rotaviruses, coxsackie viruses), particularly in patients who have had a bone marrow transplant.
- When carcinoid is the suspected cause of diarrhea, determine urine 5-HIAA (serotonin metabolite) level.
- Radiographic evaluation (supine and upright) with contrast, endoscopic exploration, and biopsy are reserved for ruling out mechanical obstruction and ileus, finding possible causes of persistent diarrhea that is refractory to intervention, or for ruling out conditions requiring tissue diagnosis.
- Ultrasound and/or computed tomography scan of the abdomen and pelvis are performed if an extraluminal site is suspected. Barium enema and endoscopy are recommended if an intraluminal site is suspected.

6. What assessment instruments are used most often to document severity of bowel dysfunction and its effects on quality of life ?
- The National Cancer Institute (NCI) Common Toxicity Criteria for Adverse Events (CTC-AE) are commonly used tools (four point grading scales) to measure diarrhea and constipation in the clinical setting. However, the scale for diarrhea is more detailed, measuring the number of loose stools per day along with accompanying symptoms and therapeutic requirements. The constipation scale is less definitive about stool frequency and consistency and relies more on the patient's requirement for therapeutic intervention. Both scales, presented on the opposite page can be accessed via the NCI website.
- The FACT–G (Functional Assessment of Cancer Therapy–General) and FACT-D (Functional Assessment of Cancer Therapy–Diarrhea) questionnaires as well as the LASA (Linear Analogue Scale) can be used to measure quality-of-life dimensions.
- Because both diarrhea and constipation are subjective self-report symptoms, use of a daily or weekly log can provide invaluable information that helps in problem analysis. The tool on the opposite page is for patients with constipation but could be customized for diarrhea or a general bowel function log.

NCI diarrhea grading scale

Adverse event	1	2	3	4
Diarrhea	Increase of < 4 stools per day over baseline; mild increase in ostomy output compared to baseline	Increase of 4-6 stools per day over baseline; IV fluids indicated < 24 hrs; moderate increase in ostomy output compared to baseline; not interfering with ADL	Increase of ≥ 7 stools per day over baseline; incontinence; IV fluids ≥ 24 hrs; hospitalization; severe increase in ostomy output compared to baseline; interfering with ADL	Life-threatening consequences (e.g., hemodynamic collapse)

NCI constipation grading scale

Adverse event	1	2	3	4
Constipation	Occasional or intermittent symptoms; occasional use of stool softeners, laxatives, dietary modification, or enema	Persistent symptoms with regular use of laxatives or enemas as indicated	Symptoms interfering with ADL; obstipation with manual evacuation indicated	Life-threatening consequences (e.g., obstruction, toxic megacolon)

Seven-day stool diary

Date
Time of bowel movement
Straining (yes/no)
Feeling of incomplete evacuation (yes/no)
Stool consistency (1-7, from Bristol Stool Scale)
Urge (yes/no)
Digital maneuvers (yes/no)
Drug therapies (including over-the-counter)

DIARRHEA

7. How prevalent is diarrhea in cancer patients?

Cancer-related diarrhea occurs in up to 10% of patients with advanced cancer, 20% to 49% of patients undergoing abdominopelvic irradiation, 50% to 87% of patients receiving fluoropyrimidines (e.g., 5-fluorouracil [5-FU]) and topoisomerase inhibitors (e.g., irinotecan), 43% of patients undergoing bone marrow transplant, and 80% of patients with carcinoid tumors. As newer antineoplastic agents (e.g., platinum analogues, targeted therapies) and higher dosages of drugs and radiation therapy are introduced into treatment regimens, it is anticipated that diarrhea prevalence will rise. A significant number of patients receiving supportive care with nasogastric feedings, high-osmolar compounds, and antibiotic therapy also experience diarrhea.

8. What pathophysiologic mechanisms occur with diarrhea?

Diarrhea occurs when the balance between intestinal secretion and absorption is disrupted so that the total secretion of fluid and electrolytes overwhelms the absorptive capacity of the bowel. These processes are influenced by a number of mechanical and biochemical factors. Increased secretion may occur in response to the release of endogenous secretagogues (inflammatory mediators, neurotransmitters) and bacterial endotoxins, which overstimulate ion transport processes. Decreased absorption results from defects in villus absorptive processes (e.g., reduced number of villi secondary to bowel surgery), osmotically active agents in the lumen of the bowel (e.g., blood from intestinal hemorrhage, enteral feeding solutions), or increased intestinal motility. (See table on pp. 377-379 for types of diarrhea and specific causes).

9. What is the difference between acute and chronic diarrhea?

- **Acute** diarrhea is characterized by sudden onset and duration of 7 to 14 days. Especially high stool output (i.e., 8-10 L/day) may occur in patients who have undergone allogeneic stem cell transplant and developed graft-versus-host disease (GVHD). Frequently, patients with acute diarrhea also experience abdominal cramping. In patients with neutropenia, fever may also accompany diarrhea. This triad of symptoms (diarrhea, abdominal cramping, and fever) is referred to as gastrointestinal syndrome and requires immediate intervention. Untreated, acute diarrhea can produce life-threatening dehydration and electrolyte disturbances.
- **Chronic** diarrhea has a more gradual onset and persists beyond 2 weeks in spite of antidiarrheal treatment. In addition to dehydration, chronic diarrhea may contribute to the development of malnutrition and an array of other problems.

10. What pharmacologic agents are most often associated with diarrhea?

Diarrhea onset, severity, and duration depend on many factors, including the pharmacologic agent being taken, its use in combination with other diarrhea-producing drugs or therapies (such as combination chemotherapy and biotherapy regimens or abdominopelvic radiation therapy), and dosages. Opiate withdrawal and the overuse of laxatives are also implicated.

- Agents associated with the highest risk for chemotherapy-induced diarrhea (CID) are 5-FU (especially in high doses or in combination with leucovorin, methotrexate, or interferon), actinomycin D, the topoisomerase inhibitors (irinotecan, topotecan), paclitaxel (Taxol), and high doses of cisplatin or cyclophosphamide. Administration of 5-FU in lower doses as a continuous infusion is associated with a lower incidence of diarrhea than treatment with higher doses given as a weekly bolus. Other agents that cause diarrhea (~10%) are fludarabine, cytarabine,

Text continued on p. 380.

Pathophysiologic mechanisms, causes, and clinical manifestations of cancer-related diarrhea

Type of diarrhea	Pathophysiologic mechanisms	Causes	Clinical manifestations
Osmotic	Mechanical disturbance Characterized by large-volume influx of fluid and electrolytes into intestinal lumen that overwhelms absorptive capacity of bowel Osmotic forces responsible for drawing substrates across the intestinal epithelium are interrupted by direct contact with hyperosmolar stimuli.	Ingestion of hyperosmolar preparations and substances Nonabsorbable solutes (e.g. sorbitol, magnesium-based antacids) Enteral feeding solutions Intestinal hemorrhage Intraluminal blood, acting as osmotic substance	Large-volume, watery stools that resolve with withdrawal of causative agent
Malabsorptive	Combined disturbance of mechanical and biochemical mechanisms responsible for maintaining absorptive processes Secondary to factors that alter luminal mucosal integrity and nature Reduction in available mucosa or membrane permeability disrupts enterohepatic circulation of bile salts; unabsorbed osmotically active substances then can enter colon, exerting direct bowel stimulatory effects	Enzyme deficiencies that prevent complete digestion of fats Lactose intolerance Pancreatic insufficiency due to obstruction by cancer or pancreatectomy Morphologic/structural changes resulting in decreased absorptive capacity Surgical resection of intestine Mucosal changes that alter membrane permeability	Large-volume, foul-smelling steatorrhea-type stools

Continued

Pathophysiologic mechanisms, causes, and clinical manifestations of cancer-related diarrhea—cont'd

Type of diarrhea	Pathophysiologic mechanisms	Causes	Clinical manifestations
Exudative	Characterized by discharge of mucus, serum protein, blood into bowel Results from inflammation or ulceration of bowel mucosa	Radiation to bowel mucosa; incidence and severity are dose-dependent Acute effects are caused by depletion of crypt stem cells Late or chronic radiation enteritis secondary to mucosal atrophy and fibrosis	Variable volume (< 1000 ml/day) but high frequency stools (> 6 stools/day); associated with hypoalbuminemia, anemia from cumulative protein, blood loss
Secretory	Primarily biomechanical disturbance with mechanical responses Characterized by intestinal hypersecretion stimulated by an array of endogenous mediators that exert primary effect of intestinal transport of water and electrolytes, resulting in accumulation of intestinal fluids	Endocrine tumors can produce excessive quantities of peptide secretagogues VIPoma, carcinoid, gastrinoma, insulinoma, glucagonoma Enterotoxin-producing pathogens irritate bowel wall, stimulating intestinal secretion Associated with antibiotic-induced change in microbial flora that permits growth of *C. difficile*	Large-volume, watery stools (> 1000 ml/day) that persist despite fasting; osmolality equals plasma concentration

| Dysmotility-associated | Mechanical disturbances characterized by deranged intestinal motility resulting in rapid transit of stool through small/large intestine
Peristaltic dysfunction (enhancement of suppression) in response to alteration in variety of mechanical stretch or neural stimuli | Clinical problems (e.g. irritable bowel syndrome, narcotic withdrawal symptoms)
External factors such as ingestion of peristaltic stimulants (food, fluid, or medication) or psychoneuroimmunologic effects of stress, anxiety, and fear | Frequent small, semi-solid/liquid stools of variable volume and frequency |
| Chemotherapy-induced | Combined mechanical and biochemical disturbances stimulated by chemotherapeutic effects on bowel mucosa
Characterized by cascade of events; mitotic arrest of intestinal epithelial crypt cells followed by superficial necrosis and extensive inflammation of bowel wall resulting in production of mucosal, submucosal factors (leukotrienes, cytokines, free radicals) that subsequently stimulate oversecretion of intestinal water and electrolytes
Destruction of brush border enzymes responsible for carbohydrate and protein digestion further adds to excessive gut-wall secretion | Chemotherapy-induced gut wall toxicity
Although many agents are associated with diarrhea, most common include fluoropyrimidines (e.g., 5-FU) and topoisomerase inhibitors (e.g., CPT-11) | Frequent watery to semisolid stools; onset occurs within 24-96 hours after chemotherapy administration |

From Rutledge DN, Engelking C: Cancer-related diarrhea: Selected findings of a national survey of oncology nurse experiences. *Oncol Nurs Forum* 25.862, 1998.

idarubicin, mithramycin, mitoxantrone, pentostatin, oxaliplatin, and floxuridine. Severe diarrhea occurring with administration of 5-FU and floxuridine is a sign of toxicity and requires cessation of therapy until resolution of diarrhea. With other agents, dose reduction on subsequent cycles or discontinuation may be indicated, depending on the chemotherapy schedule and severity of diarrhea.

- Biotherapy drugs: interleukin-2, interleukin-4, interferons, multikinase inhibitors
- Antibiotics: especially ampicillin, clindamycin, and broad-spectrum antibiotics that alter normal gastrointestinal flora or inflame the intestinal mucosa
- Other agents: antacids (especially magnesium-containing compounds), selected cytoprotectants (e.g., mesna), antiemetics (e.g., metoclopramide), antihypertensives, potassium supplements, diuretics, caffeine, theophylline, NSAIDs, antiarrhythmic drugs

11. What are some unique drug- or treatment-induced mechanisms that result in diarrhea and what is the best practice for management?

- **Camptosar (irinotecan)** produces both an early-onset cholinergic syndrome (during or within 24 hours of drug administration) and late-onset diarrhea (2-10 days after drug administration).
  - The early-onset cholinergic syndrome is an infrequent response in which diarrhea is generally a sudden occurrence accompanying other symptoms (e.g., abdominal cramping, diaphoresis, flushing, salivation, nasal congestion, rhinorrhea) that readily resolves after treatment with atropine, 0.25 to 1.0 mg intravenously or subcutaneously, but requires close patient monitoring.
  - Late-onset diarrhea occurs most commonly during the second week after treatment with a median duration of 3 days. It may be severe (grades 3 or 4) and last up to 7 days. Its occurrence may be related to the accumulation and deconjugation of SN-38 (the active metabolite of irinotecan) in the intestine and its damaging effect on the mucosa. Management involves recognition of high-risk patients and prophylaxis. Before drug administration, patients should be taught to self-administer high-dose loperamide, beginning with a loading dose of 4 mg po, followed by 2 mg at 4-hour intervals.
- **Fluoropyrimidines** can produce severe diarrhea if the patient has dihydropyrimidine dehydrogenase (DPD) deficiency, which should be suspected if the patient experiences sudden onset of diarrhea accompanied by significant mucositis and myelosuppression. This occurs in approximately 3% of adult patients with cancer. DPD is the rate-limiting enzyme that allows clearance of 5-FU. Patients who have congenital DPD deficiencies are at risk for severe adverse drug reactions after exposure to 5-FU. Recognition of this pharmacogenetic syndrome is essential to prevent the risk of severe and potentially fatal reactions to fluoropyrimidine therapy, such as cerebellar ataxia, encephalopathy, and coma.
- **Antibiotics,** particularly ampicillin, cephalosporins, and clindamycin, can cause *Clostridium difficile* diarrhea. *C. difficile* makes enterotoxins that produce watery diarrhea associated with pseudomembranous colitis. Symptoms range from mild diarrhea to life-threatening illness. *C. difficile* causes more than 50% of nosocomial infectious diarrhea. After a patient has tested positive for *C. difficile* and toxin A, precautions should be taken to prevent nosocomial transmission. When treating infectious diarrhea, it is important for the patient to avoid taking anticholinergic agents or opiates because they slow peristalsis and inhibit elimination of toxins from the gastrointestinal system, causing prolonged and severe symptoms. *C. difficile* diarrhea usually is treated with metronidazole or oral vancomycin. Note: Because of recent genetic changes in the *C. difficile* bacteria, oral vancomycin is emerging as the drug of choice.

- **Laxative dependence.** The natural defecation reflex, which empties the large bowel from the descending colon downward, is triggered when the sigmoid colon and rectum are full. The reflex is not triggered again until the colon segments are refilled. Unlike the natural reflex, large-bowel irritant purgatives (anthraquinone derivatives such as senna, and diphenylmethane derivatives such as bisacodyl and phenolphthalein) clear the entire colon. As a result, the interval to refill the sigmoid colon and rectum lengthens. During this time, patients become concerned that they are constipated and need a laxative to move their bowels. Thus, they use the laxative repeatedly; repeated use continues to empty the entire colon; and a vicious cycle begins. It is important to instruct patients to expect a "compensatory pause" after discontinuing laxative therapy. In addition, an actual physiologic bowel inertia may result from laxative-induced hypokalemia, leading the person to mistake decreased peristalsis for constipation and to reinitiate laxative therapy.
- **Radiation-induced diarrhea.** Abdominopelvic, lower thoracic, and lumbar radiation can result in mild to severe diarrhea, depending on dose, schedule, and volume of bowel included in the radiation field. Radiation causes inflammation, ulceration, and sloughing of intestinal epithelium, thus shortening the intestinal villi and reducing the functional mucosal surface necessary for the adequate transport of fluids and electrolytes. In addition, lactase, the enzyme necessary for disaccharide digestion, may be decreased or absent, and patients may become lactose-intolerant. Nonabsorbable lactose in the small intestine causes an osmotic fluid shift which results in accelerated movement of contents and cramping abdominal pain. A lactose-free diet may be recommended until healing occurs. Acute enteropathy due to crypt stem cell depletion is an immediate response (within 1-3 weeks) that develops frequently in patients receiving a dose of 45 Gy or greater. In contrast, chronic radiation enteritis, which occurs in 5% to 15% of patients undergoing abdominopelvic radiation, has an onset of at least 6 to 12 months or up to years after radiation. It results from mucosal atrophy and fibrosis secondary to damaged endothelial cells in the blood vessels and connective tissues. Ischemic enteritis may result from chronic radiotherapy; however, this complication is rare with current radiation techniques.

12. What are standard pharmacologic interventions for managing diarrhea?

Please see the table on pp. 382-385.

13. What are guidelines for the management of cancer treatment-induced diarrhea?

The newest guidelines (Benson, 2004) address the management of cancer treatment-induced diarrhea (CTID) according to whether it is uncomplicated or complicated. Please see the box on pp. 386-387.

- Uncomplicated diarrhea is grade 1-2 without risk factors or complicating signs/symptoms.
- Complicated diarrhea is grade 3-4 or grade 1-2 diarrhea with one or more of the following risk factors: nausea, vomiting (grade 2 or greater), neutropenia, fever, sepsis, abdominal cramping, frank bleeding, and dehydration.

14. What nonpharmacologic interventions are used to prevent and manage diarrhea?

Although most nonpharmacologic interventions are anecdotal rather than evidence-based, they are important adjuncts and, if used aggressively, can be effective in preventing bowel disturbances or minimizing their severity. Since most are self-management interventions, educating patients and their families is critical to a successful prevention and management plan.

Text continued on p. 388.

Antidiarrheal agents

Drug and dosage	Mechanism of action	Contraindications	Adverse effects	Drug interactions	Administration tips
Opioids					
Lomotil (2.5 mg diphenoxylate with 0.025 mg atropine sulfate tablet): May load: 10 mg, then 1-2 tablets tid or qid. Maximal dose: 20 mg/day *Loperamide* (2-mg capsules. May load: 4-8 mg po, then 2 mg after each loose stool Maximal dose: 16 mg/day *Codeine*: 15-60 mg po every 4-6 hr as needed *Opium tincture*: (10% opium liquid: 10 mg morphine/ml with 19%	*All opioids* act as agonists at opiate receptors in smooth muscle of GI tract, reducing secretion and peristalsis; also increase ileocecal valve and anal sphincter pressure, improving continence *Atropine* (in Lomotil) blocks muscarinic receptors, inhibiting peristalsis and reducing gastric secretions. It is added for prevention of abuse more than	*All opioids*: parasitic or bacterial infections accompanied by fever, obstructive jaundice *Diphenoxylate* (in Lomotil): advanced liver disease (e.g., cirrhosis) may precipitate hepatic coma *Lomotil* and *Imodium*: not recommended in children younger than 2 years *Paregoric*: convulsive states	*Atropine* (in Lomotil): limited use due to dry mouth, urinary retention, blurred vision *Imodium*: uncommon effects include cramping, gastric upset, dry mouth, skin rash, dizziness, drowsiness *All opioids*: potential constipation, abdominal and bowel distention, nausea	*Diphenoxylate* (in Lomotil), *codeine*, *paregoric*: potentiate CNS depressants *Diphenoxylate* (in Lomotil): increases risk of hypertension with monoamine oxidase inhibitors; increases risk of paralytic ileus with antimuscarinics	*Lomotil*: favored for partial bowel obstruction due to shorter action *Atropine*: useful in diarrhea associated with painful cramping *Imodium*: drug of choice for nonspecific antidiarrheal therapy; unlike codeine and diphenoxylate, it has no central opioid effect at therapeutic doses; titrate to effect; treat overdose with naloxone *Opium tincture*: for severe diarrhea; prolonged use may result in dependence; measured by drops; must be diluted in juice or water

alcohol): 0.3-1 ml every 2-6 hr until controlled Maximal dose: 6 ml/24 hr *Paregoric:* (0.4 mg morphine/ml with 45% alcohol): 5-10 ml po 1-4 times/day, or 4 ml every 4 hr	treatment of diarrhea				*Oral equianalgesic doses:* Imodium: 4 mg/day Lomotil: 10 mg/day Codeine: 200 mg/day

Adsorbents

Bismuth subsalicylate (Pepto-Bismol): chewable tablets: 262 mg, and suspensions: 262 mg/15 ml or 524 mg/15 ml (maximal strength). Usual dose: 524 mg every 30 min up to 5 gm/day	Absorbs (binds) toxins produced by bacteria and other GI irritants, allowing them to be inactivated or eliminated; direct antimicrobial effect on *E. coli*	Aspirin sensitivity	Impaction	Potentiates oral anticoagulants and hypoglycemics Reduces uricosuric effects of probenecid and sulfinpyrozone Decreases absorption and bioavailability of tetracyclines Can interfere with radiologic exams because it is radiopaque	Prophylaxis for traveler's diarrhea, but large doses limit utility Useful in secretory diarrhea for enterotoxic bacteria, radiotherapy, prostaglandin-secreting tumors (acts as mucosal antiprostaglandin) Indicated for mild diarrhea

Continued

Antidiarrheal agents—cont'd

Drug and dosage	Mechanism of action	Contraindications	Adverse effects	Drug interactions	Administration tips
		Adsorbents			
Kaopectate (5.85 gm kaolin and 130 mg pectin per 30 ml suspension). Usual dose: 2-6 gm every 6 hr as needed	Pectin produces a viscous colloidal solution with both adsorbent and absorbent properties	Obstructive bowel lesions Children younger than 3 yr	May increase K+ loss or interfere with absorption of nutrients and drugs	Decreases absorption of many drugs	Indicated for mild diarrhea
Cholestyramine (Questran)	Nonabsorbable resin: absorbs bile salts/acids, which cause diarrhea by effect on large intestine; adsorbs *C. difficile*		Constipation	Binds with and decreases absorption of many drugs (e.g., warfarin sodium, aspirin, thyroxin, digoxin, phenobarbital)	Helpful in radiation-induced diarrhea and ileal surgery Give with meals; use limited by taste; onset of action: 12-24 hr

Anticholinergics

Drug	Mechanism	Contraindications	Side effects	Drug interactions	Comments
Atropine *Dicyclomine* (Bentyl) *Propantheline* (Pro-Banthine) (15 mg po 3-4 times/day)	Muscarinic agonists: inhibit GI secretions and peristalsis; decrease spasm of small intestine lining	Closed angle glaucoma Prostate hypertrophy Heart disease Obstructive bowel disease	Decreased memory and concentration Drowsiness, dry mouth, urinary retention, tachycardia	Antacids interfere with absorption of these drugs	Useful in diarrhea due to peptic ulcer disease or irritable bowel syndrome and refractory diarrhea

Somatostatin analog

Drug	Mechanism	Side effects	Comments
Octreotide acetate (Sandostatin) 50-200 mcg 2 or 3 times/day subcutaneously	Inhibits GI hormone secretion, thus prolonging intestinal transit time and increasing net sodium and water absorption	Nausea, abdominal cramps, flatulence, steatorrhea Biliary sludge and gallstones after 6 months Transient deterioration in glucose tolerance at start	Useful in secretory diarrhea associated with endocrine tumors, AIDS, graft vs. host disease, GI resection, diabetes

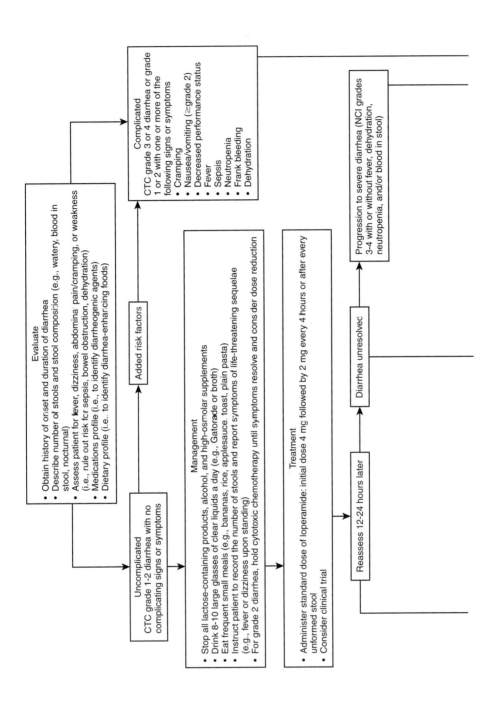

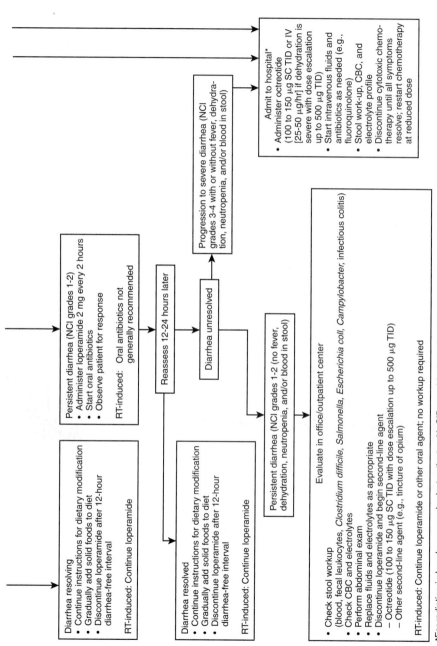

Diarrhea resolving
- Continue instructions for dietary modification
- Gradually add solid foods to diet
- Discontinue loperamide after 12-hour diarrhea-free interval

RT-induced: Continue loperamide

Persistent diarrhea (NCI grades 1-2)
- Administer loperamide 2 mg every 2 hours
- Start oral antibiotics
- Observe patient for response

RT-induced: Oral antibiotics not generally recommended

Reassess 12-24 hours later

Diarrhea resolved
- Continue instructions for dietary modification
- Gradually add solid foods to diet
- Discontinue loperamide after 12-hour diarrhea-free interval

RT-induced: Continue loperamide

Diarrhea unresolved

Progression to severe diarrhea (NCI grades 3-4 with or without fever, dehydration, neutropenia, and/or blood in stool)

Persistent diarrhea (NCI grades 1-2 (no fever, dehydration, neutropenia, and/or blood in stool)

Evaluate in office/outpatient center

- Check stool workup
  (blood, fecal leukocytes, *Clostridium difficile*, *Salmonella*, *Escherichia coli*, *Campylobacter*, infectious colitis)
- Check CBC and electrolytes
- Perform abdominal exam
- Replace fluids and electrolytes as appropriate
- Discontinue loperamide and begin second-line agent
  – Octreotide (100 to 150 µg SC TID with dose escalation up to 500 µg TID)
  – Other second-line agent (e.g., tincture of opium)

RT-induced: Continue loperamide or other oral agent; no workup required

Admit to hospital*
- Administer octreotide (100 to 150 µg SC TID or IV [25-50 µg/hr] if dehydration is severe with dose escalation up to 500 µg TID)
- Start intravenous fluids and antibiotics as needed (e.g., fluoroquinolone)
- Stool work-up, CBC, and electrolyte profile
- Discontinue cytotoxic chemotherapy until all symptoms resolve; restart chemotherapy at reduced dose

*For radiation-induced cases and select patients with CID, consider intensive outpatient management, unless the patient has sepsis, fever, or neutropenia.

From Benson III AB, Ajani AJ, Catalano RB, et al: Recommended guidelines for the treatment of cancer treatment-induced diarrhea, *J Clin Oncol* 22(14):2918-26, 2004.

- Change to a low-residue diet by avoiding foods that stimulate or irritate the GI tract:
  - Whole grain products, dried legumes, nuts, seeds, popcorn
  - Alcohol, caffeine-containing products, and tobacco
  - High-fat spreads or dressings, rich pastries, candied fruits or coconut, chocolate
  - Greasy, spicy (curry, chili powder, garlic), and fried foods
  - Raw vegetables, pickles, relishes, and other high fiber foods
- Add foods that build stool consistency:
  - Pectin-based foods (bananas, unspiced applesauce, or peeled apples)
  - White rice, plain pasta, baked potato without the skin
- Increase fluid intake:
  - Consume 3 L/day (i.e., water, weak decaffeinated tea, broths).
  - Vary the type of fluids used for rehydration to avoid water toxicity. Water lacks the necessary electrolytes (e.g., potassium) and vitamins. Carbonated caffeine drinks have low electrolyte content and extremely high osmolality which may worsen acute diarrhea.
  - Sound choices for fluid and electrolyte replacement include bouillon, fruitades, cranberry juice, grape juice, Gatorade or other sport drinks, weak tepid tea, and gelatin. Fluids with glucose are useful because glucose absorption drives sodium and water back into the body, supporting oral rehydration therapy. (**Note:** Because of their high osmolality, rehydration fluids, such as Pedialyte or Gatorade, may stimulate osmotic diarrhea).
- **Maintain a lactose-free diet or use lactobacillus preparations** to aid digestion in lactose-intolerant patients. Patients taking oral nutritional supplements also may benefit from lactose-free preparations (e.g., Vivonex T.E.N., Osmolite). Use lactose-free isotonic (300 mOsm/kg water) enteral feeding formula with dilution to at least 75 mOsm/kg and administer at room temperature.

Note: Patients experiencing nausea and vomiting or significant/refractory diarrhea may require parenteral replacement. Often bowel rest is recommended to allow the GI tract to heal. Patients are then started on a liquid diet, with a gradual increase in low-residue foods as tolerated (usually proteins first, then fats).

15. What "red flags" alert patients with diarrhea and their family members to the need for immediate medical assistance?

- Fever and/or shaking chills
- Excessive thirst, rapid pulse
- Dizziness with or without palpitations
- Severe abdominal cramping and/or rectal spasm
- Watery and/or bloody stool
- Diarrhea that continues for more than 12 hours despite antidiarrheal treatment

CONSTIPATION

16. How prevalent is constipation in cancer patients?

Constipation occurs in approximately 50% of cancer patients, over 75% of patients who are terminally ill, and 90% of patients receiving opioid therapy for pain control. It is more common in women and the elderly and most common among patients receiving palliative or hospice care.

17. What pathophysiologic events lead to constipation?

Constipation is related to biochemical (e.g., hypokalemia and hypercalcemia) and sensorimotor alterations, which can: (1) reduce peristalsis, (2) decrease sensory awareness of rectal filling, and (3) reduce motor control of the anal sphincter. Peristalsis, which is required to move the fecal mass through the gut, is slowed when bowel innervation is interrupted or diminished. Subsequently, stretch receptors may not trigger muscle action.

18. Describe acute constipation.

Acute constipation generally occurs insidiously over time, producing significant stool evacuation difficulty along with bloating sensation, low abdominal or rectal pain, and tenesmus. Sometimes liquid stool is eliminated around impacted hardened stool giving the appearance of diarrhea but is actually a sign of impaction (i.e., obstipation). It is important to distinguish between the two conditions to intervene appropriately.

19. Which drugs commonly cause constipation in patients with cancer?

- **Vinca alkaloids** are responsible for causing constipation in 20% (vinblastine) to 35% (vincristine, vinorelbine) of patients by damaging the myenteric plexus of the colon. Both vincristine and vinblastine may cause neurotoxicity involving smooth muscles of the GI tract, which leads to decreased peristalsis and, ultimately, paralytic ileus. The bowel effects of vinca alkaloids may be unaccompanied by peripheral nerve dysfunction. Combinations of a laxative and stool softener may be used prophylactically with the vinca alkaloids to avoid constipation.
- **Opioids** affect the bowel by activation of specific opioid receptors in both the GI tract and central nervous system, resulting in increased tone, nonpropulsive motility in the ileum and colon, increased transit time, and water absorption. Opioid-induced insensitivity to rectal distention further contributes to slowed defecation.
- **$5HT_3$** antagonists and other **antiemetic agents** (e.g., phenothiazines)
- **Other supportive agents:** anticholinergics, calcium and aluminum-based antacids, iron and calcium supplements, antidiarrheals, tricyclic antidepressants, diuretics, calcium channel blockers, anticonvulsants, and some sleep medications

20. What are standard pharmacologic interventions for managing constipation?

Please see the table on pp. 390-394.

21. Why are combination laxatives, such as Senokot-S or Peri-Colace, better than Colace alone for opioid-induced constipation?

Docusate (Colace) softens the stool but usually does not provide the peristaltic stimulation needed to counteract opioid-induced constipation. Combining the softening action of docusate with the peristaltic stimulant effect of the anthraquinone derivatives (e.g., senna concentrate, casanthranol) is more often successful in managing opioid-induced constipation. Patients need to be instructed to consume adequate fluids while using these medications. Senokot-S (senna concentrate and docusate sodium) and Peri-Colace (casanthranol and docusate sodium) are agents that combine mechanisms.

22. How is opioid-induced constipation managed?

To prevent opioid-induced constipation, many algorithms suggest the use of a senna concentrate and docusate sodium in combination at dose ranges of 1 to 4 tablets orally at bedtime or twice daily, and titrating to the optimal dose. Clinical trials show promising results for the opioid antagonists, methylnaltrexone and alvimopan (Entereg), in relieving opioid-induced constipation.

23. What laxatives can be used if combination laxatives are not effective in relieving constipation?

If Senokot-S or Peri-Colace are not effective, consider an osmotic agent: lactulose, sorbitol, or polyethylene glycol with electrolytes (GoLYTELY) or without electrolytes (MiraLax).

Text continued on p. 395.

Constipation medications: laxatives and cathartics

	Drug	Mechanism of action	Contraindications	Adverse effects	Drug interactions
Bulk formers	Psyllium (Metamucil) Methylcellulose (Cologel, Citrucel) Polycarbophil Onset of effect: 12 hrs-3 days	Nondigested plant cell walls absorb water in feces; softens; increases stool size, thus increasing peristalsis; acts in large and small intestines	Intestinal strictures, partial or total bowel obstruction or fecal impaction, phenylketonuria Advanced cancer with early satiety, nausea, anorexia Caution in diabetics due to sugar content	Flatulence, erratic habits, abdominal discomfort or irritation	May decrease effects of tetracycline, anticoagulants, digitalis glycosides or salicylates, nitrofurantoin
Diphenylmethanes					
Bowel stimulants	Bisacodyl (Ducolax): 5 mg enteric-coated tablet po 1-3 times/day; 10-mg suppository (single dose as needed) Onset of effect: 6-10 hr; Rectally: 15-60 min	Directly stimulates nerve plexus of colon Irritates smooth muscle of intestine, stimulating peristalsis First metabolized in liver, then colon; effect may be prolonged	Bowel obstruction Abdominal pain	Cramps, urgency, incontinence	Decreases effect of warfarin

Anthraquinones

Oxidative laxatives	Senna (Senokot, X-Prep): 187 mg tablet; daily maximum of 8 tablets or 4 tsp granules (326 mg)/day Cascara sagrada (aromatic): 5 ml or 1 tablet (325 mg) at bedtime as needed. Casanthranol (cascara derivative): 30 mg, usually in combination with docusate Onset of effect: 6-12 hours	Exact mechanism unknown; may stimulate colon and myenteric plexus Senna stimulates submucosal nerve plexus and peristalsis in transverse and descending colon; decreases sodium and water absorption and produces semiliquid or formed stool. Cascara sagrada directly irritates intestinal mucosa; results in motility and changes in fluid and electrolyte secretion	Bowel obstruction	Cathartic colon, may result in intestinal atony Fluid and electrolyte disturbances	Cascara decreases effect of oral anticoagulants
	Lactulose (Cephulac): 30-45 ml 3 or 4 times/day, or hourly to induce rapid effect in initial phase Chronulac: 15-30 ml/day; may increase to 60 ml/day	Lactulose/sorbitol: nonabsorbable sugars; exert osmotic effect mostly in large bowel Lactulose also used to treat hepatic encephalopathy to lower serum ammonia	Lactulose/sorbitol: avoid with fecal impaction or intestinal obstruction Caution with severe cardiopulmonary and renal impairment (contraindicated in anuria) May cause elevations in blood glucose levels in	Lactulose: cramps, flatulence, nausea, vomiting; excessive use may cause electrolyte losses, diarrhea Chronulac: gas from bacterial degradation Sorbitol: edema, nausea, vomiting,	Decreased effects of neomycin, other antiinfectives, and antacids

Continued

Constipation medications: laxatives and cathartics—cont'd

Drug	Mechanism of action	Contraindications	Adverse effects	Drug interactions
Anthraquinones				
Sorbitol: 3-150 ml/day (70% solution) Onset of effect:		diabetes	diarrhea, abdominal discomfort, potential fluid and electrolyte loss	
Lactulose: 24-48 hr				
Polyethylene glycol electrolyte solution (Colyte, GoLYTELY): 8 oz po every 15 min as tolerated for 3-4 hr until 1 L taken or diarrhea results	Catharsis by strong electrolyte and osmotic effects	GoLYTELY: do not give with bowel obstruction (high risk for perforation), toxic colitis, megacolon, gastric retention, bowel perforation	Nausea, abdominal fullness, bloating, cramps	Do not give oral medications within 1 hr of GoLYTELY
Also available without electrolytes (Miralax) Onset of effect: Polyethylene glycol: first bowel movement within 1 hour				
Glycerin: rectal suppositories,	Lubricates and softens Stimulates defecation	Abdominal pain, nausea, vomiting	May cause rectal irritation if used	

	Dosage	Mechanism	Contraindications	Adverse effects	Drug interactions
	1-2/day as needed, or 5-15 ml as enema Onset of effect: within 30 min of use	osmotically; sodium stearate in suppository may irritate rectal membranes		too frequently; headache	
Lubricants	Mineral oil: 15-40 ml/day po (once or in divided doses); as retention enema: 60-150 ml/day as single dose Onset of effect: within 8 hr	Lubricates intestinal mucosa and feces; softens stool by preventing loss of water from feces	Known reflux, dysphagia (risk of lipid pneumonia or aspiration pneumonitis, especially in older adults)	Excessive use may lead to anal leakage and irritation Chronic use reduces absorption of fat-soluble vitamins Lipid pneumonitis with aspiration	Docusate sodium increases absorption and risk of lipid granuloma of gut wall Alters absorption of antibiotics, anticoagulants, oral contraceptives, digitalis glycosides Increases mineral oil absorption Decreases effect of Coumadin and aspirin
Detergent laxatives	Docusate: 50-500 mg/day in 1-4 doses Docusate sodium (Colace) Docusate calcium (Surfak) Onset of effect: 24-72 hr	Decreases surface tension and allows water and fat penetration of hard stool Mucosal contact effect decreases electrolyte and water reabsorption in small and large intestines	Intestinal obstruction, acute abdominal pain, nausea, or vomiting	Diarrhea, abdominal cramps Prolonged use may lead to dependence or electrolyte imbalance	
Saline laxatives	Magnesium (Mg) salts:	Mg increases gastric, pancreatic, small	Fecal impaction, intestinal obstruction,	Mg salts: excessive use may cause	Effects of Mg counteracted by

Continued

Constipation medications: laxatives and cathartics—cont'd

Drug	Mechanism of action	Contraindications	Adverse effects	Drug interactions
		Anthraquinones		
Mg citrate: $\frac{1}{2}$–1 full bottle (120–300 ml) po as needed	intestine secretion and motor activity of small and large intestines	nausea, vomiting, abdominal pain	electrolyte losses, hypermagnesemia, diarrhea, cramps, pain	aluminum salt in many antacids
Mg hydroxide (e.g., Milk of Magnesia Regular Strength): 30–60 ml/day po or in divided doses	Mg and Na salts are poorly absorbed and draw water into lumen, thus increasing stool water content and frequency	Avoid Mg salts in renal failure, myocardial damage, heart block, hepatitis, ileostomy, colostomy	Na salts: nausea, vomiting, diarrhea, edema, hypotension; excessive use may cause dependence	Milk of Magnesia decreases absorption of tetracyclines, digoxin, indomethacin, or iron salts
Sodium (Na) salts: Sodium phosphate Fleet Phospho-soda: 20–30 ml as single dose		Avoid Na salts in cardiac or renal disease, hyperphosphatemia, hypernatremia, hypocalcemia; use with caution if diet is sodium-restricted		Na phosphate: do not give with Mg or aluminum-containing antacids or sucralfate; they may blind with phosphate
Fleet enema: 4.5 oz enema; may repeat				
Onset of effect: Mg citrate: 30 min–6 hr, depending on dose Mg hydroxide: 4–8 hr Sodium phosphate: po 3–6 hr; Rectal: 2–5 min				

Polyethylene glycol is more expensive than lactulose, but may cause less bloating from gas and be more effective. See the table on pp. 390-394 for other choices, such as Milk of Magnesia or bisacodyl). If constipation continues, consider referral to a gastroenterologist. **Note:** It is usually best to allow 2 days for the intervention to work. Titrate the regimen to produce a bowel movement every 1 to 2 days. For patients who have not had a bowel movement in 3 days, a rectal exam may be indicated. Digital disimpaction, followed by suppositories or enemas, may be necessary.

24. What nonpharmacologic interventions are used to prevent and manage constipation?

- **Increase fluid intake**. Drinking approximately 6 to 8 glasses of water/day (1-2 L) helps to keep stool soft. Suggest carrying a water bottle at all times to sip fluids (especially between meals).
- **Increase dietary fiber content**. Warn patients that that they may experience abdominal discomfort, flatulence, or erratic bowel habits in the first few weeks after increasing fiber intake. Avoid tolerance by slowly titrating fiber content upward to 6 to 10 gm/day, starting with the addition of 3 to 4 gm/day. Use one tablespoon psyllium in 8 oz fluid daily followed by 8 oz fluid in patients without structural bowel blockage. Every 3 days, increase daily psyllium and fluid in 1-teaspoon increments until stools are consistently soft and formed. Continue this dose as maintenance.
- **Discourage** drinking coffee, tea, and grapefruit juice because they act as diuretics. However, some form of warm liquid before an attempt at defecation may be helpful. Patients have reported that drinking 2 to 4 ounces of prune juice before meals may be helpful.
- **Establish routine toileting**. Regular toilet activities after breakfast are most productive because propulsive contractions in the intestine are strongest. The use of raised toilet seats, footstools, and bedside commodes may be helpful. Ensure privacy.
- **Increase exercise**. Gastrointestinal motility is diminished by immobility and stimulated by regular exercise (e.g., 30-minute walk/day). Teach patients simple diaphragmatic breathing and abdominal muscle exercises to strengthen and increase muscle tone, which is necessary for defecation.

25. Are prunes or prune juice the best choices for increasing dietary fiber?

Contrary to popular belief, prunes contain only 2 gm of fiber, and prune juice contains very little. Prunes also contain phenolphthalein and may cause cathartic colon (narrowing of the ileum and proximal colon in addition to loss of colonic muscle tone) with prolonged use. The best high-fiber foods are wheat bran (in breads and cereals), beans, broccoli, sweet potatoes, carrots, and dried apricots.

High-fiber foods

Food	Dietary fiber
Wheat bran (3 tbsp)	10 gm
Bran flakes (100 gm)	2.7-6.5 gm
Whole wheat bread (1 slice)	1-2 gm

26. Are enemas safe for cancer patients?

Enemas are used to clear impactions or to manage refractory acute constipation that is producing significant discomfort. All enemas need to be used cautiously because they may place the patient at risk for bowel perforation. Avoid enemas, rectal exams, and suppositories in myelosuppressed patients because they are at high risk for infection and bleeding.

27. What commonly recommended enemas may be used?

- Gentle tap water or saline enemas
- Water-soluble lubricant enema
  - Fill a 60-ml syringe with water-soluble lubricant (Surgilube), replace plunger, and attach rectal tube to syringe. Lubricate tip of tube and place tip inside rectum. Slowly inject, as for retention enema. Retain for 30 minutes.
- Milk and molasses enema*
  - 1 L of warm water + 1 cup of powdered milk + 1 cup of molasses or corn syrup
  - Put 8 oz of warm water and 3 oz of powdered milk into a plastic jar

Close the jar and shake until the water and milk appear to be fully mixed. Add 4.5 oz of molasses, and shake the jar again until the mixture appears to have an even color throughout. Pour the mixture into enema bag. Administer the enema high by gently introducing the tube about 12 inches into the rectum. Do not push beyond resistance. Repeat every 6 hours until good results are achieved.

*From Bisanz A: Managing bowel elimination problems in patients with cancer. Oncol Nurs Forum 24:683, 1997. By permission.

28. Why are certain types of enemas avoided?

- Fleet enemas are reported to cause tissue necrosis and are not safe for patients with renal or cardiac disease.
- Soap suds enemas are no longer used because of the risk of acute colitis (usually self-limiting). More serious potential complications include anaphylaxis, hemorrhage, and rectal gangrene.

 Key Points

- Diarrhea and constipation are relatively high incidence problems in patients with cancer; both are underreported and often mismanaged.
- Uncontrolled diarrhea can result in volume depletion, significant loss of potassium and bicarbonate, perianal irritation and denuding with secondary infection, and may affect tumor response by producing treatment dose reductions and delays, thus limiting the total dose patients are able to receive.
- Undertreated or untreated constipation can lead to obstipation (fecal impaction) severe enough to require surgical intervention. Reluctance or refusal to take opioids, because of constipating effects, can result in poor pain control.
- Prevention is the key to effective management of diarrhea and constipation and usually involves pharmacologic management.
- Most nonpharmacologic interventions are important adjuncts and, if used aggressively, can be effective in preventing bowel disturbances or minimizing their severity.

Internet Resources

Multinational Association of Supportive Care in Cancer:
   http://www.mascc.org
Cancer Therapy Evaluation Program:
   http://ctep.cancer.gov/forms/CTCAEv3.pdf
National Cancer Institute:
   http://www.cancer.gov/

Acknowledgment

The author wishes to acknowledge Leslie Tuchmann, RN, MS, HNC, for her contributions to the chapter on constipation and diarrhea published in the first and second editions of *Oncology Nursing Secrets*.

Bibliography

Arnold RJA, Gabrail N, Raut M, et al: Clinical implications of chemotherapy-induced diarrhea in patients with cancer. *J Support Oncol* 3:227-232, 2006.

Avila JG: Pharmacologic treatment of constipation in cancer patients. *Cancer Control: Journal of the Moffit Cancer Center,* May/June, 11(3): 10-18, Supplement 1, 2004.

Benson AB III, Ajani JA, Catalano RB, et al: Recommended guidelines for the treatment of cancer treatment-induced diarrhea. *J Clin Oncol* 22(14):2918-26, 2004.

Bisanz A: Managing bowel elimination problems in patients with cancer. *Oncol Nurs Forum* 24:679-688, 1997.

Engelking C: Diarrhea. In Yarbro CH, Frogge M, Goodman M, editors: *Cancer symptom management,* ed 3, Boston, 2004, Jones and Bartlett.

Goldberg Arnold RJ, Gabrail N, Raut M, et al: Clinical implications of chemotherapy-induced diarrhea in patients with cancer. *J Support Oncol* 3:227-232, 2005.

Kornblau S, Benson AB III, Catalano R, et al: Management of cancer treatment-related diarrhea: Issues and therapeutic strategies. *J Pain Symptom Manage* 19:118-129, 2000.

Lembo, C: Chronic constipation. *N Engl J Med* 349:1360-1368, 2003.

Massey RL, Haylock PJ, Curtiss C: Constipation. In Yarbro CH, Frogge MH, Goodman M, editors: *Cancer symptom management,* ed 3, Boston, 2004, Jones and Bartlett.

Rutledge DN, Engelking C: Cancer-related diarrhea: Selected findings of a national survey of oncology nurse experiences. *Oncol Nurs Forum* 25:861-872, 1998.

Salz LB: Understanding and managing chemotherapy-induced diarrhea. *J Support Oncol* 1:35-41, 2003.

Sykes NP: The pathogenesis of constipation. *J Support Oncol* 4(5):213-219, 2006.

Thomas JR: Management of constipation in patients with cancer. *Support Cancer Ther* 2(1):47-51, 2004.

Fatigue

Stacey Young-McCaughan and Lillian M. Nail

1. Define cancer-related fatigue.

Cancer-related fatigue (CRF) includes sensations of physical tiredness, mental slowness, and lack of emotional resilience. It fluctuates in intensity over the course of the day, often exhibits a pattern that it is tied to administration of treatment, and can be overcome in an emergency. Although patients with CRF may experience muscle weakness, CRF is not synonymous with weakness. In contrast to patients with neurologic problems, patients with CRF may have normal muscle strength and endurance and still experience an overwhelming feeling of tiredness.

2. Is fatigue a major problem for patients with cancer?

CRF is the most frequently reported side effect of treatment. All types of treatment produce CRF, and the most severe, dose-limiting form occurs with biologic response modifiers (e.g., interferons, interleukins). The percentage of patients experiencing CRF as a side effect of cancer treatment ranges from 15% to 95%, depending on the type of treatment, dose of therapy, and method used to measure fatigue. CRF is poorly understood and often ignored in clinical practice. Although many people attribute fatigue to "having cancer," research focuses on fatigue as a treatment side effect, and most studies of fatigue in cancer have been done with patients who have no evidence of disease.

3. How is CRF different from the fatigue experienced by healthy people?

In comparison with the fatigue experienced by healthy people, CRF is overwhelming, persistent, and relentless. Fatigue in healthy people is eventually fully relieved by sleep and rest, even if it takes more than one or two nights. In contrast, people with CRF wake up tired no matter how much rest they get. CRF also may cause patients to redefine the level of fatigue that they label as "not tired." Thus what they formerly viewed as feeling a little tired is now defined as "not tired," and a new sensation of overwhelming fatigue replaces "severe fatigue."

4. What is the impact of CRF?

Patients describe themselves as too tired to do anything, unable to concentrate, frustrated by feeling that they are not themselves, concerned that fatigue means that they are not doing well or that the cancer is progressing, and depressed because of the feeling of tiredness. The limitations imposed by fatigue are dramatic. The person experiencing CRF may not be aware of the magnitude of the negative impact on usual activities until the fatigue resolves.

5. What are the probable causes of CRF?

People with cancer are likely to experience many potential causes of fatigue, such as electrolyte imbalance, poor nutritional status, anemia, hormone shifts, volume depletion, sedation as a side effect of analgesics, hypoxia, and infection. Other contributors include sleep disruption, increased demands for physical activity, emotional strain, interpersonal demands, and increased need for vigilance and concentration.

Symptoms, side effects, anxiety, hospital noise, and interpersonal demands at home have the potential to disrupt sleep and rest. Multiple visits to health care providers, travel to appointments, physical demands of surgery and other forms of treatment, processing information about treatment options to make an informed decision, establishing relationships with new health care providers, explaining the diagnosis and treatment to friends and family members, and monitoring the care provided by others are potential contributors to fatigue that are not fully understood by health care providers or friends and family.

6. What physiologic mechanisms are responsible for CRF?

Except for chemotherapy-induced anemia, the physiologic causes of CRF are unknown. Multiple causes are likely, given the variation in the intensity and characteristics of CRF experienced with different types of treatment. Various hypotheses have been proposed, including toxic effects of accumulated products of cell death, neurohormonal changes, depletion of essential neurotransmitters, bone marrow suppression, and accumulation of cytokines. Few of these mechanisms have been studied.

7. What other symptoms are associated with CRF?

CRF can be one of a cluster of symptoms experienced by cancer patients. Symptoms associated with CRF may be related to the cancer (which can cause obstruction, pain, coughing, dyspnea, pruritus, etc.), the cancer treatment (which can cause dry mouth, stomatitis, nausea, vomiting, constipation, diarrhea, etc.), the side effects of cancer treatment (e.g., infection and fever, sleep disturbance, hot flushes and flashes, hypothyroidism), and/or the experience of having cancer (e.g., depression and anxiety). Assessment and treatment of symptoms related to the cancer or cancer treatment should be part of the treatment for CRF.

8. How does pain contribute to CRF?

Pain increases the energy needed to perform day-to-day activities, restricts mobility, disrupts sleep and rest, and constitutes an emotional burden. Pain relief should improve fatigue, although the pain management technique itself can disrupt rest (e.g., pain medication administered every 4 hours, around the clock), have sedative side effects (e.g., opioids), or require extensive energy investment (e.g., frequent changes of hot or cold packs). (See Chapter 42 for a full discussion of pain management).

9. Are CRF and sleep disturbance the same?

Although patients may initially equate sleep debt with fatigue, patients who have an accumulated sleep debt find relief with sleep, whereas patients with CRF do not report feeling rested after sleep. (See Chapter 45 for a full discussion of sleep-wake disturbances).

10. Isn't CRF just a symptom of depression?

No. Historically, the diagnosis of depression depends on the presence of vegetative symptoms, such as anorexia, sleep disturbance, decreased activity, constipation, and weight loss. All of these symptoms are likely to occur as side effects in patients undergoing treatment for cancer, potentially confounding the diagnosis of depression. Recent revisions to the diagnosis of depression state that symptoms of physical illness and side effects of treatment are not appropriate considerations in making the diagnosis. Depression in patients with cancer can be treated effectively, but CRF may interfere with attendance at support groups or participation in therapy sessions. (See Chapter 34 for a full discussion of depression).

11. How should the nurse assess CRF?

The clinical assessment of fatigue should be modeled on the approach to pain assessment. For example, "On a scale of 0 to 10 where 0 is no fatigue and 10 is the most fatigue possible, how much fatigue have you had today?" Both the time frame (now, today, during the past week, during the past month) and the reference point (highest level of fatigue, lowest level of fatigue, usual level of fatigue) can be altered to accommodate the type of treatment. Patients receiving cyclic chemotherapy often arrive for treatment on a day when they have the lowest level of fatigue during the treatment cycle. Assessment based on the "today" approach does not fully describe their experience after treatment, because the peak time of CRF is not captured. Patients assessed on the day of the next treatment should be asked about level of fatigue over the week before the previous treatment as well as "today." The average level of fatigue over each week since the previous treatment also may be assessed to evaluate rate of recovery. Weekly assessments focused on the past week and initiated the second week of treatment is appropriate for most patients receiving radiation therapy. Potential treatable causes should be evaluated, especially when: (1) the pattern of CRF is unusual for the type of treatment delivered, (2) the intensity of fatigue increases suddenly and dramatically, or (3) the impact of fatigue on quality of life is beyond the patient's level of tolerance. In addition to standard laboratory tests and physical examination, daily activity level, sleep patterns, and new demands imposed as a result of cancer should be assessed.

12. Does correcting anemia relieve CRF?

Some studies suggest that correcting anemia (returning hemoglobin levels to 12 g/dl) can relieve the fatigue associated with chemotherapy-induced anemia. However, patients with a normal or near normal hemoglobin level can still experience CRF. Anemia can be corrected by blood transfusions and treatment with hematopoietic growth factors (erythropoietin and darbepoetin alfa). Treatment with erythropoietin (epoetin alfa, Procrit, Epogen) or darbepoetin alfa (Aranesp) takes 2 to 6 weeks to raise hemoglobin levels and reduce fatigue.

13. How is exercise used in managing CRF?

Although for many years it was widely believed that CRF universally prevented patients with cancer from exercising, multiple studies have shown that the opposite is true. Of the nonpharmacological interventions recommended by the National Comprehensive Cancer Network (NCCN) practice guidelines for CRF, exercise has the strongest evidence base for treating fatigue.

14. How should exercise be prescribed for patients with cancer?

The American College of Sports Medicine (ACSM) recommends a comprehensive exercise program that includes aerobic training, strengthening, and flexibility. The exercise prescription should include: frequency, intensity, time, and type of exercise (the FITT principle). Frequency is the number of sessions per week, intensity is how hard the person is exercising, time is the duration of the exercise session, and type is the activity mode. The range for the FITT principle as recommended by the ACSM for aerobic training is a frequency of three to five sessions per week, an intensity of between 40% and 85% of heart rate reserve, and a time of 20 to 60 minutes per exercise session. As health professionals learn more about exercise in patients with cancer, more hospital-based and fitness club-based programs are being offered. However, patients can also be encouraged to pursue a safe home-based walking program, such as "Every Step Counts," developed by Victoria Mock at the Johns Hopkins University.

15. What medications are used specifically to treat CRF?

It has been very difficult to test the effectiveness of medications to relieve CRF, because fatigue rarely occurs in isolation and can be compounded by the cancer, cancer treatment, symptoms in addition to the CRF, and the psychological status of the individual. In addition to hematopoietic growth factors, various medications have been used clinically with some success.

Medications used to treat CRF

Drug	Dosage	Considerations
Stimulants		
Methylphenidate (Ritalin)	2.5-5.0 mg at 8 AM & noon	Titrate as needed; tolerance is common; avoid doses after noon.
Modafinil (Provigil)	200 mg q am	Indication for treatment of excessive sleepiness
Pemoline (Cylert)	18.75-75 mg daily or bid	Less data than with methylphenidate; associated with liver toxicity; no longer available in the United States
Steroids		
Dexamethasone	0.75-4 mg q am	Limited clinical data
Prednisone	10-30 mg q am	Limited clinical data
Miscellaneous		
Megestrol acetate (Megace)	80 mg PO tid, up to 800 mg PO once a day	

16. How can patients conserve energy and manage activity?

Although used by patients, energy conservation techniques to manage CRF have not been tested. The appeal of this approach is derived from patients' perceptions that they have a limited amount of available energy and the assumption that conserving energy allows it to be redirected to other activities. Current recommendations include assisting patients to prioritize activities by identifying those that are essential and those that are optional. Some essential activities can be delegated to others while the patient maintains involvement in activities that are highly valued. Nonessential activities that are not valued by the patient can be eliminated. Finding different ways to perform activities may also conserve energy. Examples of energy conservation techniques include sitting in a firm chair with arms to aid getting out of the chair, adding a raised toilet seat in the bathroom, using a wheelchair if walking is difficult, arranging commonly used supplies and equipment within easy reach of a workspace, and sitting rather than standing to perform repetitive tasks. Physical and/or occupational therapy referrals are important both in evaluating a patient's physical capacity and identifying appropriate energy conservation techniques.

17. Are alternative therapies helpful in treating CRF?

Vitamins, mineral supplements, herbal remedies, and hormones are used by patients with cancer. No published reports confirm the efficacy of any of these agents in preventing or ameliorating CRF.

18. Why should patients get preparatory information about the possibility of CRF?

Preparatory information helps patients to: (1) understand that CRF is a side effect of treatment, not always an indication that the cancer is progressing; (2) plan for CRF by using information about onset, pattern, and resolution in planning activities; and (3) increase confidence in dealing with CRF. Research about informational interventions in patients undergoing stressful medical procedures demonstrates that preparatory information does not cause patients to experience side effects by power of suggestion. Patients who are aware of potential side effects but do not experience them appreciate being prepared.

Key Points

- CRF negatively affects quality of life and is the most common side effect of cancer and cancer treatment.
- Fatigue experienced by "healthy" people is not the same as CRF.
- Treatment of CRF includes assessment and treatment of multiple physiological and psychological symptoms related to cancer, cancer treatment, and side effects of cancer treatment.
- Exercise is effective in reducing CRF.
- Preparatory information about CRF is helpful to patients.

Internet Resources

American Cancer Society:
    http://www.cancer.org
Lance Armstrong Foundation:
    http://www.livestrong.org
National Cancer Institute, Fatigue (PDQ):
    http://www.cancer.gov/cancertopics/pdq/supportivecare/fatigue/patient
National Comprehensive Cancer Network (NCCN):
    http://www.nccn.org
Oncology Nursing Society (ONS) *Putting Evidence into Practice (PEP)* fatigue card:
    http://www.ons.org/outcomes/PEPcard/fatigue.shtml

Bibliography

Ahlberg K, Ekman T, Gaston-Johansson F, et al: Assessment and management of cancer-related fatigue in adults. *Lancet* 362(9384):640-650, 2003. Published online, May 7, 2003 at http://image.thelancet.com/extras/02art6023web.pdf.
Curt GA, Breitbart W, Cella D, et al: Impact of cancer-related fatigue on the lives of patients: New findings from the Fatigue Coalition. *Oncologist* 5:353-360, 2000.
Dimeo FC: Effects of exercise on cancer-related fatigue. *Cancer* 92(suppl 6):1689-1693, 2001.
Mock V: Fatigue management: Evidence and guidelines for practice. *Cancer* 92(suppl 6):1699-1707, 2001.
Mock V: Evidence-based treatment for cancer-related fatigue. *J Natl Cancer Inst* 32:112-118, 2004.

Mock V, Abernath AP, Atkinson A, et al: National Comprehensive Cancer Network Clinical Practice Guidelines in Oncology – v.1.2006: cancer-related fatigue. Available at: http://www.nccn.org/professionals/physician_gls/PDF/fatigue.pdf Retrieved May 28, 2006.

Nail LM: Fatigue in patients with cancer. *Oncol Nurs Forum* 29:537-544, 2002.

Nail LM: Fatigue. In Yarbro CH, Frogge MH Goodman M, editors: *Cancer symptom management,* ed 3, Sudbury, MA, 2004, Jones and Bartlett.

Schwartz AL: *Cancer fitness: Exercise programs for patients and survivors.* New York, 2004, Simon & Schuster.

Schwartz AL, Nail LM, Chen S, et al: Fatigue patterns observed in patients receiving chemotherapy and radiotherapy. *Cancer Invest* 18:11-19, 2000.

Skirvin JA, Castanheira D: Cancer-related fatigue, US Pharm 28(7). Available at: http://www.uspharmacist.com/index.asp?show=article&page=8_1121.htm Retrieved May 27, 2006.

Stricker CT, Drake D, Hoyer KA, et al: Evidence-based practice for fatigue management in adults with cancer: Exercise as an intervention. *Oncol Nurs Forum* 31:963-974, 2004.

Winningham ML, Barton-Burke M: *Fatigue in cancer: A multidimensional approach,* Sudbury, MA, 2000, Jones and Bartlett.

Chapter 37

Lymphedema

Jean K. Smith

1. What is cancer-related lymphedema?

Cancer-related lymphedema is a chronic (incurable) stasis edema secondary to (cancer-related) lymphatic function failure in a specific area of the body. Edema occurs in both extracellular and lymphatic tissues, causing an abnormal collection of excess fluid, proteins, cell debris, and immunological cells. Over time, chronic local inflammation can cause connective tissue proliferation, including hypertrophy of adipose tissue. Gradual progression is common and can produce subcutaneous and dermal thickening and hardening.

2. How is edema different than lymphedema?

Edema is a symptom; lymphedema is a chronic disorder. Edema refers to excessive accumulation of fluid in interstitial tissues, which differs from the edema that accumulates from lymphatic function failure.

3. What is the incidence of cancer-related lymphedema?

Lymphedema can occur at any time following a cancer diagnosis. The most frequent cause of secondary lymphedema in developed countries is breast cancer treatment. There is a 20% to 28% incidence of lymphedema in breast cancer survivors who have undergone standard axillary node dissection. Addition of breast cancer radiation therapy can increase lymphedema incidence. Incidence in breast cancer patients undergoing sentinel node biopsy alone has been reported as 2% to 3%; lymphedema prevalence will require long-term research. Incidence for other cancer-related lymphedemas has begun to emerge.

Etiology of cancer-related secondary lymphedema	
Tumor-related lymphatic obstruction and/or cancer treatment	**Cancer-related complications**
Breast Cancer: standard axillary node dissection and/or radiation therapy	Primary or metastatic cancer spread
Other Implicated Cancers: head & neck; any in pelvic region (i.e., prostate, cervical), lymphoma, sarcoma, melanoma, skin cancer, lower extremity cancer, metastatic cancers	Trauma, surgery, infection, and/or deep vein thrombosis

4. How is lymphedema diagnosed?

Generally, patient history combined with physical assessment allows definitive diagnosis of cancer-related lymphedema. Imaging is occasionally important for treatment outcomes. When appropriate, lymphoscintigraphy, a nuclear medicine test, is used to evaluate lymphatic function.

5. **How do staff and patients decide when an affected limb or a high-risk limb should or must be used for intravenous therapy?**

Experts recommend that an affected limb should not be used for intravenous therapy, as much as possible, especially for chemotherapy and other irritants. Sometimes, no other reasonable option exists. Blood draw presents much less risk, but is also avoided as much as possible. Establishment of a set caregiver protocol or Lymphedema Prevention Standard of Care is recommended. Suggested criteria include: (1) venipuncture by experienced phlebotomists only; (2) required approval for IV use of an affected limb (e.g., by a physician, nurse practitioner, physician assistant, clinical nurse specialist); (3) central venous catheter consideration for patients requiring more than a few days of IV infusion; and (4) use of an established protocol for venipuncture skin preparation, and monitoring infusions in an affected limb.

6. **What is the relationship between infection and lymphedema?**

Infection is the most common precipitator and complication of lymphedema. A specific infection site may or may not be detected. Infection can cause resistance to lymphedema treatment and/or irreversible lymphatic injury. Infections may be acute with dramatic symptoms that require intravenous antibiotic therapy and possible hospitalization.

7. **Are antibiotics recommended for infection in both an area exhibiting lymphedema or one at high risk?**

With the emergence of antibiotic-resistant bacteria, the practice of early antibiotic treatment has come under scrutiny. No research, national policy, or standard of care currently clarifies this dilemma. Several studies have documented the benefit of penicillin use for lymphedema infection prevention and management. Obvious infection requires prompt medical evaluation and appropriate antibiotic therapy.

8. **Is lymphedema painful?**

Discomfort rather than pain is usually associated with uncomplicated cancer-related lymphedema. Therefore, significant pain in an area with lymphedema suggests an alternative etiology, such as infection, thrombosis or cancer metastasis. Other relevant sources of pain in cancer-related lymphedema include: (1) surgical complications, such as neuropathies, scar tissue formation, myofascial restriction, and contractures; (2) radiation therapy; and (3) unrelated pain problems, such as bursitis, arthritis, tendonitis, and fibromyalgia.

9. **What serious long-term complications can occur in people with lymphedema?**

Lymphedema complications, generally secondary to poor edema control, include recurrent infection, decreases in limb function and/or general activity, skin changes, poor body image, depression, social isolation, loss of employment, and disability.
Neglected lymphedema has also been associated with lymphangiosarcoma, a rare and generally fatal complication that occurs in 3% of patients with breast cancer and long-standing lymphedema. The median survival time for lymphangiosarcoma is 1.3 years.

10. **How helpful are diuretics in lymphedema management?**

Inadequate lymphatic transport capacity is the underlying cause of lymphedema. Diuretics decrease capillary filtration by reducing blood volume rather than improving lymphatic transport. Short-term use of diuretics help minimize symptoms during acute inflammation, infection, thrombosis, or injury. Long-term use of diuretics has not been associated with lymphedema improvement.

11. What role does exercise play in lymphedema treatment?

Gradual increases in exercise intensity, accompanied by careful monitoring of the size and condition of the area of lymphedema, are recommended by a growing number of lymphedema experts. Lymphatic function appears to be enhanced by muscle contractions and deep breathing, especially in combination with continual use of a compression product on the affected area. Ideally, patients carry out lymphedema exercises one or more times each day. However, no research has demonstrated that exercise alone is sufficient lymphedema treatment. Furthermore, excessive or rigorous exercise has been shown to increase the amount of edema in some patients. Signs of excessive exercise include increased edema, tightness, and aching or other discomfort.

12. What self-care measures should be taught to people with lymphedema?

Practical lymphedema precautions and care for people with lymphedema or who have a high risk of developing it include the following:
- Maintain ideal body weight.
- Avoid prolonged limb dependency and inactivity as much as possible. Movement increases lymph flow.
- Wash daily, dry off well, and apply moisturizing cream to skin. Inspect for signs of infection, rashes, or breaks in the skin. Signs of infection include: redness, pain, heat, puffiness, pus and/or fever.
- Avoid injury as much as possible. If a break in skin occurs, clean the area with soap and water, apply an antiseptic, and keep the wound covered with a dressing until skin is healed.
- Continue use of compression products, if at all possible.
- If bruises or blows occur in the high-risk or affected area, apply ice and observe carefully for several days. Use compression products as soon as possible. If no edema was previously present, seek medical care if edema does not resolve in several days or a week, or if signs of infection occur.
- Explore and then choose the safest method of shaving (an area at risk or with swelling): electric shaver, hand razor, or depilatory.
- Take good care of nails and cuticles. Fungus is often present on swollen toes and feet. See a podiatrist for toenail or fungus problems.
- Try to avoid blood draws or use of intravenous needles in an affected arm, although this might be necessary in emergency or unusual situations.
- Avoid tourniquet pressure in or near the affected area (elastic, tight clothing, jewelry or bands, frequent measurement of blood pressure, etc.). Occasional blood pressure measurements in a high-risk arm appear to present very little risk.
- Carry bags and purses with the unaffected arm. Watch for signs of increased swelling after carrying heavy items or participating in strenuous activities.
- Wear gloves and protective clothing when gardening, around pets, cleaning, or carrying out other jobs that risk skin injury or abrasions.
- Avoid insect bites by using insect repellent and wearing protective clothing.
- Early antibiotic treatment is often more urgent for people with lymphedema.
- Air and other long distance travel often increase swelling. Move often, drink lots of water, and consider using compression products. Some people also find it helpful to avoid salty foods.

13. What are some recommendations for skin care in patients with lymphedema?

Skin care focuses on promoting skin integrity and preventing complications from decreased tissue oxygenation. Skin care involves: daily cleansing; gentle, thorough drying; lubricating the skin; and monitoring for problems. Bland, scentless products without Vaseline or heavy oil base are recommended. Vaseline-type products can damage compression products.

14. What skin complications occur in patients with substantial lymphedema of the lower extremities?

Common complications include: dermatitis, odor, hyperkeratosis, warts, papillomas, lymphorrhea, and infection.

15. How should lymphedema be treated?

Early lymphedema treatment promotes optimal patient outcomes. External compression therapy, including bandaging, compression products, or both, is universally accepted as essential and a mainstay for lymphedema management. Insufficient research has fostered conflicting protocols for usage of compression products.

16. What is external compression?

External compression therapy refers to the provision of even pressure to skin surfaces in and around an area with lymphedema. The local effect of compression is reduction of arterial capillary filtration and increased venous uptake. Although compression does not increase local lymphatic drainage, it does decrease local fluid overload. Thus continual, safe compression offers the best assistance to a malfunctioning lymphatic system. Additional benefits of compression include protection from abrasions, sunburn, insect bites and stings, and other breaches of skin integrity.

17. What products provide external compression?

Available products include: bandages (wrapping), garments, custom-made products for unique lymphedemas, and semirigid support or other similar products. Short stretch bandaging must be distinguished from Ace-type bandages that provide long stretch elastic compression. Compression garments are either prefabricated or custom-made. Garments include sleeves, gloves, gauntlets, and stockings. (Medicare does not reimburse for external compression garments). Postoperative (TED) stockings do not provide sufficient pressure to manage lymphedema, except occasionally for patients with mild venous insufficiency-related lymphedema. Proper product fit is often a problem. Unique products are now available to assist with head, neck, genital, and trunk edema. Semirigid support products use Velcro and foam to provide adjustable, nonelastic support that appears comparable to bandaging but is much easier and more convenient to use.

18. What evidence exists regarding the use of pneumatic pumps in lymphedema care?

Despite long-established Medicare reimbursement for pneumatic pumps, research has not clarified the benefits of their use. Furthermore, complications have been reported, and there are no guidelines for the use of pumps.

Pneumatic pumps, developed in the 1980s, provide electrical inflation of a single or multi-cell chamber sleeve to compress a lymphedematous limb. As documented by lymphoscintigraphy, pumps reduce tissue fluid by decreasing the tissue capillary filtration rate. Since pumps are not used continuously, their effect is temporary. A Cochrane review of lymphedema physical therapies reported: (1) pumps are used to both reduce and control lymphedema, (2) the efficacy of pump use for lymphedema treatment is still debated, (3) pumps reduce swelling but researchers are concerned about the mechanism of swelling reduction as well as the rapid displacement of fluid elsewhere in the body, and (4) use of pumps does not eliminate the need for compression garments and *may not provide more benefit than garments alone.*

19. What are some problems associated with the use of pneumatic pumps?

Investigations report the following concerns: (1) lymphatic congestion and injury proximal to the pump sleeve; (2) increased swelling adjacent to the pump cuff in up to 18% of patients; (3) lack of benefit in all patients except those with stage I lymphedema, which is reversible and easily treated by compression alone; and (4) development of genital lymphedema in up to 43% of patients with cancer-related lower extremity lymphedema.

20. What role does surgery play in lymphedema treatment?

Surgical interventions have generally been considered a last resort in lymphedema treatment. Surgery has provided helpful cosmetic improvement in unusual lymphedemas (i.e., genitals or eyelids). Liposuction, used for patients who develop excess adipose tissue and do not respond to external compression and decongestive therapies, has been very successful in reducing breast cancer-related lymphedema. Postoperatively, lifelong, constant compression with garments is required to maintain benefit, just as lifelong compression is required for optimal outcomes in all patients with lymphedema of the extremities.

21. What is complete decongestive therapy?

Complete decongestive therapy is a four-modality treatment of extremity lymphedema consisting of:
1. Compression bandaging: requires use of a short stretch elastic bandage rather than typical long-stretch Ace bandages
2. Manual lymph drainage-type massage: manual lymph drainage (MLD) is a light touch skin-stretching massage, using principles of lymphatic anatomy and physiology to increase systemic lymph drainage
3. Lymphatic-stimulating exercises
4. Skin care routine similar to that used by persons with diabetes (see Question 13)

22. What evidence exists regarding complete decongestive therapy and manual lymph drainage in lymphedema care?

Lymphedema reduction has been reported in Europe, Australia, and the United States using MLD in combination with the other three modalities of "intensive therapy." Treatments are time and labor intensive and costly. Patients must continue long-term external compression to avoid rapid loss of treatment benefit. Research has documented: (1) garments are the optimal daytime compression modality, and (2) bandaging, with or without manual lymph drainage, produces similar outcomes in extremity lymphedema.

 Key Points

- Consistent use of external compression products is crucial to optimal outcomes for patients with lymphedema of the extremities.
- Infection is the most common precipitator and complication of lymphedema.
- Nurses improve patient outcomes by assessing for early lymphedema, assisting patients in obtaining effective treatment, and assessing long-term patient outcomes.

Internet Resources

The National Lymphedema Network (NLN):
  http://www.lymphnet.org
The British Lymphology Society (BLS):
  http://www.lymphoedema.org/bls
The International Society of Lymphology (ISL):
  http://www.u.arizona.edu/~witte/ISL.htm

Bibliography

Andersen L, Hojris I, Erlandsen M, et al: Treatment of breast cancer-related lymphedema with or without manual lymphatic drainage—a randomized study. *Acta Oncol* 39(3):399-405, 2000.

Badger C, Preston N, Seers K, et al: Physical therapies for reducing and controlling lymphoedema of the limbs. *Cochrane Database Syst Rev* Oct 18(4):CD003141, 2004.

Brorson H: Liposuction in arm lymphedema treatment. *Scand J Surg* 92:287-295, 2003.

Golshan M, Martin WJ, Dowlatshahi K: Sentinel lymph node biopsy lowers the rate of lymphedema when compared with standard axillary lymph node dissection. *Am Surg* 69(3):209-211, 2003.

Mortimer PS: Lymphoedema. In Warrell DA, Cox TM, Firth JD, editors: *Oxford textbook of medicine,* Oxford, 2003, Oxford Press.

Mortimer PS, Badger C: Lymphoedema. In Doyle D, Hank GW, Cherny N, et al, editors: *Oxford textbook of palliative medicine,* New York, 2004, Oxford Press.

Olszewski W: Episodic dermatolymphangioadenitis (DLA) in patients with lymphedema of the lower extremities before and after administration of benzathine penicillin: A preliminary study, *Lymphology* 29(3):126-131, 1996.

Smith JK: Lymphedema management. In Ferrell, B, Coyle N, editors: *The Oxford textbook of palliative nursing,* New York, 2006, Oxford University Press.

Smith JK: Treating infection as a complication of lymphedema. *Lymphedema Management: Special Interest Group Newsletter* 15(3):7-9, 2004.

Thiadens S: Eighteen steps to prevention revised: LE risk reduction practices (Medical Alert). *Lymph Link* 17(4):9, 1995.

Mucositis

Sandi Vannice

1. Define stomatitis and mucositis.

Stomatitis refers to inflammatory diseases of the mouth, including the mucosa, dentition, periapices, and periodontium. Mucositis describes an inflammatory process involving any mucous membrane. The term *mucotoxic*, rather than *stomatotoxic*, refers to treatments that cause inflammation of the mucous membranes.

2. What is the incidence of mucositis in patients with cancer?

The incidence of mucositis ranges from 40% among patients receiving standard dose chemotherapy to 100% of patients receiving radiation therapy for head and neck cancers. Approximately 80% of patients who receive a stem cell transplant develop mucositis.

3. When does mucositis occur?

Damage occurs below the epithelial surface before mucosal changes can be seen. The effects of chemotherapy on the oral mucosa begin shortly after therapy is started. Because leukocytes and oral mucosal cells have similar rates of renewal, the peak in severity of mucositis usually correlates with the neutrophil nadir around day 7 to 10 of therapy. The condition eventually resolves, usually within 2 weeks.

Oral mucosal injury has a chronic course from radiation that is administered in multiple small fractions over a period of weeks. Atrophic changes in the epithelium occur at a total dose level of 1600 to 2200 cGy. Mucositis generally appears 1 to 2 weeks after therapy is started and persists for many weeks.

4. Describe the pathogenesis of oral mucositis.

The pathogenesis of mucositis is a complex multiphase pathologic process that varies with each individual. Not all patients are susceptible to the damaging effects of chemotherapy or radiation therapy, because of varying genetic and molecular mechanisms. Both chemotherapy and radiation therapy generate free radicals that injure tissues of the submucosa and initiate a sequence of biologic processes reflected in the following five phases that may be occurring at the same time in different locations in the mouth.

Biologic phases of oral mucositis		
Phase	**Time after exposure**	**Biologic process**
Initiation	0-2 days	Direct damage to the DNA of epithelial basal cells results in cell death.

Biologic phases of oral mucositis—cont'd

Phase	Time after exposure	Biologic process
Upregulation and message generation	2-3 days	A number of biologic switches are turned on, generating an array of messages that result in damage and epithelial cell death. The mucosa starts to thin and becomes erythematous. Patients may report mild discomfort.
Amplification and signaling	2-10 days	Many of the mediators targeting tissue and causing injury also produce simultaneous "feedback," resulting in further signaling, message generation, and cytokine production, leading to further tissue damage.
Ulceration	10-15 days	Nerve endings are exposed, resulting in moderate to severe pain. The ulcerated surface is colonized by the oral microbes, releasing products that act as toxins and stimulate inflammatory cells that accumulate beneath the ulcer and generate additional cytokines. Local infection can occur, and if the patient also has neutropenia, bacteria may penetrate vascular walls and cause sepsis.
Healing	14-21 days	Eventually, healing occurs as the epithelium around the ulcer divides, cells migrate and differentiate into healthy mucosa epithelium. Once the ulcer is healed, symptoms resolve quickly.

5. Which chemotherapeutic agents are associated with mucositis?

Chemotherapeutic agents that interfere with DNA synthesis and directly affect the epithelium, such as 5-fluorouracil (5-FU) with or without leucovorin and methotrexate, are associated with mucositis. The incidence of mucositis associated with 5-FU treatment is higher with continuous infusion than with intermittent bolus infusions. (See table of Chemotherapy Side Effects in Chapter 6, Principles of Chemotherapy).

6. What are the risk factors for developing oral mucositis?

Cancer type and treatment regimen influence the development of mucositis. A chemotherapy regimen that includes mucotoxic drugs; the frequency, dose, and depth of radiation treatments; and the combination of chemotherapy with radiation therapy are major risk factors. Other risk factors include patient age (children and older adults), women, poor oral health and nutrition, smoking history, previous history of mucositis, oxygen therapy, and ill-fitting dentures. Medications, such as opioids, antidepressants, phenothiazines, antihypertensives, antihistamines, diuretics, and sedatives may cause xerostomia (dry mouth), which can allow bacterial and fungal overgrowth.

7. How is mucositis assessed?

Before each outpatient treatment or daily for hospitalized patients, the oral cavity should be assessed with a gloved hand, tongue blade, and light source. Dentures should be removed to facilitate the assessment.

- Inspect all areas of the oral cavity, including the lips, gingivae, tongue, and throat.
- Observe the appearance of any lesions and assess the color of the mucous membranes. Early signs and symptoms of oral mucositis include mild redness and swelling along the gum line and sensations of mild burning and dryness. The presence of redness or white patches may indicate a local infection.
- Note the color, amount, and consistency of saliva.
- Check for swelling, ulcerations, cracks, fissures, and bumps, both in the mouth and on the lips.
- Ask patients if they are having pain, taste changes, swallowing problems, or sore throat.

8. What tools help to assess and document the incidence of oral mucositis?

An assessment tool should be appropriate for the clinical setting, clear, easy to use, and provide the right information. The World Health Organization and the National Cancer Institute have grading tools that are easy to use and incorporate into daily practice. Scales of 0 (none) to 4 (life threatening) provide a gross indicator of the degree of mucositis. The tool can be accessed online at: http://ctep.cancer.gov/forms/CTCAEv3.pdf.

The University of Nebraska Medical Center's Oral Assessment Guide (OAG) is a commonly used tool, with demonstrated validity and reliability. The OAG contains eight categories, each with three levels of descriptive ratings. The eight categories describe quality of the voice, swallow, saliva, integrity of the lips, tongue, mucous membranes, gingivae, and teeth. The three descriptive levels rate each category from most normal (1) to most abnormal (3). In addition, the OAG includes a narrative description of each category of assessment.

9. What are the consequences of oral mucositis?

Mucositis of the oral cavity is one of the most debilitating, painful side effects of cancer treatment, resulting in:

- Disruption of function and integrity of the mucous membranes, progressing from asymptomatic erythema to painful ulcerations, bleeding, local and systemic infection, and compromised airway
- Compromised ability to talk, take oral medications, and maintain adequate nutrition and hydration
- Lack of adherence to treatment, treatment delays, and dose reductions affecting overall survival
- Bacterial, fungal, and viral infections may occur, necessitating hospitalization for treatment with IV (intravenous) antibiotics. Oral bacteria can be isolated in 25% to 64% of cases of bacteremia. Streptococcal organisms are the most common bacterial infections associated with oral mucositis.

10. Are there guidelines for the prevention and treatment of oral mucositis?

The Multinational Association of Supportive Care in Cancer and the International Society for Oral Oncology (MASCC/ISOO) created a panel to develop evidence-based guidelines for the prevention and treatment of oral and GI (gastrointestinal) mucositis. These guidelines were published in 2004 and are updated as new information regarding prevention and treatment of mucositis becomes known. The current guidelines are available online at: http://www.mascc.org.

The guidelines include the following summary of recommendations for management of oral mucositis:

- A basic oral care protocol that includes patient and staff education should be used to reduce the severity of oral mucositis. Use of a soft toothbrush that is replaced on a regular basis is recommended. There is currently insufficient evidence to recommend one oral care protocol over another.
- Patient controlled analgesia (PCA) with morphine is the treatment of choice for pain from oral mucositis in patients undergoing hematopoietic stem cell transplant (HSCT).
- Midline radiation blocks and three-dimensional radiation treatment should be used to reduce mucosal injury.
- Sucralfate and antimicrobial lozenges should *not* be used for the prevention of radiation-induced oral mucositis.
- Chlorhexidine is *not* recommended for the prevention or treatment of existing mucositis.
- Oral cryotherapy should be used for patients receiving bolus 5-FU or high dose melphalan. Placing ice chips in the mouth 5 minutes before treatment with bolus 5-FU, and continuing for a total of 30 minutes has been shown to reduce oral mucositis by 50% in clinical trials.
- Acyclovir and its analogues should *not* be routinely used to prevent mucositis.
- Keratinocyte growth factor-1 (Palifermin) should be used by patients undergoing high dose chemotherapy and total body irradiation with autologous stem cell transplant. The recommended dose to prevent oral mucositis is 60 µg/kg/day for 3 days before starting the conditioning treatment and for 3 days after transplant.
- Low-level laser therapy (LLLT) may be useful in decreasing the incidence of oral mucositis and its associated pain in patients undergoing high-dose chemotherapy or chemoradiotherapy before HSCT.

11. Summarize the MASCC/ISOO guidelines for prevention and treatment of gastrointestinal mucositis.

PREVENTION

- Amifostine may prevent radiation proctitis in patients with rectal cancer receiving standard dose radiation therapy.
- Sulfasalazine, 500 mg po twice daily, may help decrease the incidence and severity of radiation-induced enteropathy in patients undergoing external beam radiotherapy to the pelvis.
- Oral sucralfate should *not* be used for the prevention of acute diarrhea in patients with pelvic malignancies undergoing external beam radiotherapy.
- 5-aminosalicylic acid and related compounds (mesalazine and olsalazine) should *not* be used to prevent GI mucositis.
- Ranitidine or omeprazole should be used to prevent epigastric pain after treatment with cyclophosphamide, methotrexate, and 5-FU, or treatment with 5-FU with or without folinic acid chemotherapy.
- Systemic glutamine should *not* be used for the prevention of GI mucositis.

TREATMENT

- Sucralfate enemas are helpful in managing chronic radiation-induced proctitis in patients with rectal bleeding.

- If diarrhea is not relieved with loperamide, octreotide (at least 100 µg subcutaneously twice a day) should be used to control diarrhea caused by standard-dose or high-dose chemotherapy associated with HSCT.
- Amifostine should be used to decrease esophagitis related to concomitant chemotherapy and radiotherapy in patients with non-small cell lung cancer.

12. What oral care instructions should be given to a patient?

Studies show that a protocol emphasizing assessment, good oral hygiene, patient teaching, consistent documentation, and reinforcement of mouth care may decrease the severity of mucositis and associated complications. Patient education material should include the following instructions for oral care:

Oral Care

- Take care of dental problems before starting treatment
- Keep mouth and teeth clean
  - Use a soft-bristled toothbrush, a sponge-covered oral swab, or gauze covered finger if brushing is too painful. Use nonabrasive fluoride toothpaste for at least 90 seconds after each meal and at bedtime. Brush the tongue to remove bacteria.
  - Remove dentures and bridges and clean after meals.
  - Gently floss teeth with unwaxed floss only if platelet count is adequate.
  - Rinse for 30 seconds after brushing and flossing with a bland rinse (avoid alcohol-based mouthwashes). Increase the frequency of rinsing depending on the severity of mucositis (every 2-4 hours as needed is common).
  - Follow rinsing with the use of a topical anesthetic or topical antifungal as needed (these agents coat better on a clean mouth).
- Keep mouth moist
  - Use spray bottle and mist often; humidifying the room is also helpful.
  - Use commercially available salivary substitutes or supplements (e.g., Biotene, MoiStir, Oral Balance, Salagen, Salivart) for dry mouth.
  - Apply a water based lip lubricant generously.
- Maintain oral mucosa integrity
  - Eat high-protein foods and drink plenty of fluids (> 1.5 quarts a day)
  - Avoid citrus juices or foods that cause irritation, such as rough, coarse, highly spiced, or acidic foods.
  - Avoid eating foods at temperature extremes (hot coffee, ice cream).
  - Avoid tobacco and alcohol use.
- Inspect mouth daily (using a flashlight and mirror), and call your health care provider if you experience any of the following: painful mouth sores, white patches, difficulty eating or swallowing, bleeding gums, or swelling of the lips or tongue.

13. How effective are currently used rinsing agents?

The optimal agent has yet to be identified.

- **Saline** promotes healing and is a well tolerated, readily available, and cost effective rinse that is easy to use at home. A normal saline solution is prepared by adding approximately 1 teaspoon of table salt to 32 ounces of water. The patient should swish and spit the solution as often as necessary to maintain oral comfort. Saline solution can enhance oral lubrication in the presence of dry mouth, as well as stimulate salivary glands to increase salivary flow.

- **Sodium bicarbonate** has been the mainstay of nursing care for oral mucositis, yet there is evidence suggesting it increases the oral bacterial flora.
- **Multi-agent rinses** have not yet been proven effective in treating mucositis. It is important to know the ingredients in the mixture, because alcohol-based agents may cause drying, burning, and irritation.
- **Sucralfate** suspension may offer little or no benefit compared to good oral hygiene and treatment of symptoms.
- **Hydrogen peroxide** may break down new granulation tissue and disrupt the normal oral flora.
- **Povidone-iodine** solution and swabs contain a 10% concentration that should not be used at full strength. It has antiseptic activity and is well tolerated but should not be used in the presence of granulating tissue, nor should it ever be swallowed. Its clinical value warrants further study.
- **Chamomile** is inexpensive and readily available, but there are no data to demonstrate efficacy.

14. What systemic agents may be used to treat and relieve pain associated with oral mucositis?

Severe pain may require treatment with systemic opioids, such as intravenous morphine, morphine elixir, or nonsteroidal antiinflammatory drugs (NSAIDs). Pain should be controlled according to standard pain management guidelines. The dose of systemic agents and duration of use may be reduced by supplementing with topical anesthetics.

15. What topical agents may be used to relieve pain associated with oral mucositis?

- **KBX solution** (Kaopectate, Benadryl, Xylocaine (viscous 2% solution) in equal parts): 5 to 15 ml; swish for 1 minute, then spit or swallow every 2 to 4 hours as needed. Xylocaine functions as a topical anesthetic, Benadryl as a short-acting anesthetic. Mylanta may be substituted for Kaopectate. Each serves as a medium for alkalinizing oral pH, which is usually more acidic in patients with mucositis.
- **Xylocaine** (viscous 2% solution): 5 to 15 ml; swish and spit every 2 to 4 hours as needed. Topical lidocaine may sting initially but is followed by pain relief lasting 15 to 30 minutes. Taste can be altered or absent, because taste receptors are also anesthetized. The gag reflex may also be suppressed.
- **Gelclair** (polyvinylpyrrolidone, sodium hyaluronate, and glycyrrhetinic acid): a concentrated gel; rinse around mouth for at least 1 minute. This gel acts like an occlusive dressing, rapidly reducing pain with relief for 5 to 7 hours. Use 1 hour before meals.
- **Kenalog in Orabase** (triamcinolone acetonide): apply paste to mouth or lip sores 2 to 4 times/day.
- **UlcerEase** is a thick gel that coats, protects, and eases pain.
- **Zilactin** is a protective film that is applied to oral and lip lesions (burns on application).
- **Capsaicin taffy:** capsaicin is the active ingredient in chili peppers that desensitizes some of the neurons in the painful region. Patients reported less pain after the initial burning of the candy fades.

16. What are the future directions in prevention and treatment of oral mucositis?

- A better understanding of the pathophysiology of oral mucositis may reveal pathways for targeted therapies to prevent the development of mucositis before clinical symptoms occur. For example, controlled studies have shown that AES-14, a topical oral suspension that increases the uptake of L-glutamine into epithelial oral mucosal

cells 100 times more than conventional glutamine, reduces the incidence and severity of oral mucositis.
- A novel agent, benzydamine hydrochloride, a nonsteroidal antiinflammatory oral rinse, is being studied for its prolonged analgesic effects and effect in reducing the incidence and severity of oral mucositis.
- In the future, nurses may be able to choose interventions that are phase appropriate for their patients. There are almost 200 genes associated with mucositis. Studies are under way to examine more closely the role of genetics in the development of mucositis. Findings may help explain why certain patients develop this debilitating side effect of treatment.

Key Points

- Oral mucositis is an inflammation of the oral mucous membranes due to treatment with chemotherapy and/or radiation therapy.
- The pathophysiology of oral mucositis is a complex multiphase process.
- The risk factors for developing oral mucositis include type of treatment, gender and age of patient, dental health, nutrition, and neutropenia.
- The Multinational Association of Supportive Care in Cancer (MASCC) in collaboration with the International Society of Oral Oncology has developed evidence-based guidelines for managing oral and gastrointestinal mucositis that should be used in guiding clinical practice.
- The optimal agent for the prevention of oral mucositis has yet to be identified.

Internet Resources

Oncology Nursing Society:
   http://www.ons.org
Multinational Association of Supportive Care in Cancer:
   http://www.mascc.org
Common Terminology Criteria for Adverse Events v3.0:
   http://ctep.cancer.gov/forms/CTCAEv3.pdf
National Cancer Institute
   http://nci.nih.gov

Acknowledgments

The author wishes to acknowledge Janet Kemp, RN, PhD, and Harri Brackett, MS, RN, OCN, for their contributions to the Mucositis chapter published in the first and second editions of *Oncology Nursing Secrets*.

Bibliography

Avritscher EB, Cooksley CD, Elting LS: Scope and epidemiology of cancer therapy induced oral and gastrointestinal mucositis. *Semin Oncol Nurs* 20:3-10, 2004.
Brown CG, Wingard J: Clinical consequences of oral mucositis. *Semin Oncol Nurs* 20:17-21, 2004.
Cawley M, Benson LM: Current trends in managing oral mucositis. *Clin J Oncol Nurs* 9:584-592, 2005.
Eilers J: Nursing interventions and supportive care for the prevention and treatment of oral mucositis associated with cancer treatment. *Oncol Nurs Forum* 31:13-23, 2004.
Epstein JB, Schubert MM: Managing pain in mucositis. *Semin Oncol Nurs* 20:30-37, 2004.
Miller M, Kearney N: Oral care for patients with cancer: A review of the literature. *Cancer Nurs* 24:241-254, 2001.

National Cancer Institute: Oral complications of chemotherapy and head/neck radiation. Health professional version. Available at: www.cancer.gov/cancertopics/pdq/supportivecare/oralcomplications/healthprofessional. Accessed January 10, 2007.

Petersen, DE: New strategies for management of oral mucositis in cancer patients. *J Support Oncol* (suppl 1) 4:9-13, 2006.

Shih A, Miaskowski C, Dodd, MJ, et al: Mechanisms for radiation-induced oral mucositis and the consequences. *Cancer Nurs* 26:222-229, 2003.

Sonis ST: Pathobiology of mucositis. *Semin Oncol Nurs* 20:11-15, 2004.

Chapter 39

Nausea and Vomiting

Rita S. Wickham

1. How extensive is the problem of nausea and vomiting for persons with cancer?

For patients with cancer, nausea and vomiting (N&V) are often multicausal and may occur after chemotherapy, radiation therapy, and surgery, or may be related to cancer or other medical problems and medications. The risk for nausea with progressive cancer is greater than 50%, and vomiting is less common. Most antiemetic research has examined acute N&V from chemotherapy (CINV), whereas there is less research on delayed CINV, N&V from radiation therapy (RINV), postoperative N&V (PONV), and N&V from other causes. Appropriately used antiemetics can prevent acute CINV in 80% to 90% of patients. Delayed CINV is more problematic and may be compounded because most chemotherapy is administered in the clinic, and patients often do not report distressing symptoms after going home.

2. What are the consequences of poorly managed N&V?

Inadequately controlled N&V can lead to negative physical and psychosocial effects, as well as increase the risk for chemotherapy toxicities.

- Severe vomiting can lead to rapid dehydration and fluid volume deficit (FVD). A two pound weight decrease over a few days reflects the loss of one liter of body fluid, so the nurse should calculate each patient's weight loss as well as the percentage of weight lost to estimate FVD, which may range from mild (2%) to severe (8%).
- Other associated problems: anorexia and weight loss, taste changes and food aversions, and the inability or willingness to undergo rigorous therapies.
- N&V from any cause can interfere with activities a patient deems important, such as spending time with family and friends, doing work and leisure activities, and enjoying eating.

3. What is our current understanding of the physiology and pathogenesis of N&V?

Vomiting is a complex protective reflex that occurs in response to activation of the nucleus tractus solitarius, commonly called the vomiting center (VC), in the brainstem. Emetic stimuli arise in the gut, brain, bloodstream, or other organs and are transmitted by particular neurotransmitters along one or more afferent neuroreceptor pathways to the VC. For example, the peripheral pathway includes serotonin receptors—subtypes 3 and 4 ($5HT_3$ and $5HT_4$)—on the vagus (and perhaps other abdominal visceral nerves) that are stimulated or blocked by serotonin, as well as mechanoreceptor and other receptors that respond to stretch or other stimuli. Another important brain area is the chemoreceptor trigger zone (CTZ) in the area postrema that contains several neurotransmitters and receptors, including substance P and neurokinin-1 (NK_1) receptors, serotonin and $5HT_3$ receptors, dopamine (D) and D2 receptors, as well as others. The CTZ is not contained within the blood-brain barrier and detects noxious substances in the cerebral spinal fluid and bloodstream. In addition, other areas involved in N&V include higher brain centers that are associated with vision, hearing, smell, and memory; the limbic region, which is important for negative emotions and distress; the vestibular apparatus (VA); and other brain areas. The cortex is important for the realization and memory of

N&V, and the limbic region—the fight or flight part of the brain—attaches emotional meanings and responses to distressing symptoms. The VA is involved in N&V induced by motion sickness, Ménière's disease, and viral infection of the inner ear. Other neurotransmitters important for N&V include histamine, acetylcholine, and cannabinoid (and perhaps others), which bind to histamine (H_1), muscarinic cholinergic (M), and cannabinoid-1 (CB_1) receptors, respectively. We are beginning to learn about the endocannabinoid system and CB_1 receptors in brain tissues that have roles in many functions, including N&V.

4. Which pathways are most important in chemotherapy-induced N&V?

The physiologic mechanisms of acute and delayed CINV overlap but differ somewhat. The two key pathways in CINV are the peripheral and the central. The peripheral pathway is mediated by serotonin, which binds at $5HT_3$ receptors along the vagus nerve to provoke acute CINV. However, serotonin plays a lesser or small role in delayed CINV. The central N&V pathway is important in acute and delayed CINV and is mediated by substance P, which binds to NK_1 receptors in the brainstem, near the CTZ or the VC itself. Other organs and receptors that play lesser roles in acute and delayed CINV include the cortex and limbic region, and perhaps brain CB_1 receptors.

5. What is substance P and how is it involved in N&V?

Substance P, which is in the tachykinin neuropeptide class, is involved in many body functions. When substance P binds to NK_1 receptors in the brainstem, N&V ensue. Aprepitant (Emend), the only commercially available NK_1 receptor antagonist (RA) at this time, has Food and Drug Administration (FDA) approval to prevent acute and delayed CINV from highly emetogenic chemotherapy. Aprepitant, 40 mg given within 3 hours before induction of anesthesia, has recently been approved for prevention of PONV. Substance P activation at NK_1 receptors is probably an important mediator of N&V from many causes. Unfortunately, aprepitant is prohibitively expensive and has not been studied for control of N&V in palliative care.

6. Describe the role of serotonin and serotonin receptors in N&V.

Serotonin receptors of subtype 3 ($5HT_3$) located along the vagus nerve play a significant role in helping the body rid itself of perceived noxious agents, including some chemotherapy drugs and abdominal radiation that damages enterochromaffin cells. In response to perceived toxins, enterochromaffin cells in the upper gastrointestinal (GI) tract release serotonin, which binds to nearby vagal $5HT_3$ receptors and transmits the message to the VC, causing vomiting. Serotonin binding to $5HT_4$ neuroreceptors influences gastric emptying and GI transit time and may be involved in delayed N&V after chemotherapy. The vagus and other visceral nerves also have stretch receptors that respond to compression and stasis that accompanies small bowel obstruction, hepatomegaly, or extrinsic tumor compression.

7. Which chemotherapy drugs cause CINV?

Chemotherapy drugs and targeted agents are classified by their likelihood of inducing *acute* CINV. There are two current evidence-based guidelines for antiemetic management—the *National Comprehensive Cancer Network (NCCN) Practice Guidelines in Oncology – Antiemesis* and the *American Society of Clinical Oncology (ASCO) Guidelines for Antiemetics in Oncology*. Both have similarities, categorizing risk as high, moderate, low, or minimal. (See table on pp. 420-421).

Emetic potential of intravenously administered (unless stated otherwise) chemotherapy and targeted agents without antiemetics

Agent (common brand name)/guideline

High (> 90%)	AC: doxorubicin (Adriamycin) or epirubicin (Ellence) + cyclophosphamide (Cytoxan) Altretamine (Hexalen) - oral Carmustine (BiCNU) $\geq$ 250 mg/m^2 Cisplatin (Platinol) $\geq$ 50 mg/m^2	Cyclophosphamide (Cytoxan) $\geq$ 1500 mg/m^2 Dacarbazine (DTIC) Dactinomycin (Cosmegen) Mechlorethamine (Mustargen) Procarbazine (Matulane) - oral Streptozocin (Zanosar)
Moderate (30%-90%)	Aldesleukin (Proleukin) >12-15 million units/m^2 Amifostine (Ethyol) > 300 mg* Ara-C (Cytarabine) > 1 g/m^2 Arsenic trioxide (Trisenox) Azacitidine (Vidaza) - SQ Busulfan (Myerlan) > 4 mg/d Carboplatin (Paraplatin) Carmustine (BiCNU) $\leq$ 250 mg/m^2 Cisplatin (Platinol) < 50 mg/m^2 Cyclophosphamide $\leq$ 1500 mg/m^2 Cyclophosphamide (Cytoxan) - oral Dactinomycin (Cosmegen) Daunorubicin (Cerubidine)	Doxorubicin (Adriamycin) Epirubin (Ellence) Etoposide (Vepesid) - oral Idarubicin (Idamycin) Ifosfamide (Ifex) Imatinib (Gleevec) - oral Irinotecan (Camptosar) Lomustine (CeeNU) Melphalan (Alkeran) > 50 mg/m^2 Methotrexate (Mexate) 250-1000 mg/m^2 Oxaliplatin (Eloxatin) > 75 mg/m^2 Temozolomide (Temodor) - oral Vinorelbine (Navelbine)
Low (10%-30%)	Amifostine (Ethyol) < 300 mg* Ara-C (Cytarabine) 100-200 mg/m^2 Bexarotene (Targretin) - oral Bortezomib (Velcade) Capecitabine (Xeloda) - oral Cetuximab (Erbitux) Docetaxel (Taxotere) Doxorubicin-liposomal (Caelyx) Etoposide (Vepesid) Fludarabine (Fludara)	5-fluorouracil (Adrucil) Gemcitabine (Gemzar) Methotrexate (Mexate) >50 < 250 mg/m^2 Mitomycin (Mutamycin) Mitoxantrone (Novantrone) Paclitaxel (Taxol) Paclitaxel-albumin (Abraxane) Pemetrexed (Alimta) Topotecan (Hycamptin)
Minimal (< 10%)	Alemtuzumab (Campath) Alpha interferon (IntronA) Asparaginase (Elspar) Bevacizumab (Avastin) Bleomycin (Blenoxane) Bortezomib (Velcade) Busulfan (Myleran) Chlorambucil (Leukeran) - oral 2-Chlorodeoxyadenosine (Cladribine) Dasatinib (Sprycel) - oral Decitabine (Dacogen)	Hydroxyurea (Hydrea) - oral Lenalidomide (Revlimid) - oral Melphalan low dose (Leukeran) - oral Methotrexate (Mexate) $\leq$ 50 mg/m^2 Nelarabine (Arranon) Pentostatin (Nipent) Rituximab (Rituxan) Sorafenib (Nexavar) - oral Sunitinib (Sutent) - oral

Emetic potential of intravenously administered (unless stated otherwise) chemotherapy and targeted agents without antiemetics—cont'd

	Agent (common brand name)/guideline	
Minimal (< 10%)—cont'd	Denileukin diftitox (Ontak)	Thalidomide (Thalomid) - oral
	Dexrazoxane (Zinecard)*	Thioguanine (6-TG) - oral
	Erlotinib (Tarceva) - oral	Trastuzumab (Herceptin)
	Fludarabine (Fludara)	Valrubicin (Valstar)
	Gefitinib (Iressa) - oral	Vinblastine (Velban)
	Gemtuzumab ozogamicin (Mylotarg)	Vincristine (Oncovin)
		Vinorelbine (Navelbine)

*Chemoprotectant agent; *Information from ASCO (2006) and NCCN (2007)*

8. What other factors might affect the likelihood of CINV?

Antiemetic guidelines aid in antiemetic selection for chemotherapy or radiation therapy for each patient, but clinical judgment is important because of several factors:
- Patients may respond differently to particular antiemetics (better or worse, fewer or greater adverse effects) because of inherent genetic differences.
- The doses of some chemotherapy agents and dosing schedule (i.e., multiple day regimens, large single doses vs. lower divided doses vs. continuous infusion [CI] regimens) may alter individual risk.
- Poorly controlled N&V with past chemotherapy, or from other illnesses or causes might also alter risk.

9. Do patient characteristics influence risk for N&V?

Yes. Patient characteristics that *may* increase the risks of CINV, and perhaps N&V from other causes, include: female gender, low alcohol intake, poorly controlled CINV in the past, motion sickness, hyperemesis of pregnancy, and high level of anxiety. CINV may be more easily controlled in persons who regularly consume 1 to 5 alcoholic drinks per day. Patients who experienced inadequate control of CINV with previous chemotherapy may be fearful of and expect N&V with new therapy. Anxiety, past motion sickness, and hyperemesis with pregnancy do not always accurately predict poorer antiemetic control, but may be important for particular patients.

10. When is chemotherapy-induced N&V likely to occur?

CINV may be acute, delayed, or breakthrough. **Acute** CINV is arbitrarily considered to occur in the first 24 hours after chemotherapy, whereas delayed CINV persists beyond 16 to 24 hours after chemotherapy and may continue for 4 or 5 days (or more). **Delayed** nausea is more common and distressing than delayed vomiting, and may persist and worsen for days after a patient returns home. All patients who receive moderately to highly emetogenic chemotherapy regimens are at risk for delayed CINV, and may also experience **breakthrough** CINV if appropriate antiemetics are not given for the entire expected period of delayed CINV. Thus, posttherapy nursing follow-up is important.

11. What is anticipatory N&V?

Anticipatory nausea is more common than anticipatory vomiting and results when acute *or* delayed CINV are not adequately managed. Anticipatory nausea and vomiting (ANV) is a classic conditioned response, which happens because a patient experiences nausea or vomiting—an *unconditioned* response—during or shortly after their first few chemotherapy treatments. If acute and delayed CINV are poorly controlled, events associated with chemotherapy (e.g., odors in the clinic, seeing the nurse at each visit) become the stimuli that elicit the *conditioned response* of nausea. ANV is probably less common now than before the advent of effective antiemetics, but it still occurs, is difficult to manage, and may cause distress for several years after chemotherapy is completed.

12. How likely is radiation therapy to cause N&V?

Because radiation therapy (RT) is a local treatment, the risk for RINV depends on the site irradiated. Patients whose treatment field includes the upper GI tract are at greatest risk, because RT damage to enterochromaffin cells causes serotonin release and subsequent binding at $5HT_3$ receptors. In addition, large RT fields and large single doses also increase the risk for RINV. The risk of RINV is 60% to greater than 90% in patients receiving total body irradiation (TBI) before stem cell transplant, upper-body hemibody RT to control pain, or large volume RT to the abdomen. The risk for RINV is less with RT to the lower abdomen (30%-60%), chest (~20%), or head (~10%), and is rare after RT to other body areas. RINV starts within minutes of large preparatory doses for stem cell transplantation and within 60 to 90 minutes after lower doses. RINV persists for several hours after each treatment. Patients can develop ANV if RINV is not prevented each day of RT. Current evidence dictates antiemetic prophylaxis for patients at moderate to high risk for RINV.

Recommended PO and IV antiemetics for radiation therapy

Risk category	Recommended antiemetics
High: total body irradiation (TBI)	$5HT_3$ antagonist (ondansetron 8 mg po bid or tid, or granisetron 2 mg po once daily) ± dexamethasone 2 mg po tid
Moderate: radiation to upper abdomen, hemibody, abdominal-pelvic, mantle, or craniospinal regions; cranial radiosurgery	$5HT_3$ antagonist before each fraction (ondansetron 8 mg po or granisetron 2 mg po)
Minimal: radiation to breast, head, neck, cranium, or extremities	No routine recommendations As needed, use D_2 (prochlorperazine) or $5HT_3$ antagonist

Abbreviations: po = oral, IV = intravenous

13. How common is postoperative N&V?

PONV is a common complication of surgery and may prevent discharge from the hospital or surgicenter. Greater than 25% of patients who undergo surgery experience PONV, and occurrence may be almost 80% in high risk patients (i.e., women, children, nonsmokers, patients with history of motion sickness or PONV). The type and duration of surgery, type of general anesthesia used, and use of opioid analgesics also influence the likelihood of experiencing PONV. In addition, delayed return of bowel motility may exacerbate nausea. Patients with medium (2 risk factors) and high risk (≥ 3 risk factors) of developing PONV should receive prophylactic single or combination antiemetics—considered superior—before or during surgery. First-line antiemetics for PONV include a $5HT_3$ antagonist (ondansetron 4-8 mg or dolasetron 12.5 mg) plus either dexamethasone 2-4 mg, aprepitant 40 mg, or droperidol 0.625 mg. If initial antiemetics do not prevent PONV, another agent (prochlorperazine, promethazine or scopolamine) should be used. Acupuncture may also be beneficial.

14. What are other potential causes of N&V that nurses should consider?

The causes of N&V are frequently multifactorial, so nurses should assess cancer-related problems, including:

- GI causes (bowel obstruction, hepatomegaly, stomach cancer, adhesions, ileus, and severe constipation)
- Central nervous system causes (meningeal or brain metastases, increased intracranial pressure)
- Metabolic/paraneoplastic syndromes (hypercalcemia, hypernatremia, syndrome of inappropriate secretion of antidiuretic hormone [SIADH])
- Inadequately controlled pain, or side effect of taking opioids or other analgesics
- Manifestation of infection, or side effect of antibiotics or other medications

15. Are antiemetics interchangeable for N&V from all causes?

No single antiemetic can be effective for all instances of N&V, and selection should be based on presumed causes and corresponding pathogenesis, receptors, and pathways. Antiemetics are classified by their major receptor site of action (e.g., $5HT_3$ antagonists, NK_1 antagonists, D_2 antagonists) but they may bind with other receptors, which could enhance efficacy or increase side effects. For instance, chlorpromazine and prochlorperazine are phenothiazines and bind to D_2 receptors. Chlorpromazine also binds well to H_1 and alpha-adrenergic (α_1) receptors, so they may cause sedation, anticholinergic effects, dizziness, and orthostasis. Sedation might be beneficial for a terminally ill or actively dying patient with intractable symptoms, whereas it would be bothersome for other patients. (Please refer to the table on pp. 424-427).

16. Which antiemetics should be used to prevent acute and delayed CINV?

Prophylaxis of acute and delayed CINV is essential for moderately to highly emetic (30%-100%) chemotherapy, whereas prophylaxis of acute CINV is recommended for low emetogenic chemotherapy. No antiemetics are routinely recommended for CINV when risk is minimal (< 10% [see table on p 428]). *Prevention* (or on-time treatment)—not *posttherapy rescue*—is the goal for CINV (and RINV) when emetic risk is 10% or less, and antiemetics are recommended according to the emetic potential of the chemotherapy agent. Appropriate doses of antiemetics should be scheduled and given for the entire expected period of N&V. Three antiemetics, a $5HT_3$ antagonist, aprepitant, and dexamethasone, are the standard of care to prevent acute and delayed CINV from highly emetic chemotherapy, whereas a $5HT_3$ antagonist plus dexamethasone is advised for acute CINV from moderately emetic chemotherapy. A single, *lowest effective* dose of $5HT_3$ antagonist should be given before chemotherapy; oral and IV doses are therapeutically equivalent. However, interpatient variability can affect individual response to and efficacy of any $5HT_3$ antagonist. Patients who receive emetogenic chemotherapy over several days should receive appropriate antiemetics each day of therapy.

17. Why is dexamethasone recommended as an antiemetic?

Dexamethasone may effectively control some instances of CINV, RINV, PONV, and disease-related N&V (DRNV). The antiemetic mechanism of action is unknown, but there

Text continued on p. 428.

Antiemetics by class

Drug	Indications	Dose/route	Comments
NK₁ Receptor antagonists			
Aprepitant (Emend)	Acute CINV Delayed CINV PONV	125 mg PO once (day 1) 80 mg/day PO on days 2 and 3 40 mg PO ≤ 3 hrs before anesthesia	Use in antiemetic combination. Potential drug interactions: moderate inhibitor of P450 hepatic isoenzyme system CYP34A and inducer of CYP2C9
Serotonin (5HT₃) Receptor antagonists			
Ondansetron (Zofran)	Acute and delayed CINV	Acute: 8 mg (0.15 mg/kg) IV once; *or* 8 mg PO bid or 16-24 mg PO once	IV and po doses are equivalent. May continue for 2-3 days for delayed CINV Administer before RT on each day of therapy. Dose of ondansetron should be decreased for severe hepatic impairment.
	RINV	No specified doses	Little research about use of 5HT₃ antagonists for cancer-related N&V, but may be useful for metabolic, gastric stasis, hepatomegaly, drugs (not opioids), sepsis
	PONV	4-8 mg IV/PO before surgery	Ondansetron, olanzapine, and mirtazapine are available as oral dissolvable tablets (ODT). Olanzapine might induce diabetes; inform patient of possibility and check blood glucose once a week for first month or two.

Granisetron (Kytril)	Acute and delayed CINV	Acute: 1 mg (0.01 mg/kg) IV once; or 1 to 2 mg PO once	
	RINV	No specified doses	
	PONV	No specified doses	
Dolasetron (Anzemet)	Acute and delayed CINV	Acute: 100 mg (1.8 mg/kg) IV once; or 100 mg once	
	RINV	No specified doses	
	PONV	12.5 mg IV before surgery	
Palonosetron (Aloxi)	Acute and delayed CINV	0.25 mg IV once	
Olanzapine (Zyprexa)	Acute, break through and delayed CINV; DRNV: metabolic, gastric stasis, partial obstruction, hepatomegaly, uremia	2.5-5 mg PO bid	
Mirtazapine (Remeron)		15-30 mg q HS	More likely to cause sedation compared to Olanzapine.
Corticosteroids			
Dexamethasone (Decadron)	Acute CINV, low risk	4-20 mg IV/PO once	Rapid IV administration can cause perineal, perioral, or abdominal burning/itching.
	Acute CINV, mod-high risk (30-100%)	10-12 mg IV/PO once	Recommended dose with aprepitant is 12mg PO or IV
	Delayed CINV	8 mg/day for 2-4 days	May cause enhanced sense of well-being, or insomnia or anxiety
	RINV	No specified doses	
	PONV	10-20 mg IV before surgery	
	Other: GI obstruction, increased intracranial pressure (ICP), hepatomegaly, metabolic, cough	8-60 mg/day	

Continued

Antiemetics by class—cont'd

Drug	Indications	Dose/route	Comments
Dopamine (D₂) antagonists			
Metoclopramide (Reglan)	Second line: delayed CINV, RINV, PONV Other: hepatomegaly, opioids and other drugs	20-40 mg bid-qid/day No specified doses 10 mg PO tid, ↑ to 20-40 mg q 4-6 hr 10-20 mg PO or IV q 4-6 hr	Metoclopramide contraindicated if bowel obstruction suspected/confirmed ± 5HT₃ antagonist for delayed CINV (after mod-high risk chemotherapy) Risk for EPS increased in young persons Hypotension may occur with IV administration in patients who are dehydrated or have cardiac disease Haloperidol is less sedating than phenothiazines
Prochlorperazine (Compazine)	Acute or delayed CINV, RINV (minimal-low risk) Other: opioids and other drugs, bowel obstruction, hiccups, metabolic, chronic unexplained	10 mg PO or IV q 4-6 hr 1-4 mg PO, IV, or SQ q 6 hr	
Haloperidol (Haldol)		0.5-2 mg PO or IV q 4-8 hr	
Cannabinoid			
Dronabinol (Marinol)	Third-line: acute, delayed CINV Other: gastric involvement Breakthrough treatment	5 mg PO q 4 hr 2.5-5 mg PO q 4-6 hr	Start with small dose and titrate to effect (depending on adverse effects, i.e., poor concentration, mood changes, paranoia, drowsiness) Other potential side effects are orthostasis and dry mouth Dronabinol contraindicated in patients with sesame allergy Nabilone is currently a schedule II drug.
Nabilone (Cessamet)		1-2 mg PO bid	

Antihistamine / Anticholinergic

Drug	Dose	Notes
Promethazine (Phenergan)	12.5-25 mg PO or IV q 4-6 hr	Adverse effects: sedation, disorientation, and anticholinergic effects (dry mouth, constipation)
Scopolamine (Transderm Scop)	1-2 patches q 72 hr	
Hyoscyamine (Levsin)	0.125-0.25 mg PO / SL qid / ac & hs	Levsin available as tablets, solution, and ODT

Other: motion, opioids, increased intracranial pressure, liver involvement, bowel obstruction, abdominal cancer, opioids

Other

Drug	Dose	Notes
Lorazepam (Ativan)	0.5-2 mg PO / SL / IV	Lorazepam may be useful when nausea has an anticipatory component or is accompanied by anxiety

CINV, RTNV, DRNV

Abbreviations: PO = oral, IV = intravenous, bid = twice per day, tid = three times per day, qid = four times per day, ac = before meals, hs = bedtime, q = every, SL = sublingual

Recommended antiemetics for CINV

Risk category	Acute CINV	Delayed CINV
High (> 90%)	Aprepitant (Emend) 125 mg po + 5HT$_3$ antagonist, po or IV (ondansetron [Zofran] 8-16 mg, or granisetron [Kytril] 1 mg IV or 2 mg po, or dolasetron [Anzemet] 100 mg or palonosetron [Aloxi] 0.25 mg IV) + Dexamethasone 8 mg IV or 12 mg po	Aprepitant (Emend) 80 mg po days 2 & 3 + Dexamethasone 8 mg po ± 5HT$_3$ antagonist po (ondansetron 8 mg bid or granisetron 1 mg IV or 2 mg po or dolasetron 100 mg)
Moderate (30%-90%)	5HT$_3$ antagonist po or IV (ondansetron 8-16 mg, or granisetron 1 mg IV or 2 mg po, or dolasetron 100 mg, or palonosetron 0.25 mg IV) + Dexamethasone 8 mg IV or 12 mg po	
Low (10%-30%)	Dexamethasone 8 mg IV or 12 mg po	No routine antiemetic for delayed CINV
Minimal (< 10%)	No routine antiemetic for acute CINV	No routine antiemetic for delayed CINV

Abbreviations: po = oral, IV = intravenous

is a great deal of evidence for using dexamethasone, which increases control of acute CINV by about 25%. It is superior to 5HT$_3$ antagonists for treating delayed CINV. Intravenous (IV) and oral (po) doses are typically 10 to 20 mg. Dexamethasone is safe and has mild side effects when used before and for 2 to 5 days after chemotherapy. Because the plasma concentration of dexamethasone may be increased when it is co-administered with aprepitant (moderate inhibitor of cytochrome P450 hepatic isoenzyme system CYP3A4), the dose of dexamethasone is reduced by 50%.

18. Should 5HT$_3$ antagonists be used to treat delayed CINV?

5HT$_3$ plays less of a role in delayed than in acute CINV. Patients are unlikely to achieve complete control of delayed CINV with a 5HT$_3$ antagonist only. ASCO no longer recommends routine use of 5HT$_3$ antagonists for delayed CINV, whereas NCCN includes them with other antiemetics (see Question 16). One study (Hickok et al, 2005) revealed that short-acting 5HT$_3$ antagonists were no better than prochlorperazine in controlling delayed nausea caused by doxorubicin, but neither antiemetic alone acceptably prevented nausea. This small study also highlights the difficulties in preventing delayed CINV.

19. What factors are important in considering the cost of antiemetics for chemotherapy?

Practice settings usually select 5HT$_3$ antagonists based on dollar costs to the institution, availability, and ease of administration. Nurses and others should use current guidelines to develop institutional antiemetic management protocols, and should investigate medication payment concerns with the patient and family. Most pharmaceutical companies have patient assistance programs (a good inclusive site for all generic and brand name drugs is www.needymeds.com) if a third party insurer does not cover costs. Other considerations are important in calculating overall costs of CINV. Less-than-optimal antiemetics lead to poor N&V control, negative quality of life, and increased risk of N&V in the future. Furthermore, less effective antiemetic regimens may require several hours of nursing time and treatment facility use, as the patient may need to return to the treatment center for IV fluids and antiemetics.

20. What questions should nurses include in pretreatment risk and post-CINV treatment assessments?

Before therapy, the nurse should ask the patient how bothersome CINV was with past chemotherapy and identify other risk factors (see Questions 8 and 9) that might increase the likelihood of CINV. After at least the first cycle or two of a new regimen, the nurse should ask the patient the following questions regarding the second to fifth days after chemotherapy administration, which could be included in a patient diary:

- Did you vomit/throw up in the last 24 hours? How many times?
- How much nausea did you have each day/last 24 hours? Use a numerical rating scale (0 to 10) or verbal descriptor scale (none, mild, moderate, severe).
- How much did N and/or V interfere with activities important to you?
- Did anything make N and/or V worse?
- Were you able to take your antiemetic(s)? How well did it (they) work?
- Did you have any bothersome antiemetic side effects (e.g., headache, constipation, jitteriness, insomnia)?
- Did anything else make the N and/or V better?
- Were you satisfied with how well your N and/or V were controlled?

21. What are possible side effects of aprepitant, 5HT₃ antagonists, and dexamethasone?

- Aprepitant is generally well tolerated, but may cause fatigue, hiccups, and constipation. It is metabolized by hepatic cytochrome P450 enzymes that metabolize other drugs, which may alter serum levels of one or more drugs. In a small study, 25 healthy individuals took small, stable doses of warfarin and experienced an 18% decreased INR (International Normalized Ratio) on days 7 and 8 following aprepitant dosing (125 mg on day 1, 80 mg on days 2 and 3) (Depré et al, 2005). This decrease was statistically significant and might be accompanied by changes in coagulation status. Although no clinically significant bleeding events have been reported, monitoring the patient's INR from day 7 to 10 is recommended. In addition, concomitant aprepitant increases serum dexamethasone levels and decreases the effectiveness of birth control pills. Dexamethasone doses are therefore decreased 50%, and patients who could become pregnant are instructed to use barrier birth control.
- Ondansetron, granisetron, dolasetron, and palonosetron: the most common side effects are mild headache during and after administration and asymptomatic, transient, and clinically inconsequential electrocardiogram changes (e.g., minor prolongation of the ST segment). Headache may be relieved by slowing the rate of intravenous administration or by giving acetaminophen. A few patients feel dizzy or lightheaded, sleepy, or nervous. Constipation is possible, especially if a 5HT₃ antagonist is given for several doses, as with multiday chemotherapy or radiation therapy. The nurse should assess the patient's usual bowel habits, teach the patient to report subjective awareness of constipation, and initiate a prophylactic bowel program (i.e., stool softener plus laxative), when necessary.
- Dexamethasone is nonsedating and may enhance appetite and mood. However, it may also cause insomnia, dysphoria, hiccups, elevated blood glucose level, and perianal discomfort with rapid IV infusion.

22. What are possible indications for metoclopramide, dopamine antagonists, and other antiemetics?

- For treatment of CINV, RINV and PONV, metoclopramide should be reserved for patients who do not have satisfactory control with at least one of two different $5HT_3$ antagonists because of inferior efficacy and risk for sedation, diarrhea, and extrapyramidal symptoms (EPS). Most patients deem sedation disagreeable, and it may also increase the risk of falling for older adult patients. On the other hand, metoclopramide has many uses in palliative care. It increases GI motility and may alleviate N&V related to GI stasis, and is frequently used for N&V of unexplained causes. Metoclopramide should not be given to patients with confirmed or suspected bowel obstruction, in whom prochlorperazine, haloperidol, or dexamethasone would be better choices.
- Similarly, 1 or 2 scopolamine patches may relieve N&V secondary to GI obstruction, use of opioids, motion, or other causes. Transdermal administration avoids oral or parenteral administration. Patches are applied to the upper chest, which is an area of high blood flow, and not behind the ear.
- Antihistamines (hyoscyamine [Levsin], promethazine [Phenergan], diphenhydramine [Benadryl]) may also be helpful for patients with motion-induced N&V, increased intracranial pressure, and GI obstruction or compression, particularly in the presence of excessive and difficult to handle secretions.
- Benzquinamide (Emete-Con) is a useful second-line antiemetic, because it does not have dopamine antagonist activity and can be used when other antiemetics cause side effects or are not effective.

23. Why is olanzapine used as an antiemetic?

Research and clinical experience support the use of olanzapine (Zyprexa), an atypical antipsychotic agent, as an effective antiemetic for delayed and breakthrough CINV and for nausea, vomiting, and anorexia in patients with progressive cancer. Olanzapine is a 'broad-spectrum' antiemetic that binds with serotonin, dopamine, histamine, and α-adrenergic receptors. In terms of $5HT_3$ antagonism, it is almost as potent as ondansetron but has weaker binding at dopamine receptors and rarely causes extrapyramidal symptoms. Olanzapine may also increase ghrelin, a hormone that stimulates appetite and food intake, which may be advantageous in the palliation of anorexic/cachectic patients. Olanzapine may control nausea refractory to prochlorperazine, haloperidol, metoclopramide, dexamethasone and other $5HT_3$ antagonists, and may be advantageous in palliative care as a 'multipurpose' drug for multicausal nausea, may be opioid-sparing, and counter delirium or confusion, hot flushes or paroxysmal sweating. Oral immediate release and dissolvable tablets are available, and 10 mg of olanzapine costs about $8 whereas 8 mg oral ondansetron is about $40. Suggested doses for delayed CINV are 5 mg for 2 days prior to chemotherapy and then 10 mg starting on the day of chemotherapy for four days. The recommended starting palliative dose is 2.5 mg per day, and doses may be escalated every few days to 7.5 mg. Slow titration may prevent sedation. Other common side effects of olanzapine include weight gain, insomnia, and constipation, whereas diabetes, hyperglycemia, and neuroleptic malignant syndrome are uncommon. Rare case reports of olanzapine-associated neutropenia may raise concern in oncology, but a meta-analysis found none of 2500 patients taking olanzapine had neutropenia (Beasley, Tollefson, & Tran, 1997).

24. What about using marijuana for N&V?

Initial interest in marijuana as an antiemetic came about because some patients reported smoking marijuana decreased CINV after emetogenic chemotherapy. The active ingredient, tetrahydrocannabinol (THC), was subsequently isolated and formulated as dronabinol (Marinol) and nabilone (Cessamet). Cannabinoids affect nausea by acting as agonists at CNS cannabinoid subtype 1 (CB_1) receptors in the cortex, motor system, limbic system, and hippocampus. Cannabinoids may also have some pain relieving and appetite stimulating properties. Dronabinol or nabilone are later-line choice antiemetics because they may cause dysphoria or confusion, especially in elderly or debilitated patients, and are only available in oral formulations. Some patients report that smoking marijuana is more effective than taking a cannabinoid, and some clinicians support a short-term trial (< 6 months) of smoking marijuana with medical follow-up for patients with intractable nausea or pain, especially if other antiemetics have not been effective.

25. Which antiemetics can be administered by continuous subcutaneous infusion? When should this method be considered?

Continuous subcutaneous infusion (CSQI) of metoclopramide or haloperidol is generally reserved for patients with progressive or terminal cancer whose oral intake is precluded by intractable N&V, GI obstruction, or coma. Neither drug is irritating to subcutaneous tissues (as are other antiemetics), and both are compatible with morphine. Compact ambulatory infusion pumps are ideal for CSQI of these drugs, which can be concentrated to 1 mg/1ml. The upper chest and abdomen are appropriate sites for CSQI, and a small (25- to 27-gauge) IV winged or subcutaneous needle is inserted subcutaneously. Metoclopramide and haloperidol are started at low doses (i.e., 0.4-0.6 mg/hr) and titrated upward as needed to control N&V or other symptoms. CSQI needles only need to be changed every 3 to 7 days; few patients develop erythema and induration at the needle site that prevents using CSQI.

26. Are there other ways to administer antiemetics to patients without venous access devices who cannot take oral drugs?

Compounding pharmacists can formulate antiemetics and other drugs into suppositories. For example, BDR suppositories (diphenhydramine [Benadryl], dexamethasone, and metoclopramide [Reglan]) may be useful in the palliative care setting. If the patient finds rectal administration acceptable, a suppository every 4 to 6 hours may be more convenient and less expensive than parenteral medications. Hospice nurses have discovered that oral tablets can be inserted into the rectum or vagina, and absorption has been shown to be equivalent to orally administered antiemetics and analgesics. Doses of 2 tablets or less can be placed in a gel capsule. Diarrhea, bleeding, and infection may limit rectal and vaginal administration.

27. What about using other drugs to enhance antiemetic regimens?

Antiemetic regimens that include drugs with different mechanisms of action are often superior to single antiemetics. Thus, prochlorperazine or lorazepam may add antiemetic or other benefit, but the rationale for their use should be considered carefully and smaller rather than larger doses should be used to avoid distressing side effects. At best, lorazepam has modest antiemetic activity but may decrease anxiety, increase sense of control, and cause sedation, which may or may not be desirable. Sublingual administration of small doses (e.g., 0.5 mg) bypasses the GI tract and first-pass effect in the liver, leading to rapid increase in serum levels. Lorazepam can be repeated about every 15 to 30 minutes until the desired effect is achieved.

28. What are extrapyramidal symptoms and how are they treated?

Drugs that bind to dopamine (D_2) receptors (metoclopramide, prochlorperazine, promethazine, chlorpromazine, and haloperidol) can cause EPS after single large IV doses or repeated lower doses. Using more than one D_2 antagonist simultaneously can increase the risk for EPS, which may present as akathisia and dystonia. Akathisia (restless legs or dancing feet syndrome) is most common. It can range from mild akathisia (patients feel anxious or jittery), moderate (patient has difficulty in sitting still), or severe (patient cannot sit or lie still at all). Dystonia, which is uncommon, involves contraction of muscle groups in the head and neck (torticollis or opisthotonus) that may be frightening if the patient feels they cannot breathe.

Prophylactic lorazepam (Ativan) or diphenhydramine (Benadryl) may prevent EPS, whereas benztropine (Cogentin) 1 to 2 mg IV will usually rapidly reverse dystonia. Benztropine is not sedating and can be repeated if necessary.

29. What should be done if antiemetics 'fail'?

The first step is to assess whether the patient actually took the prescribed antiemetics and at the scheduled times. This can be done by telephone follow-up or patient diary, and should lead to timely changes in antiemetics. Reasons for nonadherence to the antiemetic plan should be investigated (e.g., misunderstanding, costs, or adverse effects). Reinforcement of teaching may help, as well as investigating sources of payment for antiemetics (see Question 19). Patients should also be asked about disagreeable effects from antiemetics so management or changing to a different drug can be discussed. For instance, if the first $5HT_3$ antagonist is not effective or causes distressing side effects, a trial of a second $5HT_3$ antagonist is warranted before switching to less effective antiemetics from another class.

30. Which antiemetics have a limited role for controlling N&V in patients with cancer?

Trimethobenzamide (Tigan) is a benzamide (as is metoclopramide) that is generally considered an ineffective antiemetic. Although it does not cause EPS (probably because of the small dose), it is not very effective, and EPS can develop with long-term use. Antihistamines are often limited to second- or third-line antiemetic use. For instance, hydroxyzine (Vistaril, Atarax) is not very effective and repeated parenteral administration is painful and may cause sedation. Similarly, promethazine (Phenergan) is irritating and causes dry mouth and other anticholinergic side effects.

31. What complementary measures are helpful for N&V?

The following complementary measures may decrease N&V and enhance personal control. However, they should not be viewed as alternatives to antiemetics.

- **Dietary modifications:** Limiting food intake on the day of chemotherapy may decrease the risk for developing food aversions (refer to Chapter 40).
- **Herbal remedies:** Ginger tablets, ginger ale, or ginger tea made from dried or fresh ginger root may be helpful; concerns about impaired platelet function are unfounded. Other herbal preparations that may sooth nausea are chamomile, peppermint, and slippery elm. Nurses should remind patients to inform health care providers about *all* medicine and herbs that they take.
- **Acupressure or acupuncture** can decrease N&V, but is largely unavailable and inconvenient. *Acupressure* is an alternative that might be a helpful adjunctive to antiemetics for CINV, PONV, motion sickness, morning sickness from pregnancy, and other causes of N&V. Two types of devices are available: an inexpensive band with a small button that is placed snugly over the acupuncture point for N&V and a more expensive battery-powered electronic device that stimulates the same point. The point is along the median nerve above the wrist (about 3 fingerbreadths above the lowest wrist crease between the radial and middle tendons of the dominant arm). The patient usually feels some relief within 1 hour of applying the acupressure band, and relief may last as long as it is worn.
- **Relaxation, imagery, or hypnosis** may benefit patients who have developed anticipatory nausea.
- **Aerobic exercise:** Benefits have been demonstrated by nursing research to decrease chemotherapy-related nausea.

Key Points

- Nausea and vomiting (N&V) are frequent problems for patients with cancer and may occur because of disease, therapy, drugs, or other causes.
- The physiology of N&V is complex and involves multiple organs, neuroreceptors, and neurotransmitters in peripheral body sites and the central nervous system (CNS).
- Current evidence-based guidelines can aid clinicians in managing N&V from chemotherapy, radiation therapy, or postsurgical anesthesia.
- Clinical experience and anecdotal evidence guide palliative management of N&V.

Internet Resources

Chemocare.com (patient-focused site with resources to manage CINV):
  http://www.chemocare.com/managing/nausea_vomiting__chemotherapy.asp

BioBands (commercial site; explains acupressure bands to patients):
  http://www.biobands.com/cancer_treatment.htm

NeedyMeds (resource available for people who need help with the cost of medications):
  http://www.needymeds.com

Journal of the National Cancer Institute (JNCI) Cancer Spectrum (website with resources for professionals):
  http://jncicancerspectrum.oxfordjournals.org/cgi/pdq/jncipdq;CDR0000062747

National Comprehensive Cancer Network, Clinical Practice Guidelines in Oncology—Antiemesis:
  http://www.nccn.org/professionals/physician_gls/PDF/antiemesis.pdf

OncoLink, Coping with Cancer (site for professionals and patients):
  http://www.oncolink.org/coping/coping.cfm?c=5

Oncology Nursing Society, Outcome Resources Area (continuing education program that provides evidence-based guidance on common cancer side effects: fatigue, nausea and vomiting, infection):
  http://www.ons.org/outcomes

Bibliography

Beasley CM, Tollefson GD, Tran PV: Safety of olanzapine. *J Clin Psychiatry* 1997; 58 (suppl 10), 13-17.
Depré M, Van Hecken A, Oeyen M, et al: Effect of aprepitant on the pharmacokinetics and pharmacody-namics of warfarin. *Eur J Clin Pharmacol* 61:341-346, 2005.
Glare P, Pereira G, Kristjanson LJ, et al: Systematic review of the efficacy of antiemetics in the treatment of nausea in patients with far-advanced cancer. *Support Care Cancer* 12:432-440, 2004.
Habib AS: Evidence-based management of postoperative nausea and vomiting: A review. *Can J Anaesth* 51:326-341, 2004.
Hickok JT, Roscoe JA, Morrow GR, et al: 5-hydroxytryptamine-receptor antagonists versus prochlorperazine for control of delayed nausea caused by doxorubicin: A URCC CCOP randomized controlled trial. *Lancet Oncol* 6:765-772, 2005.
Kris MG, Hesketh PJ, Somerfield MR, et al: American Society of Clinical Oncology guideline for antiemetics in oncology: Update 2006. *J Clin Oncol* 24:2932-2947, 2006.
National Comprehensive Cancer Network: NCCN Practice guidelines in oncology: antiemesis – v.1.2007. Available at: http://www.nccn.org/professionals/physician_gls/PDF/antiemesis.pdf. Accessed January 17, 2007.
Navari RM, Einhorn LH, Passik SD, et al: A phase II trial of olanzapine for the prevention of chemotherapy-induced nausea and vomiting: A Hoosier Oncology Group Study. *Support Care Cancer* 2005; 13, 529-534.

Prommer E: Aprepitant (Emend): The role of substance P in nausea and vomiting. *J Pain Palliat Care Pharmacother* 19(3):31-39, 2005.

Schwartzberg L: Chemotherapy-induced nausea and vomiting: State of the art in 2006. *J Support Oncol* 4(suppl 1):3-8, 2006.

Tipton JM, McDaniel RW, Barbour L, et al: Putting evidence into practice: Evidence-based interventions to prevent, manage, and treat chemotherapy-induced nausea and vomiting. *Clin J Oncol Nurs* 2007; 11(1) 69-78.

Wickham, R: Nausea and vomiting: Palliative care issues across the cancer experience. *Oncol Support Care Q* 1(4):44-57, 2003.

Chapter 40

Nutritional Support

Colleen Gill and Barbara Grant

1. Describe the incidence and significance of malnutrition.

Forty percent to 80% of cancer patients experience some degree of malnutrition. Not only does malnutrition contribute to increased morbidity and mortality, it has been associated with poorer performance status, response to therapy, and quality of life. When dietary intake cannot meet the body's metabolic needs, the imbalance can lead to progressive weight loss, muscle wasting, decubiti, poor wound healing, intolerance of therapy, endocrine abnormalities, electrolyte and fluid imbalances, and inadequate immune function. Weight loss is linked to decreased response to treatment, shorter survival time, and a reduction in quality of life.

2. What is cancer cachexia and what are the etiological factors?

Cancer cachexia is severe, progressive, involuntary weight loss that can result in weakness due to loss of muscle mass, anorexia, early satiety, immunosuppression, increased basal metabolic rate, and serum protein depletion. The cause of cancer cachexia is not entirely understood and may be related to the following:

- Abnormal neurotransmitter concentrations, changing levels of tryptophan and serotonin, occur with profound anorexia.
- A pro-inflammatory environment results in an inefficient utilization of nutrients.
- Cachectin (tumor necrosis factor [TNF]), a cytokine mediator, creates abnormalities in substrate metabolism and appetite.
- Increased levels of lipid mobilizing factor (LMF) and proteolysis inducing factor (PIF) lead to increased losses of both fat and muscle mass. Even when adequate calories and protein are available, muscle mass is not rebuilt.

3. Are there any nutritional interventions that can correct the metabolic abnormalities that arise in cancer cachexia?

Much of the research in this area has centered on the antiinflammatory effects of omega-3 fatty acids, offering hope that the aberrant signals produced by the tumor can be altered. When 2 grams of the omega-3 fatty acid, eicosapentaenoic acid (EPA) were provided to patients with pancreatic cancer, either as fish oil supplements or in an oral supplement drink (Novartis Nutritionals' Resource Support, or Ross Labs' ProSure), the results were as follows:

- Weight loss was limited, responding in proportion to the dose of omega-3 fatty acids, up to 2 grams a day.
- PIF and LMF levels declined; inflammatory markers normalized.
- Muscle mass increased and performance status improved.

4. When should nutritional intervention occur?

Ideally, all patients with cancer should be screened and assessed for nutritional risk at the time of diagnosis and reevaluated throughout the course of treatment and recovery. Because of the eating difficulties associated with cancer and its treatment, "catch-up" or regaining weight is more difficult than maintaining the status quo. Patients at nutritional risk will benefit from referral to a dietitian for a full nutritional assessment. If a dietitian is not available, nutritional intervention should not be delayed. Provide patients with nutrition information, such as publications and written materials from the National Cancer Institute (e.g., *Eating Hints* pamphlet), the American Cancer Society (e.g., *Nutrition for the Person with Cancer* pamphlet), or from the Oncology Nutrition Dietetic Practice Group of the American Dietetic Association (e.g., *Management of Nutrition Impact Symptoms in Cancer and Educational Handouts*).

5. What three guiding principles have been identified for nutritional management?

1. *Calories.* If there is too big a gap between the calories consumed and the calories expended, the body will go to any lengths to meet that need, including auto cannibalism (breaking down its own tissue). In this setting, the body can no longer conserve its protein reserves contained in the lean body mass (muscle).

2. *Protein.* The body must have enough protein for regeneration and synthesis to limit breakdown of muscle mass. Until adequate calories are obtained, protein will be burned as calories to meet the body's basal metabolic needs. Thus with rapid weight loss, more muscle is broken down to provide the building blocks for normal cell turnover, to make enzymes, the proteins of the immune system, and to repair tissues damaged with cancer treatment. To conserve protein reserves, the body will skimp on the proteins produced resulting in slowed wound healing, increased risk of infection, and other consequences of malnutrition. Excessive protein intake (amounts greater than estimated needs) may not be beneficial, because it may contribute undue stress to the renal and hepatic systems.

3. *Supportive care measures.* The patient needs timely and appropriate nutritional management of commonly experienced symptoms and side effects of cancer and its treatment (e.g., nausea, vomiting, bowel changes, mucositis, esophagitis, xerostomia). Other supportive care measures include medications to support nutritional intervention goals (e.g., antiemetics, antidiarrheals, supplements of pancreatic enzymes, medications for pain control).

6. Is there an evidenced-based tool for assessing nutritional risk in the oncology patient setting?

Yes. The Patient Generated–Subjective Global Assessment (PG-SGA), developed by Detsky (1987) and adapted by Ottery and colleagues (1998), is an evidence-based and easy to use nutritional assessment tool appropriate for any clinical oncology setting. The PG-SGA incorporates a section for patients and/or caregivers to complete about the patient's weight history, food intake, symptoms, and functioning. Sections completed by the nurse or member of the health care team evaluate the patient's weight loss, disease, metabolic stress, and a nutrition-related physical examination. In many practice settings, the use of the patient-generated section alone has been quite useful, and the score generated is used to determine nutrition risk, with recommendations for nutritional intervention. Studies have shown that patients identified at high nutritional risk referred to the dietitian for nutritional support had improved outcomes with lower weight loss, greater completion of their treatment courses, and fewer unplanned hospital admissions.

7. Why is weight loss such a critical marker?

Any weight loss can adversely affect nutritional reserves. Weight maintenance during cancer treatment, regardless of the extent of being overweight, is recommended. Increases in edema or ascites can obscure true weight loss. Use the following formula to calculate percent weight loss:

Percent weight loss = (usual weight − current weight) ÷ usual weight

Cancer patients were noted to have statistically increased risk of mortality and morbidity with unintentional weight losses.

Percent weight loss from baseline

Time course	Significant (%)	Severe (%)
1 wk	≤ 2.0	> 2.0
1 mo	≤ 5.0	> 5.0
3 mo	≤ 7.5	> 7.5
6 mo	≤ 10.0	> 10.0

8. What laboratory value is most commonly used to measure malnutrition and assess nutritional risk?

The serum albumin level (half-life of 20 days) reflects the availability of protein within the past month. When added to a panel of laboratory values, the test is relatively inexpensive. Albumin is measured as gm/dl; thus fluid status must be taken into account during interpretation. The value is falsely low in patients who retain fluids and falsely elevated in volume-depleted patients. Because albumin is manufactured in the liver, any liver dysfunction depresses its level. Values are laboratory-specific; check the normal range at your institution.

Albumin Levels (gm/dl)

Normal	> 3.4
Mild depletion	2.8-3.4
Moderate depletion	2.2-2.7
Severe depletion	< 2.2

9. What other laboratory values are helpful for assessing nutritional risk?

- **Prealbumin** (half-life of 3-5 days) and **transferrin** can provide more recent snapshots of protein status. Fluid status and liver function abnormalities also must be taken into account when interpreting these serum protein levels. Transferrin is inversely related to iron reserves and may be falsely elevated in patients with anemia.
- **Cholesterol** levels drop when caloric intake decreases. A low cholesterol value would support suspicions of eating problems and inadequate intake.
- **Urinary urea nitrogen (UUN)** is assessed from a 24-hour collection of urine in which the grams of nitrogen excreted from protein are measured, added to normal losses, and subtracted from nitrogen intake. Increasing negative values reflect the breakdown of lean body mass (LBM); in other words, muscle tissue is being used for calorie and protein needs.

10. How does cancer treatment affect nutritional status?

- **Surgery.** Adequate calories and protein are needed for wound healing. Transient postoperative side effects include loss of appetite, fatigue, changes in normal bowel habits, and pain. Surgeries involving the alimentary tract have specific nutritional consequences (swallowing difficulties, aspiration, dumping syndrome, maldigestion, and malabsorption), depending on the surgical site.

- **Chemotherapy** acts on tumor cells and rapidly dividing cells, including gastrointestinal (GI) tract and bone marrow, resulting in nausea, vomiting, or changes in normal bowel habits, mucositis, alterations in taste and smell, anemia, fatigue, and anorexia.
- **Radiation therapy.** Depending on the part of the GI tract that is included in the irradiated field, nausea and vomiting, mucositis, taste changes, swallowing, dry mouth, diarrhea and malabsorption, gastritis, and radiation enteritis are possible side effects. Early enteral nutritional support using percutaneous endoscopic gastrostomy (PEG) should be considered in patients receiving head and neck or esophageal irradiation, when extended mucositis, dysphagia, or odynophagia are anticipated.

11. What supportive care medications may have drug-nutrient interactions in patients with cancer?

- **Amphotericin** can impair renal function, creating possible electrolyte abnormalities, significant nausea, and decreased oral intake.
- **Antibiotics** may increase nausea and alter the natural gut flora, reducing the number of "gut-friendly bacteria" in the GI tract, resulting in bloating, gas, cramping, and diarrhea. Reinoculation with probiotics (yogurt, kefir, acidophilus milk, lactobacillus GG tablets) may be beneficial after an antibiotic course.
- **Bactrim** can cause increased folate needs; folate deficiency can affect dividing cell lines such as bone marrow. Supplementation with folic acid may be indicated. Possible decreases in the absorption of vitamin K may also be seen.
- **Cyclosporine** can cause renal insufficiency, magnesium and potassium wasting, weight gain, and increased triglyceride and cholesterol levels. Grapefruit or grapefruit juice may interfere with its metabolism, increasing serum levels of the drug into potentially toxic ranges.
- **Opioids** can cause sedation, resulting in patients sleeping through meals or snacks. Nausea with or without vomiting is common when these medications are taken on an empty stomach. Constipation must be proactively addressed as it can significantly limit oral intake and the desire to eat.
- **Steroids** can cause sodium retention with subsequent hypertension, increased protein and calcium needs, potassium wasting, glucose intolerance, and loss of muscle mass and bone density.
- **Thiazide and loop diuretics** can cause a loss of electrolytes; potassium replacement may be indicated.

12. What treatment-related medications affect nutrition in patients with cancer?

- **Aromatase inhibitors** are associated with increased bone mass loss. Bone density should be followed carefully. Appropriate supportive measures may include bisphosphonate therapy and nutrient supplementation of calcium, magnesium, and vitamin D.
- **Cisplatin** may cause decreased serum magnesium, potassium, and zinc; metallic taste.
- **5-Fluorouracil (5-FU)** may cause taste alterations. Patients should avoid pyridoxine supplements.
- **Interferon** may cause anorexia, fatigue, headache, and nausea. Increased intake of hydrating fluids (1-2 L/day) helps to minimize these symptoms.
- **Interleukin-2 (IL-2)** may cause weight loss or weight gain, hypotension, fatigue, nausea, and capillary leak syndrome.
- **Methotrexate's** effectiveness may be reduced by folic acid supplementation. Until more is known, folic acid doses > 600 mcg/day should be avoided. Methotrexate is also

linked to decreased absorption of vitamin B_{12}, fat, D-xylose and change in taste acuity (metallic).

- **Pemetrexed** may cause severe anemia; supplementation of oral folic acid (350-1000 mcg/day) and Vitamin B_{12} (1000 mcg IM every 9 weeks) is required.
- **Procarbazine** is a monoamine oxidase inhibitor. Foods high in tyramine should be avoided because they may cause a severe hypertensive event.
- **Tamoxifen citrate** may cause edema and fluid retention.
- **Vincristine sulfate and vinblastine sulfate** can cause significant constipation and taste changes.
- **Xeloda**. At very high doses, folic acid will increase the toxicity of Xeloda because Xeloda binds with folinic acid to form a calcium salt, and extra folinic acid means that Xeloda will not be excreted as rapidly as it should be. Normal levels in the diet or a multiple vitamin supplement are not a problem.

13. How are energy and protein needs estimated?

ESTIMATING ENERGY NEEDS

- Patients need 13-15 calories for each pound of current body weight to meet their daily calorie needs and avoid further weight loss. For example, if a patient weighs 160 pounds they may need 2,400 calories a day ($160 \times 15 = 2400$ calories per day).
- Patients need to add 500 calories a day to allow them to gain a pound a week ($160 \times 15 = 2400$ calories + 500 calories = 2900 calories). Encourage the patient to keep eating the extra 500 calories a day until their weight becomes stable and they have regained their weight or reached a desirable weight.

ESTIMATING PROTEIN NEEDS

The minimum amount of protein needed each day is 0.5 to 0.6 g for each pound of body weight. For example, if a patient weighs 160 pounds they would need about 80 to 96 grams of protein a day (160×0.5-$0.6 = 80$-96 g/day).

14. How can calories and protein be added to favorite foods?

Sources of Additional Calories and Protein

Milk/Dairy/Cheese

- Go up one level in fat content (e.g., from skim to 2%, 2% to whole, or from low fat to regular cheeses).
- Try Carnation Instant Breakfast (CIB), 130 calories/4 grams of protein per package.
- Make milk shakes using 1 package CIB, 4 oz half-and-half, and high calorie ice creams.
- Garnish foods such as soup, casseroles, or vegetables with cheese.
- Make soups with milk instead of water.

Meats/Main Dishes

- Bread and sauté or fry meats; add gravies or sauces to baked or broiled foods.
- Add mayonnaise, cheese, avocado, or bacon to sandwiches.

Fruits/Desserts/Snacks

- Add sour or whipped cream or coconut to fruit salads.
- Spread peanut butter on fresh fruit.

Continued

Sources of Additional Calories and Protein—cont'd

- Eat chips with dip; guacamole provides a healthy fat.
- Nuts and nut butters provide great calories and are also great snacks.

Breads/Cereals
- Add fruit, raisins, or nuts to cereals; top with sugar, half and half.
- Add CIB to hot cereal, top with maple syrup.
- Eat fruit and nut breads with cream cheese; top crackers with cheese or nut butters.

Salads/Vegetables
- Use regular, not low-fat, salad dressings; top with cheese, meat, nuts, avocado, and eggs.
- Add butter, olive oil, or sauces to cooked vegetables.

© Colleen Gill, MS, RD, University of Colorado Hospital, Denver, CO. More detailed patient education materials can be downloaded at: http://www.uccc.info.

15. Discuss the role of calorie-containing liquid nutritional supplements.

Fluids with calories are often tolerated very well, even when solids are not, and provide an easy option for between meal snacks or meal replacements.

- Start with the higher-calorie versions (355 vs. 250/can), which can be diluted if needed. Supplement samples allow patients to try the products and determine what they tolerate. Companies often will mail trial samples to the patient's home upon request.
- Chill supplements for improved tolerance.
- Offer liquid supplements that may benefit a patient's specific needs: lactose free, high protein, fiber containing, diabetic appropriate, and calorie dense.
- Be positive about supplements; a single negative comment may eliminate the patient's willingness to try.

16. What medications are useful as appetite stimulants?

- **Corticosteroids** (e.g., dexamethasone), although initially used to enhance appetite, have not been consistently effective in patients with cancer. Side effects, increased muscle breakdown, calcium loss, glucose intolerance, immune suppression, and fluid retention are counterproductive in this population.
- **Megestrol acetate (Megace)**, a synthetic progestational agent, is often effective in stimulating appetite and producing weight gain in some patients. The weight change is largely the result of increased adipose tissue and edema. An extra strength version is available (Megace ES, 625 mg dose), with an equivalent dose 5 cc/1 tsp a day, compared to 20 cc of the original formulation (800 mg), which is still available. The original version is less bioavailable when taken on an empty stomach, a problem that has been addressed in the Megace ES version. Encourage a 3-week trial of daily dosing for full efficacy. When appetite has increased, the dose may be reduced gradually to a level that remains therapeutic. Side effects include mild edema and occasionally deep vein thrombosis.
- **Remeron (Mirtazapine)**, an antidepressant, has been shown to stimulate appetite as a side effect in cancer-free populations (anorectic and older adult patients). A recent study reported slowed weight loss and improved appetite and quality of life in

patients with cancer. Its use in cancer symptomatology is not approved by the FDA at this time.

- **Dronabinol (Marinol)**, a synthetic cannabinoid, has been shown to increase appetite with a slight increase in weight, decrease nausea, and improve mood. Older patients may not appreciate its association with marijuana or its slight mood-altering side effect. Start with 2.5 mg at night, which allows patients to adjust to any side effects, increasing to 5 mg, or 2.5 mg bid (twice daily) or tid (three times/day) if helpful.
- **Marijuana** has been shown to help control nausea and increase appetite in many patients, but there are significant concerns. It is not legal in many states, and the risk of smoking (anything) may exacerbate the pulmonary toxicity of some chemotherapy regimens.
- **Metoclopramide (Reglan)**, a well-known antiemetic, may be useful for patients experiencing early satiety due to delayed stomach emptying. It increases GI transit time and may be very useful in patients with GI cancers. Monitor the patient for any increases in diarrhea. The typical dose is 10 mg taken up to four times a day.
- **Exercise**, although it is not a medication, is very helpful in improving appetite. Encourage short walks daily.

17. What medications may be used to enhance lean body mass and weight gain?

Two medications evaluated in controlled clinical trials in patients with cachexia due to cancer or AIDS have been shown to help patients maintain and rejuvenate lean body mass:

- **Juven** is a nutritional juice-flavored supplement that contains HMB (a metabolite of the amino acid leucine), glutamine, and arginine (Ross Labs). These ingredients were found to slow protein breakdown from muscle and to build lean body mass. Treatment with Juven is now covered by many insurance plans, including Medicaid.
- **Anabolic steroids (norandrolone propionate)** have shown transient improvements in appetite and weight gain (primarily fluid). Side effects include negative nitrogen balance, hyperglycemia, immune suppression, and calcium loss. Oxandrolone (Oxandrin/BTG pharmaceuticals), is an oral anabolic agent that is FDA approved for use as adjunctive therapy for weight gain. Dosage: 2.5 mg tablets, 2-4 times/day; maximal dose = 20 mg total for adults, 0.1 mg/kg total daily dose for children.

18. What are some key dietary strategies for patients experiencing nausea and vomiting?

- Cold clear liquids are often the first foods tolerated. Begin with popsicles, sherbets, sorbets, frozen ices, Jell-O, and ginger ale or dilute juices.
- Gradually incorporate soft, smooth foods, such as applesauce, mashed potatoes, oatmeal/hot cereals, fish, rice, ice cream, milk shakes, puddings, and soups.
- Ginger is a natural antinausea remedy. Have patients try flat ginger ale, a tincture of ginger, or ginger tea (made from a 1 inch piece of ginger root, chopped and boiled in 3 cups of water for 20 minutes).
- Small, frequent meals reduce distention and reflux.
- Cold or room-temperature foods decrease aroma-related nausea. Remove the lids to hot foods outside the room to decrease odors. Avoid fatty, fried foods that delay stomach emptying.

19. What do you say to patients who are concerned about frequent vomiting and inability to keep calories down?

It is helpful to tell patients that unless they lose their meals immediately after eating, they are deriving some benefit from them. The stomach empties into the intestinal tract during the 2 to 3 hours following a meal; thus, even if the food stays down for only 1 hour, about one half of its nutrients are available to the body. Unless vomiting immediately follows a meal, the clinician can reasonably recommend that the patient keep trying to eat. Vomiting often occurs independently of intake, and some nutrients will be retained. Encourage the patient to remain upright after eating to reduce aspiration risk.

20. What can you do for patients who refuse to try foods that previously caused vomiting?

Anticipatory nausea and vomiting and food aversions may develop as early as within 48 hours of the first treatment. Try a three-step process:

- **Relaxation therapy**. Arrange consultation with a therapist who can teach patients to recognize impending nausea and to use relaxation techniques to avoid vomiting.
- **Education**. Explain the typical peak nausea times after chemotherapy, and encourage patients to avoid favorite foods during this period to limit development of new aversions.
- **Reintroduction**. Retry foods that previously were associated with nausea and vomiting at a time when it is most likely to be tolerated (e.g., earlier in the day). Most patients can identify "good times" vs. times when they feel more nauseated and need to stay with "safe" foods. Good antiemetic medication coverage throughout the reintroduction process is imperative.

21. How can you enhance flavors for patients who often complain "nothing tastes good anymore"?

Patients with cancer often complain that food is absolutely tasteless (ageusia, or mouth blindness) because of widespread damage to taste buds, or that food has an "off" taste (dysgeusia) due to changes in balance among the taste centers.

- Use more strongly seasoned foods, such as Italian, Mexican, curried, or barbequed foods, unless mouth sores are a problem. Stronger flavors increase the probability that patients will sense the taste. Encourage patients to experiment with what works for them.
- Try lemon, citrus or cranberry juices, or lemon drops. Tart foods help to overcome metallic tastes.
- Marinate food in wine, fruit juice, soy or teriyaki sauce, Italian dressing, or barbeque sauce.
- Sauces and gravies help to spread taste through the mouth and add calories as well.
- Eat meats with something sweet, such as applesauce, jelly, glazes, or cranberry sauce.
- Use a multiple vitamin and mineral supplement that will limit the risk of zinc deficiency that can alter the function of the metallic based receptors in the mouth and nose. Higher doses of 50 mg of zinc daily for 2 to 3 months may be useful if intake has been limited for some time.

22. A patient with mouth or throat sores often says, "It hurts to eat." What can you do?

- Eat a liquid diet, including Carnation Instant Breakfast (CIB), commercial supplements, pasteurized eggnog, milk shakes, and blenderized foods. Fruit-flavored beverages or nectars are tolerated better than acidic juices.
- Choose foods that are soft: yogurt, puddings, cream of wheat, refried beans.
- Cool foods to room temperature rather than eating them hot (e.g., soups, mashed potatoes, eggs, quiche, cooked cereals).
- Encourage eating cold foods, because they are tolerated by most patients (e.g., milk shakes, cottage cheese, yogurt, watermelon, Jell-O, soft canned fruits, baby food). Some patients will have problems tolerating extremely cold temperatures (e.g., popsicles, ice cream, frozen yogurt, slushes/ices).

- Make food slick! Dry foods can be soaked in liquids, mixed with yogurt or sour cream, or covered with gravies or sauces to make them easier to swallow.
- Drink through a straw to bypass mouth sores.
- Tilt the head backward or forward while swallowing, if swallowing is painful.
- Glutamine is an amino acid that may limit damage to the GI tract when 10 g is mixed with fluid, swished around the mouth, and swallowed, three times a day. It may help patients who have had GI tract irradiation or some chemotherapies. It has not been useful with 5-FU based regimens. Patients with renal or hepatic dysfunction may not tolerate the high protein content.
- Use slippery elm tea or lozenges to coat inflamed tissues.
- Avoid tart, acidic, or salty foods; strong flavorings and spices; and rough, coarse, or scratchy foods (e.g., raw fruits and vegetables, dry breads, cereals, chips).

23. What dietary modifications can be instituted to decrease diarrhea?

- Try eating complex carbohydrates (e.g., applesauce, potatoes, rice, cooked vegetables, bananas), because they are particularly well absorbed and beneficial to gut healing.
- Stick to a clear liquid diet for 12 hours only if diarrhea has been severe.
- Limit high-fiber sources, such as bran, whole grains, raw fruits and vegetables, nuts, dried beans and legumes.
- Check the Cancer Nutrition Information website, http://www.cancernutritioninfo.com, for a recipe for a rice congee that is helpful.
- There are anecdotal reports that coconut macaroon cookies relieve diarrhea.
- Avoid gastric irritants such as caffeine (coffee/tea/sodas), pepper, and alcohol. These substances can also be irritating to rectal and anal tissues.
- Consider eating lactose-free products until diarrhea is resolved.
- Drink an additional cup of fluid for every episode of diarrhea. Nonacidic juices and nectars often work well. Fruitade drinks, especially those without carbonation (e.g., Hawaiian Fruit Punch), are especially well tolerated. Sport drinks (e.g., Propel, Gatorade), broth, and fruit nectars can help to replace lost electrolytes.
- For stool losses greater than 1000 ml/day, consider zinc supplementation to cover losses in the stool (12-17 mg/1000 ml stool volume).

24. What dietary changes can help patients with constipation?

- Add a fiber-containing cereal in the morning (Kashi cereals or Barbara Puffins). If needed, mix one with a familiar cereal.
- Make a fruit and bran spread with 3 parts wheat bran, 2 parts applesauce, and 1 part prune juice.
- Add stewed prunes or dried fruit to cereals, or use for snacks.
- Add ground flaxseed, oat or wheat bran (up to 3 T per day), to cereal, casseroles, breads, soups, or sprinkled on cottage cheese or salads. Start with 2 teaspoons a day and gradually increase.
- Encourage drinking 6-8 glasses of fluids/day.
- Drinking a warm beverage around the time that a bowel movement typically occurs will stimulate contractions of the GI tract.

25. How can I help the patient with an overly invested caregiver, whose "force feeding" is creating control battles?

Discuss the reality of "force feeding"—it never works! Eating is one area over which the patient exerts total control; others cannot do it on their behalf. In fact, if others attempt to take responsibility for their eating, some patients simply relinquish the responsibility altogether, which is a set-up for failure. Nutrition education must always include the patient, so that they understand the consequences of their weight loss—loss of strength and quality of life—and are motivated to eat to their best ability.

26. Why are tube feedings preferred over total parenteral nutrition (TPN)?

Tube feedings are preferred over TPN because they have a lower risk of infection, require less medical assistance, create less disruption of normal eating patterns, and are significantly less expensive. A nighttime tube feeding may improve the patient's quality of life by allowing a more normal lifestyle during the day and by lessening the pressure on the patient to "force feed" the total requirement of calories. Severe mucositis, dysphagia, esophagitis, and odynophagia can prevent both oral nutrition and placement of a nasogastric feeding tube, requiring gastrostomy tube placement.

27. What supplements are best tolerated, orally or as tube feedings?

Supplement preferences are as varied as food choices. Cost, personal taste preferences, and health considerations may influence patient choices.

- Flavored packets of instant breakfast powder, generally found in the cereal aisle, provide 250+ calories when added to 8 oz milk, with 12 g of protein.
- Smoothie recipes can provide variety. Try the Cancer Nutrition Information website at http://www.cancernutritioninfo.com.
- Scandishakes (http://www.axcanscandipharm.com) provide 440 calories and may be added to 8 oz of milk (total of 600 calories) or 6 oz of juice and ice (total of 500 calories). Using tart juices can counteract sweet aversions of many patients.
- Lactose-free supplements containing intact proteins from soy isolates or calcium caseinate, with calorie versions ranging from 220 to 560 calories/can. Flavored versions can be used orally (e.g., Ensure, Boost), whereas unflavored options are typically intended for tube feeding only (e.g., Fibersource, Jevity). Fiber-containing versions often help limit diarrhea as well as constipation.
- A food-based blenderized formula, Compleat (Novartis) often helps patients having difficulty tolerating the casein- or soy-based proteins. Home-made blenderized formulas have the advantage of lower cost; however, they are suitable only for large-diameter tubes and may require large volumes to meet calorie needs.
- Formulas containing omega-3 fatty acids can be helpful in limiting the inefficient use of macronutrients in cachectic patients. Maximal benefit is gained with the use of 2 servings a day of ProSure or Resource Support, each providing 1 g of omega-3 fatty acids per serving. They can be consumed orally or included in tube feeding regimens.

28. How can nutrition be reinstated after the gut has not been used for awhile?

The unfed GI tract atrophies within days, requiring a gradual reintroduction of feeding to avoid diarrhea and abdominal cramping. Glutamine supplementation (10 g, 3-4 times a day) may promote regeneration of gastrointestinal cells. Delayed emptying of the stomach can lead to high residuals and intolerance, and can be effectively limited with prokinetic agents, such as metoclopramide or IV erythromycin.

29. How are enteral feedings instituted?

If the gut is functional, enteral tube feedings should be used. The nasogastric or naso-duodenal (Dobbhoff) tube is used most often if the tube feeding is expected to be short term. For long-term feeding, especially in a patient who cannot be expected to take food orally for more than 1 month, a tube may be placed directly into the stomach (via percutaneous endoscopic gastrostomy [PEG]) or small bowel (percutaneous endoscopic jejunostomy [PEJ]).

30. When is total parenteral nutrition appropriate?

Common reasons for TPN implementation include extensive GI surgery, bowel obstruction, or severe malabsorption. Prolonged oral or esophageal mucositis may be an indication for short-term TPN, but if long-term support is needed, placement of a gastrostomy tube should be considered. It should be initiated only when problems prevent adequate oral intake for longer than 10 days, the patient has a life expectancy of at least 40 days, and central line access can be established.

TPN is expensive ($120-$250/day); without insurance, it is usually not financially feasible. Patients on TPN are also at increased risk of infection unless blood sugar levels are well controlled.

31. What should I say to the patient who asks about using dietary supplements?

Vitamin, mineral, and dietary supplements cannot replace a good diet, where components of foods often act synergistically in providing their benefits. Use of supplements and single nutrients at doses higher than the recommended daily intakes raises safety concerns related to toxicity and the possibility of adverse interactions with anticancer therapies. A daily multivitamin can help to ensure adequate coverage when intake is limited. Iron should not be included in the supplement unless there is a source of ongoing blood loss, such as menstruation, or where there is documented iron deficiency.

Key Points

- 40% to 80% of all cancer patients experience some degree of malnutrition.
- The metabolic abnormalities in many cancer patients can result in rapid weight loss that, without timely nutritional interventions, will quickly compromise strength and quality of life.
- Screening patients allows the early, preventative nutrition interventions that are most effective, avoiding the unplanned weight loss that is associated with decreased response to therapy and shorter survival time.
- Effective strategies exist to manage common barriers to eating.
- Families need help in defining roles and responsibilities to avoid control battles around eating.
- Reliable resources are available for professionals and patients looking for information on nutrition and cancer survivorship.

Internet Resources

American Institute for Cancer Research:
  http://www.aicr.org
  A registered dietitian is available to answer questions. Register for free weekly email recipes, free pamphlets that offer practical information and recipes for nutrition and cancer prevention.
American Cancer Society:
  http://www.cancer.org
  Educational material: *Nutrition for the Person with Cancer, a Guide for Patients and Families*

Continued

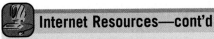

Internet Resources—cont'd

American Dietetic Association:
  http://www.eatright.org
  Patients type in a zip code to find a local dietitian with oncology experience in private practice.
Oncology Nutrition Dietetic Practice Group:
  http://www.oncologynutrition.org
Cancer Nutrition Information, LLC:
  http://www.cancernutritioninfo.com
Consumer Labs:
  http://www.consumerlab.com
Diana Dyer, MS, RD:
  http://www.cancerrd.com
National Cancer Institute:
  http://www.nci.nih.gov/cancertopics/pdq/supportivecare/nutrition
Natural Medicines Database:
  http://www.naturaldatabase.com
Office of Complementary and Alternative Medicine (NIH):
  http://nccam.nih.gov/

Acknowledgment

The authors wish to acknowledge Deborah Rust, RN, MSN, CRNP, AOCN, for her contributions to the Nutritional Support chapter published in the first and second editions of *Oncology Nursing Secrets*.

Bibliography

Brown JK, Byers T, Doyle C, et al: Nutrition and physical activity during and after cancer treatment: An American Cancer Society guide for informed choices. *CA Cancer J Clin* 53:268-291, 2003.

Detsky A, McLaughlin J, Baker J, et al: What is subjective global assessment of nutritional status? *J Parent Ent Nutr* 11:8-13, 1987.

Eldridge, B, Hamilton K: *Management of nutrition impact symptoms in cancer and educational handouts*, Chicago, 2004, American Dietetic Association.

Eldridge B, Rock C, McCallum P: Nutrition and the patient with cancer. In Coulston AM, Rock CL, Monsen ER, editors: *Nutrition in the prevention and the treatment of disease*, San Diego, 2001, Academic Press.

Gill C, Murphy-Ende K: Immunonutrition, the role of specialized nutritional support for cancer patients. In Kogut V, Luthringer S, editors: *Nutritional issues in cancer care*, Pittsburgh, PA, 2005, Oncology Nursing Society.

Glade MJ: Food, Nutrition, and the Prevention of Cancer: A global perspective. American Institute for Cancer Research/World Cancer Research Fund. *Nutrition* 15(6):523-526, 1997.

McMahon K, Decker G, Ottery F: Integrating proactive nutritional assessment in clinical practices to prevent complications and cost. *Semin Oncol* 25:20-27, 1998.

McTiernan A: Obesity and cancer: The risks, science, and potential management strategies. *Oncology* 19(7):871-881, 2005.

Moses A, Slater C, Preston T, et al: Reduced total energy expenditure and physical activity in cachectic patients with pancreatic cancer can be modulated by an energy and protein dense oral supplement enriched with n-3 fatty acids. *Br J Cancer* 9:996-1002, 2004.

Ravasco P, Monteiro-Grillo I, Vidal PM, et al: Dietary counseling improves patient outcomes: A prospective, randomized, controlled trial in colorectal cancer patients undergoing radiotherapy. *J Clin Oncol* 23(7):143-1438, 2005.

Savarese D, Savy G, Vahdat L et al: Prevention of chemotherapy and radiation toxicity with glutamine. *Cancer Treat Rev* 29(6):501-513, 2003.

Tisdale M: Cachexia in cancer patients. *Nat Rev Cancer* 2(11):862-871, 2002.

Chapter 41

Organ Toxicities and Late Effects

Brenda Ronk Martin

1. How do late effects differ from acute toxicities?

Late effects are toxicities caused by cancer therapy that appear months to years after treatment. They may be mild, severe, or life-threatening, often occurring in tissues with slowly proliferating cells, such as the heart. Acute toxicities tend to occur in tissues with rapidly proliferating cells, such as bone marrow and mucous membranes of the gastrointestinal tract, and are manifested during or shortly after treatment. Some drugs cause specific toxicities only when given in high doses or in combination with other chemotherapy agents or radiation therapy.

Some acute and late toxicities are well defined and predictable, whereas others are unpredictable and vary with dose, duration of treatment, method of administration, and patient status.

2. What is the most common dose-limiting toxicity of chemotherapy?

Depression of bone marrow stem cells or peripheral blood cell lines is caused to some degree by almost all chemotherapy agents. The acceptable degree of myelosuppression depends on the type of cancer, the duration of myelosuppression, treatment goals, and patient status. Neutropenia occurs before thrombocytopenia and anemia because the half-life of granulocytes is much shorter (6-8 hours) than the life span of platelets (5-7 days) and red blood cells (approximately 120 days). The nitrosoureas cause a late thrombocytopenia 4 to 6 weeks after administration; drugs such as ifosfamide and mitoxantrone are not as toxic to platelets. Drugs that usually do not cause bone marrow depression include steroidal hormones, bleomycin, vincristine, and L-asparaginase.

3. What are the most common late effects of cancer treatment on the major organ systems? How are they managed or prevented?

Selected late effects of therapy			
Organ system	**Late effect**	**Causative treatment**	**Prevention/ management**
Cardiovascular	Cardiomyopathy	Anthracycline-based chemotherapy regimens; risk increases with mediastinal irradiation High dose cyclophosphamide, 5-FU, paclitaxel, ifosfamide, trastuzamab	Limit dosage to lifetime maximum Cardiac function tests (baseline and periodically) Treatment of congestive heart failure Dexrazoxane: cardioprotectant

Continued

Selected late effects of therapy—cont'd

Organ system	Late effect	Causative treatment	Prevention/management
Pulmonary	Dyspnea Dry cough Decreased diffusion capacity Pulmonary fibrosis Pneumonitis	Chemotherapy drugs excreted via the lungs (bleomycin, cytarabine, high dose cyclophosphamide, carmustine, methotrexate) Lung irradiation	Limit dose Pulmonary function tests (baseline and periodically) Corticosteroids Avoid high concentrations of oxygen
Musculoskeletal	Kyphosis, scoliosis, fibrosis, joint immobility Shortening of a growing bone Osteoporosis	Radiation therapy in childhood Radiation therapy for head and neck cancers, sarcomas Women: Chemotherapy drugs (cyclophosphamide, methotrexate, fluorouracil, doxorubicin), ovarian failure, and aromatase inhibitors Men: androgen-deprivation therapies	Orthopedic rehabilitation Physical therapy Counseling about unequal length of limbs
Gastrointestinal	Chronic enteritis	Radiation therapy to pelvis	Symptomatic treatment with antidiarrheal drugs, low-residue diet
Neurologic	Chronic neuropathic pain syndromes; peripheral neuropathy Orthostatic hypotension due to autonomic nervous system defects Hearing loss (high-frequency range)	Cisplatin (usually higher doses), vinca alkaloids, taxanes Cranial irradiation	Effect may be permanent Surgical correction Audiology consultation Fit with hearing aid
Reproductive/sexual	Men: Infertility, increased fatigue, hot flashes, erectile dysfunction, decreased libido, breast swelling/discomfort, gynecomastia	Chemotherapy agents (cyclophosphamide, ifosfamide, nitrosoureas, chlorambucil, melphalan, busulfan, vinblastine, cytarabine, cisplatin, procarbazine)	Sperm banking Symptomatic treatment

Selected late effects of therapy—cont'd

Organ system	Late effect	Causative treatment	Prevention/ management
		Radiation (low-dose total body irradiation) Androgen deprivation	
	Women: Infertility Early menopause with symptoms (hot flashes, sleep disturbances, decreased libido)	Estrogen treatment Chemotherapy agents (as above)	Ovarian cryopreservation Symptomatic treatment
	Irregular menstrual cycles, oligomenorrhea, amenorrhea	Radiation therapy	
	Vaginal stenosis	Brachytherapy	
	Masculinization	Androgen therapy	

4. Which chemotherapeutic agents are cardiotoxic?

- Doxorubicin, daunorubicin, and to a lesser degree, idarubicin, epirubicin, and mitoxantrone may cause cardiac damage, commonly manifested as myocardial depression or congestive heart failure (CHF). At a cumulative dose of 450 to 550 mg/m^2, the incidence of CHF related to doxorubicin is only 0.1% to 0.2%, whereas it increases to 30% for doses above 550 mg/m^2.
- Cyclophosphamide normally has no cardiac effects at standard doses but can be cardiotoxic at high doses. Paclitaxel causes asymptomatic bradycardia, and its safety in patients with significant preexisting cardiac problems is still being investigated.
- Trastuzumab, a monoclonal antibody approved for treatment of certain breast cancers, can be cardiotoxic, causing ventricular dysfunction and CHF. Incidence and severity of cardiac dysfunction appear to be higher in patients who receive the drug in combination with anthracyclines and cyclophosphamide. Left ventricular ejection fraction (LVEF) and/or echocardiogram should be routinely monitored in all patients before, during, and after treatment with trastuzumab. Discontinue trastuzumab in patients with any significant change in left ventricular function.

5. How can cardiac toxicity be reduced or prevented?

- *Limit total life-time doses.* Numerous studies have shown that lifetime doses of anthracyclines (daunorubicin, doxorubicin) above 450 to 550 mg/m^2 are likely to produce cardiac symptoms. Dosing depends on current cardiac status, age of the patient, and amount of mediastinal irradiation. Often LVEF, which is the portion of blood in the ventricle that is ejected during systole, is measured in patients before therapy with high doses of anthracyclines. LVEF can be measured with a multigated acquisition (MUGA) blood pool scan, a radionuclide imaging study of ventricular function. Normal LVEF is greater than 50%. Measurement of LVEF before treatment assists in making decisions about the chemotherapeutic agent and dosage for persons with impaired cardiac function.

- *Use alternative drugs.* Because of the importance of dose-intensive therapy in prolonging disease-free survival, alternatives and modifications for current therapy have been developed. One such alternative is mitoxantrone, an anthracycline analog that may be less cardiotoxic than doxorubicin. Mitoxantrone may be substituted for doxorubicin for patients at risk for cardiac compromise.
- *Use a cardioprotective agent.* Cardiac toxicity may be decreased by using dexrazoxane, a cardioprotective agent that is given intravenously 30 minutes before administration of an anthracycline.
- *Vary administration schedule or infusion time.* Doxorubicin by continuous infusion or on a weekly schedule in lower doses is less toxic than the traditional higher dose given every 21 days. Cardiotoxicity can also be reduced by administering doxorubicin over 30 to 45 minutes instead of as a bolus infusion.

6. What is radiation recall?

Radiation recall is severe erythema, pain, blistering, or ulceration in areas previously irradiated. Radiation recall most commonly occurs 3 to 7 days after infusion of dactinomycin, doxorubicin, daunorubicin, or bleomycin. Other agents include mitoxantrone, idarubicin, mitomycin, fluorouracil (5-FU), methotrexate, cyclophosphamide, and paclitaxel.

7. Why are patients with pulmonary toxicity cautioned about using oxygen?

Oxygen must be used judiciously in patients with pulmonary toxicity, especially if the toxicity is produced by bleomycin or carmustine (BCNU). The pulmonary toxicity may be caused by inflammatory responses in the lung related to the formation of reactive oxygen metabolites. However, the physiologic mechanism for the relationship between high-oxygen concentrations and bleomycin-induced lung injury are not entirely clear. In such patients, high-concentration oxygen may cause acute respiratory failure that requires mechanical ventilation and exacerbates lung injury. Oxygen may be used during anesthesia as long as the patient receives the least amount needed to produce an oxygen saturation of greater than 90%. Patients should be warned to avoid scuba diving. Patients who have received high doses of chemotherapeutic agents or who have experienced pulmonary toxicity should carry identification describing their pulmonary condition and the risk of oxygen administration.

8. What are some dermatologic toxicities caused by chemotherapy?

Dermatologic effects include rashes (docetaxel, idarubicin, erlotinib), hyperpigmentation (hydroxyurea, methotrexate), nail thickening or banding, acral erythema, phlebitis, chemical cellulitis, radiation recall and enhancement, photosensitivity, reactivation of UV light-induced erythema (methotrexate), seborrheic inflammation or actinic keratoses (dacarbazine, dactinomycin, doxorubicin, cisplatin, cytarabine), scleroderma-like changes, and vasculitis (cytarabine, hydroxyurea, methotrexate).

9. Do hyperpigmentation and photosensitivity induced by 5-FU, bleomycin, or methotrexate ever resolve?

Hyperpigmentation, photosensitivity, generalized skin darkening, dermatitis, and nail changes usually occur during the course of treatment and diminish gradually once therapy has stopped.

10. What is "hand-foot syndrome"?

Palmar-plantar erythrodysesthesia (acral erythema) syndrome, referred to as hand-foot syndrome, is a painful erythema of the palms, fingers, and soles of the feet that may progress to bullae or vesicular formation and desquamation before healing spontaneously within a week. Patients with this condition may require treatment with opioids for pain relief. The condition may respond to pyridoxine treatment and cooling. Acral erythema is induced by standard and high-dose cytarabine, hydroxyurea, continuous infusion 5-FU, bleomycin, doxorubicin, methotrexate, high-dose etoposide, thiotepa, docetaxel, and capecitabine.

11. What are some hepatotoxic effects of chemotherapy, and which drugs usually require dose modification with hepatic dysfunction?

Hepatotoxic effects of chemotherapy agents include hepatocellular injury, necrosis, veno-occlusive disease, and reactivation of chronic hepatitis B virus infection. Combination chemotherapy and high-dose regimens used for autologous bone marrow transplantations have enhanced the potential for hepatotoxicity, particularly hepatic veno-occlusive disease. At conventional doses, veno-occlusive disease has been associated with cytarabine, dacarbazine, 6-mercaptopurine, and 6-thioguanine.

If there is evidence of hepatic impairment or abnormal liver function tests (e.g., bilirubin >1.5 mg/dl), the following agents should be held or reduced: doxorubicin, daunorubicin, vinblastine, vincristine, cyclophosphamide, methotrexate, 5-FU, and paclitaxel.

12. Can chemotherapy affect vision or cause other ocular complications?

Although relatively uncommon, the incidence of ocular complications has increased in accordance with increased patient survival and high-dose chemotherapy regimens. Ophthalmologic side effects include decreased or blurred vision (cisplatin, cyclophosphamide, cytarabine, mitomycin C, methotrexate); eye pain (busulfan, cytarabine, methotrexate); papilledema (cisplatin); altered color vision (cisplatin); conjunctivitis (cytarabine, 5-FU, methotrexate); tear duct stenosis and increased lacrimation (5-FU, doxorubicin, methotrexate); photophobia (cytarabine, methotrexate); optic neuropathy or blindness (vincristine); photopsia (paclitaxel); and cataracts (busulfan).

Conjunctivitis related to high-dose cytarabine may be reduced effectively with prophylactic glucocorticoid eye drops, as well as artificial tears, which probably decrease toxicity by diluting intraocular drug concentrations.

13. What is the most frequent long-term effect of radiation therapy to the head and neck?

Xerostomia (dryness of the mouth) is the most frequent chronic effect of radiation to the oral cavity. Radiation, both external beam and implanted, may produce permanent injury to the acinar cells of the salivary glands. The small amount of saliva that is produced is thick and ineffective at performing the normal salivary functions: lubricating the mouth, providing a buffer for acids, and washing food and organisms from the teeth and gums. Chronic xerostomia is a highly distressing condition. Swallowing dry foods and taking pills become difficult, and the patient frequently awakens at night with dry mouth. Artificial saliva products are available. Some patients may find relief with pilocarpine hydrochloride. Many patients find that water, hard candies, or lozenges are equally effective in relieving the sensation of dryness.

14. How are dental caries related to radiation therapy? How can they be prevented?

Inadequate production of saliva increases the risk of dental caries because there is too little saliva to clear bacteria from the mouth. In addition, patients undergoing radiation therapy may also have poor oral hygiene if they experience mucositis. These factors contribute to the development of dental caries, which may create a problem for several years. Dental caries are prevented by the following methods:

- A thorough dental evaluation before the start of therapy, with diseased teeth repaired or extracted
- Meticulous oral hygiene with frequent saline rinses, gentle toothbrushing, and fluoride application
- Provision of adequate analgesia for oral care to be performed
- Prompt treatment of any infection in the oral mucosa
- Prevention of further irritation to the oral mucosa by avoiding the use of alcohol and tobacco

15. How is the gastrointestinal tract affected by radiation therapy to the pelvis?

Proctitis and enteritis, which may be acute effects of radiation therapy, also may become chronic effects if the mucosa is permanently damaged. Radiation may produce shortening of the intestinal villi, thus preventing adequate absorption. Acutely injured mucosa may become atrophied, thickened, or ulcerated. Proctitis or small bowel enteritis results, causing diarrhea with cramping. This chronic condition is physically and psychologically debilitating. A few individuals also experience fecal incontinence. Nurses may assist patients to cope with this problem by instructing them about low-residue diets and use of antidiarrheal drugs. Steroid enemas are sometimes used. If conservative measures fail, a colostomy may be required.

16. What are some common late effects of childhood cancer treatment?

- Short stature
- Skeletal growth retardation
- Dental caries
- Intellectual deficits
- Cataracts
- Delayed sexual development
- Kyphoscoliosis
- Secondary malignancies

17. How are the late effects of therapy different in children?

Because children undergo such rapid growth and development, effects on their developing tissues are different from those seen in mature tissues. Children often receive treatment to the central nervous system (total body irradiation, brain irradiation, intrathecal chemotherapy) for leukemia or brain tumors. The most serious long-term effects are seen in children under the age of 3 years when brain development is rapid. Such patients may later manifest intellectual deficits, as well as attention and memory problems. CNS treatment also may affect endocrine function because of damage to the hypothalamic-pituitary axis. Frequently seen are growth impairment with growth hormone deficiency and delayed or arrested development of secondary sexual characteristics. Children may need exogenous hormones to grow and mature normally.

Adults who have undergone cancer treatment in childhood may also be more likely to experience chronic illness. One third of childhood cancer survivors can expect to have a life-threatening or serious chronic illness by age 45 years.

18. What are secondary malignancies?

Secondary malignancies are cancers caused by damage to the DNA of normal cells exposed to chemotherapy and/or radiation therapy. The most common secondary malignancy is acute myeloid leukemia due to therapy with an alkylating agent for

Hodgkin lymphoma, non-Hodgkin lymphoma, and multiple myeloma. Agents that may cause secondary malignancies include nitrogen mustard, procarbazine, melphalan, cyclophosphamide, busulfan, chlorambucil, and thiotepa. Radiation-induced sarcomas have occurred in patients treated for Hodgkin lymphoma and non-Hodgkin lymphoma. The period of highest risk for developing secondary leukemia is 2 to 10 years after treatment. Secondary leukemia is one of the most serious long-term effects of therapy because it generally has a poor prognosis.

19. What late psychosocial effects may be seen in patients after treatment for cancer?

Numerous psychosocial changes may be experienced by patients who have received cancer treatment. Often they live with the fear of recurrence of cancer and death. Any change in health status may produce worry about cancer recurrence. Changes may occur in relationships with family, friends, coworkers, and sexual partners. Persons who are healthy after recovering from cancer and its treatment may still be perceived as ill or disabled, creating relationship stress and feelings of isolation. Disabilities and physical changes may require adjustment in lifestyle, employment, or family role.

20. Is there such a condition called "chemo brain"?

Yes, many patients, particularly women with breast cancer, have been reporting for years to their health care providers that they have problems with memory and concentration, which they call "chemo brain" or "chemo-fog." Other reported cognitive changes include difficulty with learning new facts, reading comprehension, working with numbers, and multitasking. Although limited, data show that there are changes in verbal and working memory following chemotherapy. This phenomenon has finally been taken seriously. Fortunately, the cognitive impairments resolve over time. Research is ongoing about prevalence, types of cognitive dysfunction, assessment methods, and therapeutic interventions.

Possible mechanisms or causes of chemo brain include progressive fatigue, anxiety, release of by-products of chemotherapy agents, injury response (release of neurotoxic cytokines), immune response, genetic factors, and reduced estrogen and testosterone levels. Although high-dose chemotherapy regimens carry more risk than standard dose, it is unclear whether one chemotherapy regimen causes more cognitive decline than others.

21. Are there any treatments for chemo brain?

Although controlled studies are lacking, some of the pharmacologic interventions currently under investigation are methylphenidate (Focalina), erythropoietin, modafinil, antidepressants, insomnia treatments, herbal remedies (*Ginkgo biloba* and ginseng), and cognitive rehabilitation.

Key Points

- Late effects are toxicities caused by cancer therapy that appear months to years after treatment.
- The most common dose-limiting toxicity of chemotherapy is myelosuppression.
- Secondary malignancies are cancers caused by damage to the DNA of normal cells exposed to chemotherapy and/or radiation therapy.
- Numerous psychosocial changes may be experienced by patients who have received treatment.

Internet Resources

National Cancer Institute, Late Effects of Treatment for Childhood Cancer:
   http://cancer.gov/cancertopics/pdq/treatment/lateeffects/healthprofessional
National Coalition for Cancer Survivorship, Palliative Care and Symptom Management:
   http://www.canceradvocacy.org/resources/essential/effects/cognitive.aspx
Leukemia and Lymphoma Society, Long-term and Late Effects of Treatment for Blood Cancers:
   http://www.leukemia-lymphoma.org/attachments/National/br_1098117804.pdf

Bibliography

Genentech: Herceptin Prescribing Information (website): http://www.gene.com/gene/products/information/
   oncology/herceptin/index.jsp. Accessed January 10, 2007.
Jacobs LA, Hobbie W, Moore IM: Late effects of cancer treatment. In Yarbro CH, Frogge MH, Goodman M,
   et al, editors: *Cancer nursing: Principles and practice,* ed 6, Boston, 2005, Jones and Bartlett.
Lasky JA, Ortiz L: Bleomycin-induced lung injury. UpToDate 2006 version 14.1 www.uptodate.com
Leung W, Hudson M, Zhu Y, et al: Late effects in survivors of infant leukemia. *Leukemia* 14:1185-1190, 2000.
National Cancer Institute: Late effects of childhood cancer therapies: http://cancer.gov/cancertopics/pdq/
   treatment/lateeffects/healthprofessional. Accessed January 10, 2007.
National Cancer Institute: Survivors of childhood cancer are likely to develop chronic illness years later:
   http://www.cancer.gov/cancertopics/coping/childhood-cancer-survivor-study. Accessed January 10, 2007.
Oeffinger KC, Mertens AC, Sklar CA, et al: Prevalence and severity of chronic diseases in adult survivors of
   childhood cancer: A report from the Childhood Cancer Survivor Study. 2005 ASCO Annual Meeting,
   Orlando, FL, 16 May 2005. *Journal of Clinical Oncology,* 2005 ASCO Annual Meeting Proceedings.
   23(16S):9, 2005
Partridge AH, Winer EP: Long-term complications of adjuvant chemotherapy for early stage breast cancer.
   Breast Dis 21:55-64, 2004.
Polovich M, White JM, Kelleher LO: *Chemotherapy and biotherapy guidelines and recommendations for
   practice,* ed 2, Pittsburgh, PA, 2005, Oncology Nursing Society.
Simon B, Lee SJ, Partridge AH, et al: Preserving fertility after cancer, *CA Cancer J Clin* 55:211-228, 2005.
Steinherz LJ, Yahalom J: Adverse effects of treatment: Cardiac toxicity. In DeVita VT Jr, Hellman S,
   Rosenberg SA, editors: *Cancer: Principles and practices of oncology,* ed 6, Philadelphia, 2001, Lippincott
   Williams & Wilkins.
Tichelli A, Socie G: Considerations for adult cancer survivors. *Hematology Am Soc Hematol Educ Program*
   2005:516-522. http://www.asheducationbook.org/cgi/content/abstract/2005/1/516. Accessed January 10,
   2007.
VonRoenn JH, editor: Adjuvant chemotherapy and cognitive dysfunction in breast cancer patients.
   J Support Oncol 4(2):66-67, 2006.

Pain Management

Regina M. Fink, Diana L. Ruzicka, and Rose A. Gates

1. What causes pain in cancer patients?

Patients with cancer have multiple sources and sites of pain due to:
- Direct tumor involvement (bones, soft tissues, muscle, and nerve structures) and related pathology (65%-80% of patients)
- Anticancer therapy and invasive diagnostic or therapeutic procedures (25% of patients)
- Unrelated to cancer or therapy; prior or concurrent painful conditions (3%-10% of patients)

2. How prevalent is pain in cancer patients?

Current estimates suggest that cancer pain occurs in:
- 20%-75% of adults at diagnosis
- 30%-50% of patients undergoing active treatment
- 75% of patients with advanced disease
- Approximately 50% of terminally ill patients during the last 48 hours of their lives

3. Can cancer pain be controlled?

Pain is well controlled by oral analgesics in 90% of patients with cancer. Surgery, radiation, and chemotherapy may be used to control pain by removing or shrinking the tumor. Drugs (nonopioids and opioids) remain the mainstay of pain treatment. Only about 10% of patients will experience pain that is resistant to traditional analgesic therapies. Patients who do not receive adequate pain relief from traditional analgesics should be promptly referred to pain specialists or anesthesiologists for consideration of modalities such as regional or local blocks, intrathecal or epidural drug administration, or spinal cord stimulation.

4. How do the types of pain differ?

Pain is classified as nociceptive (traveling along normal nerve conduction pathways) or neuropathic (caused by damage to the central or peripheral nervous system). Nociceptive pain may be further divided into somatic and visceral. Psychologic pain etiologies are uncommon.

Pain classifications

Pain type	Etiology	Descriptors	Treatment choice
Somatic (well localized)	Bone and spine metastasis; fractures, arthritis; cutaneous or deep tissue inflammation or injury	Dull Achy Throbbing	NSAIDs, steroids, muscle relaxants, bisphosphonates, ± opioids and/or

Continued

Pain classifications—cont'd

Pain type	Etiology	Descriptors	Treatment choice
			radiation therapy (bone metastasis)
Visceral (poorly localized)	Originates in deep organs; often referred to dermatomes innervated by same fibers; post abdominal or thoracic surgery; bowel obstruction, stretching, or infection; liver metastasis, ascites; blood flow occlusion	Squeezing Pressure Cramping Distention Deep	Opioids (caution must be used in the administration of opioids to patients with bowel obstruction), ± nonsteroidal anti-inflammatory drugs (NSAIDs)
Neuropathic (deafferentation)	Nerve damage by tumor or nerve plexus fibrosis (cervical, brachial, lumbar plexopathies); spinal cord compression; postherpetic neuralgia; post surgical pain syndromes; peripheral neuropathies secondary to tumor involvement, chemotherapy, and radiation fibrosis	Burning "Like a fire" Shooting Numbness Tingling Radiating Lancinating "Electrical sensation"	Antidepressants, anticonvulsants, local anesthetics, benzodiazepines, ± opioids, ± steroids
Psychologic	Psychologic disorders	All encompassing, everywhere	Support, counseling, nonpharmacologic approaches, antidepressants psychiatric medications

5. How is pain assessed?

Patients should be queried about their description of pain to include its quality, intensity, location, temporal pattern (presence of constant, intermittent, and/or breakthrough pain), and aggravating/alleviating factors (refer to Pain Assessment Guide on p. 457). In addition to assessment of pain characteristics, the effect of pain on functional and psychosocial status (e.g., activity, sleep, mood), and thorough physical and neurologic evaluations are necessary, as is a review of other concomitant symptoms (e.g., nausea/vomiting, constipation, anorexia). Cultural and ethnic backgrounds also may influence pain expression and behavior; patients should not be stereotyped.

6. How is pain intensity measured?

Four commonly used pain intensity scales are available:

- The Numeric Pain Intensity (0-10) Scale is useful in the clinical setting for patients older than 5 years. Ask the patient, "If 0 is no pain and 10 is the worst

PAIN ASSESSMENT GUIDE

TELL ME ABOUT YOUR PAIN

Words to describe pain

aching	throbbing	shooting
stabbing	gnawing	sharp
tender	burning	exhausting
tiring	penetrating	nagging
numb	miserable	unbearable
dull	radiating	squeezing
crampy	deep	pressure

Pain in other languages

itami	Japanese	dolor	Spanish
tong	Chinese	douleur	French
dau	Vietnamese	bolno	Russian

Intensity (0-10)

If 0 is no pain and 10 is the worst pain imaginable, what is your pain now? ... the last 24 hours?

Location

Where is your pain?

Duration

Is the pain always there?
Does the pain come and go? (Breakthrough Pain)
Do you have both types of pain?

Aggravating and Alleviating Factors

What makes the pain better?
What makes the pain worse?

How does pain affect

sleep	energy	relationships
appetite	activity	mood

Are you experiencing any other symptoms?

nausea/vomiting	itching	urinary retention
constipation	sleepiness/confusion	weakness

Things to check

vital signs, past medication history, knowledge of pain, and use of noninvasive techniques

REFERENCES: Jacox A, Carr DB, Payne R, et al. Management of Cancer Pain. Clinical Practice Guideline No. 9. AHCPR Publication No. 94-0592. Rockville, MD. Agency for Health Care Policy and Research, U.S. Department of Health and Human Services, Public Health Service, March 1994. — Wong, D, and Whaley, L: Clinical Handbook of Pediatric Nursing, ed. 2, The C.V. Mosby Company, St. Louis, 1986, p. 373.

pain possible, what is your pain right now …, the worst pain in the last 24 hours …, since you received your pain medication …, what level do you want your pain to be?"
- The Verbal Descriptor Scale has six numerically ranked choices of word descriptors that are given a number indicating the patient's pain intensity.
- The Wong-Baker Faces Pain Rating Scale is appropriate for children aged 3 years and older and for patients with language barriers.
- The Faces Pain Scale Revised (FPS-R) measures pain intensity by using six drawings of adult faces (no smiling or tears). Many different language versions are available.

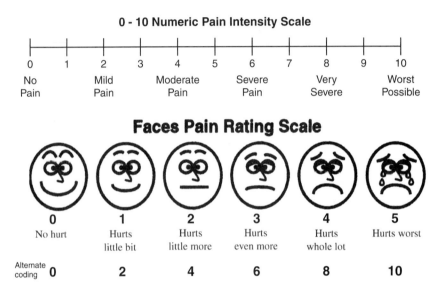

0 - 10 Numeric Pain Intensity Scale

| 0 | 1 | 2 | 3 | 4 | 5 | 6 | 7 | 8 | 9 | 10 |

| No Pain | | Mild Pain | | Moderate Pain | | Severe Pain | | Very Severe | | Worst Possible |

Faces Pain Rating Scale

| 0 | 1 | 2 | 3 | 4 | 5 |
| No hurt | Hurts little bit | Hurts little more | Hurts even more | Hurts whole lot | Hurts worst |

Alternate coding: 0 2 4 6 8 10

Brief word instructions: Point to each face using the words to describe the pain intensity. Ask the person to choose face that best describes own pain and record the appropriate number.
Original instruction: Explain to the person that each face is for a person who feels happy because he has no pain (hurt) or sad because he has some or a lot of pain. **Face 0** is very happy because he doesn't hurt at all. **Face 1** hurts just a little bit. **Face 2** hurts a little more. **Face 3** hurts even more. **Face 4** hurts a whole lot. **Face 5** hurts as much as you can imagine, although you don't have to be crying to feel this bad. Ask the person to choose the face that best describes how he is feeling.
Rating scale is recommended for persons age 3 years and older.
From Hockenberry MJ, Wilson D: *Wong's Nursing care of infants and children,* ed. 8, St. Louis, 2007, Mosby. Used with permission.

7. How often should pain be assessed?
- All cancer patients should be screened for pain at each outpatient or clinic visit, on hospital admission and at least once a shift, or on each home or hospice visit.
- The frequency of assessment is determined by the clinical situation. If the patient is having persistent or breakthrough pain, pain should be assessed routinely (every 4 hours or every shift), reassessed after analgesic administration, and after any modification of the pain management plan.

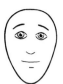

Faces Pain Scale Revised (FPS-R) (*Hicks CL, von Baeyer CL, Spafford P, van Korlaar I, Goodenough B. The Faces Pain Scale – Revised: Toward a common metric in pediatric pain measurement. Pain 2001;93:173-183. Scale adapted from: Bieri D, Reeve R, Champion GD, Addicoat L, Ziegler J. The Faces Pain Scale for the self-assessment of the severity of pain experienced by children: Development, initial validation and preliminary investigation for ratio scale properties. Pain 1990;41:139-150. From the Pediatric Pain Sourcebook. Original copyright © 2001. Used with permission of the International Association for the Study of Pain and the Pain Research Unit, Sydney Children's Hospital, Randwick NSW 2031, Australia. This material may be photocopied for clinical use. For all other purposes permission should be sought from the Pain Research Unit: contact Tiina Piira, piirat@sesahs.nsw.gov.au.*)

- If a patient has severe pain requiring upward titration of analgesics, pain assessment should be completed more frequently (e.g., every 15 minutes). Pain should be assessed approximately 15 to 30 minutes after administration of a parenteral medication and 60 minutes after oral medication.
- If pain is well controlled, pain intensity should be assessed routinely with vital signs.

8. How is pain assessed in patients who are nonverbal or cognitively impaired?

The patient's self-report of pain is the gold standard even in patients who are nonverbal or cognitively impaired. However, instruments that rely solely on verbal self-report are not appropriate for use in patients who are nonverbal, cognitively impaired, demented, delirious, or dying. Other measures must be used to determine if a nonverbal or cognitively impaired patient is having pain: knowledge of patient history, condition, and potential for pain; use of a behavioral assessment tool; observation of nonverbal pain behaviors in the patient at rest and on movement; and proxy reports or pain estimates by others (family, significant others, caregivers). A comprehensive evaluation of the various scales developed for use in nonverbal and cognitively impaired populations is included in the Position Statement with Clinical Practice Recommendations, *Pain Assessment in the Nonverbal Patient*, developed by the American Society of Pain Management Nursing, 2006. Information on currently published tools useful for assessing pain in nonverbal persons with dementia is available at http://www.cityofhope/prc/elderly.asp.

9. Who is at risk for inadequate pain assessments and the undertreatment of pain?

Individuals who have the following characteristics are at risk for inadequate assessment and undertreatment of cancer pain:
- Older adults or very young children
- Member of a minority groups or unable to speak English
- Concomitant pain from another source
- Neuropathic pain
- Female
- History of substance abuse (alcohol ± drug)
- Socioeconomically disadvantaged
- Cancer survivors with chronic pain syndromes
- Nonverbal or cognitively impaired

10. Should placebos be used to assess pain?

No. According to the Oncology Nursing Society's Position Statement on the Use of Placebos, "Placebos should not be used (a) to assess or manage cancer pain, (b) to determine if the pain is 'real,' or (c) to diagnose psychological symptoms, such as anxiety associated with pain. Nurses should not administer placebos in these circumstances even if there is a medical order." Placebos are appropriate in the context of controlled studies when patients have given informed consent. Because placebos involve secrecy, ethical tenets of truth-telling and patient autonomy are violated. Use of placebos can destroy a therapeutic relationship if the patient becomes aware of their use.

11. Are patients with cancer addicted when they keep asking for more pain medicine?

No. They are probably exhibiting signs of tolerance, an involuntary response in which the patient requires higher doses of opioids to provide the same analgesic effect. It is important to determine whether tolerance or disease progression is responsible for an increased opioid requirement. Because of incomplete cross-tolerance, opioid rotation (see Question 28) is usually recommended to treat tolerance.

12. Do signs of withdrawal mean the patient is addicted?

No. The patient is probably showing signs of physical dependence, which develops when patients take opioids for an extended period (usually 1 week or more). Like tolerance, physical dependence is a normal body response. If an opioid is abruptly stopped, the patient may experience withdrawal symptoms: nervousness, sweating, anxiety, chills alternating with hot flashes, salivation, lacrimation, rhinorrhea, diaphoresis, piloerection, nausea, vomiting, abdominal cramps, or insomnia. Reassure patients that physical dependence is not unique to opioids. For example, an abstinence syndrome occurs when patients abruptly stop taking long-term steroids. Opioids should be tapered gradually. In contrast, addiction or psychological dependence is an abnormal behavior involving an overwhelming desire to obtain the medication for its psychological effects. Addiction rarely occurs in patients with cancer (less than 1%).

13. How do I take care of pain in a cancer patient who has a problem with substance abuse?

Although there is a low prevalence of substance abuse in cancer patients, caring for the patient with concurrent drug abuse and cancer pain is a challenge. A multidisciplinary team approach with family support and the development of clear treatment goals presented in a written agreement is mandatory. (Patient agreement example: http://www.painedu.org/tools.asp?Tool=11)

Long-acting pain medications should be the basis of treatment with frequent follow-up and the inclusion of pill counts and spot urine testing as appropriate. The "4 A's" mnemonic developed by Passik and Weinreb (2000) provide a framework for nurses' evaluation of optimal therapy in the cancer patient with a substance abuse history:

- **Analgesia:** Does pain relief make a true difference in the patient's life? A successful outcome involves more than lowering pain intensity scores.
- **Activities of daily living:** Does pain relief improve functionality and stabilize psychosocial interactions?
- **Adverse events:** Is pain medication administered without concomitant adverse events or side effects?
- **Aberrant drug-taking behaviors:** Are less aberrant drug-taking behaviors (e.g., losing prescriptions, using more medication than prescribed, aggressively complaining about the need for more pain medication, injection of an oral formulation) observed?

14. How do you know which analgesic to use when a patient is experiencing pain?

The analgesic must be selected according to the type, severity, and temporal nature of the pain as well as other factors.

- **Pain type:** Opioids and nonopioid analgesics are effective for nociceptive pain. Adjuvants (antidepressants, anticonvulsants, local anesthetics, etc.) are effective for neuropathic pain.
- **Severity of pain:**
  - Pain that is severe and rated a 7-10 (0-10 scale) is considered a pain emergency and should be treated with a short-acting, immediate release opioid with rapid titration ± adjuvant analgesics as needed.
  - Pain that is moderate and rated a 4-6 (0-10 scale) is treated with a slower titration of short-acting, immediate release opioid ± adjuvant analgesics as needed.
  - Pain that is mild and rated 1-3 (0-10 scale) is treated with a nonopioid (acetaminophen or NSAID) if the patient is not already taking an opioid.
- **Temporal nature:** Successful relief of cancer pain requires around-the-clock dosing of a long acting analgesic for persistent pain with as-needed short-acting doses for breakthrough pain.
- **Other factors:** Analgesic choice should also be based on the patient's previous experience with the medication, age, physical condition (e.g., renal and hepatic function), appropriate route of administration, response to the prescribed regimen, provider recommendations, and possible interactions with current therapies.

15. How do nonsteroidal antiinflammatory drugs (NSAIDs) decrease pain?

NSAIDs may relieve bone or generalized musculoskeletal pain by decreasing subperiosteal swelling around nerve endings and inhibiting prostaglandin synthesis. Although NSAIDs may be given in higher than recommended doses, they have a ceiling effect; that is, increases above a certain dose do not provide additional analgesia.

16. How do I select and use NSAIDs?

The selection of NSAIDS is influenced by side-effect profile, patient preference, and cost (over the counter NSAIDs, such as ibuprofen, are most economical). NSAID use is limited by concerns about side effects, such as platelet dysfunction, nephritis, fluid retention, and gastrointestinal tract bleeding or ulceration. Some guidelines for using NSAIDs include:

- Switch to an NSAID from a different class if no response is demonstrated.
- Use with extreme caution in patients with thrombocytopenia, poor renal function, and in older adults.
- Do not use regularly or around the clock indefinitely, because of their side effect profile.
- Assess for potential hypersensitivity reactions. Patients with a history of aspirin or NSAID allergy, rhinitis, nasal polyps, or asthma are susceptible to development of severe respiratory reactions.
- Instruct patients not to take NSAIDs on an empty stomach.
- Use NSAIDs, such as nabumetone (Relafen), to cause less gastric distress.
- Use histamine-2 blockers or prostaglandin analogs to decrease the potential for gastric ulceration in patients who require chronic use of NSAIDs.
- Use nonacetylated salicylates when concerned about platelet aggregation or altered bleeding times; however, be aware that their analgesic effect may not be strong enough for patients with more intense pain.

Dosing for nonopioid analgesics

Nonopioid analgesic	Dose
Acetaminophen (Tylenol) or acetylsalicylic acid (aspirin)	325-1000 mg po every 4-6 hr (maximal daily dose: 4 gm)
Salsalate (Disalcid)	750-1500 mg po every 8-12 hr (maximal daily dose: 3000 mg)
Ibuprofen (Motrin)	200-400 mg po every 4-6 hr (maximal daily dose: 3200 mg)
Naproxen (Naprosyn)	375-500 mg po every 8-12 hr (maximal daily dose: 1000 mg)
Nabumetone (Relafen)	500-1000 mg po in 1 dose or 2 divided doses (maximal daily dose: 1500 mg)

17. What is the concern about too much acetaminophen?

Excessive acetaminophen can cause liver damage. The maximum daily dosage in adults is 4000 mg (1000 mg QID; 650 mg 6 times daily). Safety guidelines for using acetaminophen include:

- Lower acetaminophen dose to 2000 mg QD if the patient drinks alcohol, has liver disease, or is taking other drugs that may damage the liver.
- Use less acetaminophen in frail, older adults; liver damage may occur with 3000 mg QD.
- Look for hidden acetaminophen in other medications.

18. What are COX-2 inhibitors? How do they work?

The COX-2 inhibitors (e.g., celecoxib [Celebrex]) are NSAIDs that selectively block the cyclooxygenase-2 (COX-2) enzyme without blocking COX-1 enzymes, which protect gastric mucosa. In 2004, Celebrex use showed a 2.5-fold increased risk of major fatal and nonfatal cardiovascular (CV) events in a large NCI trial on colorectal cancer. Celebrex remains on the market because its benefits have been proven to outweigh the potential risks in properly evaluated and informed patients. As required by the FDA, Celebrex carries a boxed warning in the product labeling that includes information related to cardiovascular (CV) and gastrointestinal (GI) risks. COX-2 inhibitors are most appropriate for patients who are unable to tolerate nonselective NSAIDs, or those with a history of gastrointestinal bleeding. Health care providers are encouraged to carefully assess patients for cardiovascular risk factors before prescribing COX-2 inhibitors and to use the lowest effective dose (100 to 200 mg twice daily or 200 mg daily) for the shortest duration of time.

19. How do tricyclic antidepressants control pain?

Tricyclic antidepressants (TCAs) relieve neuropathic pain (usually described as burning or tingling) by blocking the reuptake of the neurotransmitters serotonin and norepinephrine, which is released by the pain-modulatory systems that descend from the brainstem to the spinal cord. Neurotransmitter accumulation at the synapse inhibits transmission of pain impulses. Some of the TCAs (e.g., amitriptyline) interact with endogenous opioid systems and morphine or other opioids that result in opioid-sparing effects.

Tricyclic antidepressant dosages to control pain are much lower (e.g., 10-50 mg/day) than those needed to treat depression (e.g., 100-150 mg). Although it takes weeks for a therapeutic antidepressant effect with tricyclics, the onset of analgesia is much sooner (usually 1 week). Pain may be reduced by the next morning after taking one dose of amitriptyline or nortriptyline.

20. What are limiting side effects of TCA in cancer patients?

Dose-related side effects of the tricyclics include sedation, orthostatic hypotension, mental clouding, and anticholinergic effects, particularly dry mouth. Uncommon, serious side effects include cardiac arrhythmias, obstipation, and urinary retention. Desipramine and nortriptyline are less sedating and may produce insomnia; they can be given during the day. To increase patient compliance and decrease side effects, start with low doses (10 mg in older adults or frail patients) and gradually titrate upward. (**Note:** To prevent confusion in patients, avoid increasing at the same time that opioids are increased.) After symptoms are controlled, titrate dosage downward to the lowest level that maintains pain relief (Refer to Chapter 34 for more information about antidepressants).

21. Are other classes of antidepressants effective in reducing pain?

Yes. The SSNRIs (selective serotonin and norepinephrine reuptake inhibitors), venlafaxine and duloxetine, have demonstrated analgesic effectiveness in the treatment of neuropathic pain, particularly diabetic neuropathy. Venlafaxine was shown to be effective in reducing neuropathic pain in breast cancer patients after completion of treatment.

Studies have yielded mixed results of the effectiveness of the SSRIs (serotonin reuptake inhibitors), such as paroxetine and citalopram, in reducing neuropathic pain. Buproprion, an inhibitor of neuronal norepinephrine and serotonin uptake with less potent dopamine reuptake, is effective in reducing neuropathic pain.

22. Which anticonvulsants are best to treat neuropathic pain?

- Gabapentin, a second generation anticonvulsant, is generally considered to be the first-line treatment of neuropathic pain of various types. It reduces neuronal hyperactivity associated with neuropathic pain states by inhibiting calcium influx into the neuron. Common side effects include blurred vision, dizziness, confusion, and mild generalized edema. When discontinuing gabapentin, taper slowly (10% of the daily dose/day over 10 days) because patients may experience side effects, such as anxiety, stomach cramps, and sweating. Other second generation drugs effective in treating neuropathic pain include: pregabalin, lamotrigine, and topiramate.
- First-generation anticonvulsants (e.g., phenytoin, carbamazepine, clonazepam) work by stabilizing the nerve membrane, preventing depolarization, and blocking transmission of pain impulses. They are indicated for trigeminal and postherpetic neuralgias, lancinating pains (e.g., electrical, shooting), and nerve injury caused by cancer or cancer treatment. Because of side effect limitations and potential drug interactions, the use of first-generation anticonvulsants has declined in favor of newer, second-generation agents.
- Several newer anticonvulsants (oxcarbazepine, tiagabine, levetiracetam, zonisamide) may be considered for treating refractory neuropathic pain; however, more research is needed.

Anticonvulsant indications and dosing

Anticonvulsant	Indication*	Dose
Carbamazepine (Tegretol)	Trigeminal neuralgia	Start with 100 mg po/day (Q HS); increase by 100 mg every 4 days to 500-800 mg/day in divided doses (bid)
Clonazepam (Klonopin)	Neuropathic pain; anxiety	Start with 0.25-0.5 mg po/day preferably Q HS; increase to 0.5-6 mg/day in divided doses (bid or tid)
Gabapentin (Neurontin)	Postherpetic neuralgia	Start with 100-300 mg po/day (Q HS); increase by 100-300 mg increments every 2-3 days to 600-3600 mg/day in divided doses (tid)
Pregabalin (Lyrica)	Postherpetic neuralgia; painful diabetic neuropathy	Start with 50 mg po Q HS-bid; increase by 50-75 mg every 5-7d to 150-600 mg/day in divided doses (bid)
Lamotrigine (Lamictal)	HIV-associated neuropathy	Start with 25-50 mg po/day; increase to 200-400 mg/day
Topirimate (Topamax)	Diabetic neuropathy; migraine prophylaxis	Start with 25 mg po Q HS; increase by 25 mg every 7d to 100-200 mg/day (bid)

*Not all indications are FDA approved.

23. When are local anesthetics indicated?

Local anesthetics are effective for lancinating, neuropathic pain and various neuralgias. They produce analgesia by stabilizing the nerve cell membrane, inhibiting depolarization and transmission. They also may inhibit the release of neurotransmitters centrally. Patients may be given an IV trial of lidocaine, which if effective, may indicate a response to mexiletine (oral form of lidocaine) or other oral neuropathic agents. During IV administration, the patient should be observed for slurred speech (a sign of toxicity); the dose should be adjusted accordingly. The lidocaine (5%) patch, approved for use in postherpetic neuralgia, may be applied to a painful area; systemic absorption is not significant. Up to three patches may be applied at once for 12 hours on/12 hours off. Anecdotally, a cream compounded with a mixture of lidocaine 5% and ketamine 10% has been effective in reducing painful peripheral neuropathies.

24. How do corticosteroids decrease pain?

A short course of corticosteroids helps to reduce pain due to perineural edema, visceral organ distention, infiltration of soft tissues, and bone pain in advanced disease. Typical corticosteroids include:

- Dexamethasone 4 mg po 2-4 times/day
- Prednisone 10 mg po daily or up to 3 times/day; maximal dose: 20-80 mg/day

25. How is pain due to muscle spasms treated?

Treatment for muscle spasms		
Drug	**Indication**	**Dose**
Baclofen (Lioresal)	Spasticity, neuropathic pain, organic headache, trigeminal and postherpetic neuralgias, fibromyalgias	5-20 mg po bid-tid; increase by 5 mg every 3 days to maximum of 80 mg/day
Cyclobenzaprine (Flexeril)	Spasticity	5-10 mg po tid; range: 20-40 mg/day in 2-4 divided doses; maximal dose: 60 mg/day
Methocarbamol (Robaxin)	Spasticity	Initially 1500 mg po tid-qid for 2-3 days; maintenance dose: 4-4.5 gm/day in 3-4 divided doses
Dicyclomine (Bentyl)	Abdominal cramps (colorectal cancer) and irritable bowel syndrome	10-20 mg po tid-qid to maximum of 160 mg/day
Oxybutynin chloride (Ditropan)	Bladder spasm	5 mg po bid-tid; maximal dose of 5 mg qid. Belladonna and opium suppositories (B&O Supprettes) are also effective for bladder spasms
Tizanidine (Zanaflex)	Spasticity	2-4 mg po Q HS-tid; maximal dose 8-12 mg tid
Diazepam (Valium)	Acute anxiety, spasticity	2-10 mg po/IV bid-tid

26. What is capsaicin? How is it used?

Capsaicin (Zostrix), a cream made from cayenne pepper, depletes and prevents reaccumulation of substance P in peripheral sensory neurons. Capsaicin cream is effective in some patients with chemotherapy-induced neuropathies, chronic postherpetic neuralgia, and postmastectomy pain. A thin film is applied to the affected area of intact skin 3 to 5 times/day; fewer applications per day may decrease efficacy. Onset of action may take 14-28 days. Patients need to be warned about transient burning that occurs with application but decreases within several days.

27. What agents are used for metastatic bone pain?

- Acetaminophen and antiinflammatory agents (NSAIDs and corticosteroids) are first line therapy in treating metastatic bone pain.
- Radiation therapy is the mainstay for palliation of localized bony metastases. Wide-field and hemibody irradiation have been used for diffuse bony metastasis.
- Bisphosphonates inhibit accelerated osteoclast-mediated bone resorption. Zoledronic acid 4 mg is administered over 15 minutes; pamidronate is given as a 90 mg intravenous infusion over 2 hours. Both agents are given approximately every 4 weeks.
- Calcitonin inhibits osteoclastic bone resorption by the tumor and also has been reported to be effective for bone pain and phantom limb sensation. It is given in doses of 4 IU/kg every 12 hr. The dose may be increased to 8 IU/kg every 12 hr if no

response is seen in 2 days. If this regimen produces no response in 2 days, the dose may be increased to 8 IU/kg every 6 hr.

- Strontium-89 and samarium-153, radiopharmaceuticals that follow the same biochemical pathways as calcium, are used for pain due to diffuse bony metastasis from breast or prostate cancer. Both have demonstrated 60% to 80% efficacy lasting greater than 6 months. Patients need to be warned about possibility of flare pain for a few days after administration. Response can take as a long as 2 to 3 weeks; patients must remain on analgesics during that time.

28. What is opioid rotation and why is it used?

Opioid rotation (switching from one opioid to another) is used when there is inadequate analgesia, unacceptable toxicity (e.g., myoclonus, agitation, hallucinations, pruritis, nausea/vomiting), the need for an alternative route of administration, to ensure patient adherence to the regimen, to decrease analgesic cost, or to comply with formulary requirements.

29. How do you switch from one opioid to another?

- Use an equianalgesic chart or dose conversion table as a guideline (refer to table on p. 467)
- Doses should be adjusted to the patient's age, condition, history (chronic pain or opioid naïveté) and pain intensity.
- Due to interindividual variability in response, decrease dose of new opioid by 30% to 50%, and titrate to effectiveness.
- In hepatic or renal impaired patients, opioids should be initiated at one fourth to one third of the usual dose and slowly titrated upward.
- Frequent dose adjustments may be necessary when converting from an opioid with a short elimination half-life to one with a long half-life.

30. Give an example of switching from one opioid to another, using an equianalgesic chart, considering opioid rotation principles.

Equianalgesic Conversion Equation

To convert 6 mg of oral hydromorphone every 3 hr to oral, continuous-release morphine (every 12 hour):

1. Calculate the 24-hr dose of medication that the patient currently receives:
   6 mg × 8 (every 3 hr) = 48 mg hydromorphone/24 hr
2. Review the equianalgesic chart for equivalence guidelines:
   7.5 mg oral hydromorphone is equivalent to 30 mg oral morphine.
3. Equation:
   $$\frac{30 \text{ mg oral morphine}}{7.5 \text{ mg hydromorphone}} = \frac{X \text{ mg morphine}}{48 \text{ mg hydromorphone}}$$
4. Cross-multiply to solve for X:
   48 mg hydromorphone × 30 mg morphine = 7.5 mg hydromorphone × X mg morphine
   1440 mg = 7.5 X   1440/7.5 = X   X = 192 mg oral morphine
5. Divide the dose by the number of administration times per day to obtain the interval dose.
   Continuous-release morphine (dosed every 12 hr).
   192 mg/2 = 96 mg po 2 times/day (100-mg tablet or three 30-mg tablets bid)
6. In addition to the scheduled dose, order as-needed doses for breakthrough pain; for example, morphine elixir (20 mg/ml), 20-40 mg po every 2 hr as needed.

OPIOID EQUIANALGESIC CHART (USE AS GUIDELINE ONLY)

The following equianalgesic opioid doses are for severe pain in an opioid naïve adult. When converting from one drug to another, the calculated equianalgesic dose is just an estimate, not the usual starting dose. Individualize and titrate dose according to patient age, condition, history (chronic pain), response, and the clinical situation. Reduce dose by 25-50% in the elderly; by 25% in hepatic or renal impaired patients. Unless otherwise stated, t ½ of opioids ranges from 2-3 hours.

Equianalgesic Conversion Equation

Current opioid (single conversion dose & route) = $\dfrac{\text{Total 24° dose of current opioid}}{\text{Total 24° dose of new opioid}}$
New opioid (single conversion dose & route)

Example

Patient is receiving a total 24° dose of morphine 180 mg PO.
What is the equivalent 24° dose of hydromorphone?

$\dfrac{\text{Equianalgesic Dose}}{\text{morphine 30 mg PO}} = \dfrac{\text{Total 24° dose}}{\text{morphine 180 mg PO}}$
hydromorphone 7.5 mg PO = hydromorphone X mg PO

X = hydromorphone 45 mg PO/24°. The patient will receive hydromorphone 6-8 mg PO q 4°

COMMENTS

UCH formulary items are in **BOLD**.

Comparative costs ($ least - $$$$ most).

ANALGESIC OPIOID AGONISTS	EQUIANALGESIC DOSES Parenteral (IV/IM/SQ) (mg)	Oral (mg)	Dose Interval (hours)	COMMENTS
Morphine	10	30	3-4	Active Metabolites: M6G more potent and longer half-life than morphine; M3G may accumulate in renal impairment and cause myoclonus, hyperalgesia. Sublingual: 20-30% bioavailability. Systemic vasodilation due to histamine release. Injection: **0.5, 1, 2, 4, 5, 8, 10, 15** mg/ml. Extended release liposomal encapsulated morphine (DepoDur®) for epidural injection: 10, 15, 20 mg vials. Oral tablets: 15, 30 mg. Oral solution: **10** and **20 mg/5 ml; 20 mg/1 ml**. Suppository: 5, 10, 20, 30 mg. **$$**
Morphine Sustained Release Capsules	--	30	12-24	Avinza® 30, 60, 90, 120 mg capsules every 24 hr, not PRN. Kadian® 20, 30, 50, 60, 80, 100 mg capsules every 12-24 hr, not PRN. Capsules and contents should not be chewed, crushed or dissolved but may be opened and given by gastrostomy tube or sprinkled over food (e.g. applesauce) immediately prior to ingestion. **$$$**
Morphine Controlled/Sustained Release Tablets	--	30	8-12	Do not crush. Give every 8-12 hr, not PRN. MS Contin® 15, 30, 60, 100, 200 mg; Oramorph SR® 15, 30, 60, 100 mg; Morphine Sulfate XR (generic MS Contin® **15, 30, 60, 100, 200 mg**. Other generic formulations available. **$$$**
Fentanyl	100 mcg (0.1 mg)	1000 mcg OT	0.5-1	Drug of choice in patients with renal and liver disease. Injection: **50** mcg/ml **$**. Actiq®, oral transmucosal (OT) fentanyl, approved for breakthrough pain; 200, 400, 600, 800, 1200, 1600 mcg units. Use only up to 4 Actiq doses for breakthrough pain episodes/day. Do not bite or chew Actiq®; consume one unit, may repeat at 30 minutes. Fentora®, sublingual fentanyl tablets, 0.1, 0.2, 0.4, 0.6, 0.8 mg. **$$$$**
Transdermal Fentanyl (Duragesic®)	--	--	72	Transdermal (Duragesic®) patch: **12, 25, 50, 75, and 100** mcg/hr. Change patch every 48-72 hr. Approximate equianalgesic conversion: divide total 24-hour oral morphine dose (mg) by 2 to get fentanyl dose in mcg/hr. Reaches therapeutic serum level 12-16 hr after initial application; lasts 17 hr after removal. Absorption dependent on skin thickness, subcutaneous tissues (fat), and temperature. May cause less constipation than oral controlled/sustained release opioids. Other generic formulations available. **$$$**
Hydromorphone (Dilaudid®)	1.5	7.5	3-4	No active metabolites. Injection: **1, 2, 4, 10** (high potency) mg/ml. Tablet: **2, 4, 8** mg. Suppository: 3 mg. Oral solution: 1 mg/ml. **$$**
Meperidine (Demerol®)	75	300 NR	3-4	Normeperidine (toxic metabolite) has t ½ of 15-40 hr; accumulates with repetitive doses, causing CNS excitation which may result in headaches, altered mental status, and seizures. Use should be restricted for procedural pain of short duration. Avoid use for pain longer than 48 hr; doses > 600 mg/24 hr. Contraindicated in patients with impaired renal function. Injection: 10, **25, 50, 75, 100** mg/ml. Tablet: 50 or 100 mg. Oral solution: 10 mg/ml; 10, 50 mg/5 ml. **$$**
Methadone (Dolophine®) acute use chronic use	10 2-4	20 2-4	6-8 12-24	**Warning:** Careful titration and monitoring due to long and variable t ½ of 13-100 hr; accumulates on days 2-5. High inter-patient variability in metabolism and elimination. Dose increases no sooner than every 3-5 days. For chronic pain the morphine:methadone ratio is: 4:1 if 90 mg daily morphine, 8:1 if 90-300 mg daily morphine. Injection: **10** mg/ml. Tablet: **5** or **10** mg. Oral solution: 1, 2, 10 mg/ml. **$**
Oxycodone	--	20	3-4	Tablet: **5,** 10, 15, 20, 30 mg (Oxy IR®, Roxicodone®) **5 mg + acetaminophen 325 mg** (Percocet®); 5 mg + acetaminophen 500 mg (Roxicet®, Tylox®); 5 mg + aspirin 325 mg (Percodan®). Oral solution (Roxicodone®, OxyFast®) 1 and 20 mg/ml, 5 mg/ml; 5 mg + acetaminophen/5 ml (Percocet®). Other compounded formulations are available. **$$**
Oxycodone Controlled Release Tablets	--	20	12	Do not crush. Give every 12 hr, not PRN. Oxycontin® **10, 20, 40, 80** mg. Oxycodone ER (generic) 10, 20, 40, 80 mg. **$$$**
Oxymorphone (Opana®)	1	10	4-6	Numorphan® Injection: 1, 1.5 mg/ml. Numorphan® Suppository: 5mg. Tablet: 5, 10 mg. Take on an empty stomach, at least one hour prior to or two hours after eating as the C$_{max}$ was increased by approximately 50% in fed compared to fasted subjects. Contraindicated in patients with moderate to severe hepatic impairment. Increased bioavailability with moderate to severe renal impairment; reduce dose accordingly. **$$$**
Oxymorphone Extended Release Tablets (Opana® ER)	--	10	12	Do not crush. Tablet: 5, 10, 20, 40 mg. Give every 12 hr, not PRN. Take on an empty stomach, at least one hour prior to or two hours after eating as the C$_{max}$ was increased by approximately 50% in fed compared to fasted subjects. Indicated in patients on opioids for 7 days or more. Contraindicated in patients with moderate to severe hepatic impairment. Increased bioavailability with moderate to severe renal impairment; reduce dose accordingly. Do not take with alcohol; co-ingestion with alcohol may result in increased plasma levels and fatal overdose. **$$$**
Codeine	130	200 NR	3-4	Use for mild to moderate pain; more constipating than other opioids. Injection: 15, **30,** 60 mg/ml. Tablet: 15, 30, 60 mg. **30 mg + acetaminophen 300 mg acetaminophen** (Tylenol #3®); 60 mg + 300 mg acetaminophen (Tylenol #4®). Oral solution: **2.4** mg/ml + acetaminophen 24 mg/ml. **$$**
Hydrocodone	--	30 NR	3-4	Use for mild to moderate pain. Tablet: **5 mg + 500 mg acetaminophen** (Vicodin®); 7.5 mg + 750 mg acetaminophen (Vicodin ES®); 7.5 mg + 200 mg ibuprofen (Vicoprofen®); 2.5, 5, 7.5, 10 mg + acetaminophen 500 (Lortab®, Norco®); 10 mg + acetaminophen 650 (Lorcet®); 5, 7.5, 10 mg hydrocodone + 400 mg acetaminophen (Zydone®); Lortab®, generic Elixir: 2.5 mg hydrocodone + 167 mg acetaminophen per 5 ml. Other compounded formulations are available. **$$**
Propoxyphene (Darvon®)	--	NR	4-6	**Warning:** Norpropoxyphene (toxic metabolite) accumulates; NR in elderly or renal impairment patients; long t ½ of 12 hr. Tablet/capsule: 65 mg propoxyphene hydrochloride (Darvon®); 100 mg propoxyphene napsylate (Darvon N®); 100 mg propoxyphene napsylate + 650 mg acetaminophen (Darvocet-N 100®). Other compounded formulations are available. **$$**
Tramadol (Ultram®)	--	NA	4-6	Weak opioid agonist for moderate pain. Also inhibits reuptake of norepinephrine and serotonin. Tablet: **50** mg (not to exceed 400 mg/day or 300 mg/day in patients > 75 years). Decrease dose by 50% in patients with renal impairment. 37.5 mg tramadol + 325 mg acetaminophen (Ultracet®). Ultram ER® (every 24 hr, not PRN): 100, 200, 300 mg. **Warning:** Lowers seizure threshold; consult drug reference for drug interaction seizure risks **$$$**

NR = not recommended at that dose; NA = equianalgesic dose is not available

31. How do you calculate the dose of medication for breakthrough pain?

Breakthrough pain refers to an exacerbation or transitory flare of pain, which occurs in 60% to 75% of patients who take regularly scheduled analgesics for stable or baseline pain. The recommended breakthrough dose should be 10% to 20% of the 24-hr dose administered every 2 to 4 hours or more frequently, as needed.

32. What is the relevance of plasma half-lives and steady states in opioid dosing?

The half-life is the time taken for a drug to reach half of its plasma concentration. For all drugs and routes of administration, usually 4 to 5 half-lives are necessary to reach steady state; therefore, dose changes should not be made until steady state is achieved. This approach is often not possible in patients with increasing levels of pain. In such patients, it is more advantageous to use opioids with short (2-3 hr) half-lives (morphine, hydromorphone, oxycodone) for breakthrough pain. Drugs with long half-lives (methadone, levorphanol, propoxyphene) may result in delayed or prolonged side effects, particularly in older adults or patients with liver or renal impairment.

33. How is opioid-induced sedation managed?

Tolerance to sedation usually develops within 3 to 5 days with repeated opioid doses. Decrease the opioid dose and consider an adjuvant analgesic to allow for a decrease in opioid dose. Additionally, caffeine drinks (tea, coffee, coke), antisedatives, such as dextroamphetamine (2.5-10 mg po [0.05-0.1 mg/kg in children]) and methylphenidate (2.5-10 mg po [0.1-0.2 mg/kg in children]), are helpful and should be administered in the morning or early afternoon.

34. How is respiratory depression managed?

High-dose opioids given to an opioid-naive patient may cause respiratory depression; however, tolerance to respiratory depression develops with repeated doses over several weeks. The risk of respiratory depression in a patient receiving chronic opioid therapy is less than 1%. Oversedation usually can be managed by holding or not giving the opioid dose and stimulating the patient. Naloxone (Narcan), an opioid antagonist, should be administered only to patients with significant respiratory depression or apnea. In the rare instance that naloxone is indicated, the following regimen is appropriate: (1) dilute 1 ampule (0.4 mg/ml) with 9 ml of normal saline, and (2) administer 20 mcg (0.02 mg or 0.5 ml) every 2 minutes to desired effects. The goal is to reverse the respiratory depression or sedation without reversing the analgesia.

35. Describe the management of pruritus associated with opioids.

Pruritus due to IV or oral opioids is associated with histamine release; pruritus from epidural opioids is not due to histamine release but may result from binding of the opioid to the trigeminal nerve as it spreads rostrally (e.g., facial itching). Both may be treated with diphenhydramine 12.5-25 mg po/IV every 6 hr. Mild pruritus may be treated with cool compresses or lotion. Mixed agonist/antagonists, naloxone (20 mcg or 0.02 mg IV) and nalbuphine (2.5-5 mg IV every 6 hr) have been used to reverse pruritus due to spinal opioids; however, analgesia also may be reversed. Naltrexone (a long-acting formulation of naloxone) 5 mg po has been recommended with epidural morphine to prevent pruritus. Other causes of pruritus (e.g., drug allergy) should be ruled out.

36. What drug:drug interactions are causes of concern with opioid use?

Any medication that causes sedation must be used cautiously with opioids. When phenothiazine antiemetics, muscle relaxants, benzodiazepines, anticonvulsants, antihistamines, tricyclic antidepressants, and alcohol are given with opioids, the patient should be monitored closely and the opioid dose may need to be decreased to prevent oversedation and respiratory depression. **Note:** It is safe for patients in pain to take an opioid dose along with a regularly scheduled sleeping pill.

37. Is morphine still the gold standard for cancer pain?

Morphine is still the standard of comparison for opioids used to treat severe pain. However, as knowledge about pain physiology and pharmacology translates into better analgesics or new formulations of opioids with fewer side effects, morphine may not continue to be the drug of choice. Morphine has several active metabolites, including morphine-3-glucuronide (M3G) and morphine-6-glucuronide (M6G). M3G has no analgesic activity, antagonizes morphine's analgesic effect, may induce allodynia and hyperalgesia, and causes CNS excitation and myoclonus. (The muscle relaxant, dantrolene 50 mg po tid, is effective in relieving morphine-induced myoclonus). M6G has greater affinity for mu receptors than morphine and is responsible for respiratory depression and gastrointestinal toxicities (e.g., nausea). Morphine can be eliminated in patients with renal disease, but its metabolite M6G can accumulate because of decreased clearance and prolonged elimination half-life. Because of problems related to morphine's active metabolites, the trend may be to use semisynthetic opioids, such as fentanyl, hydromorphone, and oxycodone.

38. How effective is sublingual morphine?

For patients who cannot swallow, morphine concentrate (20 mg/ml) is ideal for sublingual administration. Drug bioavailability is estimated at 20% to 30%. Problems with sublingual morphine include sour taste, dry mouth, and bitter taste.

39. What opioids are used by nebulizer?

Inhaled or nebulized morphine and fentanyl have been used as a treatment for terminal patients with pulmonary metastases to decrease air hunger and to treat dyspnea related to end-stage cancer, chronic obstructive pulmonary disease, and congestive heart failure. Approximately one third or less of nebulized morphine is bioavailable. To administer nebulized morphine, dilute 2 to 5 ml of preservative-free parenteral morphine with 2 ml of sterile water or normal saline, and nebulize via face mask for 15 minutes every 4 hours. Nebulized doses of morphine range from 5 to 30 mg (hydromorphone 1-20 mg) and are not adequate for analgesia. Fentanyl 25 mcg + 2 ml of normal saline may be nebulized every 2 to 3 hours.

40. Can any long-acting opioids be used in a gastrostomy or nasogastric tube?

Two extended-release oral morphine formulations (Avinza and Kadian) are available in capsule form. Their efficacy is not destroyed by breaking the capsule and sprinkling it over soft food (e.g., applesauce) or administering it via an enteral feeding tube (e.g., gastrostomy, nasogastric tube).

41. What are the advantages of methadone compared to morphine?

- Higher oral bioavailability and highly lipophilic (permits wide distribution in body tissues)
- Useful for opioid rotation strategies because of incomplete cross-tolerance with other opioids
- No active metabolites
- Less dose escalation compared to morphine
- Good alternative if the patient is allergic to morphine
- Lower cost
- Effective against neuropathic pain and hyperalgesia due to unique pharmacodynamic properties; in addition to agonist activity at the mu opioid receptor, it blocks

the NMDA (N-methyl-D-aspartate) receptor involved in pain processing and inhibits catecholoamine uptake

42. Why is it more complicated to use methadone?

The major disadvantages of methadone are the risks of drug accumulation related to its long and unpredictable half-life. In switching from another opioid to methadone, it is also complicated to determine accurate doses according to equianalgesic guides based on single-dose studies. Effective doses of methadone vary from 3% to 68% of the calculated equianalgesic dose.

43. What are some safe guidelines for using oral methadone to treat pain?

- Carefully monitor and titrate doses according to individual patient response.
- Administer every 6 to 8 hours. Some patients require dosing only 1 to 2 times a day.
- It may be safer to start some patients with a PRN (patient-controlled titration) regimen, rather than ATC (around the clock) dosing.
- Use safe conversion ratios when switching from oral morphine to oral methadone: for patients receiving 30 to 90 mg morphine/day, use a 4:1 ratio of morphine to methadone; 91 to 300 mg morphine/day, use a 8:1 ratio; and greater than 300 mg/day, use a 12:1 ratio (Manfredi & Houde, 2003). For example, a patient taking 60 mg of daily morphine would start at 15 mg of methadone daily. Another way is to start methadone at 10% to 20% of the total morphine dose (Shaiova, 2005).

44. What are special considerations for using fentanyl patches?

- Patients must have adequate fat stores to absorb and retain the medication to enable the patch to last 72 hr. In emaciated patients, the patch may need to be changed more frequently because of more rapid absorption.
- Because the patch takes approximately 9 to 16 hours to provide analgesia, an additional analgesic is needed. If the patient is converted from continuous-release morphine, the last 12-hr dose may be administered at the same time as the patch is applied. If the patient was receiving a short-acting analgesic, continue this medication for the next 12 hours.
- Increased absorption in febrile patients may result in oversedation.
- To secure the patch in place for diaphoretic patients, apply a transparent dressing over the patch.
- For itching at the site of application, a steroid inhaler can be sprayed over the site with complete drying prior to placing the patch (Creams should not be used on sites of application because they can affect drug absorption).

45. When is tramadol used for cancer pain?

Tramadol (Ultram) is an opioid for mild-to-moderate pain; its additional analgesic effect is related to its inhibition of serotonin and noradrenaline reuptake. Tramadol is not chemically related to morphine but is thought to bind weakly to mu opiate receptors. It is not currently scheduled by the Drug Enforcement Administration. Tramadol is effective for patients with early bone or neuropathic pain and has been used primarily to treat chronic pain.

46. How should opioids be tapered to prevent an abstinence or withdrawal syndrome when they are no longer needed?

The rate of tapering may vary with individual patients; however, the following approach is often used:

- Decrease the 24-hr total dose by 50%, and administer as divided doses on schedule for 2 days.

- Decrease the dose by 25% every 2 days thereafter until the total daily dose is equivalent to 30 mg of oral morphine/day or 0.6 mg/kg/day in a child.
- After 2 days on this final dose, stop the medication. If the patient is anxious or nervous, a clonidine patch (changed every 7 days), 0.1 to 0.2 mg/day, may be used to lessen or prevent anxiety, tachycardia, sweating, and other autonomic symptoms.

47. How do you start a patient-controlled analgesia (PCA) pump?

1. Calculate the equianalgesic IV opioid dose the patient currently receives.
2. Divide the 24-hr dose by 24 to obtain the hourly or basal dose.
3. Set the hourly rate (mg/hr), PCA or bolus dose, and interval.
4. If the patient has uncontrolled or increased pain, administer an individualized loading dose to control the pain before starting the PCA. A good starting loading dose is equal to one third, one half, or one full hour total of the patient's normal maintenance (hourly plus PCA or PRN doses).

In contrast to patients with acute postoperative pain, patients with chronic cancer pain require most of the analgesic dose be programmed into the hourly PCA infusion so that pain is prevented (similar to around-the-clock oral dosing). The PCA (breakthrough) dose is usually one half of the hourly infusion rate set at every 6 to 15 minutes. Thus, if the equianalgesic dose of IV morphine was 6 mg/hr, the pump may be set at the following values: continuous infusion, 3 to 6 mg/hr, and PCA dose, 1 to 3 mg, with a 15-minute lockout. The table below lists starting dosages for commonly used PCA opioids; after the initial setting, however, the dose should be titrated to effect.

Patient-controlled analgesia (PCA) pump medications

Opioid	Concentration	PCA dose	Continuous infusion	Onset (min)	Peak (min)
Morphine	1 mg/ml	1 mg (adults) 0.02-0.03 mg/kg (children)	1-2 mg/hr (adults) 0.01-0.02 mg/kg/hr (children)	10-20	15-30
Hydro-morphone	0.2 mg/ml	0.2 mg (adults) 0.003-0.0045 mg/kg (children)	0.2-0.4 mg/hr (adults) 0.0015-0.003 mg/kg/hr (children)	5	10-20
Fentanyl	10 mcg/ml	10-25 mcg (adults) 0.1-0.2 mcg/kg/ dose (children)	10-25 mcg/hr (adults) 0.5-1.0 mcg/kg/hr (children)	1	1-5

48. Can a PCA pump be used in patients without venous access?

A PCA pump also can be used to deliver analgesics subcutaneously. Although morphine and fentanyl can be used, hydromorphone is ideal for this purpose because it provides a high concentration of medication (high-potency preparation, 10 mg/ml) in a low volume. The lockout interval should be longer (15-25 minutes) because of the longer absorption and longer time to peak effect. Butterfly (25- to 27-gauge) or special needles for subcutaneous administration may be used (e.g., a 27-gauge, $1/4$-inch needle with extension tubing). The site is covered with a transparent dressing, and the needle needs to be changed every 3 to 7 days with routine inspection of the site for erythema, swelling, or tenderness.

49. What is the difference between intrathecal and epidural administration?

- **Intrathecal administration.** The subarachnoid fluid is bounded by the dural ligament (ligamentum flavum). Intrathecal or subarachnoid catheters are placed into the subarachnoid space, and medications are delivered directly into the spinal fluid. Because medication delivered intrathecally does not have to diffuse across the dural ligament, smaller doses are required.
- **Epidural administration.** Epidural catheters are placed just outside the dural ligament. Medication is delivered into the epidural space, located between the ligamentum flavum and dura mater. The medication diffuses across the dura mater and arachnoid mater into the cerebrospinal fluid, where it binds with opiate receptors to block pain transmission.

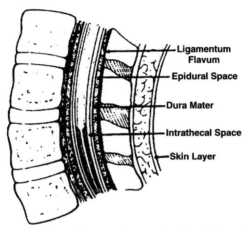

Lateral section of the spine. *(From St. Marie B:* Management of cancer pain with epidural morphine, *St Paul, MN, 1994, Pharmacia Deltec. By permission.)*

50. When should epidurals be considered for cancer pain?

The epidural route can be used to administer opioids alone, local anesthetics alone, or an opioid/local anesthetic combination. Epidurals should be considered to provide analgesia in the following settings:

- Whenever pain is not adequately controlled by other routes
- When the dose of oral or intravenous opioids reaches a point at which side effects become a significant issue; epidural analgesics are associated with fewer side effects (e.g., sedation) because the IV dose of morphine may be reduced by $1/10$ and the oral dose by $1/30$; when the intrathecal route is used, the amount of morphine is even less: the IV dose is reduced by $1/100$ and oral dose by $1/300$
- For neuropathic pain, such as tumor invasion of a nerve plexus or nerve root and scarring from radiation therapy; neuropathic pain is effectively treated with epidural or intrathecal (IT) placement of local anesthetics and clonidine, ketamine, baclofen, or midazolam
- Ziconotide, a neuronal calcium channel blocker, is an FDA-approved IT analgesic for refractory severe chronic pain

51. What effect do catheter placement and opioid choice have on epidural pain relief?

The lipid solubility of opioids is one of the major properties that influence receptor binding, systemic uptake, and rostral spread. Increased lipid solubility shortens the time needed for drug transfer through lipid barriers of blood vessels and cell membranes, resulting in a more rapid onset and shorter duration of action. The most lipophilic (lipid-soluble) opioids are sufentanil and fentanyl. Morphine is the most hydrophilic opioid; it spreads widely in the epidural and intrathecal space. Other opioids, such as hydromorphine, have intermediate lipid solubility. Because of its high lipid solubility, analgesia related to fentanyl is more segmental in nature; thus, it is more important for the epidural catheter to be placed close to the site or dermatomal area of pain.

52. What are the advantages and disadvantages of the spinal delivery of pain medications?

Advantages and disadvantages of spinal delivery of pain medications

Advantages	Disadvantages
Direct delivery to involved receptors (allows use of less medication and effective control of intractable pain)	Initial high cost if a completely implantable system is used
Effective control of neuropathic pain (e.g., intrathecal methylprednisolone for intractable postherpetic neuralgia)	Greater incidence of pruritus
Ability to use a combination of agents with minimal side effects	Risk of meningitis with intrathecal catheters
Less sedation	Risk of infection leading to epidural abscess with risk of nerve damage and paraplegia

53. What nondrug modalities are used to control pain?

Nondrug modalities include physical and psychosocial interventions, which should be introduced early to augment, not replace, pharmacologic therapy for pain management. The success of several of these modalities requires an understanding of the mind/body connection and depends on a therapeutic relationship between the nurse or health care provider and patient.

- Physical modalities used to reduce pain in patients with cancer include cutaneous stimulation (heat, cold, massage, vibration), exercise, physical therapy, joint mobilization, transcutaneous nerve stimulation (TENS), reflexology, therapeutic touch, and acupressure or acupuncture.
- Psychosocial interventions help patients to gain a sense of control by using cognitive techniques that affect how pain is interpreted and behavioral techniques that provide the patient with skills to cope with and modify responses to pain. Examples of psychosocial interventions include relaxation and imagery, meditation and deep breathing, distraction and reframing (replacing negative thoughts with more positive ones), music therapy, humor therapy, psychotherapy, biofeedback, peer support groups, hypnosis, and pastoral counseling.

54. What is important to know about controlling pain in older adult patients?

Older adult patients fail to report pain because they believe pain is expected with aging. Furthermore, health professionals may believe that elderly patients experience a lower pain level or that they are unable to tolerate high doses of opioids. Assessment is further complicated by sensory or cognitive impairments. Tips for administering or selecting analgesics include:

- Avoid opioids with long half-lives, such as methadone, propoxyphene (Darvon), or levorphanol. Drugs may have longer half-lives in older adult patients because of decreased renal clearance, decreased hepatic function, and decrease in the ratio of lean body mass to fat.
- Morphine has active metabolites (morphine 6-glucuronide) that may accumulate, resulting in nausea, confusion, and sedation.
- Avoid long-term use of NSAIDs.
- Use steroids cautiously because they aggravate osteoporosis.
- For a tricyclic antidepressant, consider nortriptyline over amitriptyline because of its lower anticholinergic effects. Start tricyclic antidepressants low at 10 mg Q HS.
- With both opioids and adjuvant medications, "start low and go slow." When the equianalgesic chart is used to convert from one agent to another, the dose of the new analgesic should be decreased by 25% to 50%.
- Increased number of medications (polypharmacy) may result in increased confusion and falls.
- Keep it simple. Avoid high-technology pumps, especially if the patient lives alone.
- Provide medication instructions to the patient and a responsible family member verbally and in writing (large print).
- Assess and treat constipation vigilantly because of elderly patients' decreased mobility, decreased fluid intake, and concomitant use of other medications.

55. Is pain treated in comatose or verbally unresponsive patients?

Yes. Comatose or verbally unresponsive patients should be placed minimally on their baseline level of analgesia, and analgesics should be administered before any painful procedure. Some patients have experienced withdrawal without the ability to express it. Health care providers should pay attention to nonverbal cues (e.g., grimacing, sighs or gasps, frowns). Significant others may be queried about their assessment of the patient's level of pain. Although they are the least sensitive, physiologic measures (elevations in pulse, blood pressure, respiratory rate) may indicate pain.

56. What new pain medications are in the pipeline?

- Ionsys (fentanyl iontophoretic transdermal system), the first needle-free, patient-activated analgesic system approved by the FDA in 2006, is indicated for acute postoperative pain in adults requiring opioid analgesia during hospitalization. Ionsys uses *iontophoresis*, a process in which a low-intensity electric field (generally imperceptible to the patient) is used to rapidly transport fentanyl across the skin and into the circulatory system. The Ionsys system adheres to the upper outer arm or chest. When pain medication is needed, the patient double-clicks the dosing button, delivering a preprogrammed 40 mcg dose of fentanyl through the skin. Each dose is delivered over a 10-minute period. More than one Ionsys system should not be applied to a patient at the same time.
- Depo-dur, a liposomal encapsulated morphine, lasts up to 48 hours
- Prialt, an intrathecal synthetic gabapentin-like drug
- Oxytrex (oxycodone + naltrexone)

Key Points

- Approximately 10% of patients will experience pain that is resistant to traditional analgesic therapies.
- The frequency of a pain assessment is determined by the patient's clinical situation.
- The patient's self-report of pain is the gold standard even in those who are nonverbal or cognitively impaired.
- The analgesic must be selected according to the type, severity, and temporal nature of the pain as well as other factors.
- Opioid rotation is used when there is inadequate analgesia, unacceptable toxicity (e.g., myoclonus, agitation, hallucinations, pruritis, nausea/vomiting), the need for an alternative route of administration, to ensure patient adherence to the regimen, to decrease analgesic cost, or to comply with formulary requirements.
- Nondrug modalities include physical and psychosocial interventions, which should be introduced early to augment, not replace, pharmacologic therapy for pain management.

 Internet Resources

American Alliance of Cancer Pain Initiatives:
    http://www.aacpi.org
American Pain Foundation:
    http://www.painfoundation.org
American Pain Society (APS):
    http://www.ampainsoc.org
American Society for Pain Management Nursing:
    http://www.aspmn.org
City of Hope National Medical Center, City of Hope Pain/Palliative Care Resource Center:
    http://www.cityofhope.org/prc
International Association for the Study of Pain:
    http://www.iasp-pain.org
Mayday Pain Link:
    http://www.edc.org/PainLink
National Comprehensive Cancer Network (NCCN) Cancer Pain Treatment Guidelines for Adult Cancer Patients and Pediatric Cancer Patients – Version I, 2006:
    http://www.nccn.org/professionals/physician_gls/PDF/pain.pdf
Oncology Nursing Society, Pain Management Special Interest Group:
    http://www.ons.org
Improving Pain Treatment by Education:
    http://www.painedu.org
Quality Improvement Guidelines for the Treatment of Acute Pain and Cancer Pain, American Pain Society:
    http://www.ampainsoc.org/whatsnew/101805_cancer.htm

Bibliography

American Pain Society: *Guideline for the management of cancer pain in adults and children,* Glenview, IL, 2005, American Pain Society.
Ashburn MA, Lipman AG, editors: *Principles of analgesic use in the treatment of acute pain and cancer pain,* ed 5, Glenview, IL, 2003, American Pain Society.

Caraceni A, Martini C, Zecca E, et al: Working group of an IASP task force on cancer pain. Breakthrough pain characteristics and syndromes in patients with cancer pain: An international survey. *Palliative Medicine* 20(2):140-148, 2003.

Coyne PJ, Viswanathan R, Smith TJ: Nebulized fentanyl citrate improves patients' perception of breathing, respiratory rate, and oxygen saturation in dyspnea. *J Pain Symptom Manage* 23(2):157-160, 2002.

Coyne PJ, Smith T, Laird J et al: Effectively starting and titrating intrathecal analgesic therapy in patients with refractory cancer pain. *Clin J Oncol Nurs* 9(5):581-583, 2005.

Fine PG, Miaskowski C, Paice JA: Meeting the challenges in cancer pain management. *J Support Oncol* 2(4):5-22, 2004.

Herr K, Bjoro K, Decker S: Tools for assessment of pain in nonverbal older adults with dementia: A state-of-the-science review. *J Pain Symptom Manage* 31(2):170-192, 2006.

Herr K, Coyne PJ, Key T, et al: Pain assessment in the nonverbal patient: Position statement with clinical practice recommendations. *Pain Manag Nurs* 7(2):44-52, 2006.

Hicks CL, von Baeyer CL, Spafford P, et al: The faces scale—revised: Toward a common metric in pediatric pain measurement. *Pain* 93:173-183, 2001.

Kolesnikov Y, Chereshnev I, Pasternak G: Analgesic synergy between topical lidocaine and topical opioids. *Pharmacology* 295:546-551, 2000.

Li S, Liu J, Zhang H, et al: Rhenium-188 HEDP to treat painful bone metastases. *Clin Nucl Med* 26(11): 919-922, 2001.

Manfredi PL, Houde R: Prescribing methadone, a unique analgesic. *J Support Care* 1(3):216-220, 2003.

Mercadante S: Dautrolene treatment of opiod-induced myoclonus. *Anesth Analg* 81:1307-1308, 1995.

McCaffery M, Ferrell BR, Turner M: Ethical issues in the use of placebos in cancer pain management. *Oncol Nurs Forum* 23:1587-1593, 1996.

McDonald AA, Portenoy RK: How to use anticonvulsants as adjuvant analgesics in the treatment of neuropathic cancer pain. *J Support Oncol* 4(1):43-52, 2006.

National Comprehensive Cancer Network: Cancer Pain Treatment Guidelines for Patients—Version II, August 2005, http://www.nccn.org/professionals/physician_gls/PDF/pain.pdf Accessed January 14, 2007.

Oncology Nursing Society: Cancer pain management, 2004: http://www.ons.org/publications/positions/documents/pdfs/CancerPain.pdf. Accessed January 14, 2007.

Passik SD, Kirsh KL: Managing pain in patients with aberrant drug-taking behaviors. *J Support Oncol* 3(1):83-86, 2005.

Passik SD, Weinreb HJ: Managing chronic nonmalignant pain: Overcoming obstacles to the use of opioids. *Adv Ther* 17:70-83, 2000.

Portenoy RK: *Cancer pain: Assessment and management,* London, 2003, Cambridge University Press.

Porter J, Jick H: Addiction rare in patients treated with narcotics. *N Engl J Med* 302:123, 1980.

Serafini AN: Samarium Sm-153 lexidronam for the palliation of bone pain associated with metastases. *Cancer* 88(suppl 12):2934-2939, 2000.

Shaiova L: The role of methadone in the treatment of moderate to severe cancer pain. *Support Cancer Ther* 2(3):176-180, 2005.

Slatkin N: Cancer-related pain and its pharmacological management in the patient with bone metastasis. *J Support Oncol* 4(2):15-22, 2006.

Sloan PA: The evolving role of interventional pain management in oncology. *J Support Oncol* 2(6):491-506, 2004.

Solomon SD, McMurray JJ, Pfeffer MA, et al: Cardiovascular risk associated with celecoxib in a clinical trial for colorectal adenoma prevention. *N Engl J Med* 352:1071-1080, 2005.

Staats PS, Yearwood T, Charapata SG, et al: Intrathecal ziconotide in the treatment of refractory pain in patients with cancer or AIDS. *JAMA* 291:63-70, 2004.

Stearns L, Boortz-Marz R, DuPen S et al: Intrathecal drug delivery for the management of cancer pain: A multidisciplinary consensus of best clinical practices. *J Support Oncol* 3(6):399-408, 2005.

Webster LR, Fakata KR: Ziconotide: For chronic severe pain. *Pract Pain Manage,* May 2005.

Wong D, Whaley L: *Clinical manual of pediatric nursing,* ed 4, St Louis, 2003, Mosby.

Disclaimer: The views expressed in this manuscript are those of the author, Diana L. Ruzicka, and do not reflect the official policy or position of the Department of the Army, Department of Defense, or the U.S. Government.

Chapter 43

Palliative Care

Sandra L. Muchka and Julie Griffie

1. What is palliative care?

The World Health Organization has defined palliative care as "an approach to care that improves the quality of life of patients and their families facing the problem associated with life-threatening illness, through the prevention and relief of suffering by means of early identification and impeccable assessment and treatment of pain and other problems, physical, psychosocial, and spiritual" (World Health Organization. Palliative care. Available at: http://www.who.int/cancer/palliative/definition/en/. Accessed March 7, 2007). The goal of palliative care nursing is to promote quality of life throughout the illness trajectory by the relief of suffering. It includes care of the dying and their family members and bereavement follow-up.

2. What is the difference between palliative care and hospice care?

The philosophies of hospice care and palliative care are identical, but there are major differences involving reimbursement, eligibility for services, and care settings. In the United States, funding for hospice care is available via the Medicare Hospice Benefit or through private health insurance to patients who have a physician-certified prognosis of less than 6 months to live and who are willing to forego life-sustaining treatments. Care is provided by Medicare-certified home hospice agencies with the goal of supporting patients and families at home. Unfortunately, limitations on reimbursement and requirements to forego certain types of therapy restrict the availability of hospice care; approximately 20% of dying patients enter a hospice program. Palliative care was first developed to "fill in the gaps," to meet the needs of dying patients and families who do not qualify for hospice care and to extend the hospice philosophy into the hospital setting or to a much wider population of patients and care settings than hospice care can provide. Today, as evidenced by the updated WHO definition, palliative care should be integrated into the care of all patients with life threatening illness. Hence, palliative care services are not limited by prognosis, types of treatments offered, or need for a hospice insurance benefit.

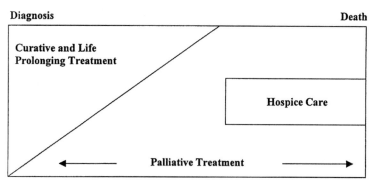

Integrated model of curative and palliative care in patients with chronic illness.

3. Who provides palliative care?

The multidisciplinary team provides palliative care. The team may include physicians, nurses, social worker, chaplain, dietitian, volunteers, and other disciplines as appropriate to meet the needs of the patient and family members. The patient and family are the unit of care. Because the nurse is the provider of the majority of direct patient care and most frequently in contact with the patient, the role of the nurse is critical.

4. List the elements of a palliative care assessment.

The palliative care assessment begins with the establishment of a relationship with the patient and family, verifying mutual goals of the encounter. Baseline health of the patient and family must be determined. Physical and psychosocial assessments are key.

A general physical assessment of the patient is followed by examination of the following:
- Distress from physical symptoms. Assess the patient's understanding of:
  o The cause of the symptom
  o Goal for relief
  o Current side effects
- Patient goals. Consider:
  o What is important to the patient?
  o How can we help the patient 'live well' in the days ahead?
  o What personal goals does the patient have that health care team members should take into consideration?
- Psychological and spiritual assessment
  o Elicit information about how the patient has coped with stressful situations in the past
  o Who does the patient turn to for support?
- Discussion of prognosis. Consider:
  o The patient's functional status
  o Major organ failure
  o Multiple symptoms
- Support systems and wishes for end-of-life care. Consider:
  o Where does the patient want to be at the time of death?
  o Who is available to assist?
  o What are the capabilities of the caregiver in relationship to the complexity of symptom management needs?

5. Why is information about prognosis important?

Patients and families need prognostic information to plan for the time ahead. The concept of time (months vs. weeks vs. days) should be communicated to the patient if the information is requested. Simply asking, "Do you need to know about time?" can begin the conversation. Prognostic information should be based on functional status, nutritional status, major organ involvement, and number of symptoms.

6. How can we open the conversation about the end of life?

Opening the conversation about dying requires maximizing personal sensitivity and communication skills. Choose a quiet time when the patient is comfortable. Sit down, when culturally appropriate, and make eye contact. Acknowledging that the situation is not going well may open the conversation. Simple statements, such as, "Things don't seem to be going as well as we would like," or the question, "How do you think things are going for you?" may open a flood of emotions and concerns. Most oncology patients recognize when they are not getting better and welcome the opportunity to talk about it.

7. Should nurses talk to patients about prognosis?

Recognition of a downhill course may first be apparent to the nurses who see patients on a regular basis. When a patient arrives in a wheelchair after months of being ambulatory, functional status and other prognostic factors should be reviewed. Nurses must be proactive in recognizing functional decline and communicating patients' goals to team members. Patients and nurses can and should discuss disease progression. Many patients have a clear idea of the time frame that is left and need our assistance to ensure that goals are met and family issues are resolved.

8. Why is goal setting important at the end of life?

Goal setting directs the plan of care. For example, if comfort is the major goal at the end of life, only measures that will add to comfort and dignity should be offered. Cardiac resuscitation does not add comfort and dignity, and should not be a part of the plan of care. If identified goals include reconciliation with a family member, escalating analgesic doses that cause sedation may not meet the patient's goals. On the other hand, if all end-of-life goals have been met and the goal is comfort above all, the side effect of sedation may be welcomed.

9. When is a family conference appropriate?

Family conferences are an excellent way of getting everyone "on the same page." A family conference may be convened to:
- Review the patient's medical condition and to establish treatment goals
- Clarify care goals
- Make decisions for nondecisional patients
- Resolve patient, family, and/or staff disagreements or conflicts

Nurses are pivotal in recognizing the need for family conferences and facilitating this important part of interdisciplinary care. For detailed information, the reader is referred to: http://www.eperc.mcw.edu/FastFact/ff_016.htm.

10. The foundation of excellent palliative care is management of what symptom?

The answer, of course, is pain. Patients consider freedom from pain to be the most important factor at the end of life. Many patients have told us over the years that physical pain is often feared more than death itself. (Refer to Chapter 42 for more information on pain management).

11. How common is dyspnea in patients with advanced cancer?

Dyspnea is one of the most prevalent symptoms among patients with advanced cancer. It is a subjective sensation defined as the perception of difficulty in breathing or as an uncomfortable awareness of breathing. Some degree of dyspnea occurs in over 70% of dying patients. In patients with advanced, incurable cancer, the sensation of dyspnea ranges from mild breathlessness to a sense of impending death from suffocation. Dyspnea can severely limit function and increase anxiety.

12. What should be included in the assessment of a patient with terminal dyspnea?

Assessment of terminal dyspnea begins with identifying the symptom. Elements of the assessment should include:
- Severity
- Onset
- Factors that exacerbate or relieve dyspnea
- Impact on daily living and quality of life
- Review of oxygen delivery system (Is the oxygen on? Is the tubing kinked?)

- Acute anxiety episode?
- Severe pain?
- Constipation?
- Urinary retention?

Understanding the goals of care is essential to guide the extent of the work-up. For example, if the patient is clearly dying and the goal of care is comfort, pulse oximetry, blood gas, and chest radiographs are not indicated.

13. How is terminal dyspnea treated?

Treatment of dyspnea in a dying patient depends on the goals of care and underlying cause. Dying patients who have severe dyspnea often need aggressive pharmacologic management. Drugs may be sedating, and often a balance needs to be found between symptom management and level of somnolence. The drugs used to treat dyspnea are directed at relieving the sensation of not being able to breathe. The major classes are opioids and anxiolytics. Adjuvant drugs include steroids, sedatives, and/or cough suppressants. It is important to include nonpharmacologic interventions in the treatment plan for terminal dyspnea. Oxygen administration, body positioning, room fans that produce tactile airflow to the patient's face, and relaxation/distraction techniques have been shown to be helpful in conjunction with pharmacologic interventions.

14. Which opioid is most commonly used to control dyspnea? How does it work?

The most commonly used opioid is morphine, which can be administered orally, intravenously (IV), subcutaneously (SC), or via nebulized aerosol. The starting dose of morphine depends on the patient's current and/or prior use. For opioid-naive patients with severe dyspnea, the recommended starting dose is 2 to 5 mg IV or SC every 5 minutes until symptoms improve.

Morphine affects dyspnea in a number of ways. First, it reduces patients' fears and anxiety. Reduction of anxiety, muscle tension, and restlessness decreases oxygen consumption, which in turn improves oxygenation and increases respiratory comfort. Morphine also improves oxygenation by reducing pulmonary edema through pulmonary vasodilation.

15. Does morphine hasten the patient's death?

A major barrier to providing adequate relief of terminal dyspnea is the fear of using opioids because of the potential for respiratory depression. Ethically, their use is appropriate as long as the intent is to relieve distress rather than shorten life. There is no ethical or professional justification for withholding symptomatic treatment to a dying patient because of fear of potential respiratory depression. It is important to understand the patient's wishes for end-of-life symptom control. Good communication with family and other caregivers about how and why drugs are administered is essential.

16. What are the treatment options for intractable nausea and/or vomiting?

Nausea may represent different sensations to different people. A thorough assessment is necessary to understand what the person is experiencing. Nausea may imply esophageal reflux, inner ear dysfunction, regurgitation, bowel obstruction, or anxiety. There is a wide variety of medications for the management of nausea and vomiting. Many times they are used in a trial-and-error fashion. Nondrug therapies include behavioral treatments such as relaxation, guided imagery, distraction, and music therapy. Nasogastric or percutaneous drainage may be indicated for gastric stasis or obstruction refractory to conservative management.

Medical management of nausea and vomiting

Cause	Indicated drug class
Movement-related nausea	Antihistamine
Anxiety	Benzodiazepine
Tumor-related elevated intracranial pressure	Glucocorticoid
Gastric stasis	Metoclopramide
Stimulation of chemoreceptor trigger zone	Dopamine antagonist, serotonin antagonist
Constipation	Laxative

Adapted from Weissman DE, Ambuel B: *Improving end-of-life care: a resource guide for physician education,* ed 3, Milwaukee, 1999, Medical College of Wisconsin.

17. **Mrs. K. is a 72-year-old woman with end-stage lung cancer. The night before discharge home to hospice care the nurse phones the doctor to report that Mrs. K. is "confused." What does this report mean?**

It is important to understand what "confusion" really means. Mrs. K. may be experiencing terminal delirium. Delirium occurs to some degree in virtually all patients before death. The cause is often multifactorial; an exact cause is not established in 40% or more of patients. Possible causes in patients with advanced cancer include drug toxicity, metabolic changes, central nervous system pathology, drug withdrawal, infections, fevers, urinary retention, and/or imminent death.

Potential causes for terminal delirium and agitation

Cause	Manifestations
Metabolic disturbances	Hypoxia, hypercalcemia, hyponatremia, hypoglycemia, liver failure, renal failure, dehydration
Central nervous system pathology	Cerebral metastases, infarction, bleeding, infection, seizures, increased intracranial pressure
Drug toxicity	Benzodiazepines, anticholinergics, opioids, steroids, illicit drugs, alcohol
Drug withdrawal	Alcohol, benzodiazepines, barbiturates, steroids, nicotine
Other causes	Systemic infections, fever, heart failure, imminent death, urinary retention, constipation, sleep deprivation, pain

---

18. **What nursing assessment is required in suspected delirium?**

1. Complete a history and physical examination, including a Mini-Mental Status Examination (MMSE; see Question 19).
2. Distinguish between delirium and dementia. Delirium refers to an altered level of consciousness with reduced attention and memory. Other characteristics of delirium include perceptual disturbances, hallucination, incoherent speech, and altered sleep/wake cycles. Dementia refers to a loss of intellectual function with diminished memory, thinking, and judgment.

3. Assess whether the patient is in danger of harming self or others.
4. Assess whether the cognitive change is distressing to the patient.
5. Review chart and medication record for recent medication changes.
6. Assess for possible physical causes (e.g., fever, urinary retention, and impaction).

Depending on the goals of care, further assessment may include a complete evaluation (e.g., brain imaging, spinal tap) to search for the underlying cause.

19. How is the abbreviated MMSE conducted?

Ask the patient the following:

1. Age
2. Birth date
3. Recognition of two persons (e.g., doctor, nurse, family)
4. Hospital or clinic name
5. Address for recall at end of test (e.g., 12 Main Street)
6. Present year
7. Current time (to nearest hour)
8. Name of current president
9. Name of first president or year World War II ended
10. Count backward from 20 to 1

Score: 9–10 = Normal   8 = Borderline   < 7 = Cognitive impairment

Adapted from Power D, Kelly S, Gilsenan J, et al: Suitable screening tests for cognitive impairment and depression in the terminally ill: a prospective prevalence study. *Palliat Med* 7:213-218, 1993.

20. It is determined that Mrs. S. is experiencing terminal delirium. What can be done?

Treatment for delirium should encompass a combination of nonpharmacologic and pharmacologic approaches. Nondrug interventions include offering the patient frequent reminders of time and date and providing a quiet, well-lit room. The presence of a family member may help to allay fears and provide patient support. Physical restraints are rarely necessary and should be applied only for a brief time while treatment is initiated.

Drug therapy is indicated for patients with agitated delirium (i.e., those who exhibit restless behaviors such as climbing out of bed or pulling out intravenous lines). The most useful agents include neuroleptics and benzodiazepines. Neuroleptics should be used as first-line agents; haloperidol (Haldol) is one of the most common choices. The recommended starting dose for haloperidol is 1 to 2 mg PO, SQ, or IV every 6 hours; a 1- to 2-mg dose should be available as needed. The dose should be titrated to meet the patient's needs.

21. Two months ago Mr. J., a 57-year-old man with advanced pancreatic cancer, was told that his survival time was estimated at 3 to 4 months. He reports a decrease in appetite and weight along with insomnia and increased fatigue. His family thinks that he is depressed. Do all patients become depressed when they find out that they are dying?

No. The incidence of depression in patients with cancer ranges from 10% to 25% and increases with higher levels of disability, advanced illness, and/or pain. Psychological distress often causes suffering in dying patients. The diagnosis of major depression in a terminally ill patient is more often related to feelings of worthlessness, hopelessness, guilt, and suicidal ideation rather than physical symptoms associated with end of life.

Always explore patients' hopes and expectations. Although there may be no hope for a cure, many patients have other hopes, such as avoidance of pain or being at home with their family. Individual and/or group counseling reduces psychological stress and depressive symptoms in patients with cancer. Nonpharmacologic interventions used to treat anxiety and depression include relaxation and distraction techniques. Antidepressants are often the first-line agents for treatment of depression in terminally ill patients. Skillful management of depression relieves suffering and is a core element of the provision of comprehensive end-of-life care.

22. One of the most frequent concerns for patients and families is loss of appetite and/or ability to drink. Does the patient suffer without food or fluids?

Loss of appetite is normal in the days or weeks before death. The loss occurs slowly. Most dying people say that the very thought of eating food is unpleasant. No pain or discomfort is associated with this feeling. After no food intake for 2 to 3 days, a chemical that suppresses the feeling of hunger accumulates in the blood. The body is shutting down and preparing to die and does not need as much energy from food. Although the feeling of hunger is usually absent in dying patients, the feeling of thirst remains. Thirst may be due to lack of water, or it may be a side effect of drugs used to provide comfort. Sips of water, juice, soda, ice chips, or lemon drops may be used to relieve thirst. A lack of fluids in the final days and weeks of life is not painful.

23. How can you reassure the family if the patient refuses to eat or drink?

It is difficult for family members to watch their loved one appear to "starve to death." Anorexia is troubling because food and drink are culturally considered nurturing and life-sustaining. Starvation in a healthy person is an awful process to watch. All dying patients will lose their appetite. The dying person who loses interest in eating is *not* starving; he or she is dying. This difference is important. A disease, such as cancer or Alzheimer's disease, may cause patients to lose their appetite, but it is the disease—not starvation—that leads to death.

24. What are the common causes of pruritus?

Pruritus, which can be among the most irritating symptoms that patients experience, may be caused by many factors. Pharmacologic agents used to treat other symptoms, such as opioids, can cause pruritus. Switching to a different opioid often relieves the discomfort. Other common causes for pruritus include jaundice and uremia.

25. How is pruritus treated?

There is no one outstanding intervention to control itching. For many patients, topical measures such as frequent baths with water at room temperature and a soap substitute or oatmeal powder can be very soothing. Other interventions include drying the skin by patting with a soft towel (no rubbing motion), applying cornstarch lightly to skin folds, and using nonalcoholic lotion after baths. Many medications are also used to control itching. Antihistamines such as diphenhydramine (Benadryl), hydroxyzine (Atarax), and loratidine (Claritin) are commonly prescribed but are frequently ineffective at nonsedating doses. Tricyclic antidepressants are sometimes effective but are frequently too toxic. Naloxone (Narcan), nalbuphine (Nubain), ondansetron hydrochloride (Zofran), and paroxetine hydrochloride (Paxil) also may have some positive effect.

26. Mr. F. is a 45-year-old man with metastatic head and neck cancer. He has a large tumor on his neck that is open, draining, and foul-smelling. He is embarrassed and has asked to have visitors limited because of the odor. What can be done to control the odor?

Odor can be highly distressing for patients and caregivers. Interventions such as frequent dressing changes and Domeboro soaks are effective in decreasing drainage and odor.

Another effective treatment is topical 0.75% metronidazole (Flagyl) gel. Other interventions include:

- Cleanse the wound with full-strength chlorhexidene (Hibiclens) for 3 minutes; then rinse.
- Administer an oral antifungal agent.
- Wash the wound with a douche powder (e.g., Massengil, 1 oz in a basin of water).
- Place a dryer fabric-softener sheet over the outside of the dressing.
- Use charcoal-filled dressings.
- Place a pan of charcoal briquettes under the bed.

27. Mrs. B., a 67-year-old woman with metastatic colon cancer, has been on the palliative care unit for 2 weeks. Yesterday she developed hiccups, which have been continuous and distressing. What can be done to relieve her distress?

The incidence of transient or chronic hiccups in terminal disease is unknown. Chronic hiccups are defined as hiccups that last 48 hours or longer or frequently recurring episodes. Complications related to chronic hiccups include fatigue, discomfort, weight loss, sleep deprivation, and depression. Various pharmacologic interventions have been reported; no one medication has been found to be most effective. Case reports support chlorpromazine hydrochloride (Thorazine), baclofen (Lioresal), metoclopramide (Reglan), haloperidol (Haldol), amitriptyline (Elavil), and carbamazepine (Tegretol). The variety of proposed treatments indicates the lack of effectiveness of any one therapy. Nonpharmacologic approaches include interventions that interrupt the vagal and/or phrenic nerve limbs of the reflex arc:

- Gargling
- Sipping ice water
- Swallowing dry bread
- Ingesting a teaspoon of granulated sugar
- Biting on a lemon
- Breath-holding
- Hyperventilation
- Breathing into a paper bag

28. When pain control results in unacceptable side effects at the end of life, what can be done?

When pain does not respond to traditional approaches, we are challenged clinically, emotionally, and ethically. When interventions no longer provide relief with tolerable side effects or the time frame required for relief is not tolerable, consideration of sedation is appropriate. Pharmacologic management of sedation at the end of life requires vigilant titration and monitoring. A policy and guidelines for the use of sedation (e.g., benzodiazepines or barbiturates) in this setting can provide support to health care providers. Consensus about sedation is essential among health care providers, patients, and family members.

29. What have family members suggested that nurses can do to help them when a loved one is dying?

Communication is perhaps the most critical component of palliative care. Family members have made clear that nurses can help them by following three critical guidelines:

- Facilitate communication between the dying patient and family members.
- Facilitate communication between the health care team and patients and family members.
- Create an environment conducive to communication.

30. What aspects of the plan of care are important to stop when death is imminent?

When the goal of care is comfort only, all aspects of the patient's care plan should be evaluated to ensure that each aspect adds to the patient's comfort:

- Diagnostic or laboratory tests should be done only if they will provide information that initiates an intervention adding to the patient's comfort. For example, finger sticks to determine blood sugar levels should be stopped when a patient is no longer eating.
- Radiologic tests providing information that will not be used to aid in the patient's comfort should be avoided.
- Implanted defibrillators should be deactivated.
- Routine measurements of vital signs, with the exception of temperature, may be stopped.
- Medications not used for symptom management may be discontinued.

31. Mr. P. is actively dying from lung cancer. His wife comes to the desk crying that Mr. P. is struggling to breathe. On entering the room you hear a coarse, rattling sound. Mr. P. appears to be struggling but is unresponsive to his surroundings. Should Mr. P. be suctioned? What is death rattle?

Death rattle is noisy breathing in terminally ill patients shortly before death as a result of uncleared upper airway or pulmonary secretions. Most likely the patient is unresponsive; family caregivers are usually more distressed than the patient. However, accumulated secretions may lead to dyspnea and restlessness in some patients. Prevention of the death rattle is one argument for not forcing hydration; excessive pulmonary secretions are less likely in dehydrated patients.

Whether to suction the secretions is determined by the level of comfort that the family and caregivers perceive in the dying patient. A family member who is distraught that the patient is suffering may be comforted by suctioning. However, suctioning also can cause trauma, bleeding, and shortness of breath. Turning and repositioning the patient to a lateral position to facilitate drainage of secretions may be helpful. Pulmonary secretions may be minimized by the use of intravenous (IV) atropine or atropine 1% eye drops given sublingually. Another option is glycopyrrolate, given PO, IV, or SQ. Hyoscine hydrobromide (scopolamine) transdermal patch is also effective at decreasing oropharyngeal secretions. One or two patches can be applied every 72 hours. Nursing judgment is critical in determining how the comfort of the patient is affected by proposed interventions. It is important to include family caregivers in the decision. Educating the family so that they can assist in decision making is critical.

32. The family tells you that the patient has died. What is expected from the nurse?

Family support is paramount. This moment will be replayed by family members many times over the next few months. Explain what you need to do. Assess the patient's condition to determine if he or she responds to verbal or tactile stimuli. Avoid overtly painful stimuli. Assess heart and lung function for absence of pulse and respiration. Look and listen for spontaneous respiration. Note the time. Advise the physician. Topics of tissue donation, autopsy, and body donation should be reviewed if not previously discussed.

Personal care should be provided for the body. The body should be bathed and dressed. Some family members may wish to assist the nurse. The body should be placed in proper alignment. The temperature in the room may be lowered if it is going to be more than a few hours until the body is moved.

33. Is it important for the nurse to contact family members in the days following the death of the patient?

Yes. Family members have many needs after the patient's death. Hearing from the nurse via telephone or written card is helpful and comforting. During contacts with family members, it is appropriate to restate enjoyable memories of the patient, what you found special in the patient, and what you will remember about the family unit. If appropriate, you may want to share information about grief support groups. Referral to a social worker may be appropriate at this time. Family members in hospice programs have the benefit of bereavement follow-up from the hospice agency.

Key Points

- Palliative care and "aggressive" disease management are not mutually exclusive paths.
- Setting patient-oriented goals early is essential to effective palliative care.
- Symptom management at the end of life can be complex. Know what resources are available in your setting to assist in symptom management.
- Good communication skills, on all levels, are essential in helping to establish and meet patient/family goals.

Internet Resources

American Academy of Hospice and Palliative Medicine:
    http://www.aahpm.org
American Alliance of Cancer Pain Initiatives:
    http://www.aacpi.org
American Pain Society:
    http://www.ampainsoc.org
Center to Advance Palliative Care (CAPC):
    http://www.capcmssm.org
Education for Physicians on End-of-Life Care (EPEC):
    http://www.epec.net
End-of-Life Physician Education Resource Center (EPERC):
    http://www.eperc.mcw.edu/
Growth House:
    http://www.growthhouse.org
Hospice and Palliative Nurses Association:
    http://www.hpna.org
Innovations in End-of-Life Care:
    http://www.edc.org/lastacts/
Last Acts:
    http://www.lastacts.org
Medical College of Wisconsin Palliative Medicine Program:
    http://www.mcw.edu/pallmed
National Hospice and Palliative Care Organization:
    http://www.nhpco.org
Oncology Nursing Society:
    http://www.ons.org

BIBLIOGRAPHY

Berry P, Griffie J: Planning for the actual death. In Ferrell R, Coyle N, editors: *Textbook of palliative nursing,* ed 2, New York, 2006, Oxford University Press.

Bruera E, Ripamonti C: Dyspnea in patients with advanced cancer. In Berger A, Portenoy R, Weissman DE, editors. *Principles and practice of supportive oncology,* 2002, Lippincott-Raven.

Centeno C, Sanz A, Bruera E: Delirium in advanced cancer patients. *Palliat Med* 18:184-194, 2004.

Glare P, Pereira G, Kristjanson LJ, et al: Systematic review of the efficacy of antiemetics in the treatment of nausea in patients with far-advanced cancer. *Support Care Cancer* 42: 432-440, 2004.

Griffie J, Muchka S, Nelson-Marten P, et al: Integrating palliative care into daily practice: A nursing perspective. *J Palliat Med* 2:65-73, 1998.

Griffie J, Nelsen-Marten P, Muchka S: Acknowledging the 'elephant': Communication in palliative care. *Am J Nurs* 104:48-58, 2004.

Jactoi A, Loprinzi C: Current management of cancer-associated anorexia and weight loss. *Oncology* 15:4,497-502. 2001.

Klinkenberg M, Willems DL, van der Wal G, et al: Symptom burden in the last week of life. *J Pain Symptom Manage* 27:5-13, 2004.

Luce J & Luce J: Management of dyspnea in patients with far-advanced lung disease. *JAMA,* 285:10,1331-1337, 2001.

Maluso-Bolton T: Terminal agitation. *J Hospice Palliat Nurs* 2(1):9-20, 2000.

Power D, Kelly S, Gilsenan J, et al: Suitable screening tests for cognitive impairment and depression in the terminally ill: A prospective prevalence study. *Palliat Med* 7:213-218, 1993.

Wilders H, Menten J: Death rattle: Prevalence, prevention and treatment. *J Pain Symptom Manage* 23:310-317, 2002.

Weissman DE, Ambuel B: *Improving end-of-life care: A resource guide for physician education,* ed 3, Milwaukee, 1999, Medical College of Wisconsin.

Chapter 44

Sexuality

Patricia W. Nishimoto

1. Define sexual health.

Over 30 years ago, the WHO (World Health Organization) declared that "sexual health is the integration of the somatic, emotional, intellectual and social aspects of sexual being in ways that are positively enriching and that enhance personality, communication, and love." In 2003, WHO defined sexual health as "not merely the absence of disease, dysfunction or infirmity. It is experienced and expressed in thoughts, fantasies, desires, beliefs, attitudes, values, behaviors, practices, roles and relationships." Sexuality is much more than sexual intercourse; it includes how persons feel about themselves as a man or woman and all aspects of intimacy from a tender touch to cuddling during late night talks, and choosing what clothes to wear or how to sit.

2. Why is there an Oncology Nursing Society standard about sexuality?

The inclusion of sexuality as a part of excellent care is recognized by the American Nurses' Association (ANA), the World Health Organization (WHO), and the Oncology Nursing Society (ONS). Standards serve as guides of nursing process to facilitate quality care. The ONS sexuality standard supports the WHO Doctrine by encouraging nurses to identify alterations in a patient's sexuality and to help that person maintain their sexual identity.

3. How does the oncology nurse meet the ONS standard?

The oncology nurse must recognize that a patient's sexual health is influenced by sexual function before diagnosis, past sexual experiences, other illnesses, medications, stage of disease, religious and cultural background, emotional and psychological status, belief about the cause of the cancer, and relationships with others. Recognition and knowledge of how these factors can affect sexuality are the keys to effective intervention.

4. How can I gain confidence in discussing sexuality?

Incorporating sexuality in your nursing care requires skills in sensitive listening and the ability to provide reassurance and understandable explanations, skills that are used in daily clinical practice. Confidence in knowing what to ask or say can be obtained by attending conferences, reading the literature, role playing, or working with an advanced practice nurse or expert mentor. Having readily available handouts from the American Cancer Society on sexuality and a listing of local resources for the patients to contact if further questions arise are also very useful. Other suggestions to increase your skills in discussing sexuality include:
- Believe that helping patients deal with changes in sexuality is an integral part of holistic nursing care.
- Obtain a basic knowledge of sexuality and how cancer and its treatments affect sexual functioning.
- Be aware of your own attitudes toward sexuality. Be careful not to impose your own beliefs.

- Have an open, accepting attitude and respect the patient's beliefs and practices.
- Avoid making assumptions and understand that sexuality is very personal and defined by each person in a unique manner.
- Be proactive in opening the discussion.

5. Why do some nurses hesitate to include sexuality counseling?

Nurses are hesitant to address sexuality for multiple and complex reasons, such as lack of time, belief that they are not qualified or that sexual counseling is someone else's job, personal discomfort, cultural backgrounds, personal values and attitudes, fear about legal liability, the absence of role models, and misconceptions about sexuality. Some misconceptions include: "cancer ends sexuality," the "focus needs to be on life-or-death issues," or the patient is not interested in sex because of their older age. Hesitation can be a natural response to not wanting to "upset," offend, or distress a frightened patient who is already dealing with multiple issues at once. Many health care professionals believe that sexual issues are not considered by patients until 'later;' however, Thewes et al. (2005) found that the first concern of women with breast cancer was how their fertility and sexuality might be affected. Nurses need to understand that their failure or hesitation to include sexuality counseling may add to the patients' anxieties and fears about future sexual activity. Nurses who are uncomfortable about discussing sexual issues should make appropriate referrals or provide written information about available resources.

6. How can I bring up the topic of sexuality in a professional, non-offensive manner?

Demonstrate your comfort with the topic and show patients that you will take the time to discuss sexuality with them. Using the BETTER mnemonic as part of nursing assessment can begin the conversation.

BETTER model to assess sexuality

"B"	Bring up the topic/initiate conversation.
"E"	Explain that sexuality is a part of life and can contribute to quality of life.
"T"	Tell the patient about resources available to them.
"T"	Timing—inform patients that you are available when they are ready to talk about sexual concerns.
"E"	Educate the patient about possible ways the diagnosis or treatment can affect sexual functioning.
"R"	Record in your nursing note that you broached the subject with the patient.

Mick J, Hughes H, Cohen MZ: Using the BETTER model to assess sexuality. *Clin J Oncol Nurs* 8(1):84-86, 2004.

---

7. What are some ways that clinics or hospitals can facilitate discussion of sexuality?

- Provide questionnaires to patients asking about symptoms that include sexuality.
- Include a space on electronic charts or assessment forms to enter information about sexuality that can create the expectation that this issue should be addressed by nurses.
- Ensure the availability of brochures and books about sexuality in waiting rooms or the patient library.
- List websites or other resources about sexuality in patient handouts.

8. What can be done if the patient is offended when sexuality is discussed?

If a nurse perceives that a comment about sexuality has offended the patient, he or she should express regret or extend an apology and reassure the patient that no offense was intended. If a degree of rapport and trust have been established before the conversation, the patient will usually recognize the sincerity of the nurse to provide information about a private and sensitive topic.

Because of cultural or religious beliefs, some patients may be uncomfortable about a direct approach about sexuality issues. The nurse can overcome initial patient embarrassment and possible offense by reassuring the patient that their unspoken fears and concerns regarding sexuality are not uncommon. Patients should be asked whether something does not fit with their religious or cultural beliefs.

9. What are the 3 L's and 1 P of sexual counseling?

The **3 L's and 1 P** are language, labeling, listening, and privacy.

Some patients may use **language** that is 'raw or earthy,' whereas others may use euphemisms or oblique sexual references. For example, a patient may ask what to do for the pain when "we do it." The problems of language and miscommunications are not one-sided. The nurse who goes into a long monologue about "strategies to prevent dyspareunia" may get a polite nod followed by the question, "But what do I do so it doesn't hurt?" Nurses need to use language that is understood by the patient and not hide behind professional jargon.

Labeling means that neither nurses nor patients should label behavior with words such as "undersexed" or "impotent."

Listening is a basic nursing skill, but it may be uncomfortable at first when patients discuss intimate topics. Role playing before working with patients can help increase the comfort level.

Privacy is having the common sense to not ask in the busy treatment room, "Hey, Mrs. S, did the lubricant help you and your husband?"

10. What may help the patient to feel more comfortable expressing sexual concerns?

- Be sincere and respectful when you ask about sexual concerns. Do not "put them down" for using slang words.
- Create a safe environment to ensure privacy. Take time to hear their concerns.
- Check your own comfort level.
- "Normalize" the discussion. Explain to patients that sexuality is part of your nursing assessment and care planning for all patients.

11. What questions about sex are most commonly asked by patients diagnosed with cancer?

- Will my partner 'catch' cancer from me?
- Will my partner leave me because I have cancer?
- Will my partner think my (ostomy, mastectomy, surgical scar) is disgusting and be 'turned off'?
- Is _____ normal?
- Will my partner still love me?
- Will anyone ever want to date me?
- Will I still be able to have sex?
- Will I ever get turned on again?
- If I am too embarrassed to ask my health care team, is there somewhere I can go to get the answers?

12. **How does the nurse intervene when the patient asks questions about sexuality?**

The PLISSIT (permission, limited information, specific suggestions, and intensive therapy) model, offers four intervention levels of sexual counseling based on the experience and expertise of the nurse. If the first level of intervention is not effective in helping the patient, the nurse then either goes to the next level if she/he has the expertise or makes a referral.

- **Permission:** The nurse gives permission for and facilitates the expression of sexual concerns or questions. An example is when a 15-year-old girl asks if French kissing caused her leukemia because her first symptom was bleeding of the gums. The nurse gives permission by sitting down to talk with the young teen about her concerns and "not blowing her off" with a curt, "Of course not." Instead the nurse asks, "What made you think it could be caused by French kissing?"
- **Limited information**: The nurse provides facts about the expressed concern or question. For example, when a 36-year-old mother with three children comments that she does not "get turned on anymore," the nurse first needs to ensure that she understands what the woman means by her comment. If it means she has low libido, the nurse can use the first level of intervention, **permission**, to reinforce that it is "normal" for women on chemotherapy to experience decreased libido. If the patient wants more information, then it may be helpful to share information about how side effects of chemotherapy, such as fatigue, stomatitis, and decreased vaginal lubrication contribute to dyspareunia that affects libido. Often, the **limited information** level of intervention will relieve the patient's concerns. Other patients may want to know what to do about the decreased libido, so the nurse will either intervene at the next level of **specific suggestions** or make an appropriate referral. The **limited information** level requires the nurse to have knowledge of how cancer and its treatments affect sexual functioning.
- **Specific suggestions:** The nurse helps the person deal with changes in sexuality. For the woman who is experiencing a decrease in vaginal lubrication due to chemotherapy, the nurse would first assess the woman's cultural/religious beliefs and current sexual practice, then provide suggestions concordant with the woman's beliefs. At this level of intervention, the nurse needs a solid knowledge of sexual behaviors and possible treatments for symptoms or concerns.
- **Intensive therapy:** The nurse provides in-depth counseling requiring more than four sessions and usually involves referral to a health care provider who specializes in sexual counseling. For example, intensive therapy is needed for the 65-year-old woman with ovarian cancer who begins to sob during a vaginal examination as she recalls childhood molestation. At this level, formal advance practice training and clinical work experience are required.

13. **What are some examples of alterations in sexuality caused by cancer treatments?**

All cancer treatments may cause fatigue that interferes with libido and stamina to engage in sexual activities. Other examples are listed below:

Alterations in sexuality caused by cancer treatments

Treatment	Alterations in sexuality
Chemotherapy	Alopecia: altered body image Fatigue: decreased libido

Continued

Alterations in sexuality caused by cancer treatments—cont'd

Treatment	Alterations in sexuality
	Cardiac/pulmonary toxicity: may affect ability to engage in strenuous sexual activity
	Thrombocytopenia: more easily bruised during sexual activities
	Neutropenia: risk of vaginal infections may increase, especially if vaginal lubrication is decreased; anal stimulation may be too risky because of potential for infection.
	Stomatitis: may make kissing or oral sex painful
	Ototoxicity: hearing the intimate whispers of a significant other may become more difficult and make aural sexual arousal more difficult
	Changes in sense of smell: body smells that used to have an aphrodisiac effect may become too strong or unpleasant; smell of food may cause nausea when on a date at a restaurant.
	Neuropathy: loss of sensation may decrease enjoyment of toe and finger sexual play; if severe, can affect gait and steadiness which would prevent sexual play while standing
	Changes in weight: altered body image (weight change of ten pounds may decrease effectiveness of diaphragms used for birth control)
	Premature menopause in female: vaginal dryness and hot flashes
Radiation to pelvis or genital areas	Delay in puberty, gonadal ablation, or complications of fistula, rectal or ureteral stricture, can affect sexual functioning.
	Changes related to therapy (e.g., vaginal lubrication, erectile dysfunction) may develop slowly over 2-3 years following completion of therapy.
	Females with cervical cancer: vaginal stenosis, shortening of vaginal vault, alopecia in radiation field, scar tissue development, skin changes in sensitivity or texture, nerve damage, and urethral irritation causing pain with intercourse
	Males: erectile dysfunction from vascular scarring; retrograde ejaculation
Surgery	Altered body image related to ostomies and loss of body part, (e.g., mastectomy, limb amputation)
	Lymphedema may affect body image, range of motion during sexual play, and may compress nerves resulting in decreased tactile sensations and pleasure.
	Changes are affected by type of surgical resection, injury to nerves, and extent of dissection.
	Women may experience dyspareunia from nerve damage and decreased vaginal lubrication from decreased blood flow.
	Women undergoing bladder surgery may have changes in vaginal diameter that affect comfort of usual sexual position.
	Hysterectomies may cause shortening of vaginal canal, and vaginal sensation may be reduced from pelvic nerve damage.
	Men may experience erectile dysfunction from nerve damage.
	Retrograde ejaculation (discharge of sperm into the bladder instead of penis) may result from retroperitoneal or pelvic surgery that affects the bladder neck.
	Men who are visually oriented may not enjoy sex as much when they cannot observe the ejaculation; their partner may miss the sensation of ejaculate during orgasm.

14. How does cancer affect phases of the sexual response cycle?

The physiological and psychological effects of cancer as well as the treatments may cause symptoms (e.g., fatigue, pain, and nausea) that affect all phases of the sexual response cycle (**libido, arousal, plateau, orgasm,** and **resolution**). Physiological effects can be caused by changes in endocrine, neurotransmitter, or central nervous systems. Additionally, the sexual response cycle is affected by other factors unrelated to cancer, such as past experiences and cultural and religious backgrounds.

Phases of the sexual response cycle in response to cancer treatments

Sexual response phase	Effect of cancer or treatments
Libido: desire or interest in sex	Stress decreases androgen, resulting in decreased desire.
Arousal or excitement	Treatments may interfere with muscle tension or vasocongestion which facilitates erection and lubrication. Damage to the periprostatic plexus from a radical retropubic prostatectomy may prevent erection. Chemotherapy may affect vaginal lubrication. After mastectomies, patients may experience the phantom sensation of nipple erection during arousal.
Plateau: continued vasocongestion and myotonia; increased pulse and/or blood pressure	Due to hypervigilance or being more attentive to bodily changes, patients may perceive normal physiological changes as "something wrong" and stop sexual activity due to fear. For example, a woman may misinterpret normal changes in the color of her labia during plateau as being abnormal.
Orgasm: sense of warmth in the pelvis and muscle contractions (3-15 seconds), increased respirations (up to 40/minute depending on age)	Use of tranquilizers may diminish the strength of pelvic muscle contractions. Surgical removal of a uterus may damage the pudendal or pelvic nerve and affect orgasm. The loss of uterine contractions during orgasm may negatively affect this phase. Some women may experience phantom uterine contractions during orgasm. (**Note:** Orgasm releases endorphins that may provide pain relief in some individuals for up to 6 hours).
Resolution (refractory period): return of body and vital signs to preexcitement level	Resolution may last longer because of fatigue from the disease or the treatments. After an orchiectomy, some men experience scrotal and groin discomfort during resolution.

15. In addition to chemotherapy, what are the most common drugs that cause sexual dysfunction? Describe their effects.

Common drugs causing sexual dysfunction

Drug	Affect on sexual function
Alcohol	Decreases libido Decreased vaginal lubrication and erection Decreased inhibitions may interfere with use of safer sex and thus increase risk for infection
Antiadrenergics	Decreases libido, vaginal lubrication, and erection May cause retrograde ejaculation
Anticholinergics	Affect arousal (decrease erection or vaginal lubrication)
Antidepressants	May temporarily decrease erection or vaginal lubrication
Antihypertensives	Affect arousal (decrease erection or vaginal lubrication)
Aromatase inhibitors and tamoxifen	May cause vaginal dryness or soreness, decreased desire and orgasmic response, hot flashes
Endocrine drugs	Hot flashes, dyspareunia due to decreased vaginal lubrication, and mood swings
Hormones	May decrease serum testosterone, which can affect sexual desire Secondary sex changes (deepening of voice, increased facial hair) may affect body image
Opioids	Less pain increases enjoyment of sex Side effect of constipation may interfere with sexual activity Long-term opioids may retard ejaculation
Recreational drugs (e.g., cocaine, marijuana)	May cause euphoria and increase self-confidence May increase tactile pleasure or may block sexual arousal and pleasure May cause extended painful erections or painful ejaculations
Tranquilizers	May decrease anxiety and improve sexual functioning Retarded ejaculation Large dose may decrease erection and vaginal lubrication Relaxation of pelvic muscles may affect orgasm (i.e., loss of muscle tension decreases pleasure of orgasm)

16. What treatments are available for women who complain of lack of desire after treatment for cancer?

Counseling is the current therapy of choice. Bibliotherapy (use of books or literature) may also be suggested; for example, the American Cancer Society pamphlet about sexuality has an excellent section about the use of the *Desire Diary*, which help a woman examine ways that she may be "turning off her libido" without realizing it. Use of erotica (nonpornographic books or movies) may also be helpful.

Many pharmacologic interventions (testosterone, bromocriptine, antidepressants) are being investigated for increasing female libido; however, results are mixed and none are considered standard of care. Transdermal testosterone patches may benefit women after oophorectomy in many phases of the sexual response cycle (i.e., increased fantasies, increased sexual activity, and higher scores of satisfaction with orgasm).

17. **How do you counsel a man who experiences painful intercourse?**

First, assess the type of pain and when it occurs. Pain on the penile shaft during intercourse is often due to skin tears that may be caused by steroids, which increase skin fragility, or be related to decreased lubrication in a partner. Lubricated condoms can protect the skin, act as a barrier to decrease possible infection, provide lubrication and protect the partner from excreted chemotherapy in body fluids the first several days after treatment. Pain with ejaculation related to postoperative orchiectomy resolves after a few months and may be relieved by lying in a warm bath.

18. **How do you counsel a woman who experiences painful intercourse?**

This is a more common occurrence in women than in men. Assess the type of pain and when it occurs. Vaginal pain may be due to decreased lubrication, stenosis following radiation therapy, shortening of the vagina from surgery, or increased sensitivity to vaginal barrel distention due to surgery or a postoperative vaginal infection. Numbness in the mons may occur because nerves were severed during surgery; it can take up to 12 months for sensation to return. Suggestions for decreasing pain include use of lubricants, use of dilators to stretch the vagina, or changes in positions during sexual activity.

19. **What types of lubricant can be used?**

There are many choices available in local drug stores, so women need not worry they will have to "mail order them or have to go to a sex shop" to buy them. Urge women to buy small samples, since each woman will find different brands better than others, and to buy nonperfumed brands that are less irritating. Suggested brands include Astroglide (Biofilm, Vista, CA) and Aqualube (Mayer Laboratories, Oakland, CA). Lubricants that help to replenish vaginal moisture but are not intended for use during coitus include Replens (Warner Wellcome, Morris Plains, NJ), Gyne-Moistrin (Health Care Products, Memphis, TN), and Lubrin (Kenwood Laboratories, Fairfield, NJ).

If using condoms, the lubricant should be water soluble. If condoms or diaphragms are not being used, a light vegetable oil placed in a small squeeze bottle can be used for lubrication. Vegetable oils are inexpensive, easily obtained, not embarrassing to buy, edible, and light enough that even with decreased vaginal lubrication, they can be flushed out and do not cause infection.

Avoid suggesting sterile lubricants that tend to 'dry' relatively quickly and result in tiny 'balls' rolling up and down in a dry vagina. Saliva and whipped cream can 'work in a pinch,' but they too dry quickly; plus the whipped cream can leave a "mess."

20. **Which positions are more comfortable?**

Patients will need to experiment with what works best for them. Guide them to books and pamphlets that demonstrate different positions and how pillows can be used for support, particularly for patients who have lost a limb due to cancer. Patients who experienced muscle tension during orgasm in their limbs may experience phantom sensations in the amputated limb. If the woman has a shortened vagina due to surgery, discuss positions where the partner's penis does not hit the posterior vaginal wall. These include having her sit or lie on top to feel more control and pleasure.

21. **What techniques help to conserve energy during sex?**

More consideration needs to be given to planning times when patients know they will be more rested and have decreased pain. To enhance comfort during sex, patients should take pain medication 30 to 45 minutes before having sex, take a warm bath to loosen tight muscles, use pillows for support, or try new sexual activities that are less tiring. Hot tubs may provide a good place for sexual play and the water supports the patient while trying different positions. However, they should be cautioned about safety issues, such as the risk of dehydration if they remain in the tub for a lengthy amount of time, risk of infection if they have neutropenia or if they have an unprotected venous access device or open wounds. Phone sex and the use of fantasy are additional ways of enjoying sex and conserving energy.

There are also alternative forms of sexual stimulation, but before discussing these, make sure that the patient is interested in exploring other options to intercourse. When making suggestions, consider how each activity may affect patients with neutropenia or thrombocytopenia.

22. How do changes in fertility affect sexual well-being?

The meaning of fertility can affect a person's perception of sexual well-being in either a positive, negative, or neutral manner. For some, not having to worry about a possible pregnancy may improve their sexual functioning. Assumptions that infertility will "always" negatively affect a person or that people over the age of 50 or who have a same sex partner will not be affected by infertility will result in a lost opportunity for the nurse to openly counsel the patient.

Multiple ethnic cultures link fertility and sexuality. For example, Puerto Ricans may believe that if a woman is unable to "give a man a child" that it is permissible to have a child with another woman. It may be considered permissible to divorce an infertile spouse to marry a woman who is fertile.

23. What chemotherapy drugs impair fertility?

Factors that affect the risk of infertility include type and dose of chemotherapy, duration of therapy, use of combination therapy, prediagnosis fertility level, and age of the patient (50% of women over the age of 35 years who receive a single alkylating agent experience permanent infertility). Alkylating agents pose the highest risk to fertility, which is also impaired by vinca alkaloids, antimetabolites, platinum agents, and others, such as procarbazine. Hormone therapy and treatment with taxanes carry the lowest risks to fertility. Drugs that affect both testicular and ovarian function include cyclophosphamide, busulfan, and nitrogen mustard. Chlorambucil, procarbazine, and nitrosoureas affect men, whereas L-phenylalanine affects women. Drugs with probable risk to testicular epithelium but unknown risk to ovaries include doxorubicin, vinblastine, cytosine arabinoside, and cisplatin. Drugs with unlikely risk to fertility for men or women include methotrexate, 5-fluorouracil, and 6-mercaptopurine. Vincristine is unlikely to affect male fertility.

For a premenopausal 40-year-old woman, combination therapy of cyclophosphamide, methotrexate, and fluorouracil can cause ovarian failure in up to 78% of women, compared to 38% with combination doxorubicin and cyclophosphamide. For men, platinum can cause prolonged azoospermia. Ablative therapy for stem cell transplantation can cause infertility risk in up to 100% of women and men; minitransplants are associated with less risk to fertility.

24. What radiation therapy factors affect fertility?

Radiation field, dose, size, fractionation schedule, location of tumor, prediagnosis fertility, and age of patient may affect risk of infertility from therapy. Radiation therapy to affected reproductive areas poses a greater risk of infertility than chemotherapy. A dose of 400 cGy can cause permanent infertility for men; lower doses can cause a temporary decrease in sperm count.

Remember that infertility may reverse as late as 4 years after completion of therapy for men. For women over the age of 40 years, doses as low as 40 cGy can cause permanent infertility. To decrease or prevent infertility related to radiation therapy, ovarian transposition (oophoropexy), lead shielding of gonads, and modifications of the fractionation schedule of radiation therapy may be considered.

25. What methods are being investigated to help prevent or decrease infertility related to cancer treatments?

Many experimental methods are not used or considered because they would cause delay in potentially life-saving therapy. Experimental therapies for women include gonadotropin-releasing hormone agonist, birth control pills, radical trachelectomy, loop electrosurgical excision procedure, ovum banking, and cryopreservation of ovarian cortical strips. If a man has retrograde ejaculation due to therapy, alpha-sympathomimetic drugs, such as imipramine and ephedrine, may improve or reverse retrograde ejaculation. Methods to retrieve sperm include transrectal electroejaculation, spinning down a urine specimen after ejaculation, and testis sperm extraction.

26. How soon after chemotherapy is pregnancy "safe"?

There is no consensus on this issue other than prevention of pregnancy during active therapy (see Chapter 54). For men, often an arbitrary period of 6 months is used, since that is the time it takes to complete the cycle from stem cell to development of mature sperm.

27. What is sperm banking? What instructions should be provided to patients?

Sperm banking is a strategy for males to cryopreserve sperm if they are receiving treatments that cause infertility. Preferably, banking is done before the initiation of therapy. If treatment needs to be started before sperm banking can be done, it is usually considered safe to bank sperm after chemotherapy is given *if* it is done within the first 10 to 14 days of the first cycle of chemotherapy. Many sperm banks recommend that donations be done at least 2 days after the last ejaculation but less than 10 days, that several donations be done to increase probability of viable and adequate number of sperm, and that tests for sexually transmitted diseases be done prior to banking.

Men need to be informed of the cost of collection and storage and the potential risk if banking causes a delay in treatment. Men with testicular cancer, Hodgkin lymphoma, or non-Hodgkin lymphoma have a low sperm count before diagnosis; however, they should still consider sperm banking because pregnancy is possible with in vitro fertilization or intracytoplasmic sperm injection. Using banked sperm does not increase the risk of congenital deformities.

28. How successful is sperm banking?

To put it in perspective for the patient, let him know that the likelihood of pregnancy from an adequately stored semen specimen is equivalent to the probability of conception from sexual intercourse. Usually less than 35% of men with cancer who bank their sperm use their specimens. Success depends on age of female partner, female fertility issues, and semen quality.

29. What other issues are relevant to sperm banking?

There are complex legal issues, such as spousal rights, involving cryopreserved sperm. Ensure that the patient is aware of possible legal ramifications before banking. If there are cultural or religious barriers to masturbation to obtain the sperm specimen, several options can be considered. If he has a partner, then a special condom without lubrication can be used to collect sperm. If there is no partner, then rectal electroejaculation can be done under anesthesia but not if the male has thrombocytopenia or leukopenia. Recent data contradict the belief that there is less risk of infertility to young boys, so parents need to discuss this issue with the oncologist before treatment. The collection of ejaculate may be painful if done soon after surgery.

30. How does a laryngectomy affect sexuality?

It is not just the change in body image but the inability to whisper softly into the ear of a partner that can dramatically affect a person's usual sexual behavior. Turning the head to kiss may no longer be possible because of the decreased range of motion of the shoulder or neck, or because this initiates coughing, and the partner cannot stand the feeling of air and sputum on their neck. The risk of getting pubic hair in the stoma during oral sex or of getting water into the stoma while having sex in the shower or hot tub may change usual sexual patterns. Enjoyment of orgasm may be diminished because it is no longer possible to hold their breath at time of orgasm.

31. What are some practical suggestions to help a person with an ostomy who is concerned about sex?

Encourage them to tell you their biggest worry of what might happen. Reassure them that many people have concerns about the appliance and how it will affect sexual activity. Allowing them to verbalize their fears, reassuring them, and then offering them suggestions are the first three levels of intervention of the PLISSIT model.

Suggestions include wearing crotchless underwear or a cummerbund to hold the appliance close to the body to conceal it; using an attractive cover over the appliance so it does not 'stick' to the skin; emptying it so there is less chance of the weight of a full appliance pulling it off the body; making sure there is a tight seal or picture framing the appliance with tape to ensure it does not fall off or emit odors; using aftershave, cologne, or appliance deodorant to increase confidence of no odor; avoiding 'gassy' or 'smelly' foods to decrease odor; and placing a towel or lining under the sheet to absorb possible spillage. Role play with the patient about what to say or do if the appliance should fall off or leak during sexual activity.

32. How does the nurse address sexual concerns of patients with same-sex partners?

Patients with same-sex partners should be treated in the same nonjudgmental manner you use with all patients. They experience the same physiologic changes from cancer and therapy, but may be even more hesitant to ask questions related to the heterosexual bias unconsciously portrayed to patients in pictures (male and female partners on covers of books), pamphlets (references to married couples), and assessment questionnaires. You can combat this bias at the beginning of your nursing assessment by asking the patient: Do you have a partner? Is your partner male or female, or do you have both? This opens up the conversation and makes this person no longer feel invisible to staff. Nurses with strong feelings about same-sex partners should make an appropriate referral.

33. What specific issues may arise with same-sex partners?

If sex toys are used, advise the patient to avoid sharing the toy or to wash the toy carefully with soap and water to decrease the risk of infection. If the patient enjoys anal stimulation (heterosexual as well as homosexual patients may enjoy this), caution the patient about how easily rectal tissue can be torn or infected. Patients should be advised to refrain from anal stimulation during therapy. However, if the patient chooses to continue, offer advice about risk-reduction strategies, such as using a liberal amount of lubricant and keeping fingernails very short.

34. **When patients are ready to resume sexual activity, what things are helpful for them to consider?**
   - Sexual behavior will not cause recurrence.
   - Expect the unexpected. Be ready to laugh when that happens. Sex does not have to be 'serious business' or a 'marathon.' It is okay to stop and rest when tired.
   - Sex should not cause pain or discomfort. If it does, do not hesitate to talk with the nurse or physician about this. Fear of pain can cause sexual dysfunction.
   - Performance anxiety can occur if the patient is hypervigilant about erection or vaginal lubrication.
   - Skin is the largest sexual organ and the brain is the most important sexual organ. Use them and the possibilities for sexual activity are limitless.
   - A diagnosis of cancer or its treatments do not dictate what a patient can or cannot do. Use creativity and a sense of play to explore new ways of pleasuring.

35. **What treatment options are available for erectile dysfunction?**
   - Counseling
   - Pelvic floor exercises
   - Intracavernous injections: papaverine, prostaglandin E, phentolamine
   - Oral medications (e.g., sildenafil)
   - Intraurethral delivery of medication
   - External vacuum constriction devices
   - Penile arterial reconstruction
   - Penile prostheses: malleable rods, hinged, inflatable

36. **What should men know about taking sildenafil citrate (Viagra) or other "pills to fix" erectile dysfunction?**
   - Consult with a health care provider about taking any medications. Because of interactions with other medications, it is not safe to "borrow" a pill from a friend or to make purchases over the internet.
   - Do not take sildenafil while taking nitrates or if allergic to the drug.
   - Precautions of other medical conditions: cardiac problems, stroke, hypotension or hypertension, retinitis pigmentosa, kidney disease, liver disease, predisposition to priapism from sickle cell anemia, multiple myeloma, leukemia, Peyronie's disease, active peptic ulcer, or bleeding disorders.
   - Do not use sildenafil with other methods of having an erection, such as intracavernous injections.
   - Sildenafil citrate works after a person becomes sexually excited; its does *not* cause engorgement if the person is not sexually excited.
   - Possible side effects: an erection lasting longer than 4 hours (because of the possibility of permanent damage, immediate medical attention is needed), headache, facial flushing, upset stomach, stuffy nose, diarrhea, temporary changes in color vision, light sensitivity, or blurred vision.

 Key Points

- Sexuality is much more than intercourse; it includes how a person feels about being a man or woman and all aspects of intimacy.
- The ONS sexuality standard encourages nurses to identify alterations in a patient's sexuality and to help that person maintain their sexual identity.

Continued

Key Points—cont'd

- The nurse's failure or hesitation to include sexuality counseling may add to the patient's anxieties and fears about future sexual activity.
- All phases of the sexual response cycle (**libido, arousal, plateau, orgasm,** and **resolution**) are affected by the physiologic and psychologic effects of cancer, its treatment, or both.
- The PLISSIT (permission, limited information, specific suggestions, and intensive therapy) model offers four intervention levels of sexual counseling based on the experience and expertise of the nurse.

Internet Resources

Fertile Hope, designed for people diagnosed with cancer with questions about fertility:
  http://www.fertilehope.org
National Breast Cancer Centre (Australia), Clinical practice guidelines for the management and support of younger women with breast cancer:
  http://www.nhmrc.gov.au/publications/synopses/cp101syn.htm
Breast Cancer, fertility, pregnancy, adoption and menopause issues addressed:
  http://www.breastcancer.org/fertility_pregnancy_adoption.html
Lavender Trust (United Kingdom), young women with breast cancer and fertility issues:
  http://breastcancercare.org.uk/content.php?page_id=70.
Susan G. Komen Breast Cancer Foundation, Fertility and Cancer research project:
  http://www.fertilityandcancerproject.org/
Gay and Lesbian Ostomates:
  http://www.glo-uoa.org/contact.htm
Pregnant with Cancer Network (newsletter):
  http://www.pregnantwithcancer.org
Sex, etc., State University of New Jersey - Rutgers (website for teens to answer questions about sex):
  http://sexetc.org

Bibliography

Annon J: The PLISSIT model: A proposed conceptual scheme for behavioral treatment of sexual problems, *J Sex Education,* 1976.

Barton D, Wilwerding MB, Carpenter L, et al: Libido as part of sexuality in female cancer patients. *Oncol Nurs Forum* 31:599-607, 2004.

Bakewell RT & Volker DL: Sexual dysfunction related to the treatment of young women with breast cancer. *Clin J Oncol Nurs* 9(6):697-702, 2005.

Brydoy M, Fossa SD, Klepp O, et al: Paternity following treatment for testicular cancer. *J Natl Cancer Inst* 97:1580-1588, 2005.

Dixon, KD, Dixon PN: The PLISSIT Model: Care and management of patients' psychosexual needs following radical surgery. *Lippincott's Case Management,* 11, 101-106, 2006.

Frumovitz M, Sun CC, Schover LR, et al: Quality of life and sexual functioning in cervical cancer survivors. *J Clin Oncol* 23:7428-7436, 2005.

Katz A: The sounds of silence: Sexuality information for cancer patients. *J Clin Oncol* 23:238-241, 2005.

Marijnen CA, van de Velde CJ, Putter H, et al: Impact of short-term preoperative radiotherapy on health-related quality of life and sexual functioning in primary rectal cancer: Report of a multicenter randomized trial. *J Clin Oncol* 23:1847-1858, 2005.

Mick J, Hughes H, Cohen MZ: Using the BETTER model to assess sexuality. *Clin J Oncol Nurs* 8:84-86, 2004.

Oktay K: Current approaches to preservation of fertility in patients with cancer. ASCO 2006 Educational Book: 42nd Annual Meeting:309-312, 2006.

Plante M, Roy M: Fertility-preserving options for cervical cancer. *Oncology* 20:479-490, 2006.

Reynolds KE, Magnan MA: Nursing attitudes and beliefs toward human sexuality: Collaborative research promoting evidence-based practice. *Clin Nurse Spec* 19:255-259, 2005.

Schover LR: Sexuality and fertility after cancer. *Hematology* 1:523-526, 2005.

Simon B, Lee SJ, Partridge AH, et al: Preserving fertility after cancer. *CA Cancer J Clin* 55:211-228, 2005.

Thewes B, Meiser B, Taylor A, et al: Fertility- and menopause-related information needs of younger women with a diagnosis of early breast cancer. *J Clin Oncol* 23:5155-5165, 2005.

Sleep-Wake Disturbances

Ellyn Matthews

1. Are sleep-wake disturbances a problem for persons with cancer?

Sleep-wake disturbances, alone or as part of symptom clusters, occur twice as frequently in persons with cancer compared with the general population. Prevalence rates for sleep-wake disturbances range from 30% to 88% across oncology populations and settings. The wide range in prevalence is likely due to differences in measurement and definition of sleep disturbance. Impairment of sleep-wake patterns occurs almost nightly, and is described as moderate to severe in the cancer population. Persons with cancer report significant sleep-wake disruptions despite increased time resting and sleeping, suggesting the problem may be sleep quality rather than quantity.

2. What physiologic mechanisms are responsible for sleep-wake disturbance?

The normal sleep-wake cycle is a highly regulated and complex process controlled by internal and external factors. Three major processes contribute to sleep regulation:
1. A homeostatic process that is evident from the increase in sleep propensity (sleep drive)
2. A circadian process that is controlled by an internal pacemaker independent of prior sleep and waking
3. An ultradian process that is responsible for the alternation of non-rapid eye movement (NREM) and rapid eye movement (REM) sleep within the sleep episode

Two main types of sleep include REM (paradoxical, dream) sleep and NREM (quiet) sleep. NREM sleep accounts for 75% to 80% of average sleep and consists of four stages: stage 1, transitional; stage 2, light sleep; stages 3 and 4, deep and slow wave sleep. The percentages of REM and NREM sleep differ at various ages. In adults, the cycles of REM and NREM sleep occur 4 to 6 times during the average 7.5 to 8 hours of a main sleep period. Many factors influence the timing and duration of sleep, including the environment, nutrition and metabolism, elimination patterns, exercise, lifestyle and habits, illness, hospitalization, sleep need, sleep architecture, or the balance between NREM and REM.

3. How is sleep measured?

- The gold standard for sleep research is polysomnography, the simultaneous recording of multiple physiologic indicators, usually done overnight in a sleep laboratory.
- Wrist actigraphy is a valid, objective, relatively inexpensive measure of motion, which allows continuous recording of sleep-wake activity in the home.
- Subjective measurements include daily sleep diaries, sleep questionnaires, visual analog scales, and interviews.

4. How are sleep-wake disturbances characterized in the context of cancer?

Sleep-wake disturbances in persons with cancer are usually insomnia or hypersomnia. According to the International Classification of Sleep Disorders (ICSD-2), **insomnias** are disorders that produce difficulty with sleep initiation, duration, consolidation, or quality, despite sufficient time and opportunity for sleep. Insomnia complaints include difficulty falling asleep and/or maintaining sleep, extended periods of nocturnal wakefulness, and insufficient amounts of quality, restorative sleep. **Hypersomnias** refer to sleep-wake disorders where the primary complaint is excessive daytime sleepiness and difficulty awakening. Excessive daytime sleepiness is the inability to stay alert and awake during major waking episodes of the day with subsequent unintentional lapses into sleep.

5. What are the risk factors associated with sleep-wake disturbance in cancer?

Cancer patients are at high risk for sleep-wake disturbances resulting from demographic, lifestyle, disease-related, and treatment-related factors.

Risk factors associated with sleep-wake disturbance	
Risk factors	**Examples**
Demographic, personal/family characteristics	Female gender, emotional characteristics (e.g. depression, anxiety), personal or family history of insomnia
Lifestyle	Environmental factors (e.g., noise, lighting, temperature), poor sleep hygiene habits
Disease-related	Emotional stress, physical symptoms, cancer pain, decrease in usual physical activity
Treatment-related	Hospitalization (routines, roommates), emotional impact (e.g., mastectomy, colostomy), chemotherapy/biotherapy side effects, radiation-related fatigue
Medication	Corticosteroids, hormones, central nervous system stimulants, antiemetics, opioids, antidepressants, hypnotic sedatives, diuretics
Side effects	Pain, fever, pruritus, anxiety, depression, delirium, night sweats/hot flashes, gastrointestinal disturbances (incontinence, diarrhea, constipation, nausea), genitourinary disturbances (urinary frequency, incontinence, retention, GU irrigation), respiratory disturbances

6. When do persons with cancer experience sleep-wake disturbances?

Sleep-wake disturbances occur in children and adults during all phases of the cancer trajectory. Years after treatment, insomnia can affect a considerable number of cancer survivors, suggesting that insomnia may develop a chronic course if left untreated.

7. What is the impact of sleep-wake disturbance?

Sleep-wake disturbances affect physical and psychological functioning, quality of life, mood, and symptom experience of patients and caregivers. Cancer diagnosis and treatments create physical and psychologic distress for patients and families. Impairment of sleep-wake patterns intensifies this burden, which can influence patient's compliance with treatment protocols, decision-making ability, and relationships. Sleep-wake disturbance in combinations with other symptoms contribute to cancer-related fatigue, often described as unpredictable and cumulative.

8. How should the nurse assess sleep-wake disturbance in the clinical setting?

Questions about sleep-wake patterns should be incorporated in initial and ongoing assessments of inpatients and during initial and follow-up visits in the ambulatory setting:

- Usual sleep schedule and daily activities including employment status (precancer and current pattern)
- Factors influencing sleep (e.g., environment, caffeine, nicotine, and alcohol)
- Total sleep time
- Perceived sleep quality and daytime sleepiness self-report
- Number of minutes to fall asleep (sleep latency)
- Number of nocturnal awakenings, time to return to sleep, and reason for awakenings
- Unusual sleep behaviors, such as snoring, irregular breathing, leg jerking
- Past strategies to improve sleep and their effectiveness
- Daytime napping (frequency and length of nap)
- Psychological stress or adjustment problems

9. What are major barriers to effective management of sleep-wake disturbance?

Barriers to effective sleep-wake management	
Health care provider	Inadequate knowledge of sleep-wake physiology, assessment and multimodal management strategies
	Concerns about the dependency and side effects of pharmacologic sleep treatment combined with the lack of knowledge of hypnotic tapering schedules
	Lack of evidence-based management and standardized assessment process guidelines
	Time pressures that prohibit effective sleep-wake assessment and management
	Belief that sleep-wake disturbance is inevitable and untreatable
	Failure to understand the negative impact of sleep-wake disturbances on treatment completion, and patient/family quality of life
Patient/family	Reluctance to report sleep-wake disturbances
	Belief that sleep-wake disturbance is part of the cancer experience and untreatable
Health care system	Failure to make sleep-wake management a research and educational priority
	Lack of systematic and collaborative sleep-wake disturbance assessment and management

10. What general principles are used to guide the management of sleep-wake disturbance?

- Treat the underlying physical and psychologic factors contributing to the sleep-wake disturbance.
- Make appropriate environmental and lifestyle modifications.
- Use a combination of nonpharmacologic and pharmacologic approaches.

11. What nonpharmacologic interventions are used to manage sleep-wake disturbance?

A variety of effective behavioral and cognitive therapies have become available in the past three decades.

Nonpharmacologic interventions for sleep-wake disturbances

Intervention	Description
Relaxation training	Muscle relaxation Guided imagery Conscious breathing Meditation
Stimulus control	Going to bed only when sleepy Avoid nonsleeping activities in bed If sleep does not come within 15-20 minutes, get out of bed and engage in relaxing activities, and return only when sleepy.
Time-in-bed restriction	Interventions limiting the amount of time spent in bed to closer approximate the amount of time asleep Restricting time in bed creates of a mild state of sleep deprivation which results in improved quality of sleep and decreased sleep latency.
Cognitive restructuring	Address and modify anxiety-producing and erroneous beliefs about sleep and sleep loss.
Environmental modifications	Minimize noise. Dim lights. Maintain a cool bedroom temperature. Consolidate patient care tasks to decrease nocturnal interruptions in the acute care setting.
Education	Sleep hygiene tips, such as: Establish consistent bedtime and wake-up time. Restrict foods and beverages containing stimulants before bedtime.

12. What practical tips help patients get a better night's sleep?

Good sleep habits seem like common sense, but patients often find it difficult to make behavioral changes; therefore, reinforcement of the following behaviors is often necessary.

Practical tips for a better night's sleep

Good sleep hygiene	Description/rationale
Fix a bedtime and an awakening time.	Choose a standard wake-up time and stick to it every day regardless of the total amount of sleep in a given night. This includes weekends.

Continued

Practical tips for a better night's sleep—cont'd

Good sleep hygiene	Description/rationale
Avoid napping during the day.	Sleeping more than 30-45 minutes during the day weakens sleep drive at night and may make it difficult to fall asleep.
Reserve the bed for sleeping.	Avoid activities such as reading, watching TV, eating, studying, using the phone, or other things that require you to be awake while you are in bed, because this unintentionally trains the body to stay awake in bed.
Avoid alcohol 4-6 hours before bedtime.	Alcohol can help you doze off, but a few hours later there is a stimulant effect, and alcohol changes the rhythm of sleep patterns.
Avoid caffeine and nicotine 4-6 hours before bedtime.	This includes caffeinated beverages, such as coffee, tea, soda, and chocolate.
Avoid heavy, spicy, or sugary foods 4-6 hours before bedtime, but have a light snack.	Warm milk and foods high in tryptophan, such as bananas and milk, help sleep onset.
Exercise regularly, but not right before bedtime.	Regular exercise, particularly in the afternoon can help deepen sleep, but vigorous exercise within 2 hours of bedtime will make it more difficult to fall asleep.
Set up a presleep ritual.	It is helpful to establish cues for slowing down such as relaxation techniques (yoga, deep breathing, warm bath), caffeine-free tea, and restful music.
Design a comfortable and familiar sleeping environment.	Invest in a comfortable mattress; use dry, unwrinkled bedding; maintain a cool (not cold) bedroom for sleep; block out distractions, noise, and light by using earplugs or sleep mask.
Get into a favorite sleeping position.	Never stay in bed at any time in the night for extended periods (> 20-30 minutes) without being asleep. Long periods of being awake in bed usually lead to tossing and turning, becoming frustrated, or worrying about not sleeping, making it more difficult to fall asleep.
Don't take worries to bed.	Do not mull over your problems, plan future events, or do other thinking while in bed. If racing thoughts can't be shut off, get up and go to another room until this thinking no longer interrupts sleep. Routinely set aside a time early in the evening to do the thinking, problem-solving, and planning.
Only go to bed/stay in bed when sleepy.	Go to bed only when feeling sleepy. Spending too much time in bed without sleeping results in a very fragmented night's sleep.

13. **When is it appropriate to use pharmacologic interventions to manage sleep-wake disturbances?**

Treatment of insomnia/sleep-wake disturbance with medications is appropriate when:
- The cause of the insomnia/sleep disturbance is known
- Insomnia/sleep disturbance is short-term or temporary
- Sleep difficulties interfere with daily activities, and/or the person is experiencing distress
- Behavioral approaches have proven ineffective or the person is unwilling to try them

14. **What are some guidelines for pharmacologic management?**

Pharmacologic treatment should:
- Begin with the lowest, effective dose
- Be used in combination with good sleep practices and behavioral approaches
- Be short-term if used nightly (4 weeks or less is recommended)
- Be intermittent if used long-term
- Be gradually tapered to avoid rebound insomnia, particularly when using hypnotics with long half-lives

15. **What pharmacologic interventions are used to manage sleep-wake disturbance?**

Treatment of insomnia in patients with cancer typically involves the use of medications, such as hypnotics, antidepressants, and antihistamines.

Medications commonly used for insomnia

Pharmacological class	Usual dose (mg)	Onset (min)	Half life (hr)	Clinical implications
Benzodiazepines (BzRA)				Cautious use in older
Triazolam (Halcion)	0.125-0.25	15-30	2-4	adults and patients
Oxazepam (Serax)	10-30	30-60	5-10	with hepatic
Temazepam (Restoril)	7.5-30	45-60	8-20	insufficiency
Flurazepam (Dalmane)	15-30	60-120	48-100	Tolerance possible
Non-BzRA				Lower risk of rebound
Zaleplon (Sonata)	5-20	20	1-1.5	insomnia and
Zolpidem (Ambien)	5-10	30	2.5-2.8	tolerance
Zolpidem CR (Ambien CR)	5-10	30	1.6-5.5	Extended dosing
Eszopiclone (Lunesta)	1-3	30	1.5-2.5	available for zolpidem and eszopiclone
Antidepressants **Tricyclics (TCAs)**				Indicated for concomitant
Amitryptline (Elavil)	10-300	30-60	14-18	depression and
Doxepin (Sinequan)	25-50	30-60	20-25	insomnia
Other				Multiple drug
Trazodone (Desyrel)	25-150	30-60	4-7	interactions with TCAs
				Cautious use in older adults

Continued

Medications commonly used for insomnia—cont'd

Pharmacological class	Usual dose (mg)	Onset (min)	Half life (hr)	Clinical implications
Antihistamines				
Diphenhydramine (Benadryl)	25-50	60-180	4-10.4	Available OTC[†]
				May cause dry mouth, constipation, urinary
Doxylamine (Unisom)	25	60-120	10	retention, and excess sedation
				Cautious use in older adults
Melatonin antagonists				
Ramelteon (Rozeram)	8	30	1-5	Associated with multiple drug interactions and must be taken with a high fat meal
				Cautious use in patients with hepatic impairment

[†]Over the counter.

16. How do I choose which medication to use to promote sleep onset and maintenance?

- Benzodiazepine receptor agonists (BzRAs) and BzRA-like medications are generally the first choice, because they disrupt REM sleep less than other hypnotics do. Temazepam, used with caution with older adult patients, is a BzRA with a relatively rapid onset, short one hour half-life, and relatively low incidence of side effects when used in low doses for short periods.
- Non-BzRA hypnotics of the imidazopyridine and pyrazolopyrimidine class with a rapid onset and short duration, such as zaleplon, zopiclone, or zolpidem are preferred because withdrawal symptoms, rebound insomnia, and tolerance are less problematic than with BzRAs. Eszopiclone, a new non-BzRA hypnotic from the pyrrolopyrazine class, has the advantages of a more rapid onset of action and a short elimination half-life.
- Tricyclic antidepressant (TCA) and selective serotonin reuptake inhibitor (SSRI) antidepressants can be used to improve sleep onset when there is concurrent depression.
- Diphenhydramine (antihistamine) enhances sleep by managing symptoms (nausea or itching) as well as decreasing sleep latency. It is inexpensive and available over the counter.
- Remelteon (Rozeram) is a new synthetic melatonin agonist that targets MT1 and MT2 receptors in the hypothalamus. Although it decreases sleep latency, it has not been shown to reduce multiple night-time awakenings.

17. How does melatonin work?

High blood levels of melatonin, an endogenous hormone secreted at night (levels normally rise at dusk, peak in the mid-dark period, and drop at dawn), is associated with the promotion of sleep by regulating circadian rhythms. Research on the use of exogenous melatonin as a dietary supplement is inconclusive because its rapid absorption and the array of doses and schedules used in recent studies confounded the findings.

18. Is there any benefit to using supplements and herbal remedies to treat sleep-wake disturbance in patients with cancer?

Increasing numbers of cancer patients use vitamins, mineral supplements, herbal remedies, and hormones to promote sleep and well-being; however, evidence of efficacy and toxicity is limited. In studies to date, the benefits from taking valerian or L-tryptophan (an endogenous amino acid) were not significantly different from that provided by placebo.

 Key Points

- Sleep-wake disturbances are a significant problem throughout the cancer trajectory, with wide reaching impact on functioning, mood, and quality of life of patients and caregivers.
- Insomnia and hypersomnia, common sleep-wake disturbances in cancer, result from demographic, lifestyle, physiologic, disease, and treatment related factors.
- Sleep is infrequently assessed in the practice setting, but a variety of sleep diaries, sleep questionnaires, and visual analog scales, among other methods, are available to evaluate sleep-wake disturbance.
- Sleep-wake disturbances can be managed through general interventions that address the underlying physical and psychologic factors, environmental and lifestyle changes, cognitive-behavioral interventions, and pharmacological treatment.
- Benzodiazepines, antihistamines, and certain antidepressants should be used with caution in older adults to treat sleep-wake disturbances.

 Internet Resources

National Cancer Institute Supportive Care Topics: Sleep Disorders:
    http://www.cancer.gov/cancertopics/pdq/supportivecare/sleepdisorders/healthprofessional/
The National Sleep Foundation (NSF):
    http://www.sleepfoundation.org/
The American Academy of Sleep Medicine (AASM):
    http://www.aasmnet.org/
AASM sleep education site:
    http://www.sleepeducation.com/
Associated Professional Sleep Societies (APSS):
    http://www.apss.org
Oncology Nursing Society: Sleep/Wake Disturbances Interventions:
    http://www.ons.org/outcomes/PEPcard/sleep.shtml
Sleep Research Society:
    http://www.sleepresearchsociety.org/site/
National Center for Sleep Disorders Research (NCSDR):
    http://www.nhlbi.nih.gov/about/ncsdr/

Bibliography

American Academy of Sleep Medicine: *International classification of sleep disorders: Diagnostic and coding manual,* ed 2, Westchester, IL, 2005, American Academy of Sleep Medicine.

Ancoli-Israel S, Moore PJ, Jones V: The relationship between fatigue and sleep in cancer patients: A review. *Eur J Cancer Care* 10:245-255, 2001.

Berger AM, Farr L: The influence of daytime inactivity and nighttime restlessness on cancer-related fatigue. *Oncol Nurs Forum* 26:1663-1671, 1999.

Berger AM, Parker KP, Young-McCaughan S, et al: Sleep/wake disturbances in people with cancer and their caregivers: State of the science. *Oncol Nurs Forum* 32:E98-E126, 2005.

Borbely AA, Achermann P: Sleep homeostasis and models of sleep regulation. In Kryger MH, Roth T, Dement WC, editors: *Principles and practice of sleep medicine,* ed 4, Philadelphia, 2005, Saunders.

Clark J, Cunningham M, McMillan S, et al: Sleep-wake disturbances in people with cancer part II: Evaluating the evidence for clinical decision making. *Oncol Nurs Forum* 31:747-771, 2004.

Edinger JD, Wohlgemuth WK, Radtke RA, et al: Efficacy of cognitive-behavioral therapy for treating primary sleep-maintenance insomnia. *JAMA* 285:1856-1864, 2001.

Lee K, Cho M, Miaskowski C, et al: Impaired sleep and rhythms in persons with cancer. *Sleep Med Rev* 8:199-212, 2004.

Lee K, Ward TM: Critical components of a sleep assessment for clinical practice settings. *Issues Ment Health Nurs* 26:739-750, 2005.

Mock V: Evidence-based treatment for cancer-related fatigue. *J Natl Cancer Inst Monogr* 32:112-118, 2004.

Redeker NS, Lev EL, Ruggiero J: Insomnia, fatigue, anxiety, depression, and quality of life of cancer patients undergoing chemotherapy. *Sch Inq Nurs Pract* 14:275-298, 2000.

Savard J, Morin CM: Insomnia in the context of cancer: A review of a neglected problem, *J Clin Oncol* 19:895-908, 2001.

Schwartz AL, Nail LM, Chen S, et al: Fatigue patterns observed in patients receiving chemotherapy and radiotherapy. *Cancer Invest* 18:11-19, 2000.

Vena C, Parker K, Cunningham M, et al: Sleep-wake disturbances in people with cancer part I: An overview of sleep, sleep regulation, and effects of disease and treatment. *Oncol Nurs Forum* 31:735-746, 2004.

Unit VI

Oncologic Emergencies

Cardiac Tamponade

Dawn Camp-Sorrell

1. What is cardiac tamponade?

Cardiac tamponade is a life-threatening emergency in which excessive accumulation (200-1000 ml) of fluid or blood between the pericardium and heart prevents an adequate amount of blood from flowing into the heart to fill the ventricles. The rate of fluid accumulation, as well as the volume, is important in causing tamponade. Cardiac tamponade results from increased intrapericardial pressure, which leads to impaired diastolic filling, and low cardiac output (the amount of blood ejected by the ventricle). As blood is increasingly unable to flow into the heart, the patient exhibits signs and symptoms of systemic venous congestion. Eventually circulatory collapse occurs. Pericardial effusion is fluid accumulation within the pericardial sac. Cardiac tamponade is fluid accumulation in the pericardial sac that is so great that normal filling and contraction fail.

2. How much fluid does the pericardial sac usually hold?

Under normal conditions the pericardium is a thin, tough, double-layered sac that encloses the heart with two distinct components: (1) visceral pericardium (covers the heart), and (2) parietal pericardium. Approximately 15 to 20 ml of pericardial fluid is located between the layers to prevent friction between the membranes during contraction and relaxation of the heart.

3. What is pericardial pressure?

Pericardial pressure is subatmospheric (negative), which allows the return inflow of low-pressure venous blood into the right side of the heart.

4. What are the common signs, symptoms, and physical examination findings of cardiac tamponade?

Small effusions usually do not cause symptoms. Larger or rapid accumulation of fluid may cause epigastric or retrosternal chest pain that is relieved by sitting up or leaning forward (pain is more severe when the patient is supine). Other signs and symptoms include chest heaviness, dysphagia, cough, dyspnea, hoarseness, increased jugular vein distention, muffled heart sounds (pericardial effusion), pericardial friction rub (when tumor is present), tachycardia, mild peripheral edema, and pulsus paradoxus.

5. Why do some patients have symptoms whereas others are asymptomatic?

Symptoms depend on how the condition develops. As small effusions begin, the pericardium stretches gradually to accommodate the fluid pressure within the sac and the patient is asymptomatic. When the effusion progresses, the patient becomes symptomatic from the increased pressure from the fluid. Rapid fluid accumulation causes a rapid decrease in cardiac output and acute symptoms.

6. List the common causes of cardiac tamponade.

- Primary cancer and/or metastasis
- Infection

- Post viral syndrome
- Cardiac conditions (heart failure, myocardial infarction, dissecting aortic aneurysm, post cardiac surgery)
- Trauma
- Central venous catheter perforation
- Autoimmune diseases
- Renal failure
- Chest irradiation
- Pharmacological agents (e.g., anthracyclines, anticoagulants, hydralazine, procainamide, interleukin-2, tumor necrosis factor)

7. What types of cancer can cause cardiac tamponade?

Autopsies provide evidence that up to 21% of all patients with cancer have metastatic disease to the heart or pericardium. Although all cancer types can affect the heart, specific cancers with higher incidence include lung cancer, breast cancer, head and neck cancers, Hodgkin and non-Hodgkin lymphomas, leukemia, lymphoma, mesothelioma, pancreatic, sarcoma, and melanoma.

8. Can pleural effusions lead to cardiac tamponade?

Yes. Cardiac tamponade may result from an increase in intrapleural pressure, which may be transmitted to the pericardial space.

9. Can cancer treatments cause cardiac tamponade?

Yes. Radiation affects the fine capillary stroma of the myocardium. Pericardial effusion may occur when up to 40 Gy is administered to the mediastinum. Chemotherapy, especially anthracyclines, may affect the myocardial fibers and thus lead to pericardial effusion.

10. What is pulsus paradoxus?

Pulsus paradoxus, often a late sign of cardiac tamponade, can be detected by assessing the blood pressure. Pulsus paradoxus results from an increase in intrathoracic pressure and is characterized by an exaggerated inspiratory fall in systolic blood pressure greater than 10 mm Hg or greater than 10%. Pulsus paradoxus is measured by inflating the blood pressure cuff until no sounds are audible (usually 10 to 20 mmHg above the normal systolic pressure). The patient is asked to breathe in and out normally. During expiration, the cuff is gradually deflated until sounds are audible, at which point the pressure is recorded. The cuff is further deflated until sounds are audible during inspiration, at which point the pressure is again recorded. The difference between the two recorded pressures should be 5 to 10 mmHg. In patients with cardiac tamponade, sounds are heard during expiration alone for a prolonged period.

11. Can pulsus paradoxus be present in other conditions?

Yes. Pulsus paradoxus may be present in patients with chronic obstructive pulmonary disease, bronchospasm, or marked shifts in intrapleural pressure. Arrhythmias may hamper the measurement.

12. Which tests are used to diagnose a pericardial effusion?

A chest radiograph reveals only an enlarged heart shadow. An echocardiogram is the definitive diagnostic tool for confirmation of pericardial disease. When effusion or tamponade are present, fluid is visible within the pericardial sac. CT or MRI cardiac imaging may be useful when echocardiogram results are indeterminate.

The electrocardiogram (ECG) provides limited information. Elevated ST segments, nonspecific T wave changes, decreased QRS voltage, and sinus tachycardia may be seen. In a small number of patients, electrical alternans may be observed. This characteristic is the alternating positive and negative deflected QRS complexes. This abnormal finding is thought to result from variations in the position of the heart at the time of electrical depolarization.

13. Describe the treatment of a pericardial effusion.

The goal of treatment is symptomatic relief. In asymptomatic patients, the treatment may be to observe the patient instead of proceeding with an invasive procedure. In an emergency, cardiac tamponade is usually relieved by percutaneous pericardiocentesis; a 16- to 18-gauge needle is placed into the pericardial sac to withdraw fluid. Surgical intervention depends on the cause of tamponade and the patient's overall condition. An indwelling pericardial catheter may be inserted to withdraw fluid or to instill medications for a pericardial sclerosis. A pericardial window may be made to allow drainage of fluid into the surrounding tissue. A total pericardiectomy may be necessary if the window is not effective in relieving the tamponade and is indicated if the patient has constriction secondary to radiation therapy.

14. What are the complications of surgical intervention?

Potential complications include puncture of the right atrium, right ventricle, or coronary arteries; infection; dysrhythmia; and pneumothorax. Indwelling catheters may cause infection, catheter blockage, dysrhythmias, and pericarditis.

15. What does *sclerosing* mean? How is it used to relieve cardiac tamponade?

Sclerosing is a method used to produce an inflammatory response that eventually obliterates the pericardial space. The intent is to prevent reaccumulation of fluid. Several sclerosing agents have been used, including tetracycline, bleomycin, doxycycline, talc, cisplatin, and thiotepa. The patient must be medicated with analgesics before the procedure, which can be very painful.

16. Is balloon pericardiotomy also used to treat cardiac tamponade?

Percutaneous balloon pericardiotomy may be used. A balloon is placed across the parietal pericardium. Inflation of the balloon creates an opening into the pericardium that allows internal drainage of the effusion into the pleural space for reabsorption.

17. Should the pericardial fluid be assayed?

To establish the diagnosis of malignancy and to rule out preexisting infection, the fluid should be assayed for presence of lactate dehydrogenase (LDH), protein, specific gravity, glucose level, cell count, cytologic findings, and pH; it also should be cultured for the presence of bacteria and fungi. Most malignant effusions are serosanguinous or bloody and have malignant cells, alkaline pH, glucose, and increased LDH level.

18. What assessment parameters must be included in the care of patients with cardiac effusion?

The assessment should include frequent auscultation of heart sounds and blood pressure; palpation of the apical pulse and peripheral pulses; observation for jugular venous distention; and checking the extremities for cyanosis, coolness, and edema. Up to 12% of patients have reoccurrence of fluid after treatment; therefore, close monitoring is indicated.

19. What is the prognosis for a patient with cardiac tamponade?

Prognosis depends on rapidity of fluid accumulation, stage of disease at time of diagnosis, presence of metastatic disease, performance status of the patient, and effectiveness of treatment. Life expectancy ranges from a few hours to years; the average duration of remission is 4 to 6 months.

20. Can radiation therapy be used to treat cardiac tamponade?

If cardiac tamponade is of gradual onset and caused by a radiosensitive tumor, such as lung or breast cancer or lymphoma, radiation therapy may be the treatment of choice. Usually 200 to 400 Gy of external radiation is delivered to the heart, pericardial structures, and lower mediastinum. In most patients who have received previous mediastinum radiation (e.g., for Hodgkin lymphoma), the maximal dose to the pericardial region has already been used.

21. What supportive care strategies can be used?

To ease the patient's suffering, the nurse can provide emotional support, administer oxygen, reposition the patient to enhance circulation, assist with all activities, administer analgesics, encourage relaxation techniques, and administer antianxiety or other medications as prescribed. Infusion of intravenous fluids is initiated to increase systolic pressure, thereby increasing effective ventricular filling pressure. Vasoactive drugs may be ordered to increase heart rate and contractility. Referral for home nursing services or hospice care should be considered as needed.

 Key Points

- Patients with cancer and those who have received radiation over the heart area are at risk for cardiac tamponade.
- Signs and symptoms of cardiac tamponade are related to the amount and rapidity of fluid accumulation. With fluid progression, symptoms increase in acuity.
- Dyspnea is the most common symptom followed by retrosternal chest pain that is relieved when the patient leans forward.
- Echocardiogram is the definitive diagnostic test for confirmation of cardiac tamponade.
- Treatment, based on the patient's symptoms and fluid accumulation, can be observation or fluid removal with instillation of medications to prevent fluid reaccumulation.

 Internet Resources

Bibliography

Bischiniotis TS, Lafaras CT, Platogiannis DN, et al: Intrapericardial cisplatin administration after pericardio-centesis in patients with lung adenocarcinoma and malignant cardiac tamponade. Hellenic *J Cardiol* 46:324-329, 2005.

Bueno R: Multimodality treatments in the management of malignant pleural mesothelioma: An update. *Hematol Oncol Clin North Am* 19:1089-1097, 2005.

Colomina MJ, Godet C, Pellise F, et al: Cardiac tamponade associated with a peripheral vein central venous catheter. *Paediatr Anaesth* 15:988-992, 2005.

Fitzgerald M, Spencer J, Johnson F, et al: Definitive management of acute cardiac tamponade secondary to blunt trauma. *Emerg Med Australas* 17:494-499, 2005.

Flounders JA: Cardiovascular emergencies: Pericardial and cardiac tamponade. *Oncol Nurs Forum* 30: E48-E55, 2003.

Kirsner KM: Cancer: New therapies and new approaches to recurring problems. *AANA J* 71:55-62, 2003.

Retter AS: Pericardial disease in the oncology patient. *Heart Dis* 4:387-391, 2002.

Disseminated Intravascular Coagulation (DIC)

Carol S. Viele

1. What is disseminated intravascular coagulation and what are the patient's presenting symptoms?

Disseminated intravascular coagulation (DIC) is an acquired process arising from various causes. It is generalized activation of the hemostatic system, which results in widespread intravascular deposition of fibrin in the microvasculature and the simultaneous consumption of coagulation factors and platelets. The presenting symptoms of patients with severe forms of DIC may be those of thromboembolic disease that may manifest as multiple organ dysfunction. The patient's symptoms may be evidence of both bleeding and thrombosis.

2. What causes DIC?

DIC does not occur in isolation; it is always a symptom of underlying disease. DIC is the direct response to the presence of specific proteins or cancer procoagulants, which may be secreted by malignant cells. Tissue factor, tumor necrosis factor (TNF), and cell proteases are among the proteins responsible for initiating DIC.

3. What is the mechanism of bleeding in DIC?

Fibrin degradation products and D-dimers are almost always abundant in DIC and frequently clump together. These fragments or clumps, particularly D-dimers, competitively inhibit the formation and action of thrombin by binding to thrombin at its fibrinogen receptor site. These fragment complexes, if soluble, may deposit indiscriminately throughout the vasculature. Others bind abnormally to preexisting, growing microthrombi, weakening clot structure. This is the clotting mechanism of DIC.

The mechanism of bleeding comes from the failure of the clotting cascade, which results in systemic release of fibrinogen, fibrin degradation products, or D-dimers. This release creates a host of circulatory disturbances, including the formation of small fragments that inhibit platelet function, large fragments that induce platelet clumping, and mixtures of soluble fragments that may increase capillary permeability, cause extravascular coagulation, and disturb endothelial activity. The result is significant bleeding throughout the vascular system. Both thrombosis and bleeding occur from many areas at the same time.

4. What types of malignancies are associated with DIC?

Both solid tumors and leukemia have been reported to cause DIC. Patients with mucin-secreting adenocarcinomas, prostate cancer, or disseminated carcinomas are at highest risk for developing DIC. In addition, all leukemias, to various extents, may induce DIC. However, promyelocytic leukemia (M3) is almost universally associated with the development of some degree of DIC.

5. What are some other causes of DIC in persons with cancer?

Infection is the most common cause of DIC. Gram-negative organisms triggering sepsis may be the culprit. DIC is also seen in gram-positive bacterial sepsis and viremias, most often involving varicella, hepatitis, and cytomegalovirus (CMV). Patients also may develop DIC from intravascular hemolysis secondary to multiple transfusions of whole blood and transfusion reactions. At times, the administration of chemotherapy may cause destruction of blast cells, releasing substances with procoagulation properties.

6. What is the difference between acute and chronic DIC?

Acute DIC develops rapidly during a few hours. The patient develops sudden bleeding from multiple sites, and it must be treated as a medical emergency. Chronic DIC may be subclinical and develop over several months. Eventually, however, it evolves into an acute DIC pattern with hemorrhage or thromboembolic episodes.

7. What are the symptoms of DIC?

The most common sign of DIC is bleeding, usually manifested by ecchymosis, petechiae, and purpura. The patient's presenting symptoms are bleeding from multiple sites, including skin, nose, gums, lungs, and central nervous system. This bleeding may range from the continuous oozing of venipuncture sites or wounds to uncontrollable hemorrhage that will lead to shock and death unless intervention is swift and effective. If DIC persists for more than a few hours, hemorrhages may be extensive and involve the pleura and pericardium. When this occurs, patients may complain of dyspnea and chest pain.

8. How is DIC diagnosed?

DIC is diagnosed on the basis of clinical presentation plus laboratory evidence of abnormalities. The activated partial thromboplastin time is a less helpful test for diagnosing DIC except in severe cases, because it may be physiologically prolonged in children and masked by elevated factor VIII in adults.

Laboratory abnormalities associated with DIC

Test	Abnormality
Platelet count	Decreased
Fibrin degradation products	Increased
Prothrombin time	Prolonged
Activated partial thromboplastin time	Prolonged
Thrombin time	Prolonged
Fibrinogen level	Decreased
Protein C levels	Decreased
Antithrombin levels	Decreased

9. How is DIC managed?

The overall management of DIC is highly controversial because few controlled studies on treatment have been done. The immediate goal of therapy is to stop the patient from actively bleeding and clotting. However, the most important component in the management of DIC is to treat the underlying disorder. Management of DIC can be divided into two categories: use of blood component therapy and use of medications.

10. Describe the use of blood component therapy.

Platelet concentrates, cryoprecipitate, and fresh frozen plasma are frequently used to attempt to control the bleeding associated with DIC. Patients should not be automatically transfused; transfusion is appropriate only when the diagnosis is well established with documented depletion of factors. The exception, of course, is a life-threatening situation with little time to establish a diagnosis. Replacements for thrombocytopenia include 10 units of random donor platelets or a single unit of donor hemapheresed platelets. Hypofibrinogenemia (e.g., fibrinogen level < 100 mg/dl) may be treated with 8 units of cryoprecipitate. A prolonged prothrombin time due to a factor deficiency may be corrected by administering two units of fresh frozen plasma. Patients with severe DIC may require fresh frozen plasma drips to maintain the prothrombin time. Depending on the severity of DIC, replacement therapy may need to be given and repeated every 6 hours or more frequently in the case of life threatening bleeding, with adjustments for platelet count, prothrombin time, activated partial thromboplastin time, fibrinogen level, and volume status. Replacements are discontinued when levels are normal or near normal.

11. Which medications may be used to treat DIC?

There are a variety of medications that can be used to manage DIC. The choice of medication depends on the patient's condition.

Heparin. Because the patient with DIC has evidence of clotting in addition to bleeding, heparin is used to prevent further clotting. It is indicated as a treatment for DIC in acute promyelocytic and acute monocytic leukemia during induction therapy. Heparin is also used to treat DIC-induced thromboembolic complications in large vessels and is given to patients with metastatic carcinoma before surgery. The recommended dose of heparin is 4 to 5 U/kg/hr by continuous infusion.

Antithrombin III (ATIII). ATIII concentrate has been used as treatment for patients with DIC, either alone or in combination with heparin. To date, no definitive studies have shown a decrease in mortality with use of ATIII.

Fibrinolytic inhibitors. Fibrinolytic inhibitors are used only in the setting of an undeniable threat to hemostasis—that is, bleeding that has not responded to any other measures. The agent most commonly used is epsilon aminocaproic acid (Amicar). Epsilon aminocaproic acid (EACA) is a protease inhibitor that is uniquely reactive with plasminogen activators. It inhibits spontaneous fibrinolytic activity. A standard loading dose of 4 to 6 g followed by 6 to 12 g/day in divided doses provides sufficient plasma concentration to preserve the fibrin of a hemostatic vascular plug. The adverse effects are gastrointestinal disturbances, muscle necrosis, impotence, and the risk of creating clots in the urinary tract and bladder in patients with renal bleeding and hemorrhagic cystitis.

12. What is the controversy over the use of heparin for DIC?

Heparin may be given to inhibit factors IX and X, enhancing the neutralization of thrombin and halting the clotting cascade. However, hemorrhage is one of the main causes of death in patients with DIC, and heparin may induce bleeding. Heparin therapy is not indicated in patients who bleed in areas that compromise important functions (e.g., intracranial or intraspinal hemorrhage). Heparin therapy should be stopped if the patient has any life-threatening bleeding episode. Sometimes physicians think it is safer to use factor replacement therapy, especially if the underlying cause, such as infection, can be treated successfully.

13. What is the prognosis of patients diagnosed with DIC?

Both DIC and the patient's underlying disorder contribute to the high mortality rate. Mortality is correlated independently with the extent of organ or system involvement.

It is also correlated with the degree of hemostatic failure and increasing age of patient at onset. Mortality rates in various studies range from 42% to 86%, regardless of whether heparin was used to treat DIC.

14. What nursing interventions are important to patients with DIC?

Nurses should assess the patient for any signs or symptoms of bleeding. A thorough and organized approach must be used when evaluating the symptoms of a patient suspected of having DIC, with a physical assessment performed at least every 4 hours. Starting with the skin, the nurse should inspect the patient from head to toe, including palms of the hands and soles of the feet, looking for petechiae or bruising. Particular attention should be paid to the sclera and buccal mucosa. The patient should also be asked about vision changes. Blurred, cloudy, or diminished vision may indicate retinal hemorrhage and should be reported to the physician immediately. The nurse also should inspect the oral cavity, evaluating for bleeding, ulcers, or hematomas. A mouth care regimen is imperative for patients with DIC because oral cavity bleeding may be significant. Both nares should be inspected for signs of bleeding; epistaxis may be a significant source of blood loss. The inspection proceeds to the chest, back, abdomen, groin area, and lower extremities. Pressure areas should be examined closely, because they are common sites of petechiae, hematomas, and ecchymoses.

15. What can be done to stop bleeding from a central line site?

Many patients with leukemia and DIC require central line dressing changes every 2 hours or more frequently because of bleeding. A patient may lose units of blood from the central line site with close to 100 ml of blood contained within each hematoma. Pressure should be applied during each dressing change for at least 5 to 10 minutes to reduce oozing. If pressure is not sufficient, Gelfoam sponges may be used at the exit site to enhance hemostasis. An alternative method is to apply topical thrombin to the Gelfoam sponges to control bleeding. Once the bleeding has stopped, do not remove the topical thrombin-soaked sponge until it falls off, or the site may again begin to bleed. The Gelfoam sponge usually falls off when clotting conditions have returned to normal.

16. What other critical areas should the nurse assess?

After a thorough inspection of the skin, the nurse should complete an assessment of the chest cavity, including the heart and lungs, and the abdominal cavity, including the liver, spleen, and bowels. Because patients with DIC may develop diffuse alveolar hemorrhage, listening for rales, rhonchi, or areas of decreased breath sounds is important. Any positive finding, in addition to signs or symptoms of respiratory distress, such as dyspnea, shortness of breath, nasal flaring, and increased respiratory rate should be reported.

17. What other medical emergencies may occur with DIC?

In some patients, cardiac tamponade may result from DIC and thrombocytopenia. Signs of tamponade may be acute and include chest pain and shortness of breath (refer to Chapter 46). Patients with DIC may have symptoms of abdominal pain due to ischemic bowel. Abdominal examination should include listening for bowel sounds in all four quadrants, noting any areas of decreased or absent bowel sounds. Evaluation also should include palpating and looking for peritoneal signs, indication of rebound tenderness, or a fluid wave due to bleeding in the abdominal cavity. The liver and spleen should be palpated and percussed to determine size and degree of tenderness. Any abnormal findings should be noted and reported to the physician. Urine and stool should be inspected for signs of blood.

Key Points

- DIC is always a symptom of underlying disease.
- Patients with mucin-secreting adenocarcinoma, prostate cancer, disseminated cancer, and all leukemias are at highest risk for DIC.
- Bleeding is the most common sign of DIC, manifested by ecchymosis, petechiae, and purpura.
- DIC is managed symptomatically with blood component therapy and medications (heparin, ATIII, fibrinolytic inhibitors).

Internet Resources

UpToDate, Clinical Features, Diagnosis, and Treatment of Disseminated Intravascular Coagulation in Adults:

http://www.utdol.com/utd/content/topic.do?topicKey=coagulat/10248&type=A&selectedTitle=1~85

eMedicine, Disseminated Intravascular Coagulation:

http://www.medscape.com/files/emedicine/disseminated-intravascular-coagulation/

Post Graduate Medicine Online, Disseminated Intravascular Coagulation:

http://www.postgradmed.com/issues/2002/03_02/messmore.htm

Bibliography

Arkel Y: Thrombosis and cancer. *Semin Oncol* 27:362-374, 2000.

Friend P, Pruett J: Bleeding and thrombotic disorders. In Yarbro C, Frogge M, Goodman M, editors: *Cancer symptom management,* ed 3, Boston, 2004, Jones and Bartlett.

Gobel BH: Disseminated intravascular coagulation. *Semin Oncol Nurs* 15:174-182, 1999.

Liebman H, Weitz I, et al: Disseminated intravascular coagulation. In Hoffman R, Benz E, Shattil S, et al, editors: *Hematology: Basic principles and practice,* ed 4, Philadelphia, 2005, Elsevier.

Levi M, de Jonge E, van der Poll T: New treatment strategies for disseminated intravascular coagulation based on current understanding and pathophysiology. *Ann Intern Med* 36:41-49, 2004.

Toh C, Dennis M: Disseminated intravascular coagulation: Old disease, new hope. *Br Med J* 327:974-977, 2003.

Hypercalcemia of Malignancy (HCM)

Gari Jensen

1. What is hypercalcemia of malignancy?

Hypercalcemia of malignancy (HCM) is a paraneoplastic syndrome characterized by a serum calcium level exceeding 10.5 mg/dl or 2.62 mmol/L of blood (normal serum calcium being roughly 8.5-10.5 mg/dl or 2.12-2.62 mmol/L). HCM is the most common syndrome associated with cancer and occurs at some point in 10% to 20% of cancer patients.

2. Why are calcium levels corrected in cancer patients?

Because many patients with advanced cancer have low albumin levels, serum calcium must be corrected relative to albumin levels. A corrected calcium level of 12 to 14 mg/dl (2.99-3.49 mmol/L) is considered moderate hypercalcemia and may or may not be associated with symptoms. Patients with severe hypercalcemia (> 14 mg/dl or 3.5 mmol/L) usually have symptoms.

3. How is ionized calcium calculated?

Corrected serum calcium is obtained by adjusting the calcium level upward by 0.8 mg for every gram of albumin under 4 g/dl or downward by 0.8 mg for every gram of albumin over 4 g/dl:
1. Subtract the albumin level from 4.0.
2. Multiply the difference by 0.8.
3. If the result is a positive number, add it to the serum calcium; if it is a negative number, subtract.
4. The answer is the corrected calcium.

Example: Serum calcium is 11.4 mg/dl and albumin level is 1.9 g/dl:
1. $4.0 - 1.9 = 2.1$
2. $2.1 \times 0.8 = 1.7$
3. $11.4 + 1.7 = 13.1$

The corrected calcium level of 13.1 mg/dl indicates moderate HCM and is significantly higher than the uncorrected serum calcium level of 11.4 mg/dl.

4. Why is HCM considered an oncologic emergency?

Without treatment, about 50% of cases progress to renal failure, severe dehydration, coma, and death within days to weeks. Patients with chronic HCM are at risk for serious complications from hypercoagulative states and widespread calcifications.

5. What are the causes of HCM?

The most common cancers associated with HCM are lung cancer, breast cancer, and multiple myeloma.
- Humoral HCM (about 80% of cases) is most commonly caused by tumor cell production of parathyroid hormone-related protein (PTH-rP). Mimicking

parathyroid hormone (PTH), PTH-rP stimulates calcium release from bone secondary to osteoclast activity and increases calcium resorption from the renal tubules. PTH-rP, however, is not regulated by the feedback mechanisms that would normally suppress PTH. Control can only be achieved by diminishing the tumor burden. Humoral HCM is typically associated with squamous cell cancers (e.g., lung, head, neck, esophagus, and cervix); breast, renal, ovarian, and endometrial cancers; and hematologic cancers.

- Osteolytic HCM (20%) involves extensive invasion and destruction of bone by cancer cells and subsequent release and generation of cytokines and other substances that stimulate further damage and release of calcium. Osteolytic HCM is associated with breast cancer and multiple myeloma.
- In addition, some lymphomas convert vitamin D to its active form (1,25-dihydroxycholecalciferol); thereby, increasing absorption from the GI tract.

6. What other factors contribute to the development of HCM?

- Immobilization results in increased resorption (release) of calcium from bone.
- Thiazide diuretics decrease renal excretion of calcium.
- Patients may continue to take calcium and vitamin D supplements, calcium-containing parenteral/enteral formulas, or calcium-based antacids without realizing that they are contributing to the development of hypercalcemia.
- Taking androgens, estrogens, and antiestrogens can also precipitate HCM. The onset is usually dramatic, within the first 2 weeks of therapy.

7. What are the presenting symptoms of patients with HCM?

The usual presenting symptoms are fatigue, lethargy, weakness, nausea and anorexia, constipation, dehydrated appearance, decreased mental functioning, thirst, and polyuria. However, patients with mild-to-moderate HCM may be asymptomatic; severity does not always correlate with symptoms.

8. What are the signs and symptoms of acute HCM and its progression?

- **Mental status:** Somnolence, depression, confusion, apathy, stupor, coma
- **Cardiovascular system:** Bradycardia, hypotension, heart block, ECG changes, cardiac arrest
- **GI tract:** Nausea, vomiting, constipation, anorexia, pain and distension, adynamic ileus
- **Skeletal system:** Bone pain, immobility, osteolysis, pathologic fractures
- **Kidneys:** Polyuria, nocturia, polydipsia, dehydration, azotemia, proteinuria, renal failure
- **Systemic symptoms:** Fatigue, lethargy, weakness, hyporeflexia

9. What should be considered when planning treatment?

- **Prognosis.** Controlling the malignancy is the most effective treatment for HCM. In patients whose disease is refractory to treatment, a bisphosphonate may be used to palliate and enhance quality of life. In some cases, withholding treatment can be a humane alternative (because of the rapid progression to a decreased state of consciousness) to prolonged suffering.
- **Patient's overall condition.** Treatment must be modified for patients with underlying medical conditions such as renal and cardiac disease.
- **Severity of HCM.** The urgency and aggressiveness of treatment should correlate with the severity of HCM.

- **Symptom control and care management.** These include comfort interventions for nausea, vomiting, constipation, and pain, as well as care provisions for weakness, lethargy, confusion, and safety.
- **Monitoring of electrolytes.**

10. What is the treatment strategy for HCM?

- **Hydration:** Intravenous hydration with normal saline is usually required to restore hydration and promote calcium excretion. Infusion rates may vary from 150 to 500 ml/hour depending on the patient's underlying cardiac status and the severity of HCM. In mild or chronic cases, forced oral fluids (3-4 L/day) may be adequate to lower calcium levels.
- **Elimination of drugs that worsen hypercalcemia** (e.g., thiazide diuretics)
- **Loop diuretics:** Loop diuretics (e.g., furosemide) can be used after dehydration has been corrected. They accelerate the elimination of calcium by blocking reabsorption in the loop of Henle and help prevent volume overload from IV hydration.
- **Intravenous bisphosphonate therapy:** The bisphosphonates have become the standard of treatment in calcium-lowering drugs. Additional benefits include decreased bone complications and pain, resulting in better quality of life. For these reasons, bisphosphonates are used prophylactically. They are given intravenously because GI side effects and poor absorption prohibit adequate oral dosing. They may be given concurrently with chemotherapy. The most common side effects are flu-like syndromes of fatigue, aches, nausea, and transient fever. Electrolyte levels and serum creatinine should be monitored closely. For patients receiving multiple maintenance infusions, dose adjustments should be made for decreased creatinine clearance (see package inserts); although initially, HCM-compromised renal function may improve with normalization of calcium levels.

11. Which bisphosphonates are currently used?

Zoledronic acid (Zometa) and pamidronate (Aredia) are the IV bisphosphonates used in the United States. They inhibit the dissolution of bone matrix, and when released from bone, decrease osteoclast activity. Response occurs within 1 to 2 days with a maximum effect in 4 to 7 days and duration of 1 to 4 weeks. Zoledronic acid is dosed at 4 mg IV over at least 15 minutes. Pamidronate is dosed 60 to 90 mg IV over 2 hours. It is recommended that a week elapse before doses are repeated. Maintenance doses are generally administered at 3 to 4 week intervals.

12. What risk should patients be informed about before starting long-term use of bisphosphonates?

Osteonecrosis of the jaw, a disabling condition resulting from temporary or permanent loss of blood supply to the bone, has recently been reported in patients receiving bisphosphonates. This condition may be caused by an alteration in bone homeostasis including inhibition of angiogenesis. It is not yet clear whether there is any causal association between taking bisphosphonates and developing osteonecrosis (dead bone). Until guidelines are established, patients receiving treatment with bisphosphonates should be advised to consult their physicians before undergoing invasive dental procedures and should be evaluated for the risk of dental complications before starting bisphosphonates.

13. What second-line agents can be used if bisphosphonates are ineffective or contraindicated?

Secondary agents for acute HCM treatment

Agent	Dose	Action	Advantages	Disadvantages
Calcitonin	4-8 IU/kg SQ every 6-12 hrs	Inhibits osteoclasts Increases renal excretion	Onset: 4-6 hr Well-tolerated May decrease pain	1-2 days duration Relatively weak Rare allergic reactions (1 unit skin test recommended)
Plicamycin (mithramycin)	25 mcg/kg IV over 4-6 hr	Toxic to osteoclasts	Effective Onset: 1-2 days Duration: up to 2 weeks	Thrombocytopenia Nausea and vomiting Vesicant Renal and hepatic toxicities
Glucocorticoids	Variable	Inhibit reabsorption Increase excretion Decrease GI absorption	Selectively effective	Side effects of steroids
Gallium nitrate	100-200 mg/m^2 over 24 hrs for 5 days IV	Decreases bone resorption	Effective	5-day dosing Renal toxicity Anemia

14. Is dietary restriction of calcium necessary?

Dietary restriction of calcium is usually unnecessary because calcium absorption from the GI tract is already decreased by negative feedback mechanisms and frequently by anorexia, nausea, and vomiting; however, tube-feeding formulas and total parenteral nutrition should be modified.

15. What instructions should be given to patients and families?

- Report early signs and symptoms of hypercalcemia, such as decreased or absent appetite, nausea, vomiting, constipation, increased fatigue, weakness, excessive thirst, frequent voiding, dry mouth and skin, and dizziness with position changes.
- Promote hydration by monitoring intake, encouraging patient to drink 2 to 3 liters (quarts)/day, keeping favorite fluids handy, and reminding the patient to sip. Give antinausea medications.
- Help the patient to stay mobile by encouraging standing or walking several times a day, or doing isometric exercises if the patient is unable to bear weight. Support the patient in performing self-care activities as much as possible. Monitor pain medications, and inform the nurse or physician if pain control is not adequate.
- Promote safety by keeping the environment uncluttered and well-lit and encouraging the patient to use safety aids, such as a walker or cane, to prevent falls. Do not allow the patient to overstress bones, and educate others to be gentle when helping. They should not pull on arms or legs or squeeze ribs. Report bone pain and have it evaluated.

Key Points

- Serum calcium results must be adjusted to the albumin level.
- The most common malignancies associated with HCM are lung cancer, breast cancer, and multiple myeloma.
- Patients with mild-to-moderate HCM may be asymptomatic; severity does not always correlate with symptoms.
- Controlling the malignancy is the most effective treatment for HCM.
- The bisphosphonates are the standard of treatment for HCM.
- Osteonecrosis of the jaw has recently been associated with bisphosphonate therapy.

Internet Resources

National Cancer Institute Hypercalcemia Overview:
   http://www.cancer.gov/cancertopics/pdq/supportivecare/hypercalcemia/healthprofessional
Health A to Z (Overview of HCM for Patients):
   http://www.healthatoz.com/healthatoz/Atoz/ency/hypercalcemia.jsp
Post Graduate Medicine (Overviews of HCM for Healthcare Professionals):
   http://www.postgradmed.com/issues/2004/05_04/inzucchi.htm
Novartis Oncology Medical Services:
   http://www.OncologyMedicalServices.com

Bibliography

Clines GA, Guise TA: Hypercalcemia of malignancy and basic research on mechanisms responsible for osteolytic and osteoblastic metastasis to bone. *Endocr Relat Cancer* 12:549-583, 2005.

Durie BGM, Katz M, Crowley J: Osteonecrosis of the jaw and bisphosphonates. *N Engl J Med* 353(1):99-100, 2005.

Faulding Pharmaceutical Company: Pamidronate Package Insert, July 2002.

Fojo A: Metabolic emergencies. In DeVita VT, Hellman S, Rosenberg SA, editors: *Cancer principles and practice of oncology,* ed 7, Philadelphia, 2004, Lippincott Williams & Wilkins.

Major P: The use of zoledronic acid, a novel, highly potent bisphosphonate, for the treatment of hypercalcemia of malignancy. *Oncologist* 7:481-491, 2002.

Marx RE, Sawatari Y, Fortin M, et al: Bisphosphonate-induced exposed bone (osteonecrosis/osteopetrosis) of the jaws: Risk factors, recognition, prevention, and treatment. *J Oral Maxillofac Surg* 63:1567-1575, 2005.

McDonnell Keenan AM, Wickham RS: Hypercalcemia. In Yarbro CH, Frogge MH, Goodman M, editors: *Cancer nursing: Principles and practice,* ed 6, Sudbury, MA, 2005, Jones and Bartlett.

National Cancer Institute: Hypercalcemia (PDQ) (website): http://www.cancer.gov/cancertopics/pdq/supportivecare/hypercalcemia/healthprofessional. Accessed January 10, 2007.

Novartis Pharmaceuticals Corporation: Zometa Package Insert, March 2005.

Steward AF: Hypercalcemia associated with cancer. *N Engl J Med* 352:373-379, 2005.

Infections in Cancer Patients

Robert H. Gates

1. What factors place patients with cancer at risk for infection?

Infections are the major cause of morbidity and mortality in many patients with cancer. Multiple factors place cancer patients at risk for infection, including factors associated with the cancer itself and with current therapy as well as previous antibiotic therapy.

Factors increasing the risk of infection in cancer patients

Factor promoting infection	Examples of associated organisms	Examples of disease states

Diminished antibody response	Encapsulated organisms
	  Pneumococci
	  Haemophilus influenzae
	  Neisseria spp.
	Staphylococci
	Streptococci
		Multiple myeloma
		Poor nutrition
		B-cell lymphomas
		Post splenectomy (Hodgkin lymphoma)
		Myelophthisis

Poor white blood cell function or number	Aerobic gram-positive organisms
	  Staphylococci
	  Enterococci
	Aerobic gram-negative organisms
	  Pseudomonas aeruginosa
	  Enterobacter spp.
	Fungi
	  Candida spp.
	  Aspergillus spp.
	  Fusarium spp.
		Leukemias
		Lymphomas
		Myelophthisis
		Chemotherapy
		Radiation therapy

Poor cellular immunity	*Listeria* spp. Herpes group virus *Mycobacterium* spp. Cryptococci *Legionella* spp. *Pneumocystis* spp.	Hodgkin lymphoma Non-Hodgkin lymphoma Poor nutrition Chronic leukemias Chemotherapy (especially fludarabine) Steroids
Skin and mucosal defects	Staphylococci *Candida* spp. Herpes group virus Aerobic gram-negative organisms	Chemotherapy Radiation therapy Vascular access devices

Factors increasing the risk of infection in cancer patients—cont'd		
Factor promoting infection	**Examples of associated organisms**	**Examples of disease states**

Environmental problems
  Construction
  Poor airflow
  Contaminated water
    supply
  Raw foods
	Aspergillus spp.
	Mycobacterium tuberculosis
	Legionella spp.
	Aerobic gram-negative
	  organisms
		Organ transplants
		Neutropenia

Anatomic mechanical
  problems
	Anaerobes
	Staphylococci
	Aerobic gram-negative
	  organisms
		Lung cancer causing airway blockage
		Skin or mucosal disruption due to
		  primary or metastatic cancer
		Bowel obstruction due to primary
		  or metastatic cancer
		Urinary obstruction due to renal or
		  cervical cancer

Prior infection with organism that has propensity to recur	*Aspergillus* spp. *Candida* spp. Herpes group virus	Not disease-specific

2. Why should patients have a dental consultation before they begin chemotherapy?

Before administering myelosuppressive chemotherapy, it is good practice to take care of sites that are actively infected and to consider preventive care for potential sources of infection. A dental site that is a minor problem in normal hosts may become a life-threatening source in neutropenic patients.

3. What is the most significant predisposing factor to infection in cancer patients?

Neutropenia. Neutrophils are mature white cells that attack and destroy invading bacteria, viruses, and fungi (particularly *Aspergillus* and *Candida* spp.). The absolute neutrophil count (ANC) is calculated by multiplying the percentage of granulocytes (neutrophils = segments + bands) by the total white blood cell (WBC) count. The risk of infection rises as the WBC count falls, with the greatest risk at neutrophil counts less than 500/mm³. Most serious infections occur in patients with neutrophil counts less than 100/mm³. In addition to presence and degree, duration of the neutropenia is also important. As the duration of neutropenia increases, the risk of infection increases, ultimately reaching 100%. A duration of 3 to 7 days is much less of a risk than a duration beyond 14 days. Currently, about one third of neutropenic patients with fever have a microbiologically proven infection (positive blood cultures), whereas about one fifth have clinically apparent infection with negative cultures.

4. What is low-risk neutropenia?

Low-risk neutropenia is a relative term used to describe neutrophil counts less than 500/mm³ but greater than 100/mm³ with an expected duration of less than 7 to 10 days. Such neutropenias are often seen after chemotherapy for solid tumors (as opposed to the neutropenia that follows therapy for leukemias or bone marrow transplant). Patients are considered at low risk because they usually respond well to initial antibiotic therapy. An oral quinolone (e.g., levofloxacin) is often used empirically because of its broad-spectrum gram-negative activity and excellent oral bioavailability.

5. Describe the management of patients with low-risk neutropenia.

Many centers use outpatient therapy for patients with low-risk neutropenia. Patients are treated entirely as outpatients or have responded well to initial inpatient treatment. Outpatient management should be done only by clinicians experienced in the management of neutropenic fevers. Candidates for outpatient therapy should be symptomatically well without hypotension, have no comorbid conditions (e.g., heart failure, kidney failure, serious chronic obstructive pulmonary disease), a responsive tumor, good outpatient support systems, and easy access for follow-up and readmission.

6. List important neutropenic precautions?

- Strict hand washing is the most important precaution.
- Routine wearing of masks by health care providers is not necessary. Providers with a transmissible respiratory disease should not care for the patient. The practice of requiring hospitalized patients to wear a mask when leaving their rooms varies by institution.
- Ideally, the airflow in the patient's room should be positive compared with the hall. The intent is to avoid exposure to airborne pathogens, such as *Aspergillus* spp.
- The patient's room should not be cleaned in a manner that causes dust to be shed (e.g., from drapes).
- Sources of gram-negative organisms should be avoided (e.g., live flowers in water, raw food).

7. What else can be done to prevent infections in neutropenic patients?

- **High-efficiency particulate air (HEPA) filtration** is used by many centers for patients who undergo organ transplantation or who are expected to have prolonged neutropenia from therapy. The intent is to remove airborne pathogens, such as *Aspergillus* spp.
- **Immunizations** should be up to date, including pneumococcal and *Haemophilus influenzae* vaccines. Special consideration should be given to patients about to undergo elective splenectomy. Such patients should receive the above vaccines as well as a meningococcal vaccine.
- **Prophylactic antibiotic** use has become a more common practice. Experience with prophylactic agents has been mixed, ranging from spectacular success with acyclovir and ganciclovir in bone marrow transplant recipients to failure with nystatin. Prophylactic regimens, especially those that include a quinolone (e.g., levofloxacin) may reduce infection-related and all causes of mortality by about 4% in afebrile neutropenic patients. Major problems of prophylactic agents are that they promote resistant bacteria and are partially responsible for the emergence of *Staphylococcus epidermidis* and enterococci as significant pathogens in neutropenic patients.
- **Granulocyte colony-stimulating factors (G-CSFs)** used proactively shorten the duration of chemotherapy-induced neutropenia, reduce complications due to neutropenia, and decrease the incidence of hospitalizations for febrile neutropenia. The cost-benefit ratio is best in patients with an expected prolonged duration of neutropenia (> 7 to 10 days) and high risk of infection with opportunistic pathogens, such as *Aspergillus* spp.

8. When is fever in neutropenic patients significant?

Fever in the presence of neutropenia is always significant and should be treated as a medical emergency. A patient may die within hours if prompt and effective therapy is not begun. In neutropenic patients, fever is usually regarded and treated as indicating the presence of bacteria in the blood (bacteremia). Clinical evidence of infection and systemic response are usually equated with sepsis; evidence of organ dysfunction (oliguria, altered mentation) indicates sepsis syndrome. If hypotension is added to the list, the result is severe sepsis. If the hypotension is not relieved by fluid resuscitation, septic shock is present. This spectrum of response to infection involves a complex and incompletely understood cascade of events triggered by the presence of bacteria, fungi, or viruses.

Although there is no universal agreement, most authorities agree that significant fever in the neutropenic patient is a single oral temperature greater than 38.3° C (101° F) in the absence of a clear cause (e.g., administration of blood products), or the presence of a temperature greater than 38° C (100.4° F) for 1 hour or more. In certain situations the febrile response may be greatly blunted, absent, or less than expected. Steroid therapy is the most common culprit. Treatment with nonsteroidal antiinflammatory drugs (NSAIDs), old age, renal failure, and overwhelming infection also may blunt the normal fever response. Unfortunately, the absence of fever does not mean that the patient does not have a potentially serious infection.

9. What should be done when the neutropenic patient becomes febrile?

- Assess vital signs and evaluate early signs and symptoms of serious infection without delay.
- Obtain appropriate cultures of blood, urine (even with no signs or symptoms), throat (in presence of abnormal findings), stool (in presence of diarrhea), stool for *Clostridium difficile* toxin assay (with current or recent antibiotic treatment), and intravenous (IV) line sites with evidence of inflammation.
- Administer antibiotic therapy promptly, ideally within 1 hour of recognizing the fever.
- Obtain other tests appropriate to the signs and symptoms. Keep in mind that without neutrophils, many of the expected signs and symptoms of inflammation may be minimal or absent. For new skin findings, consider immediate evaluation with biopsy and culture. Obtain a baseline chest radiograph in the presence of signs or symptoms attributable to the lungs. CT scans of the chest have been shown to be more sensitive than plain chest x-rays in detecting pulmonary abnormalities but unfortunately have not been shown to improve outcome. A question of sinus disease should prompt an early CT scan of the sinuses; plain radiographs are often not sensitive enough to pick up early evidence of infection.

10. What empirical antibiotics should be prescribed to neutropenic febrile patients?

In the absence of findings that may direct therapy (e.g., pus from a vascular access device (VAD) exit site with gram-positive cocci in clusters, which suggests a staphylococcal species), all broad-spectrum regimens (regimens containing antibiotics that are anticipated to be effective against the commonly found gram-negative bacteria) appear to work equally well. Initial clinical responses vary from 60% to 80%. This variation is probably due to differences in study design, patient populations in different centers, antibiotic use, and antibiotic susceptibility, according to the institution. Broad-spectrum combination antibiotic regimens may include an extended-spectrum penicillin (e.g., ticarcillin, piperacillin) plus an aminoglycoside (e.g., gentamicin, amikacin), a third-generation cephalosporin, (e.g., ceftazidime) or a carbapenem (e.g., meropenem).

Clinical trials and experience support the use of broad-spectrum monotherapy with agents that have antipseudomonal activity (e.g., ceftazidime, imipenem, meropenem). Some physicians prefer treatment with two antibiotics when the patient exhibits altered vital signs from infection. The decision usually is determined by the institution's antibiotic susceptibilities. For example, if a patient is on a medical or surgical ward with infection problems from a resistant strain of *Enterobacter* spp., initial therapy should cover the possibility that the patient is infected with this organism.

Coverage for staphylococci is not given initially unless there is reason to suspect a source for staphylococci. Other agents may be added as necessary for special circumstances (e.g., to cover anaerobes in the case of suspected typhlitis).

11. What is a Gram stain?

This valuable tool, developed over 100 years ago by Dr. Hans Gram, allows bacteria to be picked out from cellular material and debris under a microscope. It is a basic test that can be done in a few minutes at little cost. The technique consists of several sequential steps with a different staining solution (crystal violet, iodine, acetone-alcohol, or safranin) in each step. It takes advantage of the different ways that staining solutions are retained within bacteria. Bacteria that retain the crystal violet-iodine complex appear dark blue or violet. Bacteria that cannot retain this complex are stained by the safranin and appear pink under the microscope. Organisms that retain the stain and appear blue are said to be gram-positive, whereas organisms that do not retain the stain are said to be gram-negative. By making the organism visible, the Gram stain makes it possible to determine the morphology of the bacteria; that is, whether it is a coccus (spherical) or bacillus (rod-like).

12. Give examples of gram-positive and gram-negative organisms.

- **Gram-positive** organisms include: staphylococci, streptococci, enterococci, *Listeria* spp., and *Bacillus* spp.
- **Gram-negative** organisms include: *Escherichia coli, Klebsiella* spp., *Enterobacter* spp., *Pseudomonas aeruginosa,* and *Bacteroides* spp.

13. What is the source of most bacteria that infects patients with cancer?

Although some infections are acquired from the environment, about 50% of infections in neutropenic cancer patients result from bacteria that make up the patient's endogenous flora (e.g., *Escherichia coli, Enterobacter* spp., *Klebsiella* spp., other gram-negative bacteria, yeast, and anaerobes). A patient's flora may change rapidly on admission to the hospital. In immunosuppressed patients, bacterial flora can change in a matter of hours, quickly resembling the bacteria found in the hospital setting.

14. What are the risk factors that predispose a patient to fungal infection?

- Previous fungal infection
- Environmental exposure
- Treatment with broad-spectrum antibiotics and steroids
- Use of indwelling venous access devices (VADs)
- Intensive chemotherapeutic regimens
- Immunosuppressive therapies used to treat graft vs. host disease in patients with stem cell transplants
- Prolonged neutropenia

15. List the early signs and symptoms of serious infection.

- Decrease in mentation
- Decrease in urine output

- Decrease in platelet count
- Decrease or increase in body temperature
- Increase in blood glucose level
- Increase in heart rate or respiration

16. **What aspects of the physical assessment should receive particular attention in patients with suspected infection?**

Physical assessment in patients with suspected infection

System	Assessment goals
Skin	Check all current and previous IV sites New rashes: consider drug reaction, blood-borne spread of bacteria or fungi Perianal pain or inflammation: consider hemorrhoids, fissure, phlegmon (inflammation of soft tissue due to infection)
Head and neck	Headache, sinus, or jaw pain: consider sinusitis Nasal ulcers or mucosal necrosis: consider fungal involvement Cotton wool spots in front of retina: consider candidal infection Oral mucosal white patches that rub off: consider candidal infection Oral ulcers: consider herpes, gram-negative bacteria, chemotherapy Odynophagia (pain when swallowing): with oral ulcers, consider herpes virus; with thrush, consider candidal esophagitis
Lungs	Findings on exam may be minimal; may precede radiographic abnormalities
Abdomen	Rebound tenderness, especially involving the right lower quadrant: consider typhlitis

17. Define typhlitis.

Typhlitis or neutropenic enterocolitis is a necrotizing infection of the bowel secondary to a combination of factors toxic to the intestinal mucosa. The resulting mucosal damage allows bacterial invasion. The infection, usually involving the large bowel (especially the cecum), results in bowel wall edema, thinning, and perforation. The situation significantly predisposes bacterial translocation. Typhlitis is particularly common in children. Patients may develop symptoms suggesting appendicitis, such as abdominal pain, nausea and vomiting, and fever.

18. How is typhlitis diagnosed and treated?

Blood cultures may be positive despite administration of effective antibiotic therapy. In the proper clinical setting, the diagnosis may be made by CT scan, which shows a thickened bowel wall. Peritoneal lavage with a positive culture for the same organisms as the blood cultures is confirmatory. Medical therapy includes antibiotics to cover the gram-negative organisms, *Candida* spp., and anaerobic organisms. Laxatives and enemas should be avoided. Surgical intervention may be indicated. Unfortunately, surgery is usually difficult because the patients are critically ill and poor surgical risks.

19. Define ecthyma gangrenosum.

Ecthyma gangrenosum is a skin manifestation of the vascular spread of bacteria that are usually gram-negative. *Pseudomonas aeruginosa* is the most commonly involved organism.

Other organisms include staphylococci and fungi, such as *Aspergillus* and *Alternaria* spp. Blood cultures are often positive for the causative bacteria. Lesions begin as nodular papules that quickly progress to central blebs, then ulcerate with underlying induration and central necrosis. The lesions are usually erythematous, often with a violaceous hue. Not unlike petechiae, they may be somewhat hidden in skin folds, buttocks, and the perineum.

20. What are MRSA and MRSE? Why are they significant?

MRSA is methicillin-resistant *Staphylococcus aureus*. MRSE is methicillin-resistant *Staphylococcus epidermidis*. Penicillins and cephalosporins belong to the beta-lactam class of antibiotics. The beta-lactam antibiotics bind to a receptor in bacteria and interrupt the synthesis of the bacterial cell wall, leading to cell death. Shortly after the introduction of penicillin, many bacteria developed resistance by producing a beta-lactamase enzyme that destroyed a portion of the penicillin molecule (the beta-lactam ring), rendering the antibiotic inactive. Biochemists retaliated by making penicillins that were resistant to the destructive action of this enzyme (e.g., nafcillin, methicillin).

In recent years, staphylococci resistant to all antibiotics of the beta lactamase-resistant class have evolved. They have a receptor that is much more difficult for the antibiotics to bind. MRSAs are resistant to all beta-lactam antibiotics (e.g., penicillins, cephalosporins, and carbapenems). They are often susceptible to trimethoprim-sulfamethoxazole but usually are treated with vancomycin. Infection with MRSA can be deadly, and the necessity of using more vancomycin has led to increased resistance of other bacteria to vancomycin. A good example of this resistance development is the vancomycin-resistant enterococci, which have become a problem in many medical centers. Alternative antibiotics with activity include linezolid and daptomycin and they should not be used for pulmonary infections.

21. Define bacterial translocation.

Bacterial translocation is the movement of living bacteria from the gastrointestinal tract to the mesenteric lymph nodes and blood stream and thus to other organs. Every moment of our lives, bowel flora are either prevented from translocating or are quickly cleared when they try to move across the bowel wall. In the presence of neutropenia and other immunosuppression, life-threatening infections can result from mucosal disruption of the bowel wall caused by chemotherapy, invading organisms, or antibiotic suppression of normal bowel anaerobic bacteria (the predominant normal bowel flora that help to prevent translocation). Gram-negative organisms most likely to translocate include *E. coli, Klebsiella* spp., and *Pseudomonas aeruginosa*. Nutritional counseling may be important. Many authorities believe that fiber ingestion assists in mucosal preservation, thus decreasing the rate at which bacterial translocation occurs.

22. How many blood cultures should be done? How much blood is needed per culture?

Two pairs of aerobic and anaerobic blood cultures are usually enough to obtain a positive result. Because many culture systems are optimized for a given amount of blood, it is important to obtain the amount of blood required by the hospital laboratory.

23. How far apart should blood cultures be done?

The time interval between cultures need be only as long as it takes to prepare the second site after the first culture is obtained. Delaying therapy so that a second blood culture can be done in 30 or 60 minutes places the patient at needless risk.

24. Should blood be obtained from venous access devices?

Whether to draw blood through a VAD is problematic but is usually done. The advantage is that a positive culture from the VAD may suggest the catheter as the source of infection. The bad news is that it may be a contaminant from the hardware of the VAD.

If your institution has the ability, quantification of the number of colony-forming units (CFUs) of bacteria may help to decide whether the positive culture is a contaminant.

- If the central catheter and peripheral culture sites yield positive cultures and the central catheter culture has 5 times the number of CFUs as the peripheral site, the central catheter is probably the source.
- If the peripheral culture is negative and the central catheter culture colony count is low (< 100 CFUs/ml of blood), the central culture may represent contamination.
- If the culture from the central catheter is positive more than 2 hours sooner than the peripheral culture, it is likely that the central catheter is the source of infection.

25. What are the indications to remove an infected VAD?

- Lack of response to appropriate antibiotic therapy after 48 to 72 hours
- Persistent positive blood cultures
- Deteriorating patient
- Tunnel infection
- Line malfunction to include thrombosis
- Infection with organisms poorly responsive to antimicrobial therapy (e.g., *Bacillus* spp., *Corynebacterium* spp., mycobacteria, fungal species)

26. What strategies are used to guide therapy for infected VADs?

Therapeutic strategies are guided by the identity of the infecting organism and location of infection.

Therapeutic strategies based on infecting organism and location

Organism	Location	Therapy
Staphylococcus epidermidis	Exit site	Medical therapy
	Tunnel	Consider removal
	Port	Remove port
Staphylococcus aureus	Exit site	Consider medical therapy
	Line or tunnel	Remove line
	Port	Remove port
Candida spp. and *Mycobacterium* spp.	Exit site	Remove line
	Tunnel	Remove line
	Port	Remove port
Gram-negative organisms	Exit site	Try medical therapy
	Line	Remove line
	Tunnel	50% failure rate with medical therapy

In short, for all but a *Staphylococcus epidermidis* exit site infection, device removal is the preferred option. Do *not* lose sight of the patient when applying these or any other guidelines. If the patient is not doing well, even with a site or organism that should respond to medical therapy, remove the VAD. Most febrile neutropenic patients without a VAD infection can be treated successfully without removing the VAD.

27. What factors should be considered in choosing an antibiotic regimen?

- Patient drug allergies
- Route of administration

- Concomitant drugs
- Suspected organism
- Antibiotic resistance patterns
- Previous antibiotic therapy
- Previous infecting organisms
- Duration of neutropenia
- Patient exposure to pathogens

28. **Which antimicrobial agents have been used to prevent or delay infection in patients undergoing chemotherapy?**
    - **Antibiotics:** The quinolones, trimethoprim-sulfamethoxazole, oral aminoglycosides, and oral amphotericin B are used for selective bowel decontamination. The use of trimethoprim-sulfamethoxazole to prevent *Pneumocystis carinii* pneumonia is well established in marrow stem cell transplant recipients, as well as in patients receiving the monoclonal antibody, alemtuzumab, and the antimetabolite, fludarabine.
    - **Antifungal agents:** imidazoles (e.g., fluconazole)
    - **Antiviral agents:** acyclovir and ganciclovir
    - **Isoniazid** is used to prevent reactivation of tuberculosis in patients with a positive tuberculosis skin test, particularly patients with lymphoreticular cancer.

29. **Summarize the most commonly used antibiotics in neutropenic febrile patients.**

Common antibiotics in neutropenic febrile treatment

Class	Examples	Spectrum/Activity	Cautions
Penicillins	Ticarcillin Piperacillin	Streptococci Gram-negative anaerobes	Allergic reactions Potassium loss Rash with allopurinol Drug-induced neutropenia
Cephalosporins	Ceftazidime	Streptococci Gram-negative organisms	Allergic reactions Drug-induced neutropenia
Quinolones	Ciprofloxacin Levofloxacin	Gram-negative organisms *Legionella* spp.	GI absorption decreased by aluminum, magnesium, iron, zinc, sucralfate
Aminoglycosides	Gentamicin Tobramycin Amikacin	Gram-negative organisms	Avoid with cisplatin Avoid with cyclosporine Ototoxicity Nephrotoxicity Avoid with amphotericin B
Sulfonamides	Sulfamethoxazole (with trimethoprim)	Gram-negative organisms *Pneumocystis carinii*	Allergic reactions Marrow suppression
Glycopeptides	Vancomycin Teicoplanin	Gram-positive organisms	Red neck, red man syndrome Drug-induced neutropenia
Imidazoles	Fluconazole Voriconazole	*Candida* spp. *Aspergillus* spp.	*Candida* spp. resistance Multiple potential hepatic drug interactions
Echinocandins	Caspofungin	*Candida* spp.	Intravenous use only

30. Why is it necessary to review the patient's previous antibiotic regimens?

Antibiotics used for previous infections can greatly affect the likely organisms currently infecting a neutropenic patient. If an antibiotic that kills or suppresses one kind of bacteria is given, other bacteria or fungi that are resistant to the agent will try to take over the niche left by the killed bacteria. In treating a patient with a quinolone antibiotic, beware of anaerobic bacteria and yeast. Vancomycin therapy leaves gram-negative organisms without the usual competition from gram-positive organisms. Broad-spectrum antibiotics give a free hand to fungi. Even the imidazole class of antifungal agents (ketoconazole, fluconazole, itraconazole) may allow growth of fungi that are resistant to the imidazoles.

31. How long should antibiotics be continued?

In general, antibiotics are continued for the duration of the neutropenia. Guidelines to consider include the following:
- **No fever and > 500/mm³ neutrophils**
  - No source of infection: stop antibiotics
  - Known source of infection: give course appropriate for source
- **No fever and < 500/mm³ neutrophils**: continue antibiotics for up to 14 days
- **Fever and ≥ 500/mm³ neutrophils**: consider changing or stopping therapy after evaluation for:
  - Hidden site of infection
  - Abscess or catheter-related infection
  - Resistant bacteria, fungi, or virus
  - Drug-induced fever
  - Tumor fever
- **Fever and < 500/mm³ neutrophils**: continue antibiotics and consider:
  - Fungal superinfection
  - Inadequate antibiotic dosing
  - Resistant bacteria
  - Viral infection
  - Abscess or catheter-related infection

32. What is meant by a third- or fourth-generation antibiotic?

The habit of referring to cephalosporins by generation was popularized by pharmaceutical companies and has evolved into calling an antibiotic with expanded activity the product of a new generation. The generation refers roughly to the order in which the drug was introduced and the range of bacteria against which it is active. The first-generation cephalosporins (e.g., cephalothin, cefazolin) have good activity against *Staphylococcus aureus*. The following generations tend to have less activity against staphylococci. The second- and third-generation cephalosporins (e.g., cefamandole and ceftriaxone, respectively) tend to have increased activity against gram-negative aerobic bacteria. The term fourth-generation is sometimes used to denote the extremely broad-spectrum carbapenem class of beta lactam antibiotics (e.g., meropenem).

33. What is antibiotic lock therapy?

Antibiotic lock therapy is a relatively new approach to the management of an infected catheter line. A small volume of concentrated antibiotic solution is placed in the lumen of the catheter and allowed to remain for hours. The approach is said to work poorly for candidal infections. A variation of this technique uses fibrinolytic therapy (tissue plasminogen activator) locally instilled as an adjunct to antibiotic therapy. The fibrinolytic agent is thought to exert its antibacterial effect by dissolving the fibrin layer on the interior of the catheter that promotes adherence of bacteria and development of thrombus. Caution is indicated in considering this procedure in the presence of an infected thrombus because the potentially large bacterial burden that may be released into the bloodstream may worsen signs and symptoms of systemic infection.

34. Are all fevers due to infections?

No. Fevers in patients with cancer are commonly drug-induced or related to the cancer itself (e.g., leukemias, lymphomas, renal cell cancer, liver cancer).

35. What is drug-induced fever?

Drug-induced fever is caused by the drug itself. Drugs that induce fevers include antibiotics, antifungals (e.g., amphotericin B), allopurinol, biologic response modifiers, and chemotherapy agents (e.g., bleomycin, dactinomycin, gemcitabine). The usual mechanism is production of antibody by the patient's immune system that reacts with the drug to cause fever. The diagnosis of drug-induced fever may be relatively easy or obscure and challenging.

36. What clues point to the presence of drug-induced fever?

- Timing of the fever. Drug-induced fever may occur with each administration of the drug or after 10 to 14 days of treatment (a typical time frame for the patient's immune system to develop antibodies to the drug). The time to development of drug fever may be accelerated if the patient has received the drug before and already has developed antibodies.
- Appearance of the patient. The patient often appears well. The pulse may not be elevated in proportion to the fever. Patients also may appear quite ill, with shaking chills (as in reactions to quinidine).
- Signs/symptoms. The patient may have a rash (not due to infection) and/or other evidence of drug-induced end-organ dysfunction (e.g., interstitial nephritis or hepatitis).
- No other reason for the fever.

37. Amphotericin B has a bad reputation for side effects and for causing problems with kidney and bone marrow function. Is there any truth to this reputation?

Considerable folklore surrounds the administration of amphotericin B ("amphoterrible"). Common signs and symptoms include chills and fever, phlebitis, and nausea and vomiting. Renal problems include tubular dysfunction leading to loss of electrolytes (particularly potassium and bicarbonate) and suppression of erythropoietin production by the kidney. Newer lipid formulations, amphotericin B lipid complex (Abelcet) and amphotericin B liposomal (AmBisome) are better tolerated and considerably more expensive.

38. What should be done to assist in the administration of amphotericin B?

- Extend administration period to 1 to 2 hours.
- Reassure the patient that administration of the drug usually is better tolerated with time.
- Use meperidine 25-50 mg intravenously, to terminate chills and fever. Rare intractable chills and fever may be treated with dantrolene.
- To help avoid renal toxicity, maintain adequate volume status. Saline boluses given with the infusions are often used for this purpose.
- Consider using the newer lipid-complexed and liposomal preparations of amphotericin B, which may be better tolerated and have less renal and bone marrow toxicity. Thus, larger doses may be given.

39. True or false: A patient who receives vancomycin and experiences flushing, wheezing, and hypotension is most likely allergic to vancomycin.

False. The so-called red neck or red man syndrome (from the flushed appearance of the face, neck, and upper torso) is not, strictly speaking, an allergy. Classic allergic reactions are defined by the presence of an antibody that reacts with the patient's immune system to produce the allergic response. Vancomycin directly causes release of histamine from mast cells; antibodies have no role. The histamine causes the vasodilation, flushing, and wheezing. Because histamine release from mast cells is also important in anaphylactic reactions (IgE-mediated mast-cell degranulation), it is not difficult to understand how the patient's clinical appearance suggests an allergic reaction. The patient is not allergic to vancomycin in this setting. Tolerance to infusions tends to improve with time. Do not infuse vancomycin rapidly unless you have never seen the red neck syndrome and would like to do so. Infusion times longer than 60 to 90 minutes is recommended.

40. Allogeneic marrow stem cell transplants result in severe immunosuppression in recipients. When and what infections are patients prone to develop?

The time of greatest risk for infection in marrow stem cell recipients can be divided roughly into three phases:

1. The first 30 days after transplant involve the immunosuppressant effects of a pretransplant bone marrow-eradicating regimen of irradiation and chemotherapy. After transplant, immunosuppressive medication (e.g., cyclosporine) is also used. Profound, prolonged neutropenia is present, with the increased possibility of gram-negative and gram-positive infections. Antibiotic treatment promotes common candidal infection. A striking concern is the risk for herpes simplex virus in patients who are seropositive before transplant.
2. After the first 30 days, initial engraftment of the transplanted marrow begins. Cytomegalovirus infections replace herpes simplex as the major viral concern, with the potential for severe involvement of multiple organ systems. *Aspergillus* spp. replace *Candida* spp. as the major fungal pathogen.
3. After 90 to 100 days, bone marrow engraftment is completed. Unfortunately, the immune system does not completely recover for up to 1 to 2 years. The patient remains at increased risk for infections with organisms, particularly the pneumococci, that take advantage of poor immunoglobulin function. Varicella zoster replaces cytomegalovirus as the principal viral pathogen. Another major problem is graft vs. host disease, which can begin during the time of bone marrow engraftment. Graft vs. host disease may require immunosuppressive therapy, which further increases the risk of infection.

41. What are some new antibiotic drugs used in the oncology setting and how do they work?

- Linezolid (Zyvox) is the first commercially available member of a new class of antibiotics, the oxazolidinones. Linezolid acts early to block bacterial protein synthesis by preventing the binding of messenger RNA to the 30s ribosome. This mechanism of action is unique to this class of antibiotics, and cross-resistance to other antibiotics has not been reported. Although linezolid is effective against some anaerobic bacteria, the spectrum of activity is largely against gram-positive organisms, including MRSA and vancomycin-resistant enterococci (VRE). Although clinical experience is limited, linezolid appears to be better tolerated and easier to administer than quinupristin/dalfopristin (Synercid), a member of the streptogramin class of antibiotics with similar antibacterial activity. Linezolid is 100% bioavailable, which means it should work well by mouth as well as by intravenous administration. Currently, linezolid is marketed for treatment of nosocomial infections due to susceptible organisms. Hematologic toxicity may limit its use in the recovering bone marrow.

- Daptomycin (Cubicin) is a reintroduced lipopeptide antibiotic that acts by binding to and depolarizing bacterial membranes. This unique mechanism of action allows activity against a wide variety of gram-positive organisms to include MRSA and VRE. This drug is also better tolerated than quinupristin/dalfopristin but is available as an intravenous formulation only. Daptomycin is inactivated in the lung and should *not* be used to treat pneumonia.

 Key Points

- Fever in a neutropenic patient is a medical emergency.
- Outpatient treatment of neutropenic fever requires an assessment of the risk.
- Prophylactic antibiotics in afebrile neutropenic patients reduce mortality from all causes and mortality due to infection by about 4%.
- The most important precaution for people with neutropenia is strict hand washing.
- VAD infections beyond the exit site require catheter removal.

 Internet Resources

National Cancer Comprehensive Network (Treatment Guidelines for Patients): Fever and neutropenic treatment guidelines for patients with cancer, v.1. 2006: http://www.nccn.org/patients/patient_gls/_english/_fever_and_neutropenia/ 1_introduction.asp

Infectious Diseases Society of America (Practice Guidelines): Fever: neutropenic patient; Outpatient parenteral anti-infective therapy; Catheter-related infections: http://www.idsociety.org/Content/NavigationMenu/Practice_Guidelines/Standards_ Practice_Guidelines_Statements/Standards,_Practice_Guidelines,_and_Statements.htm

Centers for Disease Control and Prevention (Morbidity and Mortality Weekly Reports: Recommendations and Reports): Guidelines for the prevention of intravascular catheter-related infections: http://www.cdc.gov/mmwr/PDF/rr/rr5110.pdf

Oncology Nursing Society: Prevention of Infection Interventions: http://www.ons.org/outcomes/PEPcard/prevention.shtml

Bibliography

Forest GN, Walsh TJ: Approaches to management of invasive fungal infections in patients with hematologic malignancies. *Support Cancer Ther* 2(1):21-30, 2004.

Gafter-Gvili A, Fraser A, Paul M, et al: Meta-analysis: Prophylaxis reduces mortality in neutropenic patients. *Ann Intern Med* 142:979-995, 2005.

Hoeprich PD: Clinical use of amphotericin B and derivatives: Lore, mystique, and fact. *Clin Infect Dis* 14(suppl 1):S114–S119, 1992.

Hughes WT, Armstrong D, Bodey, GP, et al: 2002 Guidelines for the use of antimicrobial agents in neutropenic patients with cancer. *Clin Infect Dis* 34:730-751, 2002.

Kern WV: Risk assessment and treatment of low risk patients with febrile neutropenia. *Clin Infect Dis* 42:533-540, 2006.

Moore K, Crom D: Hematopoietic support with moderately myelosuppressive chemotherapy regimens: A nursing perspective. *Clin J Oncol Nurs* 10(3):383-388, 2006.

Raad I, Hanna HA, Alakech B, et al: Differential time to positivity: A useful method for diagnosing catheter-related bloodstream infections. *Ann Intern Med* 140(1):18-25, 2004.

Vento S, Cainelli F: Infections in patients with cancer undergoing chemotherapy: Aetiology, prevention, and treatment. *Lancet Oncol* 4:595-604, 2003.

Syndrome of Inappropriate Antidiuretic Hormone (SIADH)

Leigh K. Kaszyk and Jaine Jewell

1. What is the syndrome of inappropriate antidiuretic hormone?

The syndrome of inappropriate antidiuretic hormone (SIADH) is a syndrome of hyponatremia due to abnormal secretion or production of antidiuretic hormone (ADH). Despite a normal intravascular volume, the urine osmolality is inappropriately high (concentrated) compared with plasma osmolality. ADH causes water retention, which leads to decreased sodium and inability to excrete dilute urine. SIADH may also be called *dilutional hyponatremia*.

2. What physiologic mechanisms maintain normal plasma osmolality and plasma sodium concentrations?

1. ADH, also known as vasopressin, helps the body to conserve water. ADH is secreted by the posterior pituitary in response to hypotension, decreased fluid intake, and blood loss. Water is conserved when ADH is released; hence the word *antidiuretic* in its name. ADH acts on the distal renal tubules to increase permeability, resulting in increased reabsorption of water from the kidney.
2. The thirst mechanism is activated by osmoreceptors in the hypothalamus in response to dry mouth, hyperosmolality, and plasma volume depletion. A water loss of 2% of body weight or increase in osmolality activates the thirst mechanism.

3. How does ADH affect the body?

When blood levels of ADH increase, the epithelium of the cortical collecting ducts of the kidneys becomes water-permeable. Water enters the extracellular fluid through osmosis, less water is excreted, and urine osmolality increases. The results are excessive water retention and dilutional hyponatremia.

4. Why do so many cancer patients develop SIADH?

Many types of cancerous tumors and metastases (lung, prostate, and gastrointestinal cancers; thymoma; mesothelioma; and lymphomas) cause the body to release ADH. Also, some cancer patients receive drugs, such as cytotoxic agents, morphine and tricyclic antidepressants, which release or potentiate the release of ADH. In addition, certain lung conditions that are common in cancer patients (pneumonia, emphysema) may result in SIADH.

5. What other pathogenic mechanisms are responsible for SIADH?

SIADH may also be caused by other factors, such as:
- Production of atrial natriuretic peptide (ANP) from the cardiac atrial tissue
- Injury to the cells of the central nervous system (CNS) by such mechanisms as trauma, hemorrhage, infection, and Guillain-Barré syndrome

- Medications, such as:
  - Nonsteroidal antiinflammatory drugs (NSAIDS)
  - Tricyclic and monoamine oxidase antidepressants, as well as selective serotonin uptake inhibitors
  - Thiazide diuretics, barbiturates, and anesthetics
  - Antibiotics, such as azithromycin
  - Neuroleptics (e.g., antipsychotics, phenothiazines)
  - Oral hypoglycemics (chlorpropamide, tolbutamide)
  - Clofibrate, carbamazepine
- Pulmonary disorders, such as pneumonia, tuberculosis, lung abscess, empyema, cystic fibrosis, pneumothorax, chronic obstructive pulmonary disorder (COPD), asthma, positive pressure ventilation
- Nausea
- Pain
- Stress
- Cigarette smoking

6. How is SIADH diagnosed?

First, the patient must be assessed clinically (history and physical exam) to determine whether intravascular volume is normal, low, or expanded. Blood and urine specimens are obtained for assessment of sodium and osmolality. The patient has SIADH if the intravascular volume is normal or increased; urine osmolality is high compared with plasma osmolality; and renal, thyroid, and adrenal function are normal.

Observe for fluid overload: weigh patient, maintain strict input and output values, and test urine for specific gravity. To make a diagnosis of SIADH, adrenal insufficiency and hypothyroidism must be ruled out, because both may increase ADH secretion.

7. Which laboratory values should the nurse observe in patients with SIADH?

Laboratory values for SIADH treatment

Test	SIADH levels	Normal levels
Serum sodium	Low serum sodium (< 130 mEq/L)	135-145 mEq/L
Serum osmolality	Low serum osmolality (< 280 mOsm/kg)	280-300 mOsm/kg
Urine sodium	High urine sodium level (> 20 mEq/L)	40-220 mmol/L
Urine osmolality	High urine osmolality (> 1400 mOsm/kg)	200-800 mOsm/kg
Blood urea nitrogen (BUN)	Low BUN	6-23 mg/dl
Serum creatinine	Low creatinine	0.6-1.1 mg/dl
Uric acid	Low uric acid	Male: 3.4-7.0 g/dl
		Female: 2.4-5.7 g/dl
Serum albumin	Low albumin	3.4-5.0 g/dl

8. What are the early signs and symptoms of SIADH?

- Mild hyponatremia (sodium level 115-130 mEq/l)
- Fatigue and weakness
- Nausea, vomiting, anorexia, thirst, diarrhea

- Headaches, lethargy, confusion, irritability
- Decreased urine output, weight gain
- Myalgias, muscle cramping

9. What are some later signs and symptoms?

- Altered mental status
- Confusion, personality changes
- Psychosis
- Seizures
- Progressive lethargy, coma

10. How is SIADH treated?

Treatment of SIADH focuses on determination and treatment of the underlying cause. Initial interventions are aimed at correcting the sodium-water imbalance. Discontinue agents that contribute to SIADH, such as diuretics, morphine, and antidepressants. For patients with cancer, the primary goal is treatment with systemic chemotherapy.

11. How are the patients managed until these solutions take effect?

- Fluid restriction of 500-1000 ml/day for mild to moderate SIADH (sodium level > 125 mEq/l)
- Offering the patient high sodium beverages (tomato juice, V8 juice, beef or chicken broth, or Gatorade)
- IV hypertonic saline, with concurrent administration of furosemide to increase fluid excretion in the presence of life-threatening hyponatremia.

12. What nursing interventions are recommended for the treatment of the patient with SIADH?

- Restrict fluids to 500-1000 ml/day.
  - Divide the amount of fluids the patient consumes among day, evening, and night hours and post in the patient's room. Educate the patient and family.
- Rinse the patient's mouth every 2 hours, and offer sugar-free candy and gum to stimulate salivation.
- If the patient is confused, orient the patient to person, time, and place using cues, such as calendars and clocks.
- Implement seizure precautions as necessary.

13. What is done for patients with chronic or recurrent SIADH despite chemotherapy?

Chronic or recurrent SIADH is treated with drugs that inhibit the renal effects of ADH, such as demeclocycline, furosemide, and lithium.

14. What are the nursing implications of demeclocycline treatment?

Demeclocycline (Declomycin) 600 to 1200 mg daily may be prescribed for patients who are unable to comply with fluid restriction, or who have persistent severe hyponatremia. This tetracycline derivative interferes with ADH action by decreasing the renal response to ADH, causing isotonic or hypotonic urine and an increase in serum sodium. Absorption may be impaired if the drug is taken with milk or milk products. Side effects include photosensitivity, hematologic changes, azotemia, superinfection, and mild nausea or heartburn. This medication should be used with caution in patients with hepatic or renal insufficiency.

15. Does recurrent SIADH mean that the cancer is returning?

SIADH usually resolves once the cancer is treated. However, it may return during stable disease while the patient is receiving maintenance chemotherapy.

Key Points

- SIADH may also be known as *dilutional hyponatremia*.
- SIADH is commonly seen in patients with cancer.
- SIADH can be caused by either the tumor or the treatment of the tumor.
- Signs and symptoms are caused by water intoxication.
- Early signs/symptoms of SIADH include: mild hyponatremia, weight gain, decreased urine output, fatigue, headaches, muscle aches, and vomiting.
- Treatment of SIADH focuses on treating the underlying cause.

Internet Resources

Oncology Nursing Forum, Online Exclusive, Oncology Emergency Modules: SIADH:
    http://www.ons.org/publications/journals/onf/volume30/issue3/3003381.asp
Enotes, Syndrome of Inappropriate Antidiuretic Hormone:
    http://health.enotes.com/cancer-encyclopedia/syndrome-inappropriate-antidiuretic-hormone
emedicine.com, Syndrome of Inappropriate Antidiuretic Hormone Secretions:
    http://www.emedicine.com/emerg/topic784.htm
AllRefer.com, Dilutional Hyponatremia (SIADH):
    http://health.allrefer.com/health/dilutional-hyponatremia-siadh-info.html
University of Iowa Healthcare, Fluid & Electrolyte: Diagnosis and Management:
    http://www.int-med.uiowa.edu/Patients/bonemarrow/Healthpro/FluidElectrolyte/Sodium.htm

Acknowledgment

The authors wish to acknowledge Debra Adornetto-Garcia, RN, MS, for her contribution to the SIADH chapter published in the second edition of *Oncology Nursing Secrets*.

Bibliography

Arnold SM, Lieberman FS, Foon KA: Paraneoplastic syndromes. In DeVita VT, Hellman S, Rosenberg SA, editors: *Cancer: Principles and practices of oncology,* vol 2, ed 7, Philadelphia, 2005, Lippincott-Raven.
Block JB: Paraneoplastic syndromes. In Haskell CM, editor: *Cancer treatment,* ed 5, Philadelphia, 2001, WB Saunders.
McDonnell Keenan AK: Syndrome of inappropriate antidiuretic hormone. In Yarbro CH, Frogge MH, Goodman M, editor: *Cancer nursing: Principles and practice,* ed 6, Boston, 2005, Jones and Bartlett.
Peng Goh K: Management of hyponatremia. *Am Fam Physician,* 69:2387-2394, 2004.

Spinal Cord Compression

Lisa Schulmeister and Christine G. Gatlin

1. Why is spinal cord compression an oncologic emergency?

Spinal cord compression is a true neurologic emergency that develops in 5% to 10% of patients with cancer, and up to 40% of patients with preexisting nonspinal bone metastasis. Without prompt treatment, the patient may become partially or completely paralyzed. Spinal cord compression is sometimes the first presentation of undiagnosed cancer. The key prognostic factor is the neurologic status of the patient at the time of presentation. Significant neurologic deterioration at diagnosis is associated with a worse prognosis. Therefore, spinal cord compression is an oncologic emergency that requires prompt recognition and emergency treatment to relieve pain and preserve neurologic function.

2. What are the most common cancers associated with spinal cord compression?

Breast cancer is the most common cause of spinal cord compression in women. Other cancers that are commonly associated with spinal cord compression include lung and prostate cancer and multiple myeloma. Less commonly associated cancers include lymphomas, melanomas, renal cell cancers, gastrointestinal adenocarcinomas, and sarcomas. In children, sarcomas, neuroblastomas, and lymphomas have been associated with spinal cord compression.

3. What levels of the spine are most frequently involved?

Cancers associated with spinal cord compression

Spinal level	Involvement (%)	Associated cancers
Cervical	10	Lung, breast, kidney, lymphoma, myeloma, melanoma
Thoracic	70	Lung, breast, kidney, lymphoma, myeloma, prostate
Lumbosacral	20	Lung, breast, kidney, lymphoma, myeloma, melanoma, prostate, gastrointestinal

4. How does spinal cord compression occur?

The most common source of spinal cord compression in patients with cancer is metastasis to the epidural space with or without bony involvement. Tumors may also reach the epidural space by direct extension through the intervertebral foramen; in particular, this occurs with lymphomas and nerve sheath tumors. Some primary cancers may occur within the cord itself and may not be associated with pain. Regardless of the route of access, the mass effect of the tumor with associated edema compresses the cord, resulting in ischemia and neural damage. The degree of involvement and speed of compression of the cord explain the wide range of signs and symptoms.

5. Can spinal cord compression be prevented?

Spinal cord compression is often caused by bone metastasis, which is characterized by excess osteoclast number and activity. Bisphosphonates, such as zoledronic acid, pamidronate, and clodronate, inhibit osteoclast activity, differentiation, and survival. Bisphosphonates are used to treat bone metastasis; their role in preventing bone metastasis is currently being studied. Spinal cord epidural metastasis (SEM) progression also can cause spinal cord compression. A newer treatment modality, stereotactic radiosurgery, may be used to treat SEM, and if effective, may prevent the development of spinal cord compression. Lastly, several studies support irradiation of subclinical cord compression as a method of preserving neurologic function. Predictive risk models are being developed to define the population of patients who are at risk for developing cord compression and identify patients who should receive prophylactic radiotherapy.

6. What is the first symptom of spinal cord compression?

Because the dura is pain sensitive, 90% of patients with spinal cord compression report pain as the first symptom. The areas most commonly involved are the thoracic, lumbosacral, and cervical spine. The pain evolves over 4 to 6 weeks before neurologic signs, such as muscle weakness (the second most common symptom), begin to appear. However, very early symptoms of spinal cord compression may be nonspecific.

7. How is back pain caused by spinal cord compression characterized?

The pain may be localized or radicular. Local pain usually occurs at the level of the lesion and is said to be dull and constant. The pain is more severe when the patient moves, coughs, bears weight, or uses the Valsalva maneuver. Ideally, the diagnosis will be made while the patient is having only spinal axis pain—before neurologic deficits develop. Among children, the back pain is characterized as severe and persistent and is often accompanied by stiffness of the affected extremities.

8. How does dural pain from tumor compression differ from referred pain of visceral origin or musculoskeletal back pain?

Patients with cancer also may have other sources of back pain. Musculoskeletal pain, by far the more common, is accentuated by movement and improved with rest; it is not associated with imaging changes of spinal metastasis.

Visceral tumor pain may refer to the back, with a constant boring quality that worsens at rest. The pain may have fleeting sharp qualities, cause sleeplessness, and even be improved with activity. This type of pain may be seen in patients with intraabdominal tumors (pancreatic cancer, lymphoma, or sarcoma). Abdominal computed tomography (CT) scan may be diagnostic.

9. What other signs and symptoms are associated with spinal cord compression?

If the epidural lesion is not detected at the painful phase, ischemic and compressive damage to neurons may follow, often initially manifested as weakness (75%-85% of cases). Weakness may progress rapidly, adding to the clinical urgency of making a diagnosis. The weakness is typically bilateral and corresponds to the level of spinal cord involvement. Cervical lesions cause quadriparesis, whereas thoracic or lumbosacral lesions cause paraparesis. Other motor signs include spasticity, hyperreflexia, abnormal stretch reflexes, and extensor plantar responses. Patients with motor impairment are at high risk for injury. Sensory loss below the level of cord compression and autonomic dysfunction with impotency and bladder or bowel retention (or incontinence) may result. These deficits may occur in any sequence and progress rapidly.

10. How long is the interval from diagnosis of cancer to presentation with symptoms of spinal cord compression?

The interval from diagnosis to presentation depends on the biologic rate of growth of the cancer and varies from the initial presentation to years later. A longer interval from cancer diagnosis to spinal cord compression is associated with improved survival.

11. How is spinal cord compression diagnosed?

- **Physical examination.** Back pain in any patient with cancer should prompt a rapid evaluation. Palpation with gentle percussion over the vertebral spinous processes often will reveal tenderness at the site of involvement. The neurologic findings follow logically from the extent of compromise of cord function. Weakness, as noted above, is often associated with signs of upper motor neuron involvement (spasticity, hyperreflexia). A change in the patient's sensory exam is usually seen below the level of cord involvement. Decreased rectal tone and a distended bladder signal autonomic dysfunction.
- **Laboratory results.** In adults, an elevated alkaline phosphatase level may suggest bony involvement by the cancer.
- **Complete spinal images.** Magnetic resonance imaging (MRI) of the spine is the most sensitive imaging technique used to diagnose spinal cord compression. Images of the entire spine should be obtained since one third of patients have asymptomatic but radiographically evident spinal cord compression distant from the symptomatic site. Spine MRI is best performed without contrast, because contrast agents obscure differentiation between involved and uninvolved bone.

12. How is spinal cord compression treated?

Despite the high frequency of spinal cord compression, there is variation in its management and limited evidence to guide treatment decisions. The majority of patients are treated with fractionated external beam radiotherapy to all sites of compression that have been radiographically identified. Various treatment schedules produce similar functional outcomes.

Surgery for spinal cord compression is associated with a high complication rate and long convalescent period. However, it may be indicated for patients with vertebral body collapse with spinal instability. Radiotherapy is unlikely to decompress the spinal cord, so these patients are best considered for vertebral body resection and spinal reconstruction. Further, patients with compressed areas that do not respond to initial or subsequent radiotherapy may be considered for surgery. In patients with more than one neurologic sign/symptom but who are not totally paraplegic for greater than 48 hours, direct decompressive surgery plus radiotherapy was reported to improve the ability to walk more than radiotherapy alone. Depending on the location and extent of the spinal cord compression, symptoms may also be managed with nonopioid and opioid analgesics, antiinflammatory medications, and/or bisphosphonates.

13. How quickly is treatment for spinal cord compression initiated?

Radiation therapy for spinal cord compression is often initiated as an "emergency"; it is not uncommon for radiation therapy to be delivered in the middle of the night or on weekends. Expedient treatment is just as important as timely diagnosis.

14. Why are corticosteroids given to patients with spinal cord compression?

Corticosteroids (usually intravenous dexamethasone followed by oral dosing) are used in conjunction with various treatment options to reduce edema and mass effect, which lessens pain. Treatment is begun as soon as spinal cord compression is suspected.

Neuropathic pain caused by spinal cord compression is often alleviated by corticosteroid alone. Corticosteroid toxicity is both a function of dose and duration of treatment; the incidence of toxicity is minimized if duration of therapy is less than 3 weeks. However, about 25% of patients with spinal cord compression require maintenance treatment with dexamethasone for preservation of neurologic function. These patients require monitoring of potential steroid-related effects (e.g., hyperglycemia, gastrointestinal bleeding, psychosis).

15. What percentage of patients with spinal cord compression are able to ambulate after pretreatment motor dysfunction?

Pretreatment ambulatory function is the main determinant of posttreatment gait function. About 90% of patients who were ambulatory before treatment remain so; only 10% of patients who were paraplegic before treatment regain the ability to ambulate.

16. What are the options for recurrent spinal cord compression?

Approximately 80% of previously irradiated patients experience recurrent spinal cord compression at the site of previous radiation. Treatment options include surgery, systemic therapies, radiation therapy, or comfort measures alone. Although surgery is often recommended, the risk-benefit ratio may be high. Patients who experience recompression in a previously irradiated area may be considered for reirradiation, especially if 6 or more weeks have passed since the completion of radiation therapy. However, a tumor that compresses the cord in an area that has been previously irradiated may be radioresistant and additional treatments may lead to radiation myelitis.

17. What is the nurse's role in caring for a patient with spinal cord compression?

The major role of the oncology nurse is continual assessment of the patient and prompt notification of changes in pain, sensory, motor, urinary, or bowel function. Because nearly all patients report back pain as their first symptom, pain assessment and treatment are crucial. Methods of pain relief may include nonpharmacologic techniques (e.g., relaxation, distraction, massage), nonopioid and opioid analgesics, and adjuvant medications. Analgesics also are sometimes given epidurally. Nearly all patients can achieve pain control with appropriate multidisciplinary pain management.

Other important nursing roles include patient safety and interventions to preserve and maximize the patient's functional status. A bowel and bladder program may be required. It also may be necessary to provide skin care, wound care, and rehabilitation services. The nurse needs to instruct the patient about diagnostic tests, treatment and possible side effects, potential complications, and general safety measures. Emotional support for patient and family is a major focus of care, particularly if spinal cord compression is the presenting sign of a cancer diagnosis. Patients with severe neurologic deficits may require home and hospice care.

 Key Points

- Early recognition and diagnosis of spinal cord compression before the appearance of neurologic signs results in the best treatment outcome.
- Back pain in any patient with cancer should prompt a rapid evaluation.
- The patient's neurological status before initiation of treatment is the single most critical prognostic factor.
- The patient's response to treatment must be continually reassessed to promptly recognize treatment side effects and toxicity.

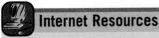
Internet Resources

Evidence-based Review of the Surgical Management of Vertebral Column Metastatic Disease:
  http://www.medscape.com/viewarticle/465373_1
Spinal Cord Compression: An Obstructive Oncologic Emergency:
  http://www.medscape.com/viewarticle/442735
Treatment of Metastatic Spinal Epidural Disease: A Review of the Literature:
  http://www.medscape.com/viewarticle/465359

Acknowledgments

The authors wish to acknowledge Linda Petersen-Rivera, RN, MSN, OCN, and Michael R. Watters, MD, FAAN, for their contributions to the Spinal Cord Compression chapter published in the first and second editions of *Oncology Nursing Secrets*.

Bibliography

Abdi S, Adams CI, Foweraker KL, et al: Metastatic spinal cord syndromes: Imaging appearances and treatment planning. *Clin Radiol* 60:637-647, 2005.
Abrahm JL: Assessment and treatment of patients with malignant spinal cord compression. *J Support Oncol* 2:377-388, 391, 2004.
Gabriel K, Schiff D: Metastatic spinal cord compression by solid tumors. *Semin Neurol* 24:375-383, 2004.
Klimo P, Thompson CJ, Kestle JR, et al: A meta-analysis of surgery versus conventional radiotherapy for the treatment of metastatic spinal epidural disease. *Neuro-Oncology* 7(1):64-76, 2005.
Lu C, Gonzalez RG, Jolesz FA, et al: Suspected spinal cord compression in cancer patients: A multidisciplinary risk assessment. *J Support Oncol* 3:305-312, 2005.
Patchell RA, Tibbs PA, Regine WF, et al: Direct decompressive surgical resection in the treatment of spinal cord compression caused by metastatic cancer: A randomized trial. *Lancet* 366:643-648, 2005.
Prasad D, Schiff D: Malignant spinal-cord compression. *Lancet Oncol* 6:15-24, 2005.
Rades D, Stalpers LJ, Veninga T, et al: Evaluation of five radiation schedules and prognostic factors for metastatic spinal cord compression. *J Clin Oncol* 23:3366-3375, 2005.
Ruckdeschel JC: Early detection and treatment of spinal cord compression. *Oncology* 19:81-86, 2005.
Schmidt MH, Klimo P, Vrionis FD: Metastatic spinal cord compression. *J Natl Compr Canc Netw* 3:711-719, 2005.

Superior Vena Cava Syndrome

Kelly C. Mack and Carolyn Becker

1. Define superior vena cava syndrome.

Superior vena cava syndrome (SVCS) is a clinical diagnosis that describes a pattern of physical findings resulting from obstruction of blood flow through the superior vena cava. The resulting engorgement of collateral veins of the thorax, head, and neck produces the classic symptoms.

2. What causes SVCS?

Obstruction of blood flow can be caused by any or a combination of the following three factors:

- **Compression.** Extrinsic pressure on the blood vessel from a tumor or enlarged lymph nodes is the most common mechanism of superior vena cava obstruction.
- **Thrombosis.** Thrombosis, usually caused by compression by a tumor or the presence of a central venous catheter or pacemaker wire, is becoming an increasingly common cause of superior vena cava obstruction.
- **Invasion.** Invasion within the superior vena cava by tumor is an unusual cause.

3. What anatomic mechanism underlies SVCS?

The superior vena cava is the major vessel for drainage of venous blood from the head, neck, upper extremities, and upper thorax. Located in the right anterior superior mediastinum, it is surrounded by rigid structures: sternum, trachea, right bronchus, aorta, pulmonary artery, perihilar and paratracheal lymph nodes, and vertebral bodies. The superior vena cava, a low-pressure, large but thin-walled, easily compressible structure, is vulnerable to any space-occupying process in its vicinity.

When the superior vena cava is fully or partially obstructed, venous return to the right atrium is diminished, resulting in increased venous pressure behind the obstruction. This increase in pressure (venous hypertension) causes venous stasis in the head, arms, and upper chest. Engorgement and dilation of superficial veins result, and extensive venous collateral circulation in the neck and thorax develops in an effort to bypass the obstruction. Other mediastinal structures, such as the bronchi, esophagus, and spinal cord, may be threatened by a growing mass within the mediastinum.

4. What are the classic signs and symptoms?

The most common **early** symptoms include dyspnea, orthopnea (ability to breathe easily only in the upright position), and facial edema. A "tight-collar" feeling with fullness in the face and upper extremity swelling is less common. Less frequently, chest pain and dysphagia are experienced.

Symptoms of **advanced** disease are rare. Examples include hoarseness, stridor, engorged conjunctiva, and symptoms of increased intracranial pressure, such as headache, dizziness, visual changes, change in mental status, respiratory distress (respiratory rate > 30/min) and seizures.

The physical findings are classic and unmistakable. Venous distention of neck, scalp, anterior and posterior chest wall, and shoulders is the hallmark of SVCS. Venous pressures in the upper body and head have been recorded as high as 200 to 500 cm H_2O. The veins become prominent, dilated, tortuous, and palpable. This sign is more evident when the patient is prone or bending forward. Veins often run a vertical or nearly vertical course. They can be distinguished from the telangiectasias of the elderly because they are more numerous, widespread, and enlarged. Other features of SVCS include facial and periorbital edema and swelling of the upper extremities, in particular the right arm. Plethora (ruddy, purple-red complexion), cyanosis, and cough are less common but still considered classic features.

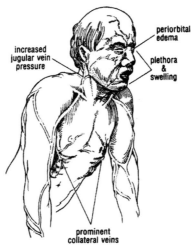

increased jugular vein pressure

periorbital edema

plethora & swelling

prominent collateral veins

Classic clinical symptoms of SVCS. *(From Miller SE: Superior vena cava syndrome. In Polomano RC, Miller SE, editors: Understanding and managing oncologic emergencies, Columbus, OH, 1987, Adria Laboratories. By permission.)*

5. What determines the severity of symptoms?

The severity of symptoms depends on the rate, degree, and location of obstruction; the aggressiveness of the tumor; and the competency of collateral circulation. A slowly developing obstruction allows time for collateral circulation to develop, and symptom severity is lessened. Conversely, rapid onset of symptoms precludes development of collateral circulation; and therefore, increases circulatory compromise. Regardless of rapidity of onset, all symptoms and physical findings are aggravated by bending forward, stooping, or lying down—anything that increases intrathoracic or intracranial pressure.

6. Who is at risk for developing SVCS?

Up to 97% of all cases of SVCS are caused by cancer. Nonmalignant causes are responsible for only 3% to 10% of cases. Although these numbers suggest that SVCS is a common disorder, in fact it is relatively uncommon. Only 3% to 4% of patients with cancer develop SVCS, usually in later stages of disease.

7. What types of malignancies are associated with SVCS?

- **Lung cancer** is responsible for 85% of all cases of SVCS. Small cell carcinoma is the most common histologic type, followed by squamous cell carcinoma of the lung.

Cancers arising in the right lung are four times more likely to cause SVCS because the superior vena cava is located in the right lung. Nonetheless, only 6% to 7% of patients with lung cancer develop SVCS.

- **Non-Hodgkin lymphoma** is the second most common malignancy to cause SVCS. Between 7% and 20% of all patients with non-Hodgkin lymphoma develop SVCS. Although Hodgkin lymphoma commonly involves the mediastinum, it is an uncommon cause of SVCS.
- **Breast cancer** is the most common metastatic disease causing SVCS. Rarely, thymoma, germ cell tumors, and Kaposi's sarcoma also may cause SVCS. Metastatic cancers are responsible for 5% to 10% of all cases of SVCS.

8. What are the nonmalignant causes of SVCS?

In the past, nonmalignant cases of SVCS were commonly caused by infectious agents. Currently, the most common nonmalignant cause of superior vena cava syndrome is thrombosis caused by the presence of central venous catheters or pacemakers. Mediastinal fibrosis, a narrowing or stricture of the superior vena cava, may be caused by radiation therapy to the mediastinum; this cause is exceedingly rare. Other non-malignant causes include goiters, histoplasmosis, and idiopathic mediastinal fibrosis.

9. How is the diagnosis of SVCS made?

Clinical signs and symptoms, along with imaging studies such as chest radiograph or chest computed tomography (CT) scan (currently the gold standard), are usually sufficient to make the diagnosis. Current practice demands a tissue diagnosis before instituting treatment unless the patient has a malignancy known to cause SVCS. The only exception to this dictum is when respiratory and neurologic status are so compromised that a delay in treatment would pose a threat to life; this situation is rare.

10. Because SVCS is listed among oncologic emergencies, is there an urgency to begin treatment?

SVCS has long been considered a potentially life-threatening medical emergency. Only patients with airway compromise, cardiovascular collapse, or increased intracranial pressure are at high risk and require emergent treatment. Whenever possible, the standard of care demands that time is taken to establish a histologic diagnosis so that proper treatment may be initiated.

11. What is the goal of treatment?

The treatment goal is to decrease the size of the tumor or obstruction, thereby relieving the pressure and restoring normal venous drainage. This strategy brings rapid resolution of symptoms. Secondarily and simultaneously, the goal is to attempt a cure of the primary malignant process. Small cell lung carcinoma, non-Hodgkin lymphoma, and germ cell tumors constitute 85% of the malignant causes of SVCS and are potentially curable.

12. Describe the treatment for SVCS.

Treatment varies, depending on the underlying cause:

- **Small cell lung cancer (SCLC)** is chemosensitive. If there is no response or if disease progresses, radiation therapy is used. The mean time to symptom resolution is 7 days. In this setting, presence of SVCS is not an adverse prognostic factor; SVCS develops quickly because of the characteristic rapid doubling time of SCLC.
- **Non-small cell lung cancer**. The initial treatment is radiation therapy. The likelihood of relieving symptoms is high, but overall prognosis is poor.

- **Non-Hodgkin lymphomas** (diffuse large cell or lymphoblastic lymphoma) are considered chemosensitive and curable in the earlier stages. A complete staging work-up is initiated before treatment if time permits. Local consolidation with radiotherapy may be beneficial in patients with bulky mediastinal disease (tumor > 10 cm or > one third the transverse diameter of the chest on chest radiograph). Chemotherapy follows and is used to treat systemic disease. Chemotherapy alone is mandated if the patient has already undergone previous mediastinal radiation. Complete symptomatic relief is usually achieved within 2 weeks after beginning treatment.
- If obstruction is caused by a **thrombus**, fibrinolytic therapy with streptokinase or recombinant tissue-type plasminogen activator (tPA), a highly selective fibrinolytic agent) is a common intervention. Another alternative is to remove the catheter that induced thrombus formation with simultaneous anticoagulant therapy to prevent embolization. Thrombus removal by surgery is rare.

13. When and how is thrombolytic therapy used?

In the past urokinase was the most commonly used thrombolytic therapy. Because urokinase is unavailable, tPA (alteplase, Activase), administered as a continuous infusion, has met with great success. tPA has selective action on a clot and can be used safely when thrombolytic therapy is administered systemically. The total dose (1.25 mg/kg) is administered over 3 hours; 60% is given in the first hour and the remaining 40% over 2 hours. Compared with urokinase, tPA is less likely to cause hemorrhagic complications, has a shorter time to clot lysis, and is more likely to dissolve a clot formed more than 5 days before the start of the infusion. These advantages must be balanced against the added cost of tPA. As always, thrombolytic therapy is contraindicated in patients with cerebral metastases or a risk for intracranial hemorrhage.

14. What monitoring is required for thrombolytic therapy?

- Vital signs are monitored every 15 minutes for the first hour, then every 30 to 60 minutes for the duration of the infusion, depending on the clinical situation.
- Monitoring for bleeding complications should continue beyond the discontinuation of thrombolytic therapy, because the effects last for several hours.

15. What other drugs may be used to treat SVCS?

Compression of the superior vena cava by tumor or adenopathy can be complicated by a secondary thrombosis. Venous stasis distal to the obstruction may allow a clot to form. For this reason, heparin (infusion or subcutaneous), enoxaparin (Lovenox), or oral anticoagulants may be used to reduce the extent of thrombus formation and prevent progression.

16. What is the role of surgery in the treatment of SVCS?

Surgery is rarely needed for malignant SVCS. It is considered when the obstructive process progresses rapidly. Generally, it is reserved for patients with chronic or recurrent SVCS who have a good prognosis and in whom all other treatment options have been exhausted. There are two types of surgical procedures:

- Endovascular stent placements provide immediate symptom relief for both malignant and benign causes. The use of this procedure is increasing because of its low morbidity and complication rate.
- Superior vena cava bypass graft creates a new vessel that circumvents the obstruction and is rarely done. At long-term follow-up, 80% of bypass grafts remained patent up to 15 years, and most patients were symptom-free.

17. Are steroids used to treat SVCS?

Corticosteroids may reduce symptoms associated with tumor necrosis, inflammation, and respiratory distress.

18. What is the role of radiation therapy?

Radiation therapy may be used if inserting a stent is not possible and the patient's clinical status is deteriorating. This situation, however, is exceedingly rare. In a true emergency, the bronchus is likely to be obstructed. Other critical structures, including the esophagus, trachea, vocal cords, and pericardium, may be involved. Initially, 2 to 4 large daily fractions (300-400 cGy) are followed by conventional fractionation (180-200 cGy/day). The radiation field includes gross tumor with appropriate margins plus mediastinal, hilar, and supraclavicular lymph nodes. Usually, improvement is seen within 24 to 72 hours.

19. What important nursing interventions are involved in the care of patients with SVCS?

- **Maintain airway patency.** Bed rest with the head of the bed elevated (Fowler's position) plus use of supplemental oxygen may temporarily relieve dyspnea and other symptoms caused by decreased cardiac output and increased venous pressure.
- **Monitor fluid and electrolyte balance.** Overhydration may exacerbate symptoms of SVCS. Although diuretic therapy and reduced salt diets have been used to decrease edema, their efficacy has not been demonstrated. Conversely, dehydration and the associated increased risk of thrombosis should not be ignored.
- **Monitor vital signs and level of consciousness.** The patient should be observed for signs of respiratory stridor and changes in mental status. Respiratory and neurologic changes may signal onset of a true emergency (extension of thromboses to cerebral veins).
- **Avoid accessing veins of the involved extremity** (usually the right arm) because of the risk of poor circulation, venous stasis, phlebitis, thrombosis, and hemorrhage. Postprocedural bleeding as a result of venous engorgement is a major concern. If chemotherapy is administered, decreased circulation may result in local accumulation of drug with poor absorption into the systemic circulation. This tendency is of particular concern when vesicant or irritant drugs are used. The safety of administering chemotherapy into the peripheral veins of lower extremities is controversial. Therefore, surgical cannulation of the femoral vein with a Broviac or Hickman catheter is recommended.
- **Avoid wearing invasive or constrictive clothing on the involved extremity and use other limbs for medical procedures.** Rings and restrictive clothing should be removed. Blood pressure measurement can be done on the thigh. Venipunctures can be done on the lower extremities.
- **Reduce anxiety.** A calm, restful environment with support from family or friends is helpful. Analgesics and tranquilizers may be administered for discomfort and anxiety. Interventions to avoid the Valsalva maneuver (e.g., stool softeners, cough suppressants, antiemetics) may be indicated to keep intrathoracic pressure as low as possible.
- **Assist with medical intervention.** Coagulation profiles should be monitored if anticoagulants are used. Emergent treatment must be instituted for symptoms of cerebral edema, decreased cardiac output, or airway obstruction.
- **Assess teaching needs.** For some patients, malignancy is diagnosed after the onset and diagnosis of SVCS. Such patients must deal with the emergency of SVCS as well as the unexpected diagnosis of malignancy and need information about the disease process, treatment of SVCS, treatment of the malignancy, and body image changes.

The nurse should stress that changes in physical appearance are temporary; body image changes secondary to facial edema and plethora subside with successful treatment.

- **Manage side effects** from chemotherapy and radiation therapy used to treat the underlying malignancy.

20. What is the prognosis of SVCS?

Positive outcomes strongly correlate with prognosis of underlying disease. Important prognostic variables include underlying malignancy (histologic findings), extent of the primary tumor (stage), responsiveness of the tumor to radiation therapy or chemotherapy, patient's performance status at the time of diagnosis, treatment history, and availability of remaining treatment options. The prognosis for lymphoma is better than that for lung cancer. For untreated malignant SVCS, survival is often less than 6 weeks.

21. What is the risk of recurrence after successful treatment of SVCS?

Recurrence of SVCS is rare in patients with non-Hodgkin lymphoma; unfortunately, it is more common with small cell carcinoma of the lung. Patients with SVCS related to malignancy have an approximately 10% to 19% chance of recurring SVCS.

 Key Points

- Superior vena cava syndrome is rarely a true emergency. It is important to establish an underlying diagnosis if the clinical situation permits.
- Treatment of superior vena cava syndrome is aimed at treating the underlying cause of the obstruction.
- The most common cause of superior vena cava syndrome is lung cancer. The highest risk is associated with small cell lung cancer and squamous cell carcinoma.
- Placement of endovascular stents is becoming an important intervention for treating superior vena cava obstruction; it can bring immediate relief of symptoms.

 Internet Resources

Association of Cancer Online Resources, Superior Vena Cava Syndrome:
  http://www.acor.org/cnet/62749.html#_24
National Cancer Institute, Cardiopulmonary Syndromes PDQ, Superior Vena Cava Syndrome:
  http://www.cancer.gov/cancertopics/pdq/supportivecare/cardiopulmonary/Patient/page5

Bibliography

Flounders JA: Superior vena cava syndrome. *Oncol Nurs Forum* 30(4):E84-E90, 2003.
Miller SE: Superior vena cava syndrome. In Polomano RC, Miller SE, editors: *Understanding and managing oncologic emergencies,* Columbus, OH, 1987, Adria Laboratories.
Moore, S: Superior vena cava syndrome. In Yarbro CH, Frogge MH, Goodman M, editors: *Cancer nursing: Principles and practice,* ed 6, Boston, 2005, Jones & Bartlett.
Yahalom J: Oncologic emergencies: Superior vena cava syndrome. In DeVita V, Hellman S, Rosenberg SA, editors: *Cancer: Principles and practice of oncology,* ed 7, Philadelphia, 2005, Lippincott Williams & Wilkins.

Chapter 53

Tumor Lysis Syndrome (TLS)

Anne Zobec

1. What is tumor lysis syndrome?

Tumor lysis syndrome (TLS) is an oncologic emergency that occurs when a large number of tumor cells are lysed or destroyed. It is manifested by several electrolyte imbalances. Without immediate treatment, TLS can lead to severe cardiac arrhythmias, acute renal failure, and death.

2. What happens in TLS?

Chemotherapy given to fast-growing tumors causes massive necrosis of cancer cells. As tumor cells die, they release intracellular contents, including potassium, phosphorus, and nucleic acids into the bloodstream. Nucleic acids are converted by the liver into uric acid. Abnormally high levels of uric acid, potassium, and phosphorus overwhelm the kidneys. High levels of uric acid crystallize in the distal tubules and collecting ducts of the kidneys, leading to obstructions and eventually acute renal failure.

3. When does TLS occur?

TLS develops within hours to a few days after treatment. It most often occurs within the first 24 to 72 hours after chemotherapy is initiated. TLS may persist for 5 to 7 days after therapy; this is the period when the most significant tumor cell destruction occurs.

4. What kinds of cancers are associated with TLS?

TLS is seen most often in patients with large, rapidly dividing tumors, such as lymphomas, leukemia, chronic leukemia in blast crisis, and B-cell or activated T-cell phenotypes. It is seen less often in solid tumors, but can occur in small cell lung cancer, metastatic breast cancer, melanoma, and metastatic medulloblastoma. Children with hematologic malignancies are particularly at risk for TLS, because their tumors are often more aggressive.

5. Are there risk factors for TLS?

Patients with elevated levels of blood urea nitrogen (BUN), creatinine, uric acid, and electrolytes before treatment are at a greater risk of developing TLS. These abnormal findings of laboratory studies indicate that the patient may have problems with renal function or dehydration. Patients with increased levels of lactate dehydrogenase (LDH) are also at a greater risk for TLS. LDH levels are correlated with large tumor masses. Other risk factors include splenomegaly, lymphadenopathy, and high white blood cell count.

6. What are the most common metabolic abnormalities in TLS?

The four hallmark signs of TLS are hyperuricemia, hyperphosphatemia, hyperkalemia, and hypocalcemia. These abnormalities result when the kidneys are unable to process and excrete the huge amount of intracellular products and metabolites that are released when the tumor cells are destroyed.

7. What are the signs and symptoms of TLS?

Initial signs and symptoms of TLS include gastrointestinal symptoms, such as nausea, vomiting, and diarrhea. Patients may also experience shortness of breath, an irregular heartbeat, lethargy, and joint pain. Flank pain, anuria, oliguria, and cloudy, sedimented urine indicate serious problems due to hyperuricemia. If TLS is not treated, it may progress to acute renal failure, cardiac arrhythmias, seizures, loss of muscle control, and death.

8. How can TLS be prevented?

When patients are identified as being at high risk for developing TLS, special treatments should be initiated before chemotherapy. Aggressive IV hydration, medications including allopurinol or Elitek (rasburicase), and alkalinization of the urine may prevent TLS.

9. What is the role of allopurinol treatment?

Traditionally allopurinol has been used to decrease uric acid concentration. Allopurinol inhibits the enzyme xanthine oxidase, which in turn blocks the conversion of uric acid precursors into uric acid. Allopurinol reduces both serum and urine levels of uric acid. Intravenous allopurinol has been found to be safe and effective in patients who are unable to take the oral medication.

10. How does Elitek (rasburicase) reduce uric acid?

Rasburicase is a recombinant form of urate oxidase, which is a nonhuman proteolytic enzyme that oxidizes uric acid to allantoin. This form is five to ten times more soluble than uric acid. It has been shown to control hyperuricemia faster and more reliably than allopurinol.

11. Has Elitek (rasburicase) been approved for adults?

Rasburicase was approved by the FDA in 2002 for initial management of plasma uric acid levels in pediatric patients with leukemia, lymphoma, and solid tumor malignancies who are receiving anticancer therapy expected to cause tumor lysis and subsequent elevation of plasma uric acid. Studies are evaluating the use of this drug in adults.

12. What steps are taken when TLS develops?

If preventative strategies fail and TLS develops, treatments are instituted to correct the specific metabolic abnormalities (hyperuricemia, hyperkalemia, hyperphosphatemia, and hypocalcemia). Dialysis may be necessary in severe cases.

13. What are the benefits and disadvantages of alkalinization of the urine?

Uric acid is much more soluble (> 10 times) in alkaline urine than in acidic urine. When the urine is acidic, high levels of uric acid form crystals in the tubules of the kidneys. To prevent crystallization, intravenous fluids are given to hydrate the patient and to increase the amount of fluids flowing through the kidneys. Historically, sodium bicarbonate has been added to the intravenous fluids to create alkaline urine. This practice is controversial in some institutions because treatment with sodium bicarbonate increases the risk of calcium phosphate precipitation and decreases the serum concentration of ionized calcium.

14. What are symptoms of hyperkalemia?

Hyperkalemia results in cardiovascular change that may lead to atrioventricular block, ventricular tachycardia, ventricular fibrillation, or asystole. Neuromuscular effects of hyperkalemia include muscle cramps, weakness, and paresthesia. Gastrointestinal effects are nausea, vomiting, diarrhea, and intestinal colic.

15. How is hyperkalemia treated?

Aggressive IV hydration and diuretics (furosemide) are the first strategies used. Sodium polystyrene sulfonate (Kayexalate) may be given orally or as an enema to promote excretion of potassium in the bowel. Sodium bicarbonate given in IV fluids may help neutralize the effects of hyperkalemia. IV administration of calcium gluconate or insulin with D25 dextrose solution pulls potassium back into the cell, reducing the serum potassium levels. Life-threatening hyperkalemia requires dialysis.

16. List problems associated with hyperphosphatemia.

Hyperphosphatemia primarily causes renal problems such as azotemia, oliguria, edema, and anuria. Excessive levels of phosphate in the blood may reduce serum calcium.

17. How is hyperphosphatemia corrected?

Diuretics may be given to promote excretion of phosphates in the urine. Phosphate binding drugs (aluminum hydroxide, lanthanum carbonate [Fosrenol], calcium acetate) may be given to promote excretion of phosphate through the bowel. Dietary intake of phosphates may be restricted or eliminated. (Phosphorus is found in milk, meat, cheese, eggs, bread, fish, nuts, poultry, legumes, cereal, chocolate, and carbonated drinks.)

18. What happens in hypocalcemia?

Symptoms of hypocalcemia include ventricular arrhythmias, lengthened ST segment, prolonged QT interval, 2:1 atrioventricular block, and cardiac arrest. Neurologic symptoms include muscle cramping and twitching, carpopedal spasms, tetany, laryngospasm, paresthesia, confusion, delirium, and convulsions.

19. How is hypocalcemia treated?

Treatment of hypocalcemia is only indicated if a patient is having severe symptoms. Replacing calcium in a patient who has hyperphosphatemia may lead to further calcium phosphate crystal formation and hasten renal failure.

20. What is significant about the patient's fluid level?

Intravenous fluids are frequently given at rates of 150 to 300 ml/hr to ensure that the patient is well hydrated. The urine output goal should be greater than 3 to 5L in 24 hours, with or without the use of diuretics. Fluid volume overload may occur. Monitoring blood pressure and pulse at least every 4 hours, auscultating lung sounds, looking for signs of edema and cough, and checking the patient's weight every 12 to 24 hours can reveal early signs of fluid overload.

21. What should be avoided in patients at risk of TLS?

Aspirin, radiographic contrast, probenecid, and thiazide diuretics should be avoided because they block tubular reabsorption of uric acid. Angiotensin-converting enzyme (ACE) inhibitors, potassium, and heparin may cause hyperkalemia. Enteral and parenteral nutrition containing phosphate may cause hyperphosphatemia. Nephrotoxic drugs (NSAIDS, aminoglycosides, amphotericin B) should be avoided.

Key Points

- Tumor lysis syndrome can be prevented.
- Elitek (rasburicase) is a new drug that is highly potent and fast acting in treating TLS.
- Careful monitoring of IV fluids, fluid intake and output, electrolytes, and weight are essential for all patients receiving chemotherapy for aggressive tumors.

Internet Resources

Ohio State University Center for Continuing Medical Education, Tumor Lysis Syndrome:
  http://ccme.osu.edu/cmeactivities/onlineeducation/ondemand/program/index.cfm?id=156
Prevention and Treatment of Hyperuricemia in Hematologic Malignancies:
  http://www.medscape.com/viewarticle/430764_34
Tumor Lysis Syndrome:
  http://www.emedicine.com/ped/topic2328.htm
Tumor Lysis Syndrome:
  http://www.emedicine.com/med/topic2327.htm
Lymphomation.org, Tumor Lysis Syndrome: Side Effects:
  http://www.lymphomation.org/side-effect-tumor-lysis.htm

Bibliography

Altman A: Acute tumor lysis syndrome. *Semin Oncol* 28(2 suppl 5):3-8, 2001.
Baird-Powell S: Hypocalcemia/hypercalcemia. In Camp-Sorrell D, Hawkins RA, editors: *Clinical manual for the oncology advanced practice nurse,* second edition, Pittsburgh, 2006, Oncology Nursing Society, pp. 1019-1029.
Bosly A, Sonet A, Pinkerton CR, et al: Rasburicase for the management of hyperuricemia in patients with cancer. *Cancer* 98:1048-1054, 2003.
Cantril CA, Haylock PJ: Tumor lysis syndrome. *Am J Nurs* 104(4):49-52, 2004.
Cheson BD, Dutcher BS: Managing malignancy-associated hyperuricemia with rasburicase. *J Support Oncol* 3(2):117-124, 2005.
Cope D: Tumor lysis syndrome. *Clin J Oncol Nurs* 8(4):415-416, 2004.
Davidson M, Thakkar S, Hix J, et al: Pathophysiology, clinical consequences, and treatment of tumor lysis syndrome. *Am J Med* 116(8):546-554, 2004.
Del Toro G, Morris E, Cairo M: Tumor lysis syndrome: Pathophysiology, definition, and alternative treatment approaches. *Clin Adv Hematol Oncol* 3:54-61, 2005.
Doane L, Gobel B: Tumor lysis syndrome: Pathophysiology, signs, and symptoms. *ONS News* 19(suppl 9):43-44, 2004.
Kaplow R: Pathophysiology, signs, and symptoms of acute tumor lysis syndrome. *Semin Oncol Nurs* 18(suppl 3):6-11, 2002.
Sallan S: Management of acute tumor lysis syndrome. *Semin Oncol* 28(2 Suppl 5):9-12, 2001.

Caring for the Person with Cancer

Cancer and Pregnancy

Linda U. Krebs

1. How common is cancer associated with pregnancy?

Although generally considered a rare event, the incidence of cancer associated with pregnancy is increasing. Cancer is one of the most common diagnoses and the second leading cause of death during the reproductive years. Approximately 1 of every 1000 pregnancies will be complicated by a cancer diagnosis.

2. Why is the incidence of cancer associated with pregnancy increasing?

As women delay childbearing until later in life (into their 30s to mid 40s), the likelihood of having concomitant pregnancy and cancer is increased. In addition, the incidence of some of the more common types of cancer (e.g., breast cancer, cervical cancer) appears to be increasing in younger women. The combination of delayed childbearing and younger incidence of specific cancers has led to this increase.

3. What is the time frame for pregnancy associated with cancer?

Most authors include not only the 9 months of pregnancy but also the 6 months before becoming pregnant or after delivering in the time frame for a pregnancy-associated cancer. Some authors suggest that the time frame is 1 year before conception and up to 2 years after delivery.

4. What are the predominant types of cancer diagnosed during pregnancy?

In descending order, the cancers most commonly diagnosed during pregnancy are breast cancer (1:3,000), cervical cancer (1:400), ovarian cancer, colorectal cancer, lymphoma, and leukemia. The majority of cervical cancer cases are not invasive but rather carcinoma in situ. Pregnancies associated with colorectal cancer, Hodgkin lymphoma, non-Hodgkin lymphoma, leukemia, and malignant melanoma are even less common.

5. Is cancer arising during pregnancy more aggressive than the same type of cancer in a nonpregnant woman?

Cancer arising during pregnancy was previously believed to be more aggressive because the stage of disease was likely to be advanced (stage III or IV) at diagnosis. However, in depth review of the stage of disease at diagnosis, treatment regimens, and overall survival statistics has shown that women at equivalent stages and receiving equivalent treatments have similar survival statistics, regardless of pregnancy. The most likely cause for advanced disease appears to be delay in making the diagnosis. This delay is due, in part, to the difficulty of recognizing the signs and symptoms of cancer in pregnant women.

6. Is therapeutic abortion beneficial in the management of cancer associated with pregnancy?

Scientific studies have not shown therapeutic abortion to be of any benefit in controlling disease or prolonging survival. In general, the pregnancy does not affect the outcome of the cancer, and the cancer does not affect the pregnancy. Therapeutic abortion may be of benefit if the planned treatment would be detrimental to the fetus and altering treatment to spare the fetus would have a negative impact on the mother's survival. The decision to have a therapeutic abortion should not be made until the risks of maintaining the pregnancy while providing optimal cancer treatment have been identified and comprehensively explained and discussed with the pregnant woman and her significant others.

7. Is it difficult to differentiate between body alterations found with routine pregnancy and signs and symptoms of cancer?

Making the diagnosis of cancer during a pregnancy may be difficult because of similarities among common symptoms associated with pregnancy and the signs and symptoms often associated with cancer. Nausea and vomiting, constipation, breast changes, changes in moles, fatigue, backache, and other constitutional symptoms are common to specific types of cancer and pregnancy. A breast mass is often believed to be related to a plugged milk duct, whereas the changes in the size and pigmentation of a mole may be believed to be part of normal changes in the skin during pregnancy (although more recent evaluations have suggested that normal moles do not commonly grow during pregnancy).

8. What diagnostic methods can be safely used in pregnant patients?

- Radiography should be used sparingly, if at all, in pregnant patients. When they are necessary, adequate fetal shielding must be used. Chest radiographs deliver minute doses of radiation and, with appropriate shielding, appear to be safe during pregnancy.
- Mammography may be safely undertaken if the abdomen is adequately shielded. However, it is not considered highly reliable because of increased breast density, decreased fatty tissue, and increased water content of the breasts during pregnancy.
- Ultrasound and magnetic resonance imaging may be safely used.
- Fine-needle aspiration, Papanicolaou test, and colposcopy are considered safe. Biopsy under local or general anesthesia is also safe if adequate fetal oxygenation and circulation are maintained.
- Cone biopsy may be undertaken; however complication rates may be as high as 30%. Loop electrode excision procedure (LEEP) has been suggested as an alternative to the complications known to occur with cone excision. However, LEEP has been associated with an increased incidence of cervical hemorrhage and premature membrane rupture, and thus may not be safer than cone biopsy.
- Computed tomography and isotope studies are not recommended. It has been suggested that the use of Technetium-99m (Tc-99m) sulfur colloid, used in sentinel lymph node mapping, is safe during pregnancy, although no definitive studies in pregnant women are available.
- Tumor markers (e.g., alpha-fetoprotein, beta-human chorionic gonadotropin, lactate dehydrogenase, CA-125) are of limited benefit because many markers are routinely elevated during pregnancy.

9. How should cancer associated with pregnancy be treated?

As a rule, a woman diagnosed with cancer during pregnancy should receive the same treatment options as a nonpregnant woman with the same malignancy. Management considerations should include the effect of the cancer on the pregnancy, the effect of the pregnancy on the cancer, and the effect of the chosen therapies on the pregnancy. Some modifications may be necessary to minimize fetal exposure to chemotherapy or radiation. In some instances, definitive therapy may be delayed until after delivery with little or no risk to the patient. In other instances, therapeutic abortion may be undertaken to provide aggressive therapy that could be potentially lethal to the fetus. In all cases, therapeutic decisions should be individualized. Recommendations for specific cancer types include the following:

Breast cancer. Modified radical mastectomy with lymph node sampling remains the standard treatment, although recently more women are selecting lumpectomy with lymph node sampling. Radiation therapy is not recommended for pregnant patients and is usually delayed until after delivery. Adjuvant chemotherapy may be safely given after the first trimester or may be delayed until after delivery if breast cancer is diagnosed closer to term.

Cervical cancer. For carcinoma in situ, the pregnancy can be allowed to continue, with definitive therapy delayed until after delivery. Close follow-up with intermittent biopsy is imperative. For invasive disease, radical surgery or radiation therapy, without therapeutic abortion, is recommended. If the patient is near delivery, viability can be awaited, the infant delivered by cesarean section, and definitive therapy then completed.

Ovarian cancer. Early-stage disease may be safely managed by unilateral oophorectomy and biopsy of the contralateral ovary. The pregnancy can be continued. For advanced disease, treatment consists of a radical hysterectomy, omentectomy, node biopsies, and peritoneal washings. The uterus is removed without prior evacuation of the fetus.

Colorectal cancer. Definitive therapy with a colectomy or abdominoperineal resection can generally be undertaken in the first 20 weeks of gestation without hazard to the fetus. For more advanced disease, involving the uterus or impeding access to the rectum, radical hysterectomy may need to be included. For the second half of gestation, viability is awaited, if possible, with definitive therapy after delivery. If an obstruction is present, a colostomy may be performed in the interim. Adjuvant chemotherapy should be delayed until the second trimester while adjuvant radiotherapy should be delayed until after delivery.

Lymphoma. Combination chemotherapy is generally the treatment of choice. In the first trimester, a therapeutic abortion is recommended for aggressive disease. In the second and third trimesters, chemotherapy may be given, or if the fetus is near viability, treatment may be delayed until after delivery. A recent study has suggested that rituximab may be given during the first trimester without subsequent fetal abnormalities; however, this result needs further investigation.

Leukemia. Treatment with chemotherapy should be instituted without delay. If the fetus is viable, delivery should occur as soon as possible. Therapeutic abortion is suggested for patients in the first trimester. Combination chemotherapy has been given with increased fetal abnormalities after the first trimester.

Malignant melanoma. Primary treatment consists of wide local excision with skin graft, if necessary. Lymph node dissection remains controversial; however, sentinel node biopsy is recommended. The benefits of adjuvant therapy with chemotherapy and biologics have not been adequately demonstrated.

10. **Is the survival rate of pregnant patients with cancer different from that of nonpregnant patients?**

Comparisons at all stages of disease reveal no difference in survivorship between pregnant and nonpregnant patients diagnosed with cancer, regardless of the type of cancer.

11. **What are the effects of cancer treatment on the fetus?**

- **Surgery**. Maternal surgery involves minimal risk to the fetus if hypotension is prevented and adequate oxygenation is ensured. General anesthesia is well tolerated after the first trimester. Pelvic surgery is more easily achieved during the second trimester.
- **Radiation therapy**. Fetal damage is unlikely at doses less than 50 cGy. Radiation doses greater than 250 cGy have been associated with fetal damage, including spontaneous

abortion, mental retardation, microcephaly, sterility, cataracts, and skin changes. Radiation exposure during the first trimester is of greatest concern. Even with adequate shielding, radiation scatter may be sufficient to cause harm or fetal demise. Radiation therapy should be avoided if possible; however, the use of the gamma knife for lesions in the brain appears to be safe.

- **Chemotherapy**. Chemotherapy during the first trimester has been associated with low birth weight, fetal malformations, and fetal demise. The incidence may be minimized or avoided by careful selection of agents or combinations of agents and/or delaying chemotherapy until after the first trimester. The fetus may experience unexpected or more severe toxic effects because of alterations in individual drug pharmacokinetics due to the normal physiologic changes associated with pregnancy. This is particularly important if chemotherapy is administered close to delivery. The neonate's metabolism and excretion of chemotherapeutic agents may not be sufficient when its primary mechanism of drug excretion, the placenta, is no longer present; thus, increased exposure to drugs and their toxic effects may result.
- **Biologic therapies/Targeted therapies**. Most biologic/targeted therapies are contraindicated during pregnancy because of lack of definitive studies to support their use. Case studies exist suggesting that rituximab, imatinib, interferon-alpha, and trastuzumab may be safely used; however, a case study links trastuzumab treatment with a decrease in amniotic fluid levels. Further studies are warranted before specific recommendations can be made.

12. What is the incidence of malformation in fetuses exposed to chemotherapy during gestation?

Fetal malformation is estimated to be less than 10%. Examples of malformation include skeletal malformations, hydrocephalus, atrial/septal defects, cranial dysostosis, various limb deformities, and cerebral anomalies. Methotrexate and aminopterin (a folic acid antagonist developed before methotrexate) have been most commonly implicated; however, alkylating agents and other antimetabolites may also cause malformations. Because of known limb deformities, pregnancy is contraindicated at any time for those receiving thalidomide. The incidence is higher when combination therapy is given, highest when chemotherapy is given in the first trimester (14% to 19%), and lowest when chemotherapy is given in the second or third trimester (~1%). The incidence of major congenital malformations in all births in the United States is approximately 3%, whereas it may reach as high as 9% for minor malformations.

13. Does the mother's cancer ever spread to the fetus?

Maternal-to-fetal spread is extremely rare, although scientific reports have included malignant melanoma, non-Hodgkin lymphoma, leukemia, breast cancer, lung cancer, and gastrointestinal malignancies. A variety of single case reports also can be found in the literature. In all instances, the mothers had widely disseminated disease. In most reported series, malignant melanoma is the most common form of cancer associated with fetal spread. In some instances, only the placenta is involved; in other instances, the cancer spreads to the fetus. Some infants have died of the disease.

14. What are the specific recommendations about delivery?

The type of delivery, vaginal versus cesarean section, is controversial for women with cervical cancer. Some health care professionals are concerned that, in the presence of active disease, vaginal delivery will spread the cancer or cause infection or hemorrhage; thus cesarean section is recommended. Others report that vaginal delivery does not increase risk of disease dissemination, hemorrhage, or infection, and, in fact, may be associated with increased maternal survival. Five cases of recurrence of disease in the vaginal episiotomy have been reported. The definitive answer for cervical cancer remains unclear. Careful follow-up for recurrence is mandatory in all women who have vaginal deliveries. Cesarean section is the method of choice if the woman is to undergo radical hysterectomy after delivery.

For all other cancer types, the type of delivery depends on disease status, fetal gestation, immediacy of delivery, and whether definitive treatment requiring an abdominal incision, is to be done after delivery. For ovarian cancer, treatment is often undertaken at delivery; a cesarean section is performed, followed by radical hysterectomy.

If possible, delivery should be timed so that patients receiving chemotherapy will have recovered from bone marrow suppression and other therapy-related toxicities. A complete blood count and other appropriate laboratory parameters should be evaluated before delivery, and extra precautions to minimize bleeding and infection should be taken as necessary.

15. What types of neonatal monitoring should occur at delivery?

The fetus exposed to chemotherapy may be premature and may weigh less than expected for gestational age. Because of the potential for increased toxicities, particularly if treatment is given close to delivery, laboratory evaluation should include a complete blood count. The neonate should be evaluated carefully for chemotherapy-induced malformations, including skeletal and internal organ abnormalities. The placenta and neonate also should be evaluated for signs of metastatic involvement, particularly if the mother has disseminated disease. Because abnormalities and disease related to placental transmission may not be apparent until months after birth, the child should be closely monitored for at least 12 to 24 months.

16. Is it possible to breast-feed an infant during or after treatment for cancer?

Breast-feeding is contraindicated when the mother is receiving chemotherapy or undergoing tests that use radioactive materials; these agents or their metabolites can be found in breast milk and may be detrimental to the infant. Breast-feeding can be safely recommended for all other patients. Women with breast cancer who have received breast radiation may have diminished or absent lactation on the radiated side. They are generally discouraged from attempting to breast-feed on the radiated side because of an increased risk of developing mastitis.

17. Are future pregnancies possible or recommended after a diagnosis of cancer?

The ability to become pregnant after a diagnosis of cancer depends on the primary site, stage of disease, type and extent of therapy, and age of the woman. For women who wish to conceive and remain physically capable of doing so, there are no known contraindications; although controversies exist for both breast cancer and malignant melanoma. Most clinicians recommend a waiting period of 1 to 5 years after completion of therapy, depending on stage of disease, age of the woman, and patient/family preferences. This recommendation minimizes the possibility of recurrence during the future pregnancy and allows the woman to regain physical and emotional health before undergoing the rigors of pregnancy.

18. What are the specific recommendations for prevention and early detection of cancer while a woman is pregnant?

All initial prenatal visits should include a Papanicolaou test and a thorough breast examination. Women should be instructed to do breast and skin self-examinations monthly throughout pregnancy. A thorough history for cancer risks should be obtained, and special precautions and evaluations should be included in prenatal care as appropriate. Pregnant women should be encouraged to discuss all abnormal findings or concerns with health care providers.

19. What is known about the long-term survival and future cancer risk of children exposed to cancer treatment in utero?

There appear to be no alterations in long-term survival and no increased risk of cancer, beyond those related to heredity, in children exposed to cancer treatment in utero. Rare abnormalities with no obvious pattern have been shown in long-term studies of children exposed to chemotherapy. Long-term effects of low-dose radiation are currently unknown. Follow-up of children exposed to higher doses of radiation is limited. Concerns for such children remain, and follow-up over many generations will be necessary to determine the exact effects.

20. Is nursing management of pregnant women with cancer any different from management of a woman who has cancer or a woman who is pregnant?

Nursing management for pregnant women with cancer is much more complex. Primary nursing roles include assessment, physical care, emotional support, and provision of information and education. The team approach, involving oncology, obstetrics, neonatology, and various support services, is essential. In addition to routine medical and nursing management strategies, educational, psychosocial, and ethical interventions need to be incorporated into the plan of care. Because of disease, treatment, fears for the fetus, concerns about survival, and numerous other anxieties, normal activities of pregnancy may be deferred or prevented. Ethical dilemmas may occur as treatment needs are weighed against fetal survival. Emotional support is essential and can take its toll on the health care provider as well as on the patient and family.

Key Points

- Cancer occurs in about 1 of every 1000 pregnancies.
- Most cancers do not adversely affect pregnancy; however, treatment may adversely affect the fetus, mother, or both.
- There is no evidence that termination of pregnancy will stop or retard cancer growth, or that hormonal and immunologic changes of pregnancy enhance cancer growth.
- Most clinicians recommend deferral of future pregnancies for at least 1 year (usually 1-5 years) following completion of therapy.

Internet Resources

Cooper University Hospital, Cancer and Pregnancy:
   http://www.cooperhealth.org/content/pregnancyandcancer.htm
Consortium of Cancer in Pregnancy Evidence (Canada), MotherRisk:
   http://www.motherisk.org/cancer
Fertile Hope:
   http://www.fertilehope.org
People Living with Cancer, Sexual and Reproductive Health:
   http://www.plwc.org/portal/site/PLWC/menuitem.724de8b96edd64acfd748f68ee37a01d/?vg
   nextoid=d1a7ea97a56d9010VgnVCM100000f2730ad1RCRD&vgnextfmt=default
Pregnant with Cancer Network:
   http://www.pregnantwithcancer.org

Internet Resources—cont'd

Young Survival Coalition, Pregnancy and Breast Cancer:
   http://www.youngsurvival.org/young-women-and-bc/bc-faqs/pregnancy/
About.com, Cancer in Pregnancy:
   http://pregnancy.about.com/od/cancerinpregnanc/

Bibliography

Brown D, Berran P, Kaplan KJ, et al: Special situations: abnormal cervical cytology during pregnancy. *Clin Obstet Gynecol* 48:178-185, 2005.

Germann N, Goffinet F, Goldwasser F: Anthracyclines during pregnancy: Embryo-fetal outcome in 160 patients. *Ann Oncol* 15:146-150, 2004.

Gwyn K: Children exposed to chemotherapy in utero. *J Natl Cancer Inst Monogr* 34:69-71, 2005.

Kal HB, Struikmans B: Radiotherapy during pregnancy: Fact and fiction. *Lancet Oncol* 6:328-333, 2005.

Keleher A, Wendt R, Delpassand E, et al: The safety of lymphatic mapping in pregnant breast cancer patients using Tc-99m sulfur colloid. *Breast J* 10:492-495, 2004.

Krebs LU: Sexual and reproductive dysfunction. In Yarbro CH, Frogge MH, Goodman M, et al, editors: *Cancer nursing: Principles and practice,* ed 6, Boston, 2005, Jones and Bartlett.

Leslie KK: Chemotherapy and pregnancy. *Clin Obstet Gynecol* 45:153-164, 2002.

Meirow D, Schiff E: Appraisal of chemotherapy effects on reproductive outcome according to animal studies and clinical data. *J Natl Cancer Inst Monogr* 34:21-25, 2005.

Mesquita MM, Pestana A, Mota A: Successful pregnancy occurring with interferon-alpha therapy in chronic myeloid leukemia. *Acta Obstet Gynecol Scand* 84:300-301, 2005.

Minter A, Malik R, Ledbetter L, et al: Colon cancer in pregnancy. *Cancer Control* 12:196-202, 2005.

Pavlidis NA: Coexistence of pregnancy and malignancy. *Oncologist* 7:279-287, 2001.

Schover LR: Motivation for parenthood after cancer: A review. *J Natl Cancer Inst Monogr* 34:2-5, 2005.

Tolar J, Neglia JP: Transplacental and other routes of cancer transmission between individuals. *J Pediatr* 25:430-434, 2003.

Ward RM, Bristow RE: Cancer and pregnancy: Recent developments. *Curr Opin Obstet Gynecol* 14:613-617, 2002.

Woo JC, Yu T, Hurd TC: Breast cancer in pregnancy. *Arch Surg* 138:91-98, 2003.

Chapter 55

Culture and Ethnicity

Patricia W. Nishimoto and Joanne Itano

1. What is the difference between culture and ethnicity?

- **Culture** refers to the values, beliefs, norms, and practices of a particular group that are learned and shared to guide thinking, decisions, and actions in a patterned way. Culture is largely unconscious, all encompassing, and exerts powerful influences on health promotion and illness prevention; the causation, detection, and treatment of illness; the care of ill and well people; whom to ask for assistance; and the social roles, relationships, and expectations that guide encounters between members and health care providers.
- **Ethnicity** refers to groups whose members share a common social and cultural heritage passed on to successive generations. The members of each ethnic group feel a sense of identity. It is frequently used interchangeably with the term *race;* however, ethnicity includes more than biological identification. The patient's ethnic background contributes to a patient's culture, but so do the patient's work, gender, hobbies, state of residence, and culture associated with the patient's health care facility, diagnosis, and treatment.

2. Is it always better that nurses have a similar ethnicity to their patients?

No, the presumption that having similar ethnicity will facilitate nurse-patient interactions falls short of the goal of cultural competency, which is much more than having the same ethnic background. An 80-year-old first generation woman may have much more ease communicating with a 20-year-old white female nursing student than with a 35-year-old male nurse of her same ethnic background. Institutions may try to meet the goal of *Healthy People 2010* to eliminate health disparities by hiring nurses of diverse ethnic backgrounds, but this assumes that having a similar ethnic background will address the issues. The cultural sensitivity and competency of the nurse has a greater impact on quality of care than the nurse's culture or ethnicity.

3. How does lack of cultural sensitivity affect patient care?

A nurse who is not attuned to cultural nuances of her/his patient is more likely to miss essential patient care cues. For example, not being aware that some Filipino patients may describe a variety of symptoms as feeling "dizzy" may result in unnecessary tests and a diminished ability to help the patient. The risk of not fully incorporating culturally sensitive care into one's practice can result in outcomes between two extremes. A nurse who believes that it is "impossible" to know all about patients' cultures may as a consequence spend less time with the patient, fail to advocate for patient needs because of lack of understanding, and may become resentful of the cultural barriers as causing additional work. Conversely, a nurse may adopt an oversimplified approach that "everyone is really the same at heart" and decide to "follow the Golden Rule" to treat all patients as she/he would want to be treated. The "Golden Rule" approach may impede optimal care when the nurse fails to collaborate with the patient in developing a cancer care strategy based on the patient's desires. For example, a well-meaning nurse's efforts to reach out and touch an American Indian patient may have undesirable consequences as some American Indian tribes reserve touching for very close friends or family.

4. How does the nurse learn to be culturally competent?

Culturally competent care is facilitated by:

- Being self-reflective
- Embracing an approach of cultural curiosity rather than trying to memorize a litany of cultural "facts" and trying to "predict" in a cookie cutter approach what a patient might believe culturally
- Developing sensitivity to the uniqueness of each individual and avoiding stereotyping that all members of a cultural/ethnic group will have the same beliefs and behaviors
- Changing from an authority figure to a learner
- Learning key words in the patient's language and being aware of how to contact and properly use an interpreter
- Being flexible with openness to new experiences
- Engaging in cultural immersion
- Developing institutional support to provide culturally sensitive care, such as additional staff for the extra time it will take to communicate. For example, the Western medicine culture of short appointment times is not conducive to "storytelling," a nonlinear communication style of some American Indians or some Asian or Pacific Islander patients. A culturally aware institution will provide access to professional interpreters, computer software that enables you to print out patient instructions in the patients' native language, and educational opportunities to learn more about developing cultural awareness.
- Engaging in self-evaluation of values and beliefs
- Using a cultural model to provide care
- Collaborating with the patient in the development of a care strategy in the context of the patient's culture to mediate health care values with the patient's experiences.

5. What cultural phenomena should nurses be aware of when caring for diverse patients?

The following six cultural phenomenon may affect health care (Giger, Davidhizar, 2004):

- Communication: verbal, nonverbal, and written words (e.g., nonverbal communication is valued by Eskimos, who may want time to sit quietly before starting to talk)
- Space: encompasses the relationship among the individual, physical body, surrounding environment, and objects within the environment
- Social organization: includes family structure and organizations, religious values and beliefs, behaviors for significant life events (e.g., birth, death, illness)
- Time: orientation towards present, past, or future
- Environmental control: includes perceptions/activities about how to control nature or environmental factors and beliefs about health, causes of illness, and health behaviors (e.g., magicoreligious health beliefs, use of holy words or charms, folk medicine)
- Biologic variations: involves differences in physical characteristics (e.g. skin, mucous membrane, amount of body hair, body size), enzymatic and genetic variations affecting metabolism of drugs and alcohol (e.g., Chinese males require less propranolol to treat hypertension than white males), risks for certain diseases (e.g., Jewish ancestry and Tay-Sachs disease; sickle cell disease in African Americans), and dietary practices

6. What is the ethnic distribution in the United States and what will be the consequences on nursing practice?

Until recently, the cultural diversity of the United States was limited largely to white immigrants from Europe. In the 1950s, nine out of every ten Americans were of European descent.

In the 1990s, one out of every four adults and one out of every three children were of African, Latin American, or Asian origin. The U.S. Census Bureau projects that by the year 2050, the population distribution will be as follows: white, 52.5%; Hispanic/Latino, 22.5%; black, 14.4%; Asian and Pacific Islander (API), 9.7%; and American Indian (AI), 0.9%.

As a group, nurses are a relatively homogenous group, with 90% of registered nurses being white and English speaking; whereas, the population being served is heterogeneous. With projected changes in the composition of the potential patient population, nurses will care for patients from diverse cultures. Without an awareness of the importance of the patient's culture in treatment and a framework to incorporate culture into patient assessment and treatment, nurses will not be able to provide holistic and appropriate nursing care to ethnically diverse patients.

7. How are ethnic groups categorized?

A person's ethnic group should be described as he or she identifies it. The U.S. government uses the following categories and definitions for race and ethnicity:

- **American Indian (AI) or Alaska Native (AN)**. A person having origins in any of the original peoples of North and South America (including Central America), and who maintains tribal affiliation or community attachment.
- **Asian**. A person having origins in any of the original peoples of the Far East, Southeast Asia, or the Indian subcontinent including, for example, Cambodia, China, India, Japan, Korea, Malaysia, Pakistan, the Philippine Islands, Thailand, and Vietnam.
- **Black or African American**. A person having origins in any of the black racial groups of Africa. The term *Haitian* can be used in addition to *Black* or *African American.*
- **Hispanic or Latino**. A person of Cuban, Mexican, Puerto Rican, South or Central American, or other Spanish culture or origin, regardless of race. The term *Spanish origin* can be used in addition to *Hispanic* or *Latino.*
- **Native Hawaiian or Other Pacific Islander**. A person having origins in any of the original peoples of Hawaii, Guam, Samoa, or other Pacific Islands.
- **White**. A person having origins in any of the original peoples of Europe, the Middle East, or North Africa.

8. Summarize the differences in cancer incidence and mortality among cultural groups.

Overall cancer incidence and mortality rates vary among ethnic groups.

- African American men have the highest incidence and mortality rates for all cancers combined when compared with other ethnic groups. The most commonly diagnosed cancers in African American men are prostate, lung, and colorectal cancer. African American women have the second highest incidence and highest mortality rates for all cancers. Breast, lung, colon, and rectal cancers are the most common and account for most of the mortality rates.
- Cancer incidence and risk factors vary among Hispanics, depending on their country of origin (U.S. or foreign-born) or heritage, degree of acculturation and socioeconomic status. They have a lower incidence for all cancers combined, except for the incidence and mortality of cancers of the stomach, liver, uterus, cervix, and gallbladder.
- Asian and Pacific Islanders have the fourth lowest incidence for all cancers and have the lowest mortality rate compared with other ethnic groups. This is a very diverse group. Data from the state of Hawaii, which has a high concentration of Asians and Native Hawaiians, indicate that cancer incidence and mortality is highest for Hawaiians when compared to Filipinos, Chinese, whites, and Japanese.

Japanese men have the highest rate of stomach and rectal cancers in Hawaii, Hawaiian women have the highest rate of lung and breast cancers, and Filipino women have the highest rate of thyroid cancer.

- American Indians/Alaskan Natives (AIs/ANs) have the lowest cancer incidence and lower mortality rates for all cancers combined. The poverty rate for AI/AN in 2001 was 24.5%, highest among the five ethnic groups, and AIs/ANs were also less likely to have health insurance than any other ethnic group.

9. Describe the major types of health beliefs affected by culture.

- **Magicoreligious view:** belief that health and illness are controlled by supernatural forces. Illness is seen as punishment for misbehavior or opposing God's will.
- **Scientific or biomedical view:** view that life and life processes are controlled by physical or biochemical processes that can be manipulated by humans.
- **Holistic view:** view that the forces of nature must be maintained in balance or harmony to maintain health.

10. What is folk medicine and why do cancer patients consult folk healers?

Folk medicine is a type of healing practice in which beliefs and practices related to illness and health are derived from cultural traditions rather than from a scientific base. Folk healing is regarded as more comfortable and less frightening than traditional Western medicine. It is thought to be more humanistic and holistic because healing is a restoration of a person to a state of harmony between body, mind, and spirit.

People may consult folk healers first because they understand the problem within a cultural context, speak the same language, and share a similar world view as the patient. The consultation and treatment take place in the community of the patient, usually in the home of the healer. The folk healer is often a woman in the community who is knowledgeable about home remedies or a spiritualist who combines rituals, spiritual beliefs, and herbal medicines. The healer typically prepares the treatment, and frequently either the healer or the patient performs some type of ritual practice.

Because cancer may be viewed as an unnatural illness caused by supernatural or sinful behavior, some cultures may have a fatalistic view that cancer cannot be treated effectively with Western medicine and prefer to use folk medicine. Consulting with a folk healer before seeing a traditional Western practitioner may delay early diagnosis and affect outcome.

11. Summarize common differences in healing practices among cultural groups.

Do NOT use the following information as a "cookbook approach"; instead, use it to stimulate conversation and exploration to learn more.

Common differences in healing practices among cultural groups

Asian Pacific Islanders	Hispanic/Latino	American Indians (500 tribes)
Holistic view of health	Fatalistic view of health	Harmony with nature
Healing practices: herbs, traditional healers, healing ceremonies, cupping, coining	Healing practices: home remedies, folk healer, massage, charms for protection	Healing practices: healer, healing ceremonies, herbs, prayers, medicine wheel

Continued

Common differences in healing practices among cultural groups—cont'd

Asian Pacific Islanders	Hispanic/Latino	American Indians (500 tribes)
Cancer = 'cold illness' so treat with 'hot' methods (e.g., foods, herbs, healing ceremonies)	Cancer = 'cold condition' so treat with hot therapies	Cancer = not a Native word Translated = 'disease for which there is no cure' or 'disease that eats the body'
Folk illnesses = *amok* (dissociative episode), *hwa-byung* (anger illness), *latah* (easily frightened), *shen kui* (anxiety, panic due to loss of semen), *wind illness* (fear of wind/cold exposure)	Folk illnesses = *susto* (fright which causes loss of soul), *mal de ojo* (evil eye), *mal puesto* (witchery), *caidade la mollera* (fallen fontanelles), *empacho* (blocked intestines), *antojos* (unusual cravings)	Folk illnesses = *iichi'aa* (*Navaho,* dissociative episode*), ghost sickness* (preoccupation with death/deceased*), hi-wa itch* (*Mohave,* insomnia, depression), witching (results in bad luck, illness, death)

12. How is screening affected by ethnicity or cultural beliefs and fatalism?

Ethnic background, health beliefs, and fears as well as level of education, acculturation, age, and insurance coverage affect and prevent screening practices. For example, Hispanic/Latino women who may believe that caressing the breast, injury to the breast, or having multiple sexual partners increase the risk of breast cancer as a punishment from God may not participate in screening because they do not want to know. Women who are not sexually active may believe screening is not necessary until a partner touches their breasts. Screening is not a customary event for West Indians, Hmongs, Puerto Rican men, and American Indians who follow traditional healing practices. Blacks may think that there is no need for screening or treatment because God's will determines whether you live or die; everything is left in God's hands. They also may believe that cancer is caused by not following God's will.

Fear that all cancers are fatal promotes the belief that there is "no use" in screening. The incidence of fatalism is reported to be higher in women of all ethnic origins, Blacks, some Asian and Pacific Islander groups, and people with low income and low educational levels. The sense of fatalism can be decreased in people who have a strong spiritual core, through the interventions of ministers, prayers, and prayer groups.

Fatalistic beliefs about screening can delay diagnosis, resulting in advanced stage of disease at presentation. This scenario reinforces the impression of the community that cancer is an automatic death sentence: "My auntie was feeling poorly and three weeks after she saw her doctor, she was lying in her coffin."

People who are fatalistic may interpret breast self-examinations as a monthly stressor. Studies reporting that the behavior of breast cancer at the molecular level is affected by ethnicity can reinforce the belief that ethnicity alone predicts survival. It is the role of the nurse to answer patients' questions honestly while helping them to interpret the statistics that they may have read.

13. What can be done to increase screening in different ethnic groups?

People from all ethnic groups need to understand the rationale for the screening test and to feel the concern and respect of the health care provider who asks them to participate in screening. This is particularly true for Arab Americans, Cambodians, Central Americans, Cubans, Filipinos, Gypsies, Iranians, Haitians, Japanese-Americans, Koreans, Vietnamese, and Samoans.

When West Indians are agreeable to screening, be extremely cognizant of their high level of modesty and need for privacy. This also holds true for Samoans, Puerto Rican women, Mexican Americans, Koreans, Filipinos, Ethiopians/Eritreans, Chinese Americans, and Cambodians. Matching the provider's gender to the patient's may help.

A strategy to help increase screening among Puerto Rican men is to get their wives to encourage them to go for screening. Screening of many Brazilians, Russians, and Hmongs can be accomplished when they visit the office for an illness or other symptoms. It is uncommon for them to come for screening while they are feeling well. American Indians may comment that they do not believe in "silent disease," and Brazilians may avoid screening to prevent hearing "bad news."

Other strategies include involving trusted and respected members of the community/ethnic group in the planning and delivery of the screening services; developing culturally sensitive patient education materials, considering preferred language, preferred method (video, written, oral tradition/story telling, group or one-on-one teaching); keeping the educational message simple; and considering communication styles (e.g., how to address the person, space and eye contact values).

14. What is the relationship between poverty and cancer?

Poverty accounts for a 10% to 15% lower survival rate from cancer in many ethnic groups. Ethnic minority groups are overrepresented in the poor of America. Poverty contributes to increased cancer incidence and mortality through risk factors of poor nutrition, occupational exposure through unskilled jobs, early initiation into sex and multiple sex partners, smoking tobacco products, and alcoholism. Less education and a greater focus on survival needs often decrease participation in screening and early detection activities by the poor.

Those patients who experience poverty may have a sense of pride or fierce independence that results in not accepting "handouts" or government subsidized treatment. Illegal aliens may be prevented from accepting government sponsored health care because of fears of being discovered and sent back to their native home. Older patients with less financial resources have a triple jeopardy of poverty, minority status, and age.

15. How does culture affect the family and its decision-making?

Our nursing culture's value of autonomy can be incongruent with cultures that value family decision-making or even cultures that value the family making the decision for the patient. Some American Indians may regard a diagnosis of cancer as shameful or even see the patient as "contagious with the cancer spirit." To insist that family be included in decision-making may result in some American Indians believing that they are inviting evil spirits or death into their bodies. Other American Indians may find it important to have family included in decision making until the discussion begins to include death. Some American Indians commonly have family meetings but do not discuss a terminal prognosis.

16. How does culture affect the process of informed consent?

If language is a barrier or if English is a second language, the patient may not be able to understand commonly used but complicated Western medical terminology of informed consent. If using translated forms, request that back-translations be used to prevent simplistic or culturally inappropriate translation errors or misinformation.

Informed consent includes possible and uncommon side effects. If your patient is an Asian/Pacific Islander who believes in bachi (bad luck that makes the thing feared actually happen), the completion of the informed consent form may be viewed as causing the side effects because they were stated in the informed consent form as possible consequences.

17. Does ethnicity affect participation in clinical trials?

Yes, there is underrepresentation of minorities in clinical trials despite overrepresentation of the incidence of cancer. If patients from an American Indian tribe believe surgical removal of a body part prevents the person from moving to the "other side" after death to be with ancestors, they may refuse to be in a clinical trial that includes surgery. Because of the additional time to complete the informed consent process, busy health care staff may hesitate to offer participation in clinical trials.

Barriers to Clinical Trial Participation

- Lack of access to health care
- Racial discrimination
- Ineligible because of desire to use native herbs

- Lack of expert translator

- Lack of trust in health care professionals
- Lack of time

- Language barriers
- Cultural beliefs/myths
- Few minority health care professionals

- Belief clinical trial = last resort

- Worry about being a "guinea pig"

- Concerns how data will be used

- Lack of insurance
- Costs of tests/treatments
- Complexity of medical information (education level)
- Lost wages from participation
- Misunderstanding of "randomization"
- Family argues against being in clinical trial

Facilitators to Clinical Trial Participation

- Desire to help future family members
- Perceive no other treatment options
- Acknowledgement and incentives to participate

- Trust and confidence in health care professionals
- Community collaboration

- Cultural competency of the study design/implementation

- Provides sense of "purpose"

- Cultural translators involved in the study
- Consent forms written in native language

18. How does culture affect support group attendance?

Age, gender, ethnicity, and levels of acculturation, education, and socioeconomic status may affect support group attendance. There are many anecdotal experiences about who will or will not attend support groups, but do not assume based on your understanding about cultural beliefs that some patients may not want to attend a support group. Support group attendance can be facilitated when language barriers are addressed and groups are customized to meet the needs of the people who will be attending (e.g., *Us, Too* support group for men structured as an inclusive educational opportunity). One report revealed that success with support groups was facilitated by redefining group membership in Chinese women of Hong Kong descent. Many Chinese people view others as belonging either to *Zijiren*, an in-group composed of family, or *Wairen*, an out-group composed of nonfamily. The Hong Kong women developed a support group where women with a similar diagnosis were redefined as *Zijiren* because of their similar experiences.

19. How do culture and ethnicity affect pain expression?

One third of patients with metastatic cancer from a nondominant ethnicity do not receive adequate pain management in accordance with World Health Organization (WHO) guidelines. Cultural barriers between providers and patients can result in an underestimation of the patient's pain level.

Many Asian patients see it as causing shame for health care providers to tell them that the pain medication they prescribed is not effective. Thus, they may nod their head or respond in the affirmative to the health care provider's question about the prescribed pain medication to help the physician or nurse to 'save face,' but not mention that they are bearing unacceptable levels of pain. Japanese may describe this as *gaman*, to silently endure the pain. This is in contrast to other cultural groups, such as Puerto Rican, Egyptian or Colombian, who may openly express their pain.

Each culture may interpret pain uniquely, such as thinking that there is a need to suffer before dying, or that if the pain goes away, it may mean impending death. Some American Indians may believe that if they bear the pain, the rest of the community will be spared the pain. Stoicism is considered a positive trait for American Indians, Japanese, Vietnamese, Chinese, Koreans, Mexicans, and Filipinos. Some Chinese may believe they need to suffer while on earth so they will not have to suffer forever in the afterlife. If cancer is believed to be caused by "sin" or the "devil," it may be necessary to experience the pain to be "cured of the sin" and to make the devil leave the body.

Language as part of culture can affect how pain is expressed or explained. "It hurt so much; I'd have liked to have died." Some Hispanic patients will describe pain as "suffering," in contrast to some African Americans who may describe it as "hurting." Some Ethiopians may not be able to describe the level of pain by using a pain scale. Language barriers can result in misunderstandings of how to properly take medications. Cultural groups who fear addiction may not use the pain medication prescribed.

20. What factors contribute to ethnic differences in the metabolism of pain medications or other drugs?

Research has shown that metabolism of drugs is genetically determined (genetic polymorphism); thus, ethnicity or a person's race may affect responses to drugs. Other factors contributing to the various reactions to drugs among ethnic groups include environment (e.g., diet, smoking, use of alcohol) and cultural values and beliefs. Although ethnopharmacology may help to individualize treatments, a potential downside is the risk of prejudice in not treating someone with a potentially helpful medication. Using ethnicity alone as a proxy to decide on therapy can be less than helpful if accuracy of participant ethnicity in the studies was not precise, resulting in flawed findings.

21. Give examples of genetic polymorphisms.

Genetic polymorphism highlights the need to consider ethnicity as well as age, gender, and weight in the type and dosages of drugs that are prescribed. Three types of genetic polymorphism have been identified with many drugs metabolized via these pathways: acetylation polymorphism, debrisoquine polymorphism, and mephenytoin polymorphism. Japanese and Inuit populations have more rapid acetylators than slow acetylators. Poor metabolizers of debrisoquine (an antihypertensive compound) are found in approximately 3% to 9% of whites in the United States, Canada, Britain, Denmark, Sweden, and Switzerland;

the lowest percentage (0%-2%) of poor metabolizers are from China, Japan, Malaysia, and Thailand. Some opioids, antihypertensives, antipsychotics, and antidepressants are metabolized similarly to debrisoquine. For example, codeine is more likely to be effective in Chinese or Japanese patients than in patients from Sweden. There is a higher percentage (about 20%) of poor metabolizers of mephenytoin (anticonvulsant agent) in China and Japan than in other countries. Drugs metabolized via the mephenytoin pathway include various barbiturates and diazepam.

22. What factors should be considered in addressing advance directives with different cultural groups?

Autonomy includes choosing not to choose. Again it is not helpful to stereotype, so ask questions and do not assume. Instead of trying to convince patients what they "should choose," invite them to teach you more about their values so you can help them. Inquire about what degree of autonomy the patient desires in decision-making, or who the decision-makers are in the patient's family.

Some Chinese may believe there needs to be a "waiting period" before death. If they believe they need time to atone for sins and to suffer before dying, then a DNR order may be rejected. Be cognizant that some Muslim Iranians and Orthodox Jews may feel a DNR directive is against their religious beliefs.

23. How do you facilitate cross-cultural communication?

To be a cultural broker, it is important to understand that everyone is different and to openly communicate with each patient that you need their help to communicate to you their cultural beliefs, priorities, and needs.

- Be continually reflective about your own values and biases.
- Learn to speak key phrases in the patient's native language to convey your sincerity in wanting to accomplish cross-cultural communication.
- Become more knowledgeable about differences in communication patterns in other cultures; for example, lack of eye contact is a form of respect, not an indication of apathy or rudeness in Hispanic/Latino or API patients. Shaking hands with the opposite sex is not acceptable for some Orthodox Jews or Muslims.
- Do not ask if they understand what you have said; instead ask them to tell you in their words what they understand you told them.
- Be careful using gestures when motioning patients to sit or come closer because in some cultures, holding your palm up, as opposed to palm down, may be the gesture for calling a dog. In other cultures, giving the OK sign by touching the tips of your thumb and index finger may be an obscene gesture. Which hand you use to give written handouts or medications can interfere with communication because using the left hand is considered unclean by some.
- Clarify the roles of family members, particularly those who are the decision-makers or spokespersons.
- Empower patients by telling them that they can help with the quality of their care by teaching you what culturally-associated actions might interfere with the provision of care that you want to give and they want to receive. Help patients understand that good communication will help to increase their satisfaction with their care, prevent misdiagnosis and complications, improve adherence to treatments, and lead to better outcomes.

24. What are some guidelines for the effective use of interpreters?

- If possible, do not use family members; use professional interpreters who will translate what you say and not "filter" the information. Professional interpreters can cue you in to cultural "mistakes."

- Pay attention to other variables that can affect translation, such as dialect, rivals, gender (usually same-sex interpreter is desired), age (usually older interpreter is desired), religion (Christian Egyptian – Muslim Egyptian), and cultural class (untouchable). Lack of cultural sensitivity can result in requesting a "Filipino or Chinese" translator but Filipino and Chinese are not languages. If the patient is Filipino, does he/she speak Tagalog, Ilacano, or another dialect?
- Remember to speak to the patient, not the interpreter.
- Make allowance for the additional time it takes to use an interpreter. Use short sentences and a normal tone of voice when speaking. Do not try to "hurry;" take the time to "talk story" before asking personal questions. Allow the patient to repeat back to you what they understand of the discussion. If the patient smiles throughout and keeps nodding their head in agreement, it may be due to politeness and not actual agreement or understanding.

Key Points

- Culture refers to the values, beliefs, norms, and practices of a particular group that are learned and shared to guide thinking, decisions, and actions in a patterned way.
- Culture exerts powerful influences on health promotion and illness prevention; the causation, detection, and treatment of illness; the care of ill and well people; whom to ask for assistance; and the social roles, relationships, and expectations that guide encounters between members and health care providers.
- Ethnicity encompasses more than biological identification; it refers to groups whose members share a common social and cultural heritage passed on to successive generations.
- Culturally competent care is facilitated by developing sensitivity to the uniqueness of each individual and avoiding stereotyping that all members of a cultural/ethnic group will have the same beliefs and behaviors.
- Use professional interpreters, not family members, to translate what you say and ensure that information is not "filtered" by the family. Professional interpreters can cue you to cultural "mistakes."

Internet Resources

American Cancer Society:
   http://www.cancer.org
American Nurses Association, Ethics and Human Rights Position Statements: Cultural Diversity in Nursing Practice:
   http://www.nursingworld.org/readroom/position/ethics/etcldv.htm
Babel Fish Translation:
   http://babelfish.altavista.com
EthnoMed (University of Washington, Harborview Medical Center):
   http://www.ethnomed.org
Hispanic Health Websites:
   http://www.hogarhispano.homestead.com/HispanicHealth.html
National Cancer Institute, Cancer Information Service:
   http://cis.nci.nih.gov/
Intercultural Cancer Council (ICC):
   http://iccnetwork.org

Continued

Internet Resources—cont'd

National Center on Minority Health and Health Disparities (NCMHD):
   http://ncmhd.nih.gov/
National Coalition of Ethnic Minority Nurse Associations (NCEMNA):
   http://www.ncemna.org
National Asian Women's Health Organization (NAWHO):
   http://www.nawho.org
Centers for Disease Control and Prevention, Office of Minority Health:
   http://www.cdc.gov/omh/
Office of Minority Health Resource Center:
   http://www.omhrc.gov
Oncology Nursing Society:
   http://www.ons.org
Multicultural Toolkit:
   http://www.ons.org/clinical/special/Toolkit.shtml
Transcultural Nursing Society:
   http://www.tcns.org

Bibliography

Barr DA: The practitioner's dilemma: Can we use a patient's race to predict genetics, ancestry, and the expected outcomes of treatment? *Ann Intern Med* 143:809-815, 2005.

Burhansstianov L, Olsen SJ: Cancer prevention and early detection in American Indian and Alaska native populations. *Clin J Oncol Nurs* 8:182-186, 2004.

Coffman MJ: Cultural caring in nursing practice: A meta-synthesis of qualitative research. *J Cult Divers* 11:100-109, 2004.

Collins KS, Hughes DL, Doty MM, et al: *Diverse communities, common concerns: Assessing health care quality for minority Americans,* New York, 2002, Commonwealth Fund.

Dhruva A, Cheng J, Kwong Luce JA, et al: Contrasts, conflicts, and change: A case in cultural oncology. *J Support Oncol* 4(6):301-304, 2006.

Freeman HP: Poverty, culture and social injustice: Determinants of cancer disparities. *CA Cancer J Clin* 54:72-77, 2004.

Giger JN, Davidhizar RE: *Transcultural nursing: Assessment and intervention,* ed 4, St Louis, 2004, Mosby.

Hernandez B: Highlights of cancer incidence data in Hawaii. *Hawaii Med J* 62:17-18, 2003.

Itano J: Coping: Cultural issues. In Itano J, Taoka K, editors: *Core curriculum for cancer nursing,* ed 4, Philadelphia, 2005, Elsevier.

Itano J: Cultural diversity of individuals with cancer. In Yarbro CH, Frogge MH, Goodman M, editors: *Cancer nursing: Principles and practice,* ed 6, Boston, 2005, Jones and Bartlett.

Jemal A, Siegel R, Ward E, et al: Cancer statistics, 2007. *CA Cancer J Clin* 57:43-66, 2007.

Juckett G: Cross-cultural medicine. *Am Fam Physician* 72:2267-2274, 2005.

Lillie-Blanton M, Rushing O, Ruiz S: *Key factors: Race, ethnicity and medical care,* Menlo Park, CA, 2003, Kaiser Family Foundation.

Office of Management and Budget, the Executive Office of the President. Revisions to the standards for the classification of federal data on race and ethnicity (website): http://www.whitehouse.gov/omb/fedreg/ombdir15.html. Accessed February 10, 2006.

Purnell LD, Paulanka BJ: *Transcultural health care: A culturally competent approach,* ed 2, Philadelphia, 2003, FA Davis.

Smedley BD, Stith AY, Nelson AR: *Unequal treatment: Confronting racial and ethnic disparities in health care,* Washington, DC, 2003, National Academies Press.

Spector R: *Cultural diversity in health and illness,* ed 6, Upper Saddle River, NJ, 2004, Pearson Education.

Taylor R: Addressing barriers to cultural competence. *J Nurs Staff Dev* 21:135-142, 2005.

Tu S, Chen H, Chen A, et al: Clinical trials: Understanding perceptions of female Chinese-American cancer patients. *Cancer* 104(suppl 12):2999-3005, 2005.

U.S. Department of Health and Human Services, Agency for Healthcare Research and Quality, 2005 National healthcare disparities report, AHRQ Publication No. 06-0017. Rockville, MD, 2005, U.S. Department of Health and Human Services.

Religion and Spirituality

Julie R. Swaney

1. What is the difference between religion and spirituality?

Spirituality is not necessarily religion. Many more people are spiritual than religious. Religion is a type of spirituality that refers to a disciplined, dogmatic set of beliefs usually set forth in writings (Quran, Bible, Creeds, and Confessions) and institutions (synagogues, churches). Spirituality refers to "an individual's essence as a person" (Belcher, 2006, p. 9) and to patterns or habits pertaining to ultimate meaning and purpose in life. Spirituality has to do with meaning-making.

2. What is the importance of religion and spirituality in illness?

Religion and spirituality provide the interpretive lens through which people make sense of living and dying. Cancer patients and their caregivers often believe in something that helps to maintain hope: chemotherapy, radiation therapy, doctors, vitamins, special diets, God's faithfulness to them, superstitious ritual, or their immune system. What they believe in provides a way of making sense of themselves and their experiences. When people are coping with cancer, what they believe about themselves—what they hold in their spirits—profoundly affects their experience. Many studies indicate a positive correlation between spirituality and illness as well as spirituality and healing. Patients who are able to identify meaning in their experiences may have increased physical and psychological well-being, less symptom distress, increased optimism, and better long-term cognitive adjustment.

3. What are the spiritual needs of cancer patients?

Spiritual needs include the need to:
- Make sense of the illness
- Find purpose and meaning in the midst of illness
- Have spiritual beliefs acknowledged, respected, and supported
- Transcend the illness and the self
- Feel in control and give up control
- Feel connected and cared for
- Acknowledge and cope with the notion of dying and death
- Forgive and to be forgiven
- Be thankful in the midst of illness
- Have relief of suffering
- Find hope

4. How do religious beliefs help people cope with terminal illness?

Healthy faith helps some people to better face reality, maintain hope, tolerate uncertainties, and retain their self-esteem and dignity. "Being religious" does not guarantee better coping but may reduce some sources of suffering. Religious beliefs that promote the constancy of God's presence help patients to realize their significance and permanence and to accept the ambiguity of God's ways. Prayer and meditation can reduce anxiety and strengthen coping skills. Certain beliefs answer the question, "Why?" whereas other beliefs provide comfort in the midst of the question itself.

The crisis of cancer prompts questions about meaning and existence. How much do I want to live? Why did this happen to me? What did I do or not do? Why does God allow this? Why do I have to suffer? Is God punishing me? Where is God? If I promise to go to church, will God heal me? Many people understand their existence in relation to God, whereas others do not. These existential questions of the human spirit are significant because they affect coping skills. Certainly "being religious" does not guarantee survival, but it can make a qualitative difference in the experience of cancer.

5. How does spiritual care contribute to healing?

Spiritual care is an important component of today's health care milieu. Spiritual care criteria has been articulated by the Joint Commission on Accreditation of Healthcare Organizations (JCAHO), providing a framework to help guide nurses' spiritual caregiving. The most powerful healing emotion is expectant faith. Healing is the product of a human bond between caregiver and patient. Faith, hope, respect, compassion, trust, and empathy are essential elements of bonds that contribute to healing. The heart of nursing or caring is a healing relationship, and the heart of healing relationships is trust, acceptance, and empathy.

To cure (Latin: *curare*) means to take care of, to take charge of. It implies successful medical treatment. To heal (Anglo-Saxon: *haelen*) means to make or become whole, to recover from sickness, to get well. Helping someone to become whole is accomplished through a healing relationship as well as technical competence. Both are important. Healing is a process and comes from the same root word as *holy*. Both refer to wholeness. To facilitate healing is to facilitate greater wholeness. Through relationships and skills, the nurse can facilitate healing, wholeness, and even that which is holy in patients. It is hoped that nurses can experience the same processes in themselves.

6. Can beliefs impede the healing process?

What people believe to be true may be what they will experience. Belief systems centered on punishment and guilt or even satanic forces may impede the healing process. Such beliefs lead people to think that they "deserve" the cancer and cannot be well again, whereas beliefs centered on forgiveness and hope facilitate healing and wholeness. Unhealthy faith provides an escape from reality and hinders adaptation to the experience.

7. What are the common religious beliefs and rituals related to illness and death?

Because a religion's stated positions may influence individual medical decisions, it is important to be familiar with some of the beliefs of particular religions, as outlined below. The nurse may ask patients about their beliefs and make use of religious authorities to assist them.

Common religious beliefs and rituals

Buddhism (Tibetan)	
Illness rituals	Prayer and meditation
Meaning of illness	Natural part of life
Faith healing	Possible through prayer and meditation

Common religious beliefs and rituals—cont'd

Sacraments	Respect intermediate state; preparation for death very important
	Death signals entry into intermediate state of great intensity
	Do not interrupt period of great concentration as deceased travels through intermediate state
	Environment to be peaceful, focused, and intimate for terminally ill or deceased
	Do not move body for 72 hours after death
	Spiritual goal: extinction
Autopsy	Permissible
Burial	Cremation
Meaning of death	Enlightenment

Roman Catholicism

Illness rituals	Baptism, Reconciliation, Sacrament of the Sick, Eucharist, prayer
Meaning of illness	Natural part of life; preserve dignity of patient; some suffering considered meaningful
Faith healing	Possible through prayer, Sacrament of the Sick (anointing)
Sacraments	Sacrament of the Sick
Autopsy	Permissible
Burial	Burial or cremation
Meaning of death	Release to God

Christian Science

Illness rituals	Prayer
Meaning of illness	Mental concept that can be destroyed by altering thoughts and discovering "spiritual truth"
	Use Christian Science practitioners
Faith healing	Primary means of healing; emphasize spiritual healing
Sacraments	None
Autopsy	Unlikely, but permissible
Burial	Burial or cremation
Meaning of death	Return to God

Mormon (Church of Jesus Christ of Latter-Day Saints)

Illness rituals	Prayer
Meaning of illness	Natural part of life; revelation of meaning through individual visions
Faith healing	Laying on of hands for divine healing
Sacraments	Adult baptism essential, even after death; preach gospel
	Wash body; dress body in white robe
Autopsy	Permissible
Burial	Burial; no cremation
Meaning of death	Death a blessing; return to God

Hindu

Illness rituals	Prayer
Meaning of illness	Punishment
Faith healing	Possible through prayer and meditation

Continued

Common religious beliefs and rituals—cont'd

Sacraments	Tie thread of blessing
	Pour water in mouth
	Washing of body
	Particular about who touches body
Autopsy	Permissible
Burial	Cremation (Ganges)
Meaning of death	Death an endless passage through cycles of life; natural part of life
	Hope for better existence in next life
	Death is liberation

Islam

Illness rituals	Prayer, visitation, assistance to families essential
	Many birth and death rituals
	Same gender treatment important
	At death, closing eyes, washing of body (Ghusl)
Meaning of illness	Everything happens by Allah's will and knowledge
	Allah is all powerful and all must seek his mercy and help
Faith healing	Healing will happen at Allah's will
	Everything is predetermined
	Destiny of all already known to Allah
Sacraments	When death approaches, it is customary to recite "the declaration of faith"
	Sick person should be turned onto his/her right side
Autopsy	Prohibited
Burial	Cremation forbidden
	Body is cleaned, scented, covered with a clean cloth for burial
	Body should be buried by Muslims as soon as possible
Meaning of death	Believe in life after death; return of soul to Allah

Jehovah's Witness

Illness rituals	Prayer
Meaning of illness	Natural part of life; strong sanctity of life
Faith healing	Possible through prayer
Sacraments	None
Autopsy	Acceptable; body intact
Burial	Burial or cremation
Meaning of death	Natural part of life

Judaism (Orthodox)

Illness rituals	Prayer
Meaning of illness	Natural part of life; strong sanctity-of-life ethic requiring all possible medical care to preserve life
Faith healing	Demand medical attention; possible through prayer
Sacraments	Goses, Shiva, Yetziat Neshamah, Kevod Hamet
Autopsy	Rarely permissible; consult rabbi
Burial	No cremation; quick burial
Meaning of death	Natural part of life; no afterlife

Common religious beliefs and rituals—cont'd

Presbyterian (Protestant)

Illness rituals	Prayer
Meaning of illness	Natural part of life; quality of life valued over quantity of life
Faith healing	Prayer, communion
Sacraments	Baptism, communion, anointing, prayer
Autopsy	Acceptable
Burial	Burial or cremation
Meaning of death	Resurrection into afterlife

8. How do religious beliefs affect ethical decision-making?

At times of uncertainty, people often turn to their moral or religious community for guidance in ethical decision-making. What appears to others to be nonbeneficial or "futile" treatment may, in fact, be perceived by a patient to be beneficial as defined by the religious community or doctrine to which he or she belongs. A Muslim patient may demand what appears to be "futile" treatment because the tenets of Islam dictate that life must be prolonged. A patient who is a Jehovah's Witness may refuse blood, even if the outcome is death, because of religious tenets. Other common religious beliefs that affect ethical issues are outlined below.

Religious beliefs that affect ethical issues

Buddhism

Drugs, blood, artificial life support	Acceptable
Organ donation	Allowed if enhances possibility of enlightenment
Termination of treatment	Allowed
Withholding/withdrawing life support	Allowed
	Death is natural, to be accepted
	Avoid unnatural intrusion of dying process
Active euthanasia	Prohibited

Roman Catholicism

Drugs, blood, artificial life support	Acceptable
Organ donation	Justified
Termination of treatment	Allowed except in cases of pregnancy
Withholding/withdrawing life support	Allowed
	"Ordinary but not extraordinary" duty to prolong life; importance of dignity
	Exception: pregnancy
Active euthanasia	Prohibited

Christian Science

Drugs, blood, artificial life support	Unacceptable
Organ donation	Unlikely

Continued

Religious beliefs that affect ethical issues—cont'd

Termination of treatment	Allowed
	Rely on faith healing
Withholding/withdrawing life support	Allowed
	Unlikely to accept in first place; unlikely to prolong dying process
Active euthanasia	Prohibited

Mormon (Church of Jesus Christ of Latter-Day Saints)

Drugs, blood, artificial life support	Acceptable
Organ donation	Individual decision
Termination of treatment	Allowed
Withholding/withdrawing life support	Allowed
	Inevitable death viewed as a blessing
Active euthanasia	Prohibited

Hindu

Drugs, blood, artificial life support	Acceptable
Organ donation	Permissible
Termination of treatment	Allowed
Withholding/withdrawing life support	Allowed
	Death is liberation
Active euthanasia	Prohibited

Islam

Drugs, blood, artificial life support	Acceptable
Organ donation	Not permitted
Termination of treatment	Allowed if death is imminent; orthodox position would not allow
Withholding/withdrawing life support	Sometimes allowed
	Orthodox position more strict: "No soul can die except by Allah's permission." (Quran 3:185)
Active euthanasia	Prohibited

Jehovah's Witness

Drugs, blood, artificial life support	Some drugs; no blood or blood products; life support acceptable
Organ donation	Forbidden
Termination of treatment	Allowed
Withholding/withdrawing life support	Allowed
	Rely on individual conscience in this decision
	Duty not to accept blood or blood products
Active euthanasia	Prohibited

Judaism (Orthodox)

Drugs, blood, artificial life support	Acceptable
Organ donation	Consult rabbi
Termination of treatment	Not allowed
	Consult rabbi

Religious beliefs that affect ethical issues—cont'd

Withholding/withdrawing life support	Not allowed
	Consult rabbi
Active euthanasia	Prohibited

Presbyterian (Protestant)

Drugs, blood, artificial life support	Acceptable
Organ donation	Acceptable
Termination of treatment	Allowed
Withholding/withdrawing life support	Allowed
	Quality of life valued over quantity of life
	Importance of dignity
Active euthanasia	Prohibited

9. How do I understand a belief system different from my own?

Listen intently. *Ask* with sincerity. *Respect* what you hear. Some people have specific religious views to fashion their understanding, whereas others have their own theology, which may not fit any particular religious tradition. Even if you do not agree with all of a patient's beliefs, you can still help the patient by allowing him or her to articulate personal beliefs. It is not appropriate to try to convert patients to your belief system during vulnerable times.

10. What is spiritual nursing care?

Spiritual nursing care is "an intuitive, interpersonal, altruistic, and integrative expression that is contingent on the nurse's awareness of the transcendent dimension of life but that reflects the patient's reality" (Sawatzky and Pesut, 2005, p. 23). The following steps can assist in the provision of spiritual nursing care:

1. Assess your own view of the role and importance of spirituality and religion in health and illness. Person-centered nursing requires tending to the human spirit.
2. Assess your personal comfort level with addressing spiritual issues. The nurse who is uncomfortable with such issues should refer the patient to someone else.
3. Offer yourself in a genuine, honest, empathic way. Listening empathically and respecting the patient's questions and views are more important than providing answers.
4. Do a spiritual assessment.

11. How can a nurse perform a spiritual assessment?

Discussion about spiritual or religious concerns may be initiated by asking questions, such as: What meaning does your cancer have for you? What gives you strength during difficult times? While there are many ways to do a spiritual assessment, one recommended approach is the FICA spiritual assessment tool. This tool simply asks:

F (FAITH):	Do you consider yourself to be spiritual or religious?
	What things do you believe in that give meaning to your life?
I (IMPORTANCE):	Is faith important to you?
	How have your beliefs influenced your behavior during this illness?
C (COMMUNITY):	Are you part of a spiritual or religious community?
	Is there a person or a group of people who are really important to you?

A (ASSESSMENT):   How would you like me, your health care provider, to address these issues in your health care?

Answers to these questions will help you to understand your patient's spiritual state, including recent changes, and need for any special religious resources.

12. What are key nursing interventions to promote the spiritual well-being of patients?

Spiritual interventions described by the Oncology Nursing Society Spirituality Special Interest Group include presence (standing with another), meditation, prayer, use of arts (music, art, and dance), storytelling, journaling, bibliotherapy (use of literature), and humor. Other ways nurses can promote spiritual well-being include:

- Actively listen to patients talk through their problems.
- Offer genuine concern and empathy in eliciting the patient's spiritual strengths, beliefs, doubts, and confidences.
- Assist patients in discovering and using their own beliefs.
- Facilitate patients' spiritual practices or rituals; provide privacy to do so.

13. What is spiritual distress?

Spiritual distress occurs when a person experiences or is at risk of experiencing a disturbance in a belief or value system that provides strength, hope, and meaning to life. Ways of interpreting life ("I always thought God would protect me"), of making sense, of finding meaning, fall apart. Sources of spiritual distress may be the crises of illness, suffering, or death itself; the inability to practice spiritual rituals; or conflict between beliefs and treatment regimen.

14. List common signs of spiritual distress.

Signs of spiritual distress range from obvious expression to subtle clues:

- Statement of spiritual distress or crisis
- Withdrawal, depression
- Anger
- Crying
- Loneliness, loss of self-esteem
- Hopelessness, helplessness
- Changes in reading or not reading religious literature
- Expression of feeling abandoned by persons and God
- Inability to cope with illness or treatment
- Refusal of or demand for treatment
- Praying for a miracle
- Tenacious grip on a rigid set of beliefs

15. What are nursing interventions for spiritual distress?

- If spiritual distress is related to the inability to practice spiritual rituals, the nurse may help by addressing the disruptive factors and enabling the patient to engage in important (health-aiding) rituals.
- When spiritual distress is related to the crisis of illness, suffering, or dying, the nurse can help the patient verbalize a sense of meaning, sense of forgiveness, and sense of belonging and love. Such distress may be expressed in such questions as "Why is this happening to me?" (meaning), "What did I do to deserve this?" (forgiveness), or "Why do I feel so alone?" (love/relatedness). The nurse can help patients use their own inner resources to address such questions and may also enlist the help of external resources (clergy, family, friends, literature, health care professionals).

- Spiritual distress related to conflict between religious or spiritual beliefs and the prescribed health regimen can be relieved by providing thorough and accurate information for informed consent or informed refusal. The health care team should support the patient in his or her stated wishes and goals.

16. What is the difference between suffering and pain?

Bodies do not suffer; people do. Pain refers to a physical sensation, whereas suffering refers to the quest for meaning, purpose, and fulfillment. Although pain is often a source of suffering, suffering may occur in the absence of pain. It is an existential state in which persons experience themselves to be fragmenting and disintegrating in terms of personal significance. Suffering may occur when a person perceives illness or death as meaningless or as a form of personal disintegration. People who have not made the most of their lives often have a hard time facing death.

Other sources of suffering are the effects of disease and treatment, such as change in identity, loss of control, isolation, not feeling understood, perception of a foreshortened future (i.e., "nothingness," death), and threats of losing relationships, mobility, independence, finances, control, and self-worth. Theologically and existentially, suffering occurs when we are threatened by something not in our control. In this sense, some suffering is inevitable, because we are always facing things we cannot control. Suffering is more bearable when we remain centered, when we can plumb the depths of our suffering to discover life's ultimate meaning for us.

17. What difference does faith make in the experience of pain and suffering?

How people view their pain and suffering affects their healing or dying process. Many people still believe that pain and suffering are meaningful signs of God's presence and must be endured. Others are outraged by the pain and suffering that they endure and demand alleviation. Both positions may be more than simple attitudes; they may be deep religious convictions. The nurse may verify patient's beliefs and give the patient permission to verbalize personal points of view. When in doubt, the nurse should err on the side of alleviating pain and suffering.

18. What is the connection between prayer and healing?

"The science of prayer" has generated much debate and controversy. Prayer seems to be effective, but how and why? Why does prayer "work" for some people and not for others? To answer this question, as well as to define the relationship between prayer and healing, we must remain open to the mystery and ambiguity of healing, and perhaps of God.

Both theologians and physicians are enlarging their frameworks for understanding the connection between faith and healing. Historically, all physicians were priests, nurses were nuns, and religious orders ran hospitals. Spiritual and physical healing were recognized as intimately connected. Early 19th century rationalism, with its mechanical view of the body, increasingly separated the body from the mind and spirit. Religion left medicine, and medicine left the church. Yet there remained a holistic notion of persons that emphasized the integration of body, mind, and spirit.

Prayer is one way of attending to the spirit. Prayer grounds people in what gives them meaning and in their relationship with God. Prayer puts important words to their experiences. Prayer also evokes important feelings for healing—safety, hope, love, seeing oneself as one is seen by God, personal worth and self-esteem, and feeling cared about and "not alone." Prayer helps people to face reality; to tolerate ambiguity and uncertainty; and to confront the unknown, which is so constant in illness. At the very least, prayer helps to reduce anxiety, to remain centered, to remember that one is part of God's greater order;

it helps patients to relax. And at the very most, prayer is an expression of a profound and empowering relationship with God.

19. What if someone is praying for a miracle?

Many people say that they are "praying for a miracle." A miracle is a purposeful intervention from God that is often a process and not an instant. Praying for a miracle does not relieve one of continuing personal responsibility, such as pursuing treatment or making difficult decisions. Miracles happen as part of God's order, not our magical wishes for situations to change. It is fine for people to pray for miracles as long as they also face the reality before them.

20. When should a chaplain be called?

Chaplains are frequently called for deaths, although religion and faith are not just about death. The goal of pastoral care is healing of the spirit, whether a person is living or dying. As nurses become acquainted with the hospital chaplain, they come to know how he or she approaches the nuances of a patient's concerns. Very often this is accomplished through an empathic relationship that encourages and allows patients to use their own inner resources to affect healing and strength.

Chaplains generally represent all denominations and faith traditions—Protestant, Catholic, Jewish, Hindu, Islam, and so on. Staff chaplains can assist the nurse in finding a representative from a particular faith. Chaplains are available for sacramental purposes such as baptism, communion, anointing, weddings, funerals, and confession. They are also available for pastoral purposes such as counseling, prayer, support, and assistance in decision-making. Although there are many times and reasons to call a chaplain, some of the most common are when the patient:

- Uses religion as a source of support
- Is withdrawn, depressed, restless, complaining, or irritable
- Is anxious (notably preoperatively)
- Worsens, becomes terminally ill, or dies
- Expresses interest or curiosity about religious questions or issues
- Reads scripture and other religious literature
- Is struggling with loss or grieving
- Exhibits spiritual distress
- Has ethical dilemmas, decisions to make
- Asks to see a chaplain, asks about worship services, desires a Bible
- Has no visitors, cards, or flowers in room
- Expresses a desire for sacraments

21. What does a chaplain do during a visit?

Chaplains respond to the presenting need (e.g., fear of dying, anxiety about procedures, grief over a diagnosis, hopelessness of ongoing treatment, need for prayer and reassurance, anger at God). One of the most valuable pastoral interventions is to offer an empathic relationship. This means entering into the world of the patient and listening to his or her experience, conflict, dilemma, or fear. Chaplains encourage a person's inner strengths. They assist persons in finding hope when they feel hopeless and help persons to recover or discover for the first time who they are in relationship with God. Because of the intimacy of the process of illness, dying, and death, many chaplains perform funerals and memorial services for patients who have died. Chaplains also assist in discussions about code status, requests for organ donation, and mortuary arrangements.

22. Are chaplains available to staff?

Most chaplains are available to staff members as well as patients and families. Oncology nurses must take care of themselves, allow themselves to suffer with their patients, acknowledge their own pain and losses, and use supportive people around them. Chaplains are also available for support, clarification, encouragement, and hope. Chaplains may offer periodic memorial services for the staff to gain closure in regard to patient deaths.

23. What is a parish nurse?

A parish nurse is a registered nurse licensed to practice within the state whose practice setting is the congregation. The parish nurse is available to congregation members as a personal health counselor, health educator, resource referral agent, volunteer facilitator, and integrator of faith and health. With roots in the Judeo-Christian tradition, the mission of parish nursing is to combine the practice of faith with the practice of nursing to help individual's achieve wholeness through faith. Oncology and parish nurses can work together as partners in providing health care to oncology patients along the continuum of care from the health care institution to the community.

 Key Points

- Religion and spirituality are not necessarily the same thing. Both are a way of finding or making meaning.
- There is a correlation between spirituality and health.
- Religious and spiritual beliefs can affect ethical decisions.
- Spiritual assessment is a way to elicit important aspects of patient beliefs, hopes, and expectations.
- The most important nursing intervention is to offer active listening, genuine concern, and empathy in eliciting the patient's spiritual strengths, beliefs, doubts, and confidences. Nurses should not impose their beliefs on patients.
- The goal of pastoral care is healing of the spirit.

 Internet Resources

The Pluralism Project:
  http://www.pluralism.org
Spirituality and Cancer Care:
  http://www.cancer.gov/cancertopics/pdq/supportivecare/spirituality/HealthProfessional/
  page9/print
Mind/Body Medical Institute:
  http://www.mbmi.org
Center for Spirituality, Theology and Health (research on effects of religion on health):
  http://www.dukespiritualityandhealth.org
International Parish Nurse Resource Center:
  http://ipnrc.parishnurses.org
Spiritual Care Special Interest Group (SIG) Toolkit:
  http://www.spiritualcaresig.org
Spiritual Care SIG Toolkit:
  http://www.spiritualcaresig.org

Bibliography

Belcher AE: Should oncology nurses provide spiritual care? *ONS News* 21(5):9-10, 2006.

Cassell E: The nature of suffering and the goals of medicine. *N Engl J Med* 306:639-645, 1982.

Gall TL, Cornblat MW: Breast cancer survivors give voice: A qualitative analysis of spiritual factors in long-term adjustment. *Psychooncology* 11:524-535, 2002.

Koenig H: *Spirituality in patient care: Why, how, when and what.* Philadelphia, 2002, Templeton Foundation Press.

Kristeller JL, Zumbrun CS, Schiller RF: 'I would if I could': How oncologists and oncology nurses address spiritual distress in cancer patients. *Psychooncology* 8:451-458, 1999.

Marty M, Vaux K, editors: *Health/medicine and the faith traditions: An inquiry into religion and medicine,* Philadelphia, 1982, Fortress Press.

Meraviglia M: Effects of spirituality in breast cancer survivors. *Oncol Nurs Forum* 33(1):E1-E7, 2006.

Post-White J, Ceronsky D, Kreitzer MJ, et al: Hope, spirituality, sense of coherence, and quality of life in patients with cancer. *Oncol Nurs Forum* 23(10):1571-1579, 1996.

Puchalski CM: Taking a spiritual history: FICA. *Spirituality and Medicine Connection* 3:1, 1999.

Sawatzky R, Pesut B: Attributes of spiritual care in nursing practice. *J Holist Nurs* 23:19-33, 2005.

Stefanek M, McDonald PG, Hess, SA: Religion, spirituality and cancer: Current status and methodological challenges. *Psychooncology* 14:450-463, 2005.

Tartaro J, Luecken L, Gunn HE: Exploring heart and soul: Effects of religiosity/spirituality and gender on blood pressure and cortisol stress responses. *J Health Psychol* 10(6):753-766, 2005.

Tartaro J, Roberts J, Nosarti C, et al: Who benefits? Distress, adjustment and benefit-finding among breast cancer survivors. *J Psychosoc Oncol* 23(2/3):45-64, 2005.

Chapter 57

Family and Caregiver Coping

Karen J. Stanley

1. Describe the typical family response to a diagnosis of cancer.

Because patients and families respond to news of life-threatening illness according to individual and family-centered coping methods, there is no typical response. Shock, anger, fear, denial, disbelief, generalized anxiety, and feelings of helplessness and vulnerability are common initial responses. While some individuals may withdraw, others respond by seeking as much information as possible from the health care team and external sources. A family's ability to cope with the unexpected stressors of a cancer diagnosis is predicated on various factors, including educational background, cultural expectations and norms, communication techniques, established coping mechanisms, family dynamics (including dysfunctional behaviors), prior history and/or experience with life-threatening illness, and confidence in the ability to be an effective caregiver. Each family employs a set of behavioral norms that may not be verbalized or readily apparent. Healthy families may use humor, good communication techniques, and willingness to be flexible to deal with unexpected happenings, but the health care provider may need to coach families who do not have such skills.

2. What is the appropriate professional approach to a patient or family who denies or refuses to discuss the diagnosis and its implications?

Because illness is a patient-defined subjective experience, a professional approach involves individualized interventions based on a thorough psychosocial assessment that targets patients and families at high risk for inadequate coping; identifies periods of time when intervention is most needed; and reflects a multicultural perspective that supports a broad range of response to the illness experience and a sensitive dialogue among all interested parties. Denial can be initially healthy because it provides a "buffer zone" or respite for the patient and significant others to absorb the reality of the diagnosis and its implications. The denial is healthy as long as it is temporary, intermittent, and does not influence major decisions.

3. What are some guidelines to help families who deny or refuse to discuss the patient's diagnosis and its implications?

- Do not confront the patient, family, or friends when they are not prepared to integrate difficult information. Confrontation at this time can be harmful and permanently destroy the chance for an ongoing therapeutic relationship.
- Use a nonintrusive, supportive approach. It is important to confirm what patients and families understand to be true and work from that point.
- Reinforce realistic goals, but avoid agreeing with unrealistic goals or hopes.
- Include family members in planning and delivering the patient's care to allow them to see the extent of the illness and also provide comfort to those who desire help.
- Remind family members that their refusal to discuss the diagnosis can isolate the patient and increase anxiety, fear, and sadness.
- Make every effort to ease the way for family members to participate in what the patient may view as essential dialogue. Encourage family members and friends to

"practice" difficult discussions with each other and with health care professionals. Give them permission to try and fail without fear of censure.

- Remind family members that their personal grieving and bereavement may be positively enhanced by the knowledge that they were able to have meaningful conversations with the patient over the illness continuum.

4. How can a health care professional balance appropriate and effective communication with a patient's need for and right to control the flow of information?

Multiple issues are involved in the patient's right to control how, when, and to whom information is conveyed. Privacy may be a priority for the patient who requests that others not be told of the diagnosis, prognosis, or treatment plan without permission. In such instances, health care providers must refer family and friends to the patient when questions are asked. Of equal importance are circumstances in which family members request that patients not be told their diagnosis for fear that they will become depressed or lose hope. It is not appropriate for a health care professional to promise a family member or friend that the patient will not be told the circumstances of the illness. The health care provider has an ongoing responsibility to confirm repeatedly with the patient the amount of information that the patient requires. Patients may delegate a family member or friend to receive the information and make decisions for them. When patients ask for information, it is always appropriate to explore exactly what they would like to know and respond accordingly.

5. What warning signs might family members exhibit suggesting they may require assistance in coping with the stressors of the patient's illness?

Maladaptive Family Coping Mechanisms

- Persistent anger, hostility, resentment, or denial
- Conflict between patient and caregiver(s)
- Missed health care appointments for patients dependent on others
- Caregiver illness or health problems
- Decreased patient self-care abilities accompanied by increasing caregiver responsibilities
- Signs of caregiver burden (e.g., weariness, depression, physical complaints)
- Inadequate or inappropriate caregiving
- Inadequate number of caregivers in relationship to care required
- Detachment or withdrawal at any stage of illness

Adapted from Frey JH: Family coping. In Harkreader H, editor: *Fundamentals of nursing: Caring and clinical judgment*, Philadelphia, 2000, Saunders.

6. Identify issues and stressors that can emerge in families across the illness continuum.

There may be weeks and/or months of disruption and emotional upheaval throughout the treatment process. Family roles and responsibilities are restructured to fill the void left by the individual who is ill. These changes can exacerbate preexistent dysfunctional relationships that in turn increase emotional distress. Resentment frequently grows if there is a perception that the burden may not be equally shared by family members and friends. Patients and caregivers (parents, spouses, children, other family members, or friends) may become overprotective or distance themselves from significant family and friends in the constellation.

7. How may families be helped to adapt to the rigors of the diagnosis and caregiving?

Supporting Adaptation and Coping in Family Systems During Diagnosis and Treatment

Present Informed, Consistent, and Honest Information in a Culturally Sensitive Way
-Treatment options and expected side effects
-Right to solicit a second opinion
-Ongoing assessment/discussion of patient's response to treatment, pending diagnostic assays
-Clarification of misinformation or misunderstanding of previous discussions
-Review of options in unexpected circumstances (e.g., lack of response to therapy or recurrent disease)

Give Concrete Instructions About Physical Care Requirements
-Informed description of what to expect from a physiologic perspective
-Detailed instruction (both written and verbal) regarding medical appointments, management of side effects of illness and treatment regimen, medication administration, use of infusion devices or other equipment

Provide Emotional Support
-Encourage patient to articulate health care choices and prepare an advance health care directive
-Acknowledge actual and potential losses
-Be emotionally available to listen and assist with problems
-Encourage realistic goals and hopes
-Assist family members and friends to understand psychologic sequelae to illness
-Make sure to pay consistent attention to family members who may otherwise be neglected
-Offer to hold family conferences, when necessary
-Offer to keep friends and family members informed (with patient and family's permission)

Offer Practical Assistance
-Assist family members to redefine roles and organize personal responsibilities
-Make referrals to outside resources for legal or financial issues
-Make referrals to other health care providers as appropriate (e.g., chaplain, social worker, community volunteer agencies)

8. How can families be assisted to extend their informal support network?

Because families often need significant encouragement to ask for help, it is useful to them to draw up lists of tasks that can be delegated to others. It may also be helpful to ask a close family friend to coordinate requests for help and relieve the family of both the emotional and physical burdens of acknowledging need. Community agencies that offer assistance, such as Meals on Wheels, American Cancer Society or other cancer support organizations, and faith communities, can be welcome sources of much needed help.

9. How may nurses ease the transition for patients and families from active treatment to palliative care?

Decisions that have life and death implications for patients and families should not be made in isolation. The nurse may need to provide assistance by outlining options and explaining the consequences of various choices. Patients and families need to hear repeatedly that they will not be abandoned, that attention to symptom management will be meticulous and professional, that the health care team is committed to maximizing the patient's quality of life, and that all involved in care are privileged to participate. Most importantly, the health care provider must listen and learn.

10. What have patients and families identified as important contributors to quality end-of-life care?

Patients have singled out the following issues: adequate pain and symptom management, no inappropriate prolongation of dying, promoting a sense of control, relieving the burden on families and caregivers, and strengthening relationships with loved ones.

11. How should nurses respond to the concerns of patients and families about quality end-of-life care?

- Empower patients and families to ask for and receive adequate pain and symptom management when the need arises.
- Encourage families to have frank discussions with the patient about desired health care interventions over the illness continuum, most particularly at the end of life. These discussions should clarify and validate how much control the patient chooses to have over personal circumstances and whether the patient chooses to relinquish control to another family member or friend at any point during the illness.
- Encourage families to explore at length and on repeated occasions the patient's perception of burden to the caregivers. This particular concern may be monumental to the patient, and planned interventions to provide respite or relief to family and friends may provide as much, if not more, comfort to patients than to caregivers.
- Strengthen relationships with loved ones at all times. Many patients regard the time remaining to them as a gift, a time in which to make amends, to enjoy precious time with family and friends, to do what is most meaningful to them, and to live every day to the fullest. If the people nearest the patient share and/or understand this outlook, the potential for the richest life possible can be realized. Active storytelling from patients and family members is a way of honoring the life that has been lived.
- Encourage communication with the patient's religious or spiritual community when appropriate; and assist in the translation of what is heard, seen, and experienced, while respecting individual expressions of grief as distinct and worthwhile. In specific circumstances it can be useful to encourage family members and friends to discuss what the future will be like after the patient has died. . . .this allows fear, resentment, and unspoken feelings to emerge. Knowledge of the widest possible landscape of feelings strengthens the grieving process for all concerned.

 Key Points

- Cancer is a family diagnosis.
- There is no typical patient/family response to a cancer diagnosis.
- There are warning signs of maladaptive family coping.
- A cancer diagnosis disrupts family roles and responsibilities and can diminish the physical health of caregivers.
- Family-centered care supports open and honest communication.

Internet Resources

National Family Caregivers Association (self-advocacy and self-care for caregivers):
http://www.nfcacares.org
CareGivers.com, (problem solving for older adults):
http://www.caregivers.com
Rosalynn Carter Institute for Caregiving:
http://www.RosalynnCarter.org
People Living with Cancer (coping with cancer for patients and families):
http://www.plwc.org/portal/site/PLWC
Oncology Nursing Society, Patient Education (for families of patients with cancer):
http://www.ons.org/PatientEd

Bibliography

Bush NJ: Coping and adaptation. In Carroll-Johnson RM, Gorman LM, Bush NJ, editors: *Psychosocial nursing care along the cancer continuum,* Pittsburgh, 2006, Oncology Nursing Society.

Duhamel F, Dupuis F: Guaranteed returns: Investing in conversations with families of patients with cancer. *Clin J Oncol Nurs* 8:68-71, 2004.

Frey JH: Family coping. In Harkreader H, editor: *Fundamentals of nursing: Caring and clinical judgment,* Philadelphia, 2000, Saunders.

Gorman, LM: Denial. In Carroll-Johnson RM, Gorman LM, Bush NJ, editors: *Psychosocial nursing care along the cancer continuum,* Pittsburgh, 2006, Oncology Nursing Society.

Nail LM: I'm coping as fast as I can: Psychosocial adjustments to cancer and cancer treatment, *Oncol Nurs Forum* 6:967-970, 2001.

Northouse LL: Helping families of patients with cancer. *Oncol Nurs Forum* 32:743-750, 2004.

Stanley KJ: The healing power of presence: Respite from the fear of abandonment. *Oncol Nurs Forum* 29:935-940, 2002.

Stephenson PS: Understanding denial. *Oncol Nurs Forum* 31:985-988, 2004.

Weekes DP: Cultural influences on the psychosocial experience. In Carroll-Johnson RM. Gorman LM, Bush NJ, editors: *Psychosocial nursing care along the cancer continuum,* Pittsburgh, 2006, Oncology Nursing Society.

Survivorship

Susan A. Leigh and Debra Thaler-DeMers

1. Why should nurses who care for patients in a hospital or clinic be interested in cancer survivors?

Historically, a diagnosis of cancer has elicited feelings of fear, dread, terror, doom, mutilation—words that describe the underlying notion that the person surely will die of the disease. This myth about cancer can psychologically paralyze the person who receives the diagnosis; it can also evoke negative reactions from nurses and other caregivers. Negative reactions from nurses can decrease the sense of hopefulness and future orientation that is vitally necessary during the early stages of survival. The knowledge that people survive different types of cancer—many are cured whereas others live for long periods with cancer as a chronic illness—helps nurses to introduce the potential for survival, to decrease the sense of helplessness, and to transform a passive acceptance of fate into a proactive sense of control. Thus, quality of life is improved for both survivor and caregiver.

2. How long after diagnosis is a patient considered a survivor?

The term *survivor* is defined in more than one way. Historically, the traditional medical definition used the quantitative landmark of 5 years free of disease as the transition point from patient to survivor. Yet, when the National Coalition for Cancer Survivorship (NCCS) was founded in 1986, the founding members crafted a definition that focused on the qualitative aspects of survival: "From the time of its discovery, and for the balance of life, an individual diagnosed with cancer is a survivor." With this definition, one becomes a survivor with the initial diagnosis of cancer.

3. What does cancer survivorship mean?

Survivorship can be defined either as a process or a stage of survival. S*urvivorship* was first paired with cancer by the founders of NCCS. Initially, the term was defined as a process of survival rather than a fixed point in time, that is, *how* we survive the experience of living with cancer, adapting to it as a part of the life process, and incorporating it into the broader perspective of overall life experiences. Quality of life throughout the continuum of cancer became the framework to describe this concept.

Many oncology health care providers view survivorship quite differently. Some researchers and clinicians define survivorship as a distinct stage of survival. A 2005 report from the Institute of Medicine (IOM) entitled *From Patient to Survivor: Lost in Transition* recognizes the discrepancies in definitions, yet the report focuses on a much neglected stage of survival. This stage follows the initial diagnosis and treatment and continues until disease recurrence or death. Although rehabilitation previously defined this stage, it is now a component of survivorship continuum.

4. How many cancer survivors are there in the United States?

The most recent estimate is that approximately 10.1 million people in the United States have histories of cancer. About half are considered long-term survivors because they have survived for 5 or more years, and approximately 14% of the total number has survived for over 20 years. Considering all types of cancer, the relative 5-year survival rate (the ratio of observed survival rate for survivors vs. the expected survival rate of the general population) has reached 64%, according to the latest Surveillance, Epidemiology, and End Results (SEER) data from the National Cancer Institute (http://seer.cancer.gov). Although this percentage is much higher for some cancer survivors and much lower for others, depending on the specific type and stage of cancer, it means that over half the number of people diagnosed with cancer today will be long-term survivors.

5. What stages describe cancer survival?

One of the most recognized models that describe stages along the cancer continuum was first introduced by Mullan in 1985. His essay in the *New England Journal of Medicine* was entitled *Seasons of Survival*, and includes the acute, extended, and permanent stages. More recently, end of life has been added as the fourth stage.

- **Acute survival** begins with the diagnosis of cancer. During this period the survivor's life is dominated by the illness. The focus is on medical treatment, whether it be surgery, radiation, chemotherapy, or biotherapy. Survivors may be feeling sick and considering their mortality. It is also a time when the survivor has more access to support services.
- **Extended survival** begins when the survivor enters remission or discontinues routine treatment, reintegrating into everyday activities. The focus shifts from the medical environment to the community. Survivors may return to work, school, or the responsibility of managing a household, and may benefit from referral to community support groups or resource centers, legal services, or professional counseling services. An increasing number of national organizations offer a variety of services specific to different cancer types.
- **Permanent survival** is sometimes equated with the word *cure*; cancer is no longer a major focus of the survivor's life. During this sustained remission, the cancer experience is integrated into the broader experience of the survivor's entire life. Ideally, cancer survivors would remain in contact with the medical community, although who is most qualified to follow this population is yet to be determined. Psychologic, legal, economic, and insurance issues may also arise or continue to be a problem. Referral to appropriate resources may be helpful, but fewer programs or agencies focus on long-term survivors.
- **End of life** (see Chapter 59, Hospice Care)

Nurses should keep in mind that no one progresses through these stages in the same way. A person may move back and forth between stages or may never experience one or more of the stages. As with any model, the stages act as guidelines.

6. Who is addressing the needs of long-term survivors?

NCCS has advocated for continued attention to long-term survivors since 1986, and in 1996 published Imperatives for Quality Cancer Care. Shortly after the release of this report, the National Cancer Institute (NCI) created the Office of Cancer Survivorship to address survivorship-related issues. More recently, national reports underscoring the needs of survivors have come from the President's Cancer Panel, the Centers for Disease Control and Prevention, the IOM, and the American Journal of Nursing State of the Science Report.

7. List helpful hints for communicating information to cancer survivors.

- Repeat information numerous times; less than 50% of what is conveyed is usually retained by the survivor.
- Use a variety of settings and contexts, both to reinforce the information and to elicit questions from the survivor.

- Encourage survivors to bring a family member or friend to consultations and conferences to take notes and help recall information.
- Assess the survivor's ability to read and understand the language of printed material.
- Encourage survivors to keep a journal or log of their experiences, questions, and concerns. The journal can be kept at the bedside, so that if questions or concerns arise during the night, the survivor can write them down and deal with them later.
- Suggest using a tape recorder. Teaching sessions, consultations, and conferences with survivors and/or caregivers can be recorded. If questions arise later when the survivor returns home, the recorded information can be used as a reference. The question may have been answered during the conference, and listening to the tape saves additional phone calls to the physician's office. In addition, family members who may not have been able to attend the conference can hear the information. The tape becomes a resource for both survivors and families.

8. **What problems or barriers may cause survivors to discontinue treatment?**

   Treatment for cancer is difficult and takes its toll in many ways. Any number of problems—physical, psychologic, social, financial, cultural—can prompt survivors to interrupt or stop therapy.

Problems Prompting Discontinuation of Therapy

Physical
- Uncontrollable or unacceptable acute effects (e.g., nausea and vomiting, fatigue, pain)
- Chronic or long-term effects of treatment (e.g., peripheral neuropathy)
- Inability to concentrate or think clearly
- Increasing disability or dependence

Psychologic
- Fear of disfigurement (e.g., scarring, hair loss)
- Fear of permanent disability, including impotence
- Fear of late effects (e.g., infertility, second malignancies)
- Decreased quality of life

Social
- Lack of transportation
- Fear of losing job
- Inadequate or unaffordable child care
- Insufficient support with family responsibilities
- Decreased social interactions (e.g., dating, marriage)

Financial
- Unable to miss work or survive on reduced paycheck
- Uninsured or underinsured
- Unaffordable out-of-pocket expenses
- Ineligible for government assistance (e.g., Medicaid, Medicare, Social Security Disability)

Problems Prompting Discontinuation of Therapy—cont'd

Cultural
- Language barriers
- Lack of understanding
- Erroneous information or belief in myths
- Conflicting attitudes, beliefs, and values

9. What issues are specific to adolescent survivors and young adults?

Issues important to younger cancer survivors include fertility, cognitive deficiencies, and growth problems. Chemotherapy protocols that may preserve fertility should be used whenever possible, and young men should be encouraged to bank sperm before treatment. Fertile Hope is now available to answer questions and educate patients about fertility options (www.fertilehope.org).

Therapy involving the brain or central nervous system of a child should minimize cognitive problems after treatment. Such children may need long-term follow-up, which includes assessment for learning disabilities, memory deficit, distractibility, and decreased verbal ability and IQ scores. If children are treated before puberty, they should receive long-term follow-up with specialists who can address potential growth problems. The book *Childhood Cancer Survivors* by Keene, Hobbie, and Ruccione is an excellent resource for this population.

10. As the initial phase of treatment is completed, the extended stage of survival begins. Does life automatically return to normal?

Anticipating the end of treatment provokes an array of mixed emotions. Ambiguity defines this stage as survivors experience a mixture of joy and fear, relief and anxiety, security and uncertainty. Although no longer a patient, the survivor is not entirely healthy and tries to balance both physical and emotional recovery. This stage encompasses learning to live with the fear of recurrence, uncertainty about the future, and loss of treatment-based support systems. The survivor also must learn to assess and trust his or her body again and to resume prior family and social roles and relationships. Often this period is characterized by a feeling of being in limbo. The sense of "normal" has changed; it will never be the same as before the cancer. A "new normal" specific to the survivor must be created gradually. This process takes time; it will not happen overnight. For many survivors, the "new normal" can be better than the original.

11. How can nurses prepare survivors for potential problems once therapy is completed?

Knowledge helps to decrease fear of the unknown. As survivors complete treatment, an individualized exit interview can assist with the transition to life after therapy. Components of the interview may include information about medical follow-up appointments with specific diagnostic tests; possible late effects from therapy; symptoms that require attention or symptoms that may be expected; cancer prevention, health promotion, and wellness education; referrals for physical, psychologic, and social rehabilitation; support networks, educational programs, and survivor publications; and continued access to specific members of the health care team. A "Survivorship Care Plan" is Recommendation #2 in the IOM report.

12. When does permanent or long-term survival begin?

The long-term stage of survival begins at different times for different people. Much depends on the type and extent of the original disease and the risk for recurrence.

Although no specific time frame or event defines this stage, freedom from disease for 2 or more years begins to yield a certain level of trust, and a sense of comfort gradually returns. This stage may be labeled *sustained remission* or possibly *cure*, although the definition of cure is controversial (see Question 14).

Some survivors can breathe a little easier after 2 years, such as those who are diagnosed with testicular cancer or Hodgkin lymphoma. Others who have non-Hodgkin lymphoma or ovarian cancer may need 5 or more years to feel out of the woods. Survivors of breast cancer are watched closely for recurrence for 10 years or more. All of these numbers are arbitrary and act only as guidelines for increased vigilance; they are not meant to hinder survivors from living life to the fullest.

13. What problems are associated with long-term survival?

A lack of guidelines to optimize disease-free survival continues to be a major problem for long-term survivors. Although many survivors have no physical evidence of disease and appear fully recovered, the life-threatening experience of having had cancer takes its toll in many ways. Physically, the survivor is at risk for other malignancies and organ system toxicities/failures related to treatment; psychologically, the survivor must live with the constant fear of recurrence; socially, the survivor frequently encounters employment and insurance discrimination; and spiritually, survivors struggle with the meaning of life and the identification of new goals and priorities. Although survivors are often praised for overcoming adversity, identification of real problems can be hampered as they are reminded how lucky they are to be alive. In this age of managed care and cost-containment, long-term survivors need continued access to appropriate specialists and guidelines for systematic follow-up. Although the research community calls for evidence-based guidelines to dictate appropriate follow-up, consensus-based guidelines are needed to fill the gaps until the evidence emerges.

14. Is there any guarantee of "cure" for survivors who remain disease-free for 5 years?

The concept of being cured implies successful treatment of disease or restoration to health. Surely being cured is the ultimate hope for anyone treated for cancer. Yet no one can say for sure that a disease as ruthless and secretive as cancer will never return; thus guarantees are not realistic. Probabilities for cure can be estimated and are available in the American Cancer Society's annual publication, *Cancer Facts and Figures*. The 1960s and 1970s brought a new sense of hopefulness to researchers and clinicians who treated people with cancer. With the development of potentially curative therapies, specialists carefully followed their patients for signs of disease recurrence. Many believed that patients who remained disease-free for 5 years had a greatly increased chance of cure and a normal lifespan. Thus, many patients anxiously waited to reach the magic 5-year landmark. They were not considered survivors until they reached this point.

Unfortunately, many survivors have recurrent disease even after 5 years, or they are diagnosed with other cancers. Because there are multiple types of cancers with different stages of disease, a wide variety of treatment options, and circumstances unique to each survivor, it is impossible to guarantee cure.

15. Do survivors face employment discrimination due to their history of cancer?

Although fewer barriers now exist to impede work opportunities, many survivors still experience some type of employment discrimination. Examples include not being hired for a particular job, being selected for a company lay-off, being demoted or having duties cut back, or being denied a promotion or increase in salary. Some employers believe that cancer survivors are less productive and use more sick days than other employees use. Studies have not supported this belief. In fact, studies have shown that survivors use fewer sick days and tend to be more productive than other workers, often because they are fearful of losing their job if they appear to be sick.

16. What problems do survivors face in terms of health insurance?

Cancer survivors also experience "job lock"; that is, they feel unable to apply for a change in employment because they fear losing the health insurance benefits attached to their current employment. Survivors also may feel that they cannot accept employment from a company that does not provide adequate health insurance benefits. For this reason, they may accept employment in a position where they are overqualified to obtain needed health insurance. Recently enacted federal legislation allows cancer survivors to obtain health insurance when they change jobs without having to endure a long waiting period, but there are no restrictions as to how much this coverage will cost.

Insurance companies also tend to give survivors a higher rating designation in setting insurance premiums. The higher rate applies to both health and life insurance. Some life insurance carriers will not insure cancer survivors until they have been disease-free for 5 years or more. Others charge very high premiums. Cancer survivors should be encouraged to check with a number of insurance providers before agreeing to a premium amount. A financial planner may be able to present options other than life insurance that will serve the same purpose for survivors and their families.

Another situation finds survivors dependent upon their spouse for health insurance benefits. In most states, the survivor is no longer able to obtain insurance benefits from their former partner once a divorce takes place. Survivors may feel themselves locked into a marriage because of the need for insurance coverage. Along with an insurance consultant, an attorney specializing in family law may provide the survivor with options for obtaining individual or group insurance. Organizations such as university alumni associations, American Association of Retired People, professional associations, fraternal organizations, and other special interest groups may provide insurance to members at group rates.

17. How long should cancer survivors be followed by an oncologist after termination of treatment?

Before managed care, long-term follow-up was left to the discretion of the oncologist and survivor. Many oncologists wanted an ongoing relationship with people whom they had treated, even if it was once a year. Furthermore, many survivors felt bonded to the specialists who had helped them overcome a life-threatening disease. The establishment of trust over the years made the yearly follow-up exam easier to bear, and many oncologists still believe that they know best how to assess survivors for potential treatment-related problems.

Exorbitant costs within our current health care management system have changed this once sacred, ongoing relationship by decreasing both use of services and referrals to specialists. Oncologists now are more inclined to see the survivor for a limited number of years after therapy, as prescribed by the individual plan. They then refer the survivor to the primary care provider (PCP)—a family practitioner or internist—for long-term follow-up. On a more positive note, the sheer numbers of long-term survivors make it unrealistic to think that oncologists can follow everyone indefinitely, thus necessitating referral back to PCP's in most cases.

Because little systematic long-term follow-up has been done in adult cancer survivors, there are no guidelines for continued care. Researchers and clinicians in oncology are just now developing standards of care that can be shared with the generalist physicians who see and assess survivors. Survivors are best served through cooperation among oncologists, primary care providers, and other specialists; education of primary care providers about the special needs of this expanding population; and timely referrals to the appropriate specialist when complicated or unusual problems arise. The American Society of Clinical Oncology (ASCO) has recently created a Survivorship Task Force, and is developing guidelines for long-term follow-up.

18. How can survivors optimize their health care follow-up?

To ensure optimal long-term follow-up care, survivors are encouraged to do the following:
- Keep all medical records, including types and doses of chemotherapy, and sites and amounts of radiation.
- Develop a personalized health maintenance plan with the oncology caregiver team that covers times of check-ups, specific diagnostic tests, rehabilitation practices, and healthy behavioral modifications.
- Carefully study and select, if possible, health insurance plans that offer flexibility and choice.
- If warranted, negotiate a price for an annual follow-up visit outside the insurance plan, and pay out of pocket if the rate is affordable. Survivors must decide for themselves whether this added expense is worth the peace of mind that it may bring.
- Learn to identify and communicate needs, and obtain assertiveness training if necessary.
- Know individual rights as a health care consumer and how to take appropriate legal action if warranted.
- Advocate insurance reform and standardized guidelines.
- Petition payers to cover follow-up visits to specially-designated survivor clinics, if available.

19. What resources are available to assist survivors and families with problems and barriers?

After specific problems or barriers are identified, nurses must find the appropriate resources to help deal with them. Consultations with other professionals within the hospital or community may involve specially trained nurses, attending physicians, social workers and social services, translators, psychologists, chaplains, legal assistance, and financial and government consultants. Other resources include written publications, cancer-related videos, educational programs, online services (Internet), and support groups. Local cancer organizations also may be accessed (e.g., Leukemia and Lymphoma Society, American Cancer Society, Wellness Communities). The important point is to be aware of available resources.

 Key Points

- If the concept of survivorship is introduced early into the cancer experience, patients have the advantage of learning self-advocacy skills that can help them navigate the confusing and complicated health care system.
- Self advocacy will help survivors and their loved ones access appropriate information, find needed resources, improve communication, and increase the quality of care throughout the stages of survival.
- Life after a cancer diagnosis often progresses through stages.
- Monitoring and follow-up are highly individualized and will depend on the age of the survivor when first treated, the developmental stage at the time of treatment and at follow-up, the cancer type, the treatments received, co-morbid conditions that may affect overall health, access to resources, and social and cultural issues.
- Decreased insurability and employment discrimination continue to impede full recovery from cancer for many survivors.

Internet Resources

Selected General Resources for Cancer Survivors

Most websites link to additional and more specific resources.

National Cancer Institute (NCI)
Cancer Information Service (CIS): 800-4-CANCER
Physician Data Query (PDQ): 800-4-CANCER
CANCERFAX: 301-402-5874
  http://www.cancer.gov

National Coalition for Cancer Survivorship (NCCS)
General Information: 877-NCCS-YES
  http://www.canceradvocacy.org

Candlelighters Childhood Cancer Foundation
General Information: 800-366-2223
Local (Washington, DC): 301-657-8401
  http://www.candlelighters.org

American Cancer Society (ACS), Cancer Survivors Network
General Information: 800-ACS-2345
  http://www.acscsn.org/

Leukemia and Lymphoma Society of America
Educational Materials: 800-955-4LSA
General Information: 212-573-8484
  http://www.leukemia.org

Cancer Care, Inc.
General Information: 800-813-HOPE
Local (New York): 212-302-2400
  http://www.cancercare.org

Lance Armstrong Foundation (LAF), Livestrong Network
General Information: 512-236-8820
  http://www.livestrong.org/site/c.jvKZLbMRIsG/b.594849/k.CC7C/Home.htm

American Society of Clinical Oncology (ASCO)
General Information: 703-299-0150
People Living With Cancer Network:
  http://www.peoplelivingwithcancer.org
  http://www.asco.org

CURE Magazine
  http://www.curetoday.com

Coping Magazine
  http://www.copingmag.com

Cancer Survival Toolbox: Building Skills that Work for You
This free set of audio programs (CD format) was developed jointly by the Oncology Nursing
  Society, the Association of Oncology Social Work, and NCCS. It is available free of charge
  by calling 877-NCCS-YES or ordering through the NCCS website at:
  http://www.canceradvocacy.org/resources/toolbox.aspx

Bibliography

Centers for Disease Control and Prevention (CDC) and the Lance Armstrong Foundation (LAF): A national action plan for cancer survivorship: Advancing public health strategies, 2004. http://www.cdc.gov/cancer/survivorship/what_cdc_is_doing/action_plan_download.htm Accessed January 13, 2007.

Clark EJ, Stovall EL, Leigh S, et al: *Imperatives for quality cancer care: Access, advocacy, action, and accountability.* Silver Spring, MD, 1996, National Coalition for Cancer Survivorship.

Clark EJ: *You have the right to be hopeful.* Silver Spring, MD, 1996, National Coalition for Cancer Survivorship.

Curtiss CP, Haylock, PJ, editors: Executive summary: State of the science on nursing approaches to managing late and long-term sequelae of cancer treatment. *Am J Nurs,* 106 (Supplement 3), 2006.

Hewitt M, Weiner SL, Simone JV, editors: *Childhood cancer survivorship: Improving care and quality of life.* Washington, DC, 2003, National Academies Press.

Hewitt M, Greenfield S, Stovall E, editors: *From cancer patient to cancer survivor: Lost in transition,* Washington, DC, 2005, National Academies Press.

Hoffman B: Cancer survivors at work: A generation of progress. *CA Cancer J Clin,* 55:271-289, 2005.

Jemal A, Siegel R, Ward E, et al: Cancer statistics, 2007. *CA Cancer J Clin* 57:43-66, 2007.

Keene N, Hobbie WL, Ruccione KS: *Childhood cancer survivors: A practical guide to your future,* Sebastopol, CA, 2000, O'Reilly.

Leigh S: Defining our destiny. In Hoffman B, editor: *Cancer survivors almanac: Charting your journey,* Hoboken, NJ, 2004, John Wiley & Sons.

Mullan F: Seasons of survival: Reflections of a physician with cancer. *N Engl J Med* 313:270-273, 1985.

National Cancer Institute, President's Cancer Panel: Annual report for 2003–2004: Living beyond cancer: Finding a new balance. http://deainfo.nci.nih.gov/ADVISORY/pcp/pcp03-04rpt/Survivorship.pdf. Accessed January 13, 2007.

National Coalition for Cancer Survivorship: Cancer survival toolbox. http://www.cancersurvivaltoolbox.org/. Accessed January 13, 2007.

Hospice Care

Janelle McCallum Orozco

1. Define hospice.

Hospice is an interdisciplinary program of care focused on the relief of symptoms and suffering of the dying (life expectancy of months, not years) and support for their families. In the United States, the Medicare Hospice Benefit is the major source of funding for hospice palliative care.

2. When is hospice care appropriate?

A person is ready for hospice care whenever he or she chooses palliative, noncurative holistic care instead of aggressive, curative medical care for a life-limiting illness. Typically hospice care has been available for people with a prognosis of 6 months or less. More recently patients have been referred close to the week of death. The average length of stay for hospice patients in the United States is 59 days. The median length of stay is 26 days. Unfortunately, such late referral may preclude much of the benefit offered by the interdisciplinary team. To meet the needs of people and physicians who are reluctant to accept hospice care earlier in the course of illness, many hospices offer prehospice or palliative care services. Prehospice services are for patients who are clearly terminal but who choose aggressive palliative care interventions, such as second- or third-line chemotherapy.

3. What are typical hospice diagnoses?

In the early days the majority of hospice patients had cancer. For the past decade, many more patients with noncancer diagnoses have used hospice services. Approximately 50% of all hospice diagnoses are cancer-related. Hospice-appropriate diagnoses include:

- Organ cancers (e.g., pancreas, liver)
- Cancers with metastatic processes
- End-stage heart disease, dementia, lung disease, and kidney disease
- Life-threatening congenital defects (pediatric cases)
- Massive cerebrovascular accidents (CVAs)
- End stage chronic diseases, such as chronic obstructive pulmonary disease (COPD), multiple sclerosis (MS), amyotrophic lateral sclerosis (ALS), and acquired immunodeficiency syndrome (AIDS)
- Failure to thrive or significant weight loss secondary to debility
- Discontinuation of treatment or medications that prolong life (e.g., dialysis, antirejection medications, ventilators)
- Bone marrow transplant failure
- Patients with a do-not-resuscitate (DNR) order
- Patients with complex pain symptoms who need expert management
- Patients with repeat hospitalizations
- Patients with social, psychological, or spiritual challenges dealing with terminal illness and disease process
- Patients in whom aggressive treatment does not have a favorable outcome

- Patients with frequent changes in the treatment plan due to slow but declining status
- Patients who decline treatment or diagnostic interventions for life-threatening illness

4. Where can a patient receive hospice care?

Hospice care can be provided in almost any setting: home, apartment, assisted living facility, nursing home, hospital, specialized inpatient hospice unit, or prison.

Some people, however, need or choose an inpatient setting, including: (1) patients who have no family or caregivers, (2) patients and families who desire an inpatient setting for personal reasons, and (3) patients with extreme medical or social conditions that make it necessary to transfer to an inpatient setting.

5. Who should bring up the subject of hospice care?

This can be a tricky area in which intuition and diplomacy are warranted. As the patient's nurse, you can do the following:

1. Begin your discussion and assessment with the patient's physician.
2. Offer to be present for the physician's discussion with the patient and family.
3. Offer to present the hospice option yourself. (In many hospitals discharge planners may be given the role of discussing hospice care).

Often a hospice referral comes abruptly from the perspective of the patient and family. They believe that an aggressive curative course is under way, and the next day everything changes. The patient "suddenly" needs hospice care and, if hospitalized, must leave the hospital that same day. Proactive public education about palliative care and hospice philosophy is the key to diminishing the frequency of this scenario.

6. What if hospice care is clearly appropriate, but the physician refuses to discuss it with the patient or family?

First, discuss your concerns with the patient's physician. Try to follow Covey's axiom, "Seek first to understand, then to be understood." Perhaps more information or a more complex dynamic is involved than is readily apparent. The physician may be more open to "palliative or supportive care." In any case, consider the following questions as guides when introducing hospice or palliative care to the patient or family:

1. How are things going with your body?
2. What do you think is going on with your medical condition?
3. What do you think the future holds for you?

Depending on the patient's answer, follow the appropriate path. Let the patient know that you are open to hearing and discussing the unthinkable—dying.

7. What do I say when patients ask me if they are dying?

Be truthful. Chances are good that the patient has already been told that he or she is dying but may need to hear it again as conditions change. Approaches to answering this question include:

- What does it seem like to you? Then confirm the answer, if appropriate.
- What has your doctor told you? Then build or expand on what the patient already knows.

Reassure the patient that symptoms will be controlled. One hospice nurse emphasizes that someone given a "terminal diagnosis" often has time to do and say almost anything they want to before they die. Many people do not have this gift of time and die without saying and doing what they may have wanted. The bottom line is to follow the patient's lead.

Ask, "Do you think you are dying?" Then take the conversation from there. This question helps to discover what the person really wants to know.

8. What promises should I never make to a dying person?

The premise is simple: Don't make promises you can't keep. Remember that the dying person has less time in which to have the promises fulfilled. Examples of key promises *not* to make include:

- I promise I'll be with you when you die.
- I promise I'll see you before you go.
- I promise I'll help you die.
- I promise I won't be depressed after you die.

It is also important to encourage family members not to make promises that they cannot keep.

9. What if I'm not sad when every patient dies?

One hospice nurse recalls that when she first started taking care of hospice patients, she expected that she should be sad when every patient died. Then she realized that she was connected to some patients and families and not so connected to others. Another hospice nurse says, "It's okay not to be sad. We don't like everyone we meet in life, so we won't like everyone we meet in death." Death is the natural conclusion of life. Hospice nurses strive to make the final hours or days a period of quality time for patient and family. Hopefully when they look back on that time, the actual death will be only a small part of a greater event.

10. How can I show respect for life after the patient has died?

Handle the patient in death as you did in life—with respect and care; make no distinction. Specific interventions include:

- Allow families private time with the body, and respect families' wishes, traditions, and customs.
- Be gentle and caring when removing lines and tubes and washing the body.
- Close the patient's eyes. Cover the patient to the neck; there is no need to cover the face.
- Brush the hair off the forehead and touch the face of the deceased in a gentle, loving manner.
- Reminisce with the family about the patient.

11. What matters to families immediately after the death of the patient?

Ask the family what matters to them. Each family is different, and we must give them space to tell us what would be helpful. For example, some families want to spend lots of time with the dead body, whereas other families want the body removed as soon as possible. For some, the patient's appearance is of great concern (e.g., hair, makeup, clothing, position). However, families seem to have some fairly universal needs:

1. Show them that someone cares about them and the patient.
2. Let them know that you will take care of necessary details (e.g., with the physician, coroner, mortuary, equipment company, medications).
3. Provide a time and a place to make phone calls.
4. For deaths that occur in a private residence, it may be important to have the medical equipment (e.g., bed, wheelchair, oxygen) removed as soon as possible.
5. Explain bereavement services and leave written materials about grief for later reading.

6. Allow dramatic expressions of grief. Sedation of family members is generally not recommended.

Be sure to ask about rituals and spiritual needs. Be sensitive to cultures unlike your own. Most families want reassurance that their loved one will be treated with respect even in death.

12. What is anticipatory grief?

In the context of hospice care, anticipatory grief refers to emotions of loss and grief and even relief before the person's death. Many people expect profound anguish, but they feel guilt as they find themselves planning for the future—before the person actually dies. Hospice workers encourage anticipatory grief and help to normalize such emotions. Planning for the future is a healthy sign of anticipating life after the death of a loved one. It does not mean the survivors do not love the dying person or wish that the person would die sooner. It is what healthy people do when facing such life-changing circumstances as losing a loved one to terminal illness.

13. What can I do to help during the grieving process?

Simply stated, listen to the person's fears, ask about strategies to deal with the fears, and assist as appropriate. Ask about future plans. If the person has none, encourage thinking about the future. Reassure the person that future planning is normal and may cause some feelings of guilt. If a severely depressed survivor speaks of having no plans or future, this may be a red flag. Refer the person immediately to a social worker or chaplain.

Not all people who die are "loved ones." Be open to relief in family members or friends, who may make such statements as "He was so abusive," "We had a terrible marriage," or "I hated her." We tend to expect everyone to be sad about the patient's death, but this is not always the case. Know that even though a person may be relieved that the patient died, the associated guilt must be resolved eventually.

14. Is it professional to go to the patient's funeral and maintain contact with the family?

In an inpatient setting, if scheduling allows and you feel a need to attend the funeral for your own closure, it is appropriate to do so. Continued contact with the family is generally *not* appropriate. Refer the family to a local hospice for bereavement assistance.

In a hospice setting, staff is encouraged to attend the patient's funeral and to make bereavement follow-up. Generally the staff who knew the patient attends the funeral, and a grief counselor does the follow-up bereavement work. The goal of follow-up is to assist the grieving person to heal in a healthy way.

Continued contact by direct care staff is discouraged because it continues a relationship that was begun during a time of crisis and death. The nurse's job is to assist the patient and family along the journey to death. The journey after death is equally important and may be assisted by another caregiver (e.g., bereavement counselor). There are always exceptions to this advice, however. Be careful to consider whose needs are primary— yours or the family's. Your goal in caring for the family after death is the same as when the patient was alive: *Do what is best for the patient and family first; meet your own emotional and social needs secondarily.*

15. What is the role of the hospice in discontinuation of life-sustaining treatments?

Unfortunately, hospice staff is not consulted enough in such situations. The interdisciplinary hospice staff can be of great assistance in discussing options and supporting choices from many perspectives. They can help in determining the patient's decision-making capacity and ensuring that all parties are informed and advised. Whereas the medical model typically addresses the physical domain, the hospice model considers the physical, emotional, social, and spiritual domains as the patient and family struggle with the decisions to end life-sustaining treatment.

16. How can the hospice staff help to assess a patient's decision-making capacity with regard to discontinuation of life-sustaining treatments?

Ultimately the physician determines patient capacity, but staff can assist by asking the following questions:

- Is the patient able to communicate feelings and desires clearly to others?
- Is the patient clearly stating (via his or her method of communication) the desire for discontinuation of technical support?
- Is the patient able to articulate (via his or her method of communication) various options and consequences of actions?
- Is the patient depressed? Have antidepressant therapy and counseling been attempted?
- What are the patient's and family's spiritual concerns or understanding about discontinuation of treatment?
- Has the patient talked with others outside the health care team about this decision? If not, would this be helpful?
- Does the patient require more time for a thoughtful decision?
- Does the patient have an advance directive consistent with this decision?

17. What areas of agreement or disagreement should be addressed before discontinuing life-sustaining treatments?

- Does the patient have capacity? If not, who can make decisions for the patient?
- Are family and friends in agreement?
- Are current health care providers in agreement?
- Is there a physician's order for discontinuation?
- Which physician will preside at removal of the ventilator?
- Does the decision seem reasonable to staff who have assessed patient and family?

18. What information is needed to address the question of whether a terminally ill person can become addicted to opioids (narcotics)?

Less than 1% of people who need opioids for terminal pain actually display symptoms of true addiction. Thinking that the family member was addicted to opioids may be a stumbling block in the bereaved person's road to recovery. To alleviate the patient's and family's fears, it is helpful to understand and be able to teach the three components of the addiction scenario (tolerance, physical dependence, and psychological dependence). The myth of addiction serves only to continue the public's misunderstanding of opioids and appropriate pain management.

19. What if the patient wants to stay at home alone, but this option really is not safe?

Our job as nurses is to assess the safety and competency of the patient in whatever setting the patient resides. At times it is hard to be objective. We often think of a preferred arrangement because it would put our minds at ease. In the case of a live-alone patient, we need to identify true safety hazards and look at our own personal tolerance for marginal situations. (Refer to checklist on the following page).

Equally important as the safety assessment is whether the patient has the capacity to make decisions. It is important to note that capacity is situational. Generally, the patient needs only to understand the consequences of a decision to have capacity. A person may

Safety Evaluation for the Live-Alone Patient

Functional, Physical, and Environmental Concerns
1. Patient residence is ( ) multiple-family dwelling ( ) single-family dwelling
2. Personal emergency response system in use: ( ) Yes ( ) No

Y	N	
3. ( )	( )	Bed bound
4. ( )	( )	History of falls
5. ( )	( )	Fire hazards
6. ( )	( )	Hearing and/or vision deficits
7. ( )	( )	Home alone
8. ( )	( )	Lives alone
9. ( )	( )	Medication compliance
10. ( )	( )	Decision maker
11. ( )	( )	Transportation assistance
12. ( )	( )	Oxygen: as needed _____ continuous _____
13. ( )	( )	Smoker
14. ( )	( )	Basic utilities
15. ( )	( )	Telephone

Psychosocial Concerns

Y	N	
16. ( )	( )	Financial management
17. ( )	( )	Psychiatric problems: Current _____ Hx _____
18. ( )	( )	Alcohol/drug problems: Current _____ Hx _____
19. ( )	( )	Suicidal ideation: Current _____ Hx _____
20. ( )	( )	Violence or potential: Current _____ Hx _____

Y = obseved and/or reported; N = not observed, not reported, or denied; Hx = history.
Adapted from The Denver Hospice: *Policy and Procedure Manual:* 2002, Denver, CO, 2002, The Denver Hospice.

have capacity and make poor decisions. In the case of poor decision making that puts the patient or others at risk, a call to Adult Protective Services is probably the best course of action.

20. What if a hospice patient talks about suicide or tries to commit suicide?

Many people who have been told they have a terminal illness think about suicide at some point. Most work through it and decide that suicide is not really what they want to do. However, some continue to have a strong desire to kill themselves. In talking about suicide it is important to let the patient know three points:
1. It is okay to talk about such thoughts. (In fact, it is imperative that staff ask for more details to assess the seriousness of the threat).
2. Suicidal ideation cannot be kept a secret; other team members need to know.
3. Support and assistance will be provided to the patient to work through fears and to continue living until the illness runs its course. The patient will not be abandoned.

When a patient talks about suicide, keep the following points in mind:

- Do not be afraid to use the "s" word. For example: "Are you considering suicide?" "Have you thought about hurting yourself?" "Do you want to do something that would end things sooner?" By speaking the words aloud, you allow the person the option of responding either yes or no. If the patient says yes, ask whether the patient has a plan and get all the details. If the patient says no, ask what keeps the patient from doing it. This information is helpful to assess lethality. Find out what specifically is intolerable for the patient. Is it pain, fear of pain, anxiety, lack of support, worry about being a burden, worry about losing dignity, or some other concern? Often we can eliminate the issue that makes the patient want to leave life early.
- Explain that the discussion of suicide cannot be a secret. You will have to tell the physician and social worker, who will ask further questions and assist as possible.

21. When are invasive measures appropriate for a hospice patient?

Invasive measures are generally not used in hospice patients. However, there are exceptions. The goals of therapy are patient and family choice and optimal quality of life. Examples of invasive treatments that may be used include:

- Intravenous fluids (when used judiciously and discontinued as fluid begins to accumulate)
- Intravenous, subcutaneous, or intraspinal pain medication
- Gastric feedings or nasogastric suction
- Rectal tubes
- Paracentesis and thoracentesis (for a limited time)
- Surgery to repair fractures (often Buck's traction and pain management are used instead)
- Certain chemotherapies and radiation (to achieve palliation of symptoms)
- Total parenteral nutrition (for a limited time)

22. What do I do when the patient insists on experiencing pain, even though I know that medications and other treatments would help?

1. Listen to the patient; hear the request to decline pain medications.
2. Ask why medications and treatments are not acceptable.
3. Ask for permission to explain pain relief measures. Describe the medications, expected actions, and side effects. Remember to explain the concept of addiction and the surrounding myths.
4. If the patient still declines, accept the answer. But check again to make sure no intervention is wanted. (Suggest starting out with a very low dose or a trial time period to decrease fear and build trust).
5. Comfort the family and friends of the patient. They too find it difficult to watch their loved one suffer. In your conversation with the family use the term *declined*, as explained below.
6. Assess reasons why the patient declines pain relief. Often there is a spiritual component to why people choose to suffer (e.g., "I want to suffer the way Christ did").
7. In your charting and discussion about the patient, consider using the words *declined medication* instead of *refused*. The simple change of wording often evokes a change in the nurse. The word *refused* conjures up the image of a noncompliant patient. By the using the word *declined* we imagine a person with dignity making an informed decision. Be sure to document the teaching you have done if the patient continues to decline the offer of pain medication.

23. What about the young patient whose body just will not die?

Younger, actively dying patients tend to linger longer than older, actively dying patients. Even though the body is full of cancer, the younger person's heart can last longer. The stage called "actively dying" is the time just before a person dies when the kidneys begin to shut down, blood pressure decreases, oral intake stops, alertness diminishes (although not always), and mottling of the extremities may occur. An older patient may be in the actively dying stage for 1 to 3 days, whereas a younger person may be actively dying for days to weeks. Although longer death vigils are grueling for all involved, they seem to serve an important purpose for the patient as well as the family.

24. Who makes the decision about what constitutes palliative treatment and when it is appropriate to discontinue blood transfusions, palliative radiation, total parenteral nutrition, or enteral feedings?

Generally the patient's primary physician, in conjunction with the hospice medical director, makes the decision as to what constitutes palliative treatment. Of great importance is how we talk to the patient and family about these issues. It is helpful to describe the physiologic reasons why the treatments are not effective and are probably more uncomfortable to continue. Be sure to speak with the physician about discontinuation before discussing it with the family. Here are general rules of thumb for discontinuing treatment within a hospice context:

- When the physician believes that the treatment is no longer effective
- When the patient can no longer make the trip to the hospital or clinic (e.g., taking the patient by ambulance to receive a blood transfusion does not usually make sense); however, it is often the patient or family member who says, "You know, I'm just too tired to make the trip—even with an ambulance"
- When the patient no longer tolerates the treatment
- When the treatment causes more pain than comfort

25. What do I say to a patient's wife who is upset because her husband will not eat the food she fixes?

First, realize that loss of appetite can be traumatic for the patient's family. Eating and drinking are not only physiologic acts but also important social activities. Adjusting to an ill person's lack of interest in food and fluids can make the family feel helpless. In the previous example, acknowledge the wife's frustration and fear. Explain that the food she fixed probably did sound good to her husband, but the disease prevents him from enjoying the meal she prepared. Explain the following:

- Loss of appetite is normal in a terminally ill person. The body needs less food when a person has cancer and is inactive; eating less does not shorten a person's life in serious disease, and in this case, low food intake does not cause hunger.
- Eating may become a difficult activity for a very ill person. Food may be offered, but the person should eat only if he wants. In some cases, the person may eat more than he desires because he believes that it is expected and then feels sick afterward.
- The person who is ill may develop new food preferences because some foods may taste different or have no taste at all.

26. What do I do when a patient insists on believing in a cure or miracle?

First, listen to the patient's belief. Do not try to talk the patient out of it. However, it may be possible to reframe what a "miracle" looks like. Hope is always appropriate. People must be allowed to hope for a miracle that can save their life. It is *not* necessary that they go through all stages of death and dying and reach acceptance. Some people are in denial until the end.

It is our task to be present to patients wherever they are. In our love and support they may find that the miracle for which they had been hoping is the nurse who is an excellent pain manager and who is present in their time of suffering and need.

27. What does normal grief look like?

Grief takes time. It often takes a year or more to regain balance in life after a loss. The following are all natural and normal grief responses:
- Tightness in the throat or heaviness in the chest
- Hollow feeling in the stomach and loss of appetite
- Need to tell and retell the story of the events leading up to the death and its aftermath
- Restlessness and need to fill time with activity, but often with difficulty in concentrating and getting organized
- Feeling as though the loss is not real, that it did not really happen
- Sensing the deceased person's presence; perhaps expecting him or her to walk in the door at the usual time, hearing the voice, or seeing the face on a stranger in a crowd
- Aimless wandering, forgetfulness, trouble with finishing projects at work or home, or absent-mindedness
- Intense preoccupation with the life of the deceased
- Crying at unexpected times
- Feeling guilty or angry over things that happened or did not happen in the relationship with the deceased
- Intense anger at the deceased for leaving
- Taking on mannerisms or traits of the deceased
- Sense of relief, sometimes followed by pangs of guilt or regret
- Unpredictable, rapid, and sharp mood swings
- Avoidance of talking about feelings of loss around others
- Weakness or lack of energy

If any of the above symptoms persists for more than 2 years or is exaggerated to the point of bodily injury, refer the person to a mental health counselor.

28. What can be done to help the grieving person?

1. Normalize the person's grief experience. Grief often feels painful and overwhelming. Many people worry that they are not grieving in the 'right' way or wonder if the feelings they have are normal.
2. Encourage grieving people to tell their story. Telling the story is a major part of the healing process because the death event is so important. To embed every detail in one's memory, one must tell the story—over and over.
3. Encourage grieving people to take care of their own health and nutrition.
4. Advise them to make as few major changes in their life as possible.
5. Encourage them to ask for what they need from a few friends they can rely on.

29. How do I respond when a patient's family member rushes from the room and says, "I think he just died!"

Give the person your immediate attention. You may say, "Okay, let's go." It is important to attend to the situation immediately. As you enter the room, all of the family may be at the bedside, waiting. At times it is hard to be sure that the patient has really died. Take the necessary time to be sure that the heart has stopped and there are no respirations.

Telling the assembled family members that their loved one has died can be difficult. Do your best to "read" their expectations in terms of the language you may use. Possible phrases for telling the news include "He's gone" or "He's passed on." Often the family will ask, "Is he dead?" or "Is she gone?" Then you can affirm the question, using the words they have chosen.

In my experience, using the "d" word (dead) has not been perceived as "sensitive" by the family. It seems that at the time of death, the word "dead" rings hollow and cold. The death of the loved one is obvious, and perhaps euphemisms are appropriate comfort at this time.

30. What does it mean when a patient is discharged from hospice?

Patients that stabilize or improve as a result of team-oriented hospice care may be discharged if they no longer fit the definition of a "hospice patient" under the Medicare Hospice Benefit. The patient may be readmitted at a later date when his or her condition has deteriorated. There is no limit to the Medicare Hospice Benefit as long as the patient meets diagnostic and functional criteria. Hospices are trying to find other ways of providing palliative care without relying solely on the Medicare Hospice Benefit. However, changes in public policy and community awareness will be required to keep the Medicare Hospice Benefit from shrinking further. Other funding options for palliative care are needed.

From a patient and family perspective, discharge from hospice can be difficult. The patient and family have come to expect death and often have difficulty readjusting to "chronic illness" and the lack of interdisciplinary support to which they have become accustomed. In many ways, discharge from hospice is a "good news, bad news" scenario. The good news: you have graduated from hospice care. The bad news: you no longer have hospice services and need to get on with life without the support and quality of life that hospice helped to provide.

31. How can I remain compassionate yet not go crazy caring for dying patients and their families?

Here is how several hospice workers answer this question:

Ed: Take care of yourself. If you don't, you can't care for others. Cherish your life and all who are in it. Nurture your spiritual being to sustain you in times of need. Be aware of how this vocation can affect you. Talk about your feelings with your co-workers, and don't be afraid to seek outside help.

Jean: I get energy from the courage and love of so many of the families. I get two hugs for every one I give.

Micki: I maintain the philosophy that everyone dies, and if I can in any way facilitate meeting the patient's needs and wishes surrounding this one-time event, it is rewarding. Educating, reassuring, and guiding families is great.

Phyllis: When I close the door of the hospice inpatient unit, I am symbolically closing that part of my life until the next day. Recipe for success: do fun things, let the inner child out.

Janelle: If you're going to work with people who die, you had better learn how to live, decide what's important to you, and say what needs to be said. Every now and then, someone will wrap their soul around your heart, and it hurts when they suffer or die. This then is the essence of life.

Kay: When I feel valued and supported by the people I work for, it helps me remain focused. Use the support of other team members. Talk about what is going on.

Sandi: For me the key has been finding a clear theology for this work. Theology really helped me with "What's it all about, Alfie?" This work has given me a nonanxious paradigm about death.

Sally: Working part-time helps. I take care of myself physically (exercise and rest) and especially spiritually (meditation). I nurture friendships outside of hospice, and I spend as much time as possible with people who make me laugh.

Suzette: Have a life. Do for yourself. Forget all work issues on the weekend. Get away from your normal environment. Don't be a caregiver for all the people in your life. Have a person who listens to your problems—even a therapist. Maintain inner balance. Exercise, shop, have parties.

Paula: Don't over identify with patients and families. Know your limits. Use the support of others.

Michelle: Set limits. Take care of yourself. Have outside interests and activities. Accept the laughter and the tears. Take opportunities for closure.

 Key Points

- The nurse can initiate hospice care discussions.
- Be truthful when patients ask if they are dying.
- Don't make promises you can't keep to a dying person.
- To help grieving people, let them tell their story . . . every detail matters to them.
- Live your life with intention. It makes it possible to look into the face of the dying on a daily basis.

 Internet Resources

End of Life Nursing Education Consortium (ELNEC):
   http://www.aacn.nche.edu/elnec
Population-based Palliative Care Research Network (PoPCRN):
   http://www.uchsc.edu/popcrn
Center to Advance Palliative Care (CAPC):
   http://www.capc.org
Promoting Excellence in End-of-Life Care:
   http://www.promotingexcellence.org
Nursing Home End-of-Life Care:
   http://www.chcr.brown.edu/nhhsp
American Academy of Hospice and Palliative Medicine:
   http://www.aahpm.org
American Hospice Foundation:
   http://www.americanhospice.org
Hospice Foundation of America:
   http://www.hospicefoundation.org
Hospice and Palliative Nurses Association:
   http://www.hpna.org
Children's Hospice International:
   http://www.chionline.org
The Dougy Center for Grieving Children and Families:
   http://www.dougy.org
Growth House, Inc.:
   http://www.growthhouse.org

Acknowledgments

The author thanks the staff of the Denver Hospice, who contributed to many of these questions. Specifically, they are Phyllis Walker, Caitlin Trussell, Michelle Taylor, Bob Severin, Sally Pyle, Micki Potter, Edward Orozco, Kay Johnson, Carolyn Jaffe, Jean Fredlund, Paula Dybinski, Vicki Dodson, Sandra Daniel, Mary Curtin, and Suzette Baca. The author also thanks the patients, families, volunteers, and other staff members who provided many life lessons as they shared the journey toward death.

Bibliography

Conner SR, McMaster JK: Hospice bereavement intervention and use of health care services by surviving spouses. *HMO Pract* 3:20-23, 1996.

Covey, S: *Seven habits of highly effective people,* New York, 1989, Fireside, Simon & Schuster.

National Hospice and Palliative Care Organization: 2005 facts and figures, 2006. http://www.nhpco.org/files/public/2005-facts-and-figures.pdf Accessed January 14, 2007.

The Denver Hospice: *Policy and Procedure Manual:* 2002, Denver, CO, 2002, The Denver Hospice.

Chapter 60

Advance Directives, End-of-Life Decisions, and Ethical Dilemmas

Paula Nelson-Marten and Jane Saucedo Braaten

1. What are advance directives and advance care planning?

Advance directives include any kind of directions, either written or oral, by which the person makes his or her wishes for medical treatment known and/or appoints a surrogate to make decisions should he or she become unable to do so. Advance directives were created to help facilitate communication and to make end-of-life care a more positive experience. They are grounded in the principle of autonomy or the patient's right to choose or refuse treatment. Examples of advance directives include living wills, medical durable power of attorney, CPR directives, medical directives, values history, and any other means by which the patient makes his or her wishes known.

2. What is the difference between a living will and a medical durable power of attorney?

A **living will** is a document signed by the patient stating that he or she does not want artificial life support in the event of terminal illness. The will takes effect when two physicians agree in writing that the patient has an irreversible condition. It does not cover acute conditions, such as infection or bleeding. A living will can be used to stop tube feedings and intravenous fluids and forego CPR only if stated specifically. Two witnesses need to sign the living will. Persons who cannot witness or sign include patients or employees of the facility in which the patient receives care, any doctor or employee of the patient's doctor, the patient's creditors, or anyone who may inherit the patient's property.

A **medical power of attorney** is a document signed by the patient naming someone to make medical decisions in the patient's behalf. Anyone can act as a medical durable power of attorney as long as that person is at least 18 years of age, mentally competent, and willing to serve as the patient's agent. Examples include spouses, significant others, siblings, or parents. This type of advance directive covers more decisions than a living will and is not limited to terminal illness. A medical durable power of attorney can be effective immediately or when the patient becomes unable to make decisions. It is crucial to stress the importance of a thorough discussion of health care wishes between the patient and the person whom the patient has chosen.

3. What is surrogate decision-making or substituted judgment?

In the event that a patient becomes unable to make decisions and is critically ill, health care providers often ask the family or friends of the patient to inform them of what decision the patient would have made under such circumstances. This practice is based on a standard of substituted judgment and is accepted by many legal and medical authorities. The family and/or friends are the surrogate or substitute decision makers.

However, studies have shown that when given hypothetical health states and asked to judge if they were acceptable or unacceptable, surrogates did not accurately choose what the patient would prefer. Written advance directives have not been shown to improve accuracy. A factor that can increase accuracy is a prior discussion of end-of-life preferences between patient and surrogate. This finding illustrates three clear needs: (1) the patient is the only one who can predict what kind of care he/she would want at the end of life, (2) a written advance directive is not a guarantee that end-of-life wishes will be followed and, (3) more effective methods of communicating wishes need to be evaluated in order to improve end-of-life care.

4. What is the role of the oncology nurse in advance directives?

As the patient's advocate, it is the nurse's role to help the patient make an informed decision and to ensure that the patient's wishes are followed. The nurse should provide educational material and programs, schedule time for discussion, and communicate patient wishes to all members of the health care team. Educating patients during home and office visits and through community presentations is also important, because the best time to discuss advance directives is before a hospitalization for acute care. Most people are more likely to discuss a sensitive topic when they are in a comfortable, nonthreatening environment. Having good communication skills and addressing the topic frequently are key to a positive outcome.

5. List some general guidelines for initiating discussion with cancer patients about end-of-life care planning.

- "What do you understand about your disease and the treatment we are providing?" The nurse may begin by asking open-ended questions that reflect the patient's understanding of the disease process, prognosis, and treatment options. Give the patient sufficient time to ventilate feelings and questions; continue the dialogue if the patient can acknowledge the condition and wants further discussion.
- "What is most important to you as you think about the future?" "What makes life worth living?" "Do you have any spiritual or religious beliefs that you would like considered by your health care providers?" The nurse needs to ask questions that clarify what the patient values in life. Documents that help clarify values, such as Five Wishes (www.agingwithdignity.org), may be helpful to present at this time.
- "Knowing that your condition cannot be cured or that you may have only a short time left to live, do you want us to attempt CPR or try to bring you back when your heart stops or you stop breathing?" The nurse should be prepared to explain and clarify terms such as CPR, resuscitation, and mechanical ventilation; discuss chances of success; and discuss possible complications. The nurse also should explain to the patient that CPR is most likely to be successful in generally healthy patients with sudden and reversible conditions; but patients with serious underlying medical conditions, such as advanced cancer, have a poor chance of successful CPR and a higher chance of serious complications. The DNR order should be clarified, and the patient should be reassured that all other levels of care, including comfort care and other therapies, will continue as the patient requests.
- "To what extent do you want your loved ones involved in decision making?" At this point in the discussion it is important to explain how advance directives are communicated and discuss some of the most effective ways of ensuring that they are followed.

6. What problems related to advance directives may occur in the acute care setting?

1. Paperwork may be lost during transfer to the hospital or misplaced within the hospital.
2. Patients may not be asked about their treatment preferences because of the fast-paced, cure-oriented environment or reluctance of the health care provider.
3. Misinterpretation may result from ambiguous language used in the advance directive.

4. The patient may have no advance directive and no surrogate decision-maker.
5. Advance directives may be ignored or misunderstood by the hospital staff.
6. The advance directive may not contain details that apply to the current situation.
7. The patient may not have understood the limitations of the advance directive selected.
8. The advance directive may not be understood by the surrogate decision maker.

7. Are oral advance directives valid?

Yes. They are the most common type of advance directive in the hospital. Courts have consistently upheld decisions to withhold therapy on the basis of clear and convincing oral advance directives. However, oral directives often are vague, made long before the situation at hand, and highly subjective, especially when being recalled by another person. Family disagreement about the meaning of a patient's prior statement can also complicate the decision-making.

8. What advice can the nurse give to patients who want to ensure that their wishes will be followed?

1. Encourage patients to talk to their relatives or other potential surrogates about their wishes before illness or hospitalization. A values history may help further clarify wishes.
2. Encourage use of a combination of living will and medical durable power of attorney. This combination ensures that wishes are followed if the living will is unclear in a specific situation.
3. Use clear language and specific examples, such as "I do not wish to be placed on a ventilator if it is deemed that my disease process is terminal and it is unlikely that I would be able to survive without ventilator support." Do not use terms such as "artificial" or "extraordinary"; these terms have different meanings to different people.
4. Be sure that the primary care physician knows and agrees to carry out the patient's wishes.
5. Encourage patients to give copies of paperwork to relatives and primary care physician and also to bring copies to the hospital.

9. What factors do nurses see as obstacles and aids to their ability to provide adequate end-of-life care?

Nurses in acute care settings experience end-of-life issues with patients every day. Obstacles include: (1) time constraints; (2) staffing patterns; (3) communication challenges with family and team members; and (4) physician behaviors, such as disregarding patient wishes.

Examples of practices that nurses believe promote better end-of-life care include: (1) preserving patient dignity, (2) ensuring that the patient is not alone, (3) adequately controlling pain, (4) knowing and following end-of-life wishes, (5) educating nurses about supportive end-of-life care, (6) communicating effectively as a team, and (7) promoting earlier withdrawal of treatment or never starting aggressive treatment.

10. Do patients with a DNR order receive different nursing care from other patients?

The DNR order is defined simply as no CPR. Nonetheless, a DNR order is often thought to imply that other life-sustaining interventions such as mechanical ventilation, blood products, and dialysis are not desired. Some believe that the amount of nursing time spent in caring for the patient with a DNR order will be decreased. Sulmasy and Sood (2003) found that nurses actually spent more time with patients who had DNR orders.

Realistically, nursing care of patients with DNR orders depends on the specific wishes of the patient and has little to do with the order itself. For example, the patient or family may request comfort care or want aggressive therapy only to a certain point. Generally, such wishes are not conveyed in a DNR order and need to be explored and documented through other more specific advance directives.

11. How successful is CPR in patients with advanced illness?

CPR was originally intended for use after acute situations in otherwise healthy people. It is now widely used in hospitals despite its limited effectiveness (0%-28% survival rate to hospital discharge). Patients most likely to benefit from CPR are those with sudden circulatory or respiratory collapse in the setting of acute cardiovascular illness. Those least likely to survive are patients with multisystem organ failure, metastatic disease, age greater than 70 years, and severe chronic or acute conditions. These facts should be discussed with patients with advanced illness.

12. Is there a difference between withdrawing and withholding care?

Most ethicists agree that legally and ethically there is no difference. In either case, the decision achieves the same outcome—inevitable death. However, many health care professionals feel that there is a difference between withdrawing treatment and not starting it in the first place. It may be that withdrawing treatment is seen as taking a more active role in the death of the patient.

13. Can treatment be withheld if the patient is not terminally ill or unconscious?

Courts have allowed treatments to be withheld in various situations, including bleeding from trauma, gangrene, respiratory failure, renal failure, cancer, and quadriplegia. The patient also may refuse any and all treatment.

14. Can fluids and nutrition be withheld?

Courts have consistently declared that fluids and nutrition are to be handled as other medical interventions and may be withdrawn or withheld in appropriate circumstances. Patients can refuse these interventions through clear and convincing oral advance directives or through a durable power of attorney. A living will may specify a time frame chosen by the patient in which to administer and then withdraw tube feedings or fluids.

15. Why is the subject of end-of-life decision-making so difficult to discuss?

It is difficult to discuss because of the overwhelming societal view that death is something to be avoided at all costs. Health care providers may not want to accept the limits to their interventions. Furthermore, discussion about death and dying has not been a routine part of medical or nursing school curricula. In a recent analysis, end-of-life content was severely lacking in critical care nursing textbooks. The patient may not want to accept the fact that death is inevitable and that his or her disease process may result in death. Whatever the reasons for avoidance, death must be seen as an inevitable part of life. Planning and discussion can help make death and dying more acceptable.

16. How has end-of-life care improved?

Ten years ago, SUPPORT (Study to Understand Prognosis and Preferences for Outcomes and Risks of Treatment), a large, 4-year, multicenter study funded by grants from the Robert Wood Johnson Foundation, examined end-of-life care in hospitals and concluded that for many patients it was less than optimal. Fifty percent of patients suffered moderate or severe pain in their last days of life, 38% of patients who died spent 10 or more days in the intensive care unit and physicians did not accurately understand or ignored the patient's preferences for advance directives. Of the patients (79%) who had a written DNR order, the DNR was written within 2 days of death. Over the last ten years, many public groups, health care providers, the government, and academics have focused efforts on improvement. However, current studies show only small improvements in care in the hospital.

Patients in health care institutions still are not receiving adequate symptom control, have concerns about adequate communication, need more patient and/or family support than was provided and have concerns about "dying with dignity." The positive exception is the great satisfaction experienced when a hospice or palliative care service was involved in the end-of-life care.

17. Who determines "futility" when the family or patient wants more intervention than the health care providers think is appropriate?

Some patients and/or family members may request care that is excessive or inappropriate. A determination of medical futility can limit such requests. The problem is that medicine is not an exact science and no prognostic indicators are completely accurate. As a result, futility is usually a value judgment. Who makes this judgment—health care providers, patient and family, or the courts—is a highly controversial topic.

Proponents of determination by clinicians or hospitals argue that futility can be judged ethically and that excessive use of scarce resources can be limited. They believe that hospitals are within their rights to create guidelines or policies for futile care that include referring the patient to a different facility or clinician for the treatment that is deemed futile. Opponents argue that determination by clinicians or hospitals is an example of paternalism (deciding for the patient) and conflicts with the principle of autonomy. When these beliefs collide in an end-of-life situation, a power struggle can ensue, causing great pain and emotional trauma to both sides. When the situation cannot be resolved, it is neither the family nor clinician who makes the decision. As recent examples have shown, these cases frequently are decided by the courts. The best strategy is to avoid futility debates by providing an honest relationship with the family/surrogate and open, frequent, updates and communication.

18. Why is it important for nurses to understand ethics and use this knowledge in everyday practice?

Ethical dilemmas occur often in every aspect of nursing practice. Without a basic knowledge of ethics, the nurse will miss opportunities to advocate for patients and families and to enhance care. The nurse uses ethics in everyday nursing practice when he or she is alert to moral conflicts, identifies ethical issues, uses the ANA Code of Ethics as a basis for practice, advocates for patients, shares decision-making with patients, and helps to implement moral decisions.

19. How does the nurse distinguish an everyday dilemma from an ethical dilemma?

A dilemma occurs whenever a situation requires a choice between two equally desirable or undesirable alternatives. All people are confronted by daily dilemmas that involve choice. A dilemma acquires moral qualities when the person can justify alternative courses of action through use of fundamental moral rules or principles. An ethical dilemma arises when moral claims conflict with one another.

20. What is the difference between morals and ethics?

Morals and ethics are often used interchangeably. Each word, however, has a distinct derivation and meaning. The word *morals* is derived from the Latin word *mores*, which means custom or habit, and refers to a set of values or rules that are peculiar to each individual. These values and rules are based on conscience and cultural or religious beliefs; they serve as guides in personal decision making regarding right and wrong. The word *ethics* is derived from the Greek word *ethos,* which means customs, conduct, and character. Ethics is the study of how one determines right from wrong. The use of ethics involves a process based on the use of principles and decision-making frameworks.

21. What ethical codes provide guidance for nursing practice?

The ANA Code of Ethics includes nine provisions that define ethical responsibilities of nurses. Topics include: respect for human dignity, safeguarding the patient's right to privacy, accountability, responsibility for nursing judgment, competence, informed judgment, development of nursing knowledge, standards of practice, advancing the profession, and collaboration to meet health needs of the public.

The International Council of Nurses (ICN) Code contains statements relating to ethical practices of the nurse in five areas—with people, in practice, in society, with co-workers, and for the profession.

22. Explain the two major traditions in Western ethics.

The general perspective of **biomedical ethics** is based on justice and/or equity in distribution of resources. This tradition is commonly used in medicine. The **ethic of care** involves a perspective on relationship. Care for the individual patient becomes highly important. This ethical tradition is closely aligned with nursing. Neither tradition is gender- or discipline-based. Physicians and nurses may operate out of either tradition.

23. What are the major ethical decision-making processes in biomedical ethics?

The two major schools of thought in Western biomedical ethics, defined by philosophers in the eighteenth and nineteenth centuries, have resulted in two major ethical decision-making frameworks. Deontology or formalism (from the work of Kant) indicates that the moral agent should consider the inherent nature of an act or rule rather than the consequences. This framework is principle-based and focuses on duties and obligations. The basic ethical principles are autonomy, justice, beneficence, and nonmaleficence. Utilitarianism or teleology (from the works of Mill and Bentham) indicate that the moral agent should consider consequences of rules and acts and seek the greatest possible balance of happiness over unhappiness for the greatest number. The two basic ethical principles for utilitarianism are beneficence and nonmaleficence.

24. What are the major ethical principles in biomedical ethics?

- **Autonomy.** This principle refers to self-rule, a person's right to self-determination, freedom of action, and noninterference to a degree consistent with respect for others. When an individual exercises autonomy, he or she determines what actions to take (self-determination). Freedom to act refers to a voluntary situation in which the individual is free of coercion and manipulation. The right of noninterference means that the individual's choices are respected whether or not they are in the individual's best interest. Use of this principle for major decision making requires consideration of the individual's wishes, values, and goals. It opposes the use of paternalism, by which the health care team and/or family determine what is best for the patient.
- **Respect for persons.** This principle is broader than the principle of autonomy. It includes respect for individual autonomy and self-determination and at the same time acknowledges the interconnectedness of individuals; that is, we are all members of communities.
- **Justice.** This principle refers to fairness. In health care ethics, its meaning narrows to distributive justice, which determines equal distribution of goods and services and

addresses equality of treatment in conditions of scarcity. In using this principle, the moral agent attempts to find a balance between benefits and burdens. Current health care policies and reform represent a national effort to provide distributive justice.

- **Beneficence.** This principle asks the individual to do good and has been defined by Frankena as the four "oughts": (1) one ought not to inflict evil or harm; (2) one ought to prevent evil or harm; (3) one ought to remove evil; and (4) one ought to do or promote good.
- **Nonmaleficence.** This principle asks the individual to do no harm and relates to one of Frankena's four oughts—one ought not to inflict evil or harm.

25. What is paternalism and how should the nurse deal with it?

Paternalism, parentalism, and *maternalism* tend to be used interchangeably. All three terms refer to actions that override an individual's wishes or actions to benefit or avoid harm to the individual. Generally, paternalism occurs when two ethical principles— beneficence and autonomy—are in conflict, and the health care practitioner believes that he or she is making the best decision in relation to the patient's care. All members of the health care team are capable of paternalistic behavior, which often occurs daily in the oncology setting. Paternalism is not always negative, but needs to be acknowledged when it occurs. The nurse needs to be alert so that he or she can recognize paternalism, call it to the attention of the health care team, continue to advocate for the patient, and foster self-determination and independence. A couple of examples of paternalism would be: (1) a patient's laboratory work and computed tomographic scan show evidence of recurrent disease, and the physician tells the patient that the cancer appears to be back but that the patient should not worry because a new course of chemotherapy should bring the recurrence under control; and (2) a nurse may want to encourage the use of a pain medication that the patient rejects because of concern over the possible side effects of constipation and sedation. The nurse starts the pain medication and tells the patient, "It's important for you to get your pain under control!"

26. Why is confidentiality important?

Confidentiality, or the keeping of promises (principle of fidelity), is necessary both ethically and legally to care for the patient and to develop a relationship of trust. The ANA Code of Ethics states that the nurse should safeguard the client's right to privacy in a judicious manner that does not endanger the patient's welfare. For example, confidentiality may be violated whenever patient cases are discussed in public places or within hearing distance of others not involved in the case. The principle of fidelity needs to be considered in sharing and withholding information.

27. Explain the principle of veracity. How should this principle apply in the nursing care of newly diagnosed patients and patients with recurrent disease?

The principle of veracity (truth-telling) requires the nurse to consider whether communication is honest. At times "being truthful" may be difficult for the nurse, inconvenient for the health care team, and distressing for the patient and family. The nurse should consider four questions:

1. Does the patient have the right to know?
2. Does the patient have the right to refuse information?
3. Does the family have the right to ask the health care team not to share all of the known information with the patient?
4. Does the family have a right to know?

In general, it is assumed that the patient has the right to full and accurate information about his or her situation. Withholding information may not be beneficial and may cause the patient to distrust the health care team. In cases of cognitive impairment or mental incompetence, the patient's level of comprehension should be considered so that the information is presented in a way that can be understood. Patients who are not informed often envision situations that are far worse than reality. Newly diagnosed patients and patients experiencing recurrence can assume no control over what is happening if they have not been told the truth. The facts may need to be restated several times in a way that promotes the truth, leads to open communication, and encourages questions. The nurse needs to be the patient's advocate. The right to information may be waived if the patient has good reason for requesting that information be withheld. The patient also may request that the family not be told. When the family requests nondisclosure, the nurse and health care team need to respect the patient's right to know.

28. What ethical issues are involved in informed consent?

Informed consent involves the ethical principles of autonomy and nonmaleficence. The health care team needs to ensure that the patient has access to information and that the information is understood. The term *informed* assumes that the health care team will provide as much information as possible to the patient so that the decision is based on full knowledge. The information shared with the patient needs to be truthful. Informed consent is important in many areas of oncology—for any treatment (surgery, chemotherapy, radiation) and for participation in research (clinical trials). Patients must understand that they can withdraw from the treatment or research at any point and that withdrawal will not affect the level of medical or nursing care that they are receiving and/or need to receive. Patients may refuse to give consent, and refusal must be respected. It is a good idea to ensure that the patient gives informed refusal as well as informed consent.

29. When resources are scarce (principle of justice), who decides which patient receives priority treatment?

When oncologic resources are scarce (e.g., expensive chemotherapy, new protocols, new medications), some patients may not have access. The principle of distributive justice may assist the health care team in deciding which patient should get the scarce item. The team needs to consider the patient's illness, how the scarce item will or will not affect outcome, cost of the item, whether the patient can enter a clinical trial, and who will benefit most. The health care team must balance benefits and burdens. Sometimes there are no easy answers, but assessing all of the known facts and balancing outcomes, benefit, and burdens help the health care team to make the fairest decision possible.

30. Describe a nursing model for ethical decision-making in the caring ethics tradition.

The Shared Decision-Making Model of Bandman and Bandman (1990) encourages the nurse to be a patient advocate. The model has five basic steps, each of which has several components:

STEP 1: DEFINITION OF THE PROBLEM
- Assess the situation: does a problem exist?
- Assess the patient's perception of the situation.
- Clarify the problem in relation to the patient's lifestyle, value system, resources, family, and other personal factors.
- Decide whether further information is needed.
- Identify alternatives that are appropriate to goals.

STEP 2: ANALYSIS OF FACTORS TO FACILITATE SHARED DECISION-MAKING
- Is the patient competent to make a decision?
- Is the patient's decision fully informed and freely given?

- Are the ethical components of the decision clear?
- Does the patient/family have relevant information?
- Can the patient reverse the decision whenever he or she wishes?

STEP 3: IDENTIFICATION OF THE ETHICAL ISSUE
- Discuss ethical choices with the patient.
- Identify sources of conflict among moral principles.
- Which moral principles can be justified for use in this situation?

STEP 4: DECISION REGARDING ETHICAL CHOICES
- The patient freely makes an informed decision consistent with his or her values, moral principles, lifestyle, and goals.
- The nurse and health care team are supportive of the patient's ethical choice.
- Family members and/or significant others are supportive of the patient's choice.

STEP 5: IMPLEMENTATION OF THE MORAL DECISION
- As the patient's advocate, the nurse supports the patient's decision.

31. Define sanctity of life.

Sanctity of life, also known as sacredness of life, is similar to the principle of avoiding killing. This principle is often relevant to end-of-life decisions. According to this viewpoint, life is sacred; therefore one ought not to do anything that may hasten death, such as removing a feeding tube or discontinuing treatment. Before putting this principle into practice, one is obligated to consider the wishes of the patient and the risks/benefits of the intervention.

32. Who determines quality of life?

In the past it was common for the physician to determine the patient's quality of life (paternalism), especially in relation to the amount of remaining physical function and the likely outcome of continued interventions. From an ethical point of view, the patient should determine his or her quality of life (principles of autonomy and respect for personhood) unless the patient is not competent to assist in this determination. The family and health care team may become involved. The nurse must advocate for the patient and family and their goals for health care.

33. Explain the principle of double effect.

The principle of double effect refers to a situation in which an act intended to produce a good effect also produces a bad or unintended effect. In oncology, for example, titration of medicine to the level needed to relieve pain (a good intention) may hasten the patient's death (an unintended effect). This principle states that bad consequences of an action (i.e., giving pain medicine) are morally permissible if four conditions are met:
1. The action is good or neutral.
2. The nurse intends only the good effect (i.e., pain relief).
3. The bad effect (i.e., death) must not be a means to bring about the good effect (pain relief).
4. There must be a balance between the good and bad effects.

According to the ANA's Position Statement, Pain Management and Control of Distressing Symptoms in Dying Patients (American Nurse's Association, 2003), "nurses must use effective doses of medications prescribed for symptom control and nurses have a moral obligation to advocate on behalf of the patient when prescribed medication is insufficiently managing pain and other distressing symptoms. The increasing titration of medication to achieve adequate symptom control is ethically justified." (See http://www.nursingworld.org/readroom/position/ethical).

34. When are ethics committees needed? What is their role?

Institutional ethics committees provide a forum for review and discussion of ethical issues and dilemmas and share information as a guide for decision-making. In general, ethics committees provide advice and consultation and do not make the final decision. Any individual involved in an ethical dilemma (health care team member, patient, family member) can request a meeting of the ethics committee.

35. How does the oncology nurse advocate for the patient when the nurse does not agree with the patient's decision?

Often the nurse faces an ethical dilemma if the patient decides either that he or she does not want further treatment or that he or she wants extraordinary treatment. In such situations, the nurse should follow the principles of respect for persons and autonomy. The nurse's role is to care for the patient, including advocating for the patient. The nurse or health care team must ensure that the patient is making an informed decision and that the patient and family understand the consequences of the decision. Once the patient or family has made a decision, the nurse's role is to care for the patient in a supportive manner, regardless of outcome. Three critical factors are maintenance of open communication, respect for the decision, and the patient's and family's need not to feel abandoned by the health care team. In such situations, the health care team should discuss how each member feels about the patient-family's decision and support one another in delivering care.

36. How does the oncology nurse deal with ethnic and cultural differences from an ethical perspective?

To care adequately for a patient and family from another culture, the nurse needs to be mindful of the principle of respect for persons. To avoid offending the patient or family, the nurse should recognize and respect the ethnic and cultural traditions that influence the required care. Standards and protocols of care that incorporate cultural beliefs, rituals, and religious preferences need to be developed. An example is the development of protocols for the care of Hasidic Jewish women receiving bone marrow transplants for breast cancer.

37. When is it ethical to let a terminal patient die without violating the principle of avoiding killing?

When it becomes obvious that treatment is of no further benefit, the nurse and health care team need to consider whether active treatment should be discontinued. Palliative or hospice care may be more appropriate. The patient and family may need guidance in making this decision. The patient may not wish to quit active treatment; an example of this is a patient who has responded to therapy for acute myelogenous leukemia in the past but whose clinical condition and laboratory values show no improvement with current therapy. In such a case the doctor may be reluctant to continue aggressive treatment. The physician and nurse must be open and honest with the patient and family, explaining that the situation is now terminal and that supportive care (i.e., palliative and hospice care) is more appropriate. Supportive care should be given regardless of the patient's decision. The nurse can advocate for the patient, put shared decision-making into practice and follow the principle of respect for persons. The decision to forego active treatment can be quite difficult for both patient and family, and a supportive atmosphere is of critical importance.

38. How does the oncology nurse care for self from an ethical standpoint? Why is self-care important?

The oncology nurse needs to work at developing an ethical sense and becoming astute at recognizing ethical dilemmas with patients, team members, and self. Although the nurse must respond to many rights, he or she also has the duty to care for self. If one does not care for self, one cannot care effectively for others. At times, the nurse has an obligation to remind others that he or she needs to care for self. Often oncology nurses attempt to be all things to all people. Living a more balanced life has positive effects on all the nurse's activities.

Key Points

- A written advance directive, without a discussion of end-of-life wishes, will not ensure that wishes are followed.
- Health care professionals need to have expert communication skills and take responsibility for initiating the conversation on advance directives.
- An ethical dilemma arises when moral claims conflict with one another.
- Ethics is the study of how one determines right from wrong.
- The ANA Code of Ethics and the International Council of Nurses (ICN) Code make explicit the ethical values of the nursing profession.
- The major ethical principles are autonomy, justice, beneficence, and nonmaleficence.
- Ethics committees provide a forum for review and discussion of ethical issues and dilemmas.

Internet Resources

ANA, The Center for Ethics and Human Rights, Code of Ethics with Interpretative Statements:
  http://www.nursingworld.org/ethics/ecode.htm
ANA Position Statements on Ethics and Human Rights:
  http://www.nursingworld.org/readroom/position/ethics/
Five Wishes:
  http://agingwithdignity.org
PBS Online, WNET, *Before I Die*:
  http://www.wnet.org/bid/
National Hospice and Palliative Care Organization (NHPCO) Database:
  http://www.nhpco.org/custom/directory
NHPCO information about hospice and palliative care:
  http://www.nhpco.org
Caring Connections:
  http://www.caringinfo.org/i4a/pages/index.cfm?pageid=1.

Education Sites

End-of-Life Nursing Education Consortium (ELNEC):
  http://www.aacn.nche.edu/elnec
Education in Palliative and End-of-Life Care (EPEC):
  http://www.epec.net

Bibliography

Bandman B, Bandman EL: *Nursing ethics through the life span,* ed 2, Norwalk, CT, 1990, Appleton & Lange.

Beckstrand RL, Callister LC, Kirchhoff KT: Providing a "good death": Critical care nurses' suggestions for improving end-of-life care. *Am J Crit Care* 15(1):38-45, 2006.

Bernat JL: Medical futility: Definition, determination, and disputes in critical care. *Neurocrit Care* 2(2): 198-205, 2005.

Beauchamp TL, Childress JF: *Principles of biomedical ethics,* ed 4, New York, 1994, Oxford University Press.

Carse A: The "voice of care": Implications for bioethical education. *J Med Philos* 16:5-28, 1991.

Ditto PH, Danks JH, Smucker WD, et al: Advance directives as acts of communication: A randomized controlled trial. *Arch Intern Med* 161(3):421-430, 2001.

Frankena WK: *Ethics,* ed 2, Englewood Cliffs, NJ, 1973, Prentice-Hall.

Fried TR, Bradley EH, Towle VR: Valuing the outcomes of treatment: Do patients and their caregivers agree? *Arch Intern Med* 163(17):2073-2078, 2003.

Kirchhoff KT, Beckstrand RL, Anumandla PR: Analysis of end of life content in critical care nursing textbooks. *J Prof Nurs* 19(6):372-381, 2003.

Lo B: *Resolving ethical dilemmas: A guide for clinicians,* ed 3, Philadelphia, 2005, Lippincott Williams & Wilkins.

Moore CD: Communication issues and advance care planning. *Semin Oncol Nurs* 21(1):11-19, 2005.

Scanlon C: Ethical concerns in end-of-life care. *Am J Nurs* 103(1):48-55, 2003.

Sulmasy DP, Sood JR: Factors associated with the time nurses spend at the bedsides of seriously ill patients with poor prognoses. *Med Care* 41(4):458-466, 2003.

SUPPORT Principal Investigators: A controlled trial to improve care for seriously ill hospitalized patients: The study to understand prognoses and preferences for outcomes and risks of treatment (SUPPORT). *JAMA* 274:1591-1598, 1995.

Teno JM, Clarridge BR, Casey V, et al: Family perspectives on end-of-life care at the last place of care. *JAMA,* 291:88-92, 2004.

Veatch RM, Fry ST: *Case studies in nursing ethics,* ed 3, Sudbury, MA, 2006, Jones and Bartlett.

Caring for the Caregiver

Pamela J. Haylock

1. What is the impact of job-related stress among oncology nurses?

Nurses' abilities to provide continual, consistent, and compassionate care, the most basic tenet of the nursing profession, are impaired by burnout, compassion stress, and fatigue. Burnout, defined by Maslach (1976) as "a syndrome of physical and emotional exhaustion resulting in the development of negative job attitudes and perceptions, a poor professional self-concept, and a loss of empathic concern," can occur in any setting when job demands exceed levels of support and resources available to employees. "Compassion stress" and "compassion fatigue" relate to the burnout phenomenon among health care professionals, with these phenomena now recognized as costs of caring.

Stress among oncology nurses relates to chronic compounded grief associated with constant exposure to patients' and families' suffering, frequent crises and intense emotional experiences, transitions throughout the cancer trajectory, death among a high percentage of the people in their care, moral distress, and relationships and communication issues with co-workers and physicians. These stressors are further complicated by the health care climate characterized by a nursing shortage, limited budgets, diminished staffing levels of nurse and supportive care personnel, demands of paperwork, and increasing complexities of therapeutic modalities and related technology.

2. Why is compassion stress important for managers to consider?

The consequences of unremitting and unrelieved job stress and subsequent compassion fatigue and burnout among nurses include negative effects on organizational behavior, absenteeism, productivity, patient care, health care quality and patient satisfaction, nurse work satisfaction, recruitment and costly job turnover, and last but not least, significant physiologic changes contributing to morbidity and mortality among nurses. Most literature addressing oncology nursing burnout or compassion fatigue such as risk factors, warning signs, and intervention strategies focuses on nurses in hospital-based practice settings; there is little information about these phenomena in ambulatory, free standing, and physician-office based settings.

3. What are the warning signs of compassion stress, compassion fatigue, and burnout?

Warning Signs of Compassion Stress, Compassion Fatigue, and Burnout		
Physical signs		
* Physical fatigue	* Dry mouth	* Upper back pain
* Clammy hands	* Eating disorders	* Heart palpitations
* Diarrhea	* Halitosis	* Stiff neck or shoulders

Continued

Warning Signs of Compassion Stress, Compassion Fatigue, and Burnout—cont'd

Emotional signs

* Anxiety
* Depression
* Fear

* Frustration
* Grief
* Social isolation

* Poor self-image
* Sense of powerlessness
* Sense of worthlessness

Behaviors

* Blaming others
* Crying, irritability
* Short temper

* Overactivity
* Negative attitude

* Risk-taking
* Shortened attention span

4. **What environmental characteristics of the practice setting diminish risks of compassion fatigue among nurses?**

   Although oncology nursing is the specific focus of very little empirical evidence to date or programmatic interventions designed to minimize compassion stress, compassion fatigue, and burnout, we can deduce environmental traits conducive to minimizing risks from available nursing and organizational literature:
   - Effective communication
   - Effective nurse-physician communication and collaboration
   - Nurses have high levels of autonomy and participate in organizational decision making
   - Manageable workload
   - High levels of support from supervisors and coworkers
   - Role clarity
   - Commitment to personal and professional growth
   - Community building in the workplace
   - Incorporates stress management initiatives
   - Promotes nurses' sense of personal accomplishment
   - Maximizes work excitement factors (work arrangements, growth and development opportunities, variable work experiences, and work environment)

5. **How can compassion fatigue and burnout be prevented?**

   Stress-reduction programs aimed at creating healthier workplaces are most beneficial in reversing work-related stress. Strategies for creating a healthier workplace include:
   - Track workplace and team member conflict
   - Identify, observe, and initiate stress-reduction assistance for at-risk team members
   - Team member training in counseling, coping, and problem-solving skills
   - Ongoing work-related grief and bereavement programs
   - Ongoing support and/or discussion groups designed to promote team relations
   - Team retreats aimed at enhancing group cohesiveness
   - Stress inoculation training for all team members
   - Acknowledge team members' accomplishments
   - Acknowledge team accomplishments

6. What skills can a nurse learn and use to reduce stress in the work environment?

Every nurse can help to create and foster a supportive, healthy work environment. Any team member can be a catalyst for positive change. A first step is to learn and use appropriate self-care skills, followed by sharing successful skills with colleagues. Important self-care stress-reduction strategies include:

- Work in (or at least work towards) a role that best fits personal and professional potential and aspirations
- Set realistic personal and professional goals, and acknowledge one's own accomplishments
- Be aware of stressors in one's own life
- Work to resolve personal losses
- Clarify work-related expectations and job descriptions
- Ask for help
- Learn to say no
- Participate in efforts to develop a good social climate at work; brainstorm to develop a list of priorities and potential solutions to problems
- Actively participate in and support ways to receive assistance from colleagues
- Focus on one's own physical, emotional, and spiritual health, including finding balance in one's own life, with good nutrition, adequate sleep, exercise, and social/recreational activities
- Develop and use a sense of humor

7. What are the options when workplace issues seem impossible to change?

When a nurse faces irreconcilable differences in the work setting, walking away from the situation to gain perspective may be the best approach. Oncology nursing is rich with opportunities for nurses to change direction to a different work setting, different focus of care, and different patient populations. Active involvement in the larger professional arena dispels the notion of isolation by providing nurses with broader perspectives and an expanded network of like-minded colleagues. Involvement with professional nursing organizations also establishes a collective voice for change that can extend beyond a single workplace or institution. Career advice, career counseling, and career change within the nursing profession can be beneficial.

Additional education can be a catalyst for role change, career change, and work excitement. These strategies may well provide nurses with new opportunities to learn; acknowledge nurses' wisdom, skills, and experience; and allow nurses to actively explore career paths more conducive to work excitement and personal enthusiasm instead of enduring the consequences of work burnout.

 Key Points

- The potential for work-related stress and burnout is inherent in oncology nursing.
- Nurses' stress and burnout in oncology care settings affects patient satisfaction, patient outcomes, organizational outcomes, and nurses' health.
- Modifiable characteristics of nurses' work environments contribute to or minimize the incidence of nurse burnout.
- Self-care strategies can prepare individual nurses to cope more effectively with work-related stressors.

Internet Resources

Queendom.com, Burnout Test:
  http://www.queendom.com/tests/career/burnout1_r_access.html
ACE-Network, Compassion Fatigue Self-Test:
  http://www.ace-network.com/cfspotlight.htm
Assessment.com, Motivational Appraisal of Personal Potential:
  http://www.assessment.com

Bibliography

Armstrong J, Holland J: Surviving the stresses of clinical oncology by improving communication. *Oncology* 18:363-368, 2004.

Cohen-Katz J, Wiley SD, Capuano, T, et al: The effects of mindfulness-based stress reduction on nurse stress and burnout: A quantitative and qualitative study. *Holist Nurs Pract* 18:302-308, 2004.

Jezuit D: Personalization as it relates to nurse suffering: How managers can recognize the phenomenon and assist suffering nurses. *JONAS Healthc Law Ethics Regul* 5:25-28, 2003.

Lally RM: Nurse heal thyself: Oncology nurses share their experiences with bereavement and self-care. *ONS News,* 20(10):4,5,11, 2005.

Larrabee JH, Ostrow CL, Withrow ML, et al: Predictors of patient satisfaction with inpatient hospital nursing care. *Res Nurs Health* 27:254-268, 2004.

Maslach C. Burned-out. *Hum Behav* 5:16, 1976.

Maslach C, Leiter M: *The truth about burnout: How organizations cause personal stress and what to do about it,* San Francisco, 1998, Jossey-Bass.

McNeely E: The consequences of job stress for nurses' health: Time for a check-up. *Nurs Outlook* 53:291-299, 2005.

Medland J, Howard-Ruben M, Whitaker E: Fostering psychosocial wellness in oncology nurses: Addressing burnout and social support in the workplace. *Oncol Nurs Forum* 31:47-54, 2004.

Rivers PA, Tsai K, Munchus G: The financial impacts of the nursing shortage. *J Health Care Finance* 31:52-64, 2005.

Sabo BM: Compassion fatigue and nursing work: Can we accurately capture the consequences of caring work? *Int J Nurs Pract* 12:136-142, 2006.

Sadovich JM: Work excitement in nursing: An examination of the relationship between work excitement and burnout, *Nurs Econ* 23:91-96, 2005.

Vahey DC, Aiken LH, Sloane DM, et al: Nurse burnout and patient satisfaction. *Med Care* 42:II-57-II-66, 2004.

Index